T0297994

HANDBOOK OF ANESTHESIA

John J. Nagelhout, PhD, CRNA, FAAN
Director, School of Anesthesia
Kaiser Permanente/California State University, Fullerton
Southern California Permanente Medical Group
Pasadena, California

Karen L. Plaus, PhD, CRNA, FAAN; CEO
National Board of Certification and Recertification for Nurse Anesthetists (NBCRNA)
Chicago, Illinois

FIFTH EDITION

ELSEVIER

ELSEVIER
SAUNDERS

3251 Riverport Lane
Maryland Heights, MO 63043

HANDBOOK OF ANESTHESIA, 5TH EDITION ISBN: 978-1-4557-1125-3

Notice

Knowledge and best practice in this field are constantly changing. As new research and experience broaden our knowledge, changes in practice, treatment and drug therapy may become necessary or appropriate. Readers are advised to check the most current information provided (i) on procedures featured or (ii) by the manufacturer of each product to be administered, to verify the recommended dose or formula, the method and duration of administration, and contraindications. It is the responsibility of the practitioner, relying on their own experience and knowledge of the patient, to make diagnoses, to determine dosages and the best treatment for each individual patient, and to take all appropriate safety precautions. To the fullest extent of the law, neither the Publisher nor the Editors/Authors assume any liability for any injury and/or damage to persons or property arising out of or related to any use of the material contained in this book.

The Publisher

Library of Congress Cataloging-in-Publication Data

Nagelhout, John J.
Handbook of anesthesia / John J. Nagelhout, Karen L. Plaus.—5th ed.
p. ; cm.
Rev. ed. of : Handbook of nurse anesthesia / John J. Nagelhout, Karen L. Plaus. 4th ed. c2010.
Includes bibliographical references and index.
ISBN 978-1-4557-1125-3 (pbk. : alk. paper)
I. Plaus, Karen L. II. Nagelhout, John J. Handbook of nurse anesthesia. III. Title.
[DNLM: 1. Anesthesia—Handbooks. WO 39]

617.9'6—dc23

2012045507

Executive Content Strategist: Teri Hines Burnham
Senior Content Development Specialist: Laura M. Selkirk
Associate Content Development Specialist: Jacqueline Kiley
Project Manager: Prathibha Mehta
Designer: Margaret Reid

Printed in (name of country)

Last digit is the print number: 9 8 7 6 5 4 3 2 1

Preface

Previous editions of this handbook have been extremely popular as a quick yet comprehensive guide to answer common clinical questions that arise during busy clinical practice. Technological innovations now allow this handbook to be used in traditional as well as various electronic formats. We approach the fifth edition of the *Handbook of Anesthesia* with a clear intent to bridge these platforms while remaining true to our educational objectives. When selecting the format of this handbook, we chose not to simply produce a condensed version of our text *Nurse Anesthesia*. We believe that there is a need for a single comprehensive source containing information on common diseases, procedures, and drugs and that such a source, in a handbook format, would complement the larger text and provide an "in the operating room" guide for practice. This fifth edition of our handbook has been totally reviewed and revised to include the most up-to-date clinical information available on numerous topics. Today many clinicians practice at more than one facility and thus may be called on to provide anesthesia care in a broader spectrum of operative and diagnostic situations. A comprehensive reference guide is an essential tool for hands-on management in the modern operating suite.

We compiled the *Handbook of Anesthesia* as a single source that provides the following:

- A thorough overview of the common diseases encountered in surgical patients
- A procedure manual and set of guidelines for anesthesia management for a wide variety of diagnostic and surgical procedures
- A convenient and comprehensive drug reference for clinical use

A standardized format was designed and customized for use throughout each of the three individual parts of the handbook. The appendixes at the end of the handbook offer clinicians easy access to the guidelines for pediatric and adult drug therapy, corticosteroid replacement, hematology, preoperative laboratory tests, immunosuppressive drugs, and much more.

In the two decades since we produced the first edition of this handbook, we are consistently amazed and grateful for the professional contributions that nurse anesthetists make to academic medicine and nursing, clinical practice, and society as a whole. We are proud that this handbook has played a part in the continuous evolution of our specialty.

John J. Nagelhout
Karen L. Plaus

Acknowledgments

We are especially gratified with the comments and widespread acceptance of this handbook by the anesthesia community. Its extensive use as a clinical guide confirms our assumptions that a convenient and inclusive source such as this is essential in modern anesthesia practice. We have incorporated many of these comments in revising and updating this new edition. Each section has been thoroughly edited to include the latest information available on common diseases, procedures, and drugs encountered during daily practice.

We would also like to thank the following individuals at Elsevier who were also instrumental in the production of this handbook—Teri Hines Burnham, Executive Content Strategist; Laura Selkirk, Senior Content Development Specialist; Jackie Kiley, Associate Content Development Specialist, and Prathibha Mehta, Project Manager. Again, we would like to thank our professional colleagues, friends, and especially our families for their support.

Travis Barber
Meredith Borg
Lisa Chaps
Lisa Chong
Cameron Christensen
Kim Edick
Sass Elisha
Mariya Fair
Jeremy Heiner
Kyle Hiestand
Marissa Horst
James Jin
Min Hee Kim
Kerrie Klein
Heather Lee
Ashley Madsen
Michelle Mekpongsatorn
Jessica Michinock
Megan Nedwick
Justin Roldan
Aumnard Saiseubyat
Cathy Sayat
Maria Tang
Jennifer Thompson
Kelly Winans
Susan Yudt
Tristie Yumul
Richelle Zhou

Reviewers

Tatjana Bevans, CRNA, MSN
Anesthetist
University of Utah Medical Center
Salt Lake City, Utah

Kevin Buss, CDR, CRNA
Assistant Professor of Nursing, Uniformed Services University of the Health Sciences - Nurse Anesthesia Program (USUHS-NAP)
Director of Clinical Academics - USUHS-NAP
Director, Nurse Anesthesia Clinical Training
Portsmouth, Virginia

Mario P. Grasso, CRNA, DNAP
Staff Nurse Anesthetist and Affiliate Faculty
Medical College of Virginia
Virginia Commonwealth University
Richmond, Virginia

Table of Contents

PART 2
Common Procedures, 238

SECTION IV Head and Neck, 312

SECTION V Intrathoracic and Extrathoracic, 348

SECTION VI Neurologic System, 369

Cardiovascular System

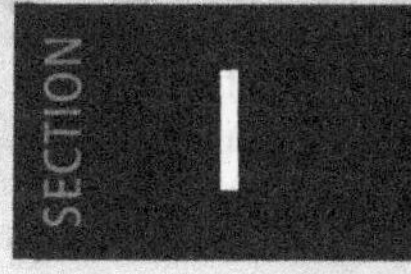

A. CARDIOMYOPATHY

Definition

Cardiomyopathies are diseases of the myocardium that are characterized by myocardial dysfunction. They ultimately affect contractile function, and life-threatening congestive heart failure (CHF) is common to all cardiomyopathies.

Etiology

Cardiomyopathies can be classified according to their pathophysiologic basis in the categories of dilated (congestive), restrictive, and hypertrophic.

DILATED CARDIOMYOPATHY

Pathophysiology

The cause of dilated cardiomyopathies can be inflammatory or noninflammatory. The inflammatory type or myocarditis usually results from infection. The noninflammatory variety results from idiopathic, toxic, degenerative, or infiltrative processes that destroy the myocardium or cardiac cytoskeleton. The primary clinical symptom is myocardial failure, which presents as ventricular dilation, elevated filling pressures, and pulmonary edema. Dilated cardiomyopathies can be acute or chronic and can lead to a decrease in myocardial contractility, often involving both ventricles. Alcoholic cardiomyopathy is an example of noninflammatory cardiomyopathy that is associated with tachycardia, premature ventricular contractions that progresses to left ventricular (LV) failure and valvular disease.

Clinical symptoms are characterized as "forward" failure or "backward" failure. Symptoms of forward failure may include fatigue, hypotension, and oliguria caused by a decreased organ perfusion.

Symptoms of backward failure may include elevated filling pressures and ventricular failure. The LV dilation and mitral regurgitation (MR) result in orthopnea, paroxysmal nocturnal dyspnea, and pulmonary edema. Symptoms of right-sided failure include hepatomegaly, jugular venous distention, and peripheral edema.

Treatment

Patients with dilated cardiomyopathy (DCM) must avoid unnecessary physical activity and must exhibit total abstinence from alcohol. Patients with CHF are treated with digoxin and diuretics. Vasodilator treatment or an inotrope with vasodilator properties (amrinone or milrinone) may also be helpful. Ventricular arrhythmias are treated with procainamide or quinidine. Because of the increased risk of pulmonary embolism, these patients may be treated with anticoagulants (not proved to be of benefit). Patients with associated collagen vascular disease, sarcoidosis, or inflammation on endocardial biopsy are treated with corticosteroids preoperatively. Tachyarrhythmias can be treated with β-blockers. Patients with CAD and DCM may benefit from coronary revascularization to improve LV function. With advanced CHF, these patients may be candidates for heart transplantation, provided pulmonary hypertension does not exist.

Anesthetic Considerations

- Avoid myocardial depression.
- Maintain normovolemia.
- Prevent increases in afterload.
- Invasive monitoring may be necessary if manipulation of pulmonary and systemic vascular resistances is needed.

Excess cardiovascular depression on induction of anesthesia in patients with a history of alcohol abuse may reflect undiagnosed DCM; however, failure of this expected response to intravenous induction agents may reflect a slow circulation time.

During maintenance, myocardial depression produced by volatile agents must be considered. Opiates exhibit benign effects on cardiac contractility but may not produce unconsciousness. In addition, an opioid, nitrous oxide, benzodiazepine technique may cause unexpected cardiac depression. Increases in heart rate associated with surgical stimulation may be treated with β-blockers. Nondepolarizing muscle relaxants that exhibit few cardiovascular effects are advised.

Cardiac filling pressures should guide intravenous fluids; therefore, a pulmonary artery (PA) catheter aids in early recognition of the need for inotropes or vasodilators. Prominent "v" waves reflect mitral or tricuspid regurgitation (TR).

Intraoperative hypotension is treated with ephedrine. Phenylephrine could adversely affect afterload as a result of increased systemic vascular resistance (SVR).

Regional anesthesia may be used in selected patients, although caution is indicated in avoiding abrupt sympathetic blockade as seen in spinal or epidural anesthesia.

Prognosis

The prognosis for patients with DCM is poor, with a 5-year survival rate of 25% to 40%. The cause of death in 75% of these patients is CHF. Pulmonary embolism or sudden death from arrhythmia is found in more than 50% of these patients on autopsy.

RESTRICTIVE CARDIOMYOPATHY

Definition

The term restrictive cardiomyopathy represents several types of pathologic conditions dependent on whether the myocardium or endomyocardial muscle layer is affected. Restrictive cardiomyopathy (RCM) can occur in the pediatric population, and it is one of the rarest forms of cardiomyopathy that occurs in children. It is associated with a high mortality rate once symptoms begin to develop.

Etiology

Causes of myocardial RCM include: genetic (e.g., familial cardiomyopathy), infiltrative (e.g., sarcoidosis), storage diseases (e.g., hemochromatosis), and endomyocardial (e.g., endomyocardial fibrosis). Furthermore, it is believed that there is a genetic predisposition for those who are more likely to develop RCM.

Pathophysiology

Infiltration of fibrous tissue and deposition into the myocardium or endomyocardium is the pathologic mechanism by which RCM develops. As a result, one or both ventricles become stiff and noncompliant, which inhibits normal diastolic filling. As a result of reduced end-diastolic volume (reduced ventricular preload) caused by restricted ventricular filling, stroke volume (SV) is decreased. An increase in the sensitivity of the troponin and tropomyosin complex calcium mediated myofilament is thought to be the cause of genetically derived RCM. Systolic ejection remains relatively normal. The atria become dilated as a compensatory response volume overload and left- and/or right-sided heart failure can occur. Significantly elevated right atrial (RA) pressures (15–20 mmHg) and PA systolic pressure (as high as 50 mmHg) can occur as the disease progresses. Signs and symptoms associated with RCM include dyspnea, fatigue, cardiomegaly, atrioventricular valve regurgitation, jugular venous distention, pulmonary hypertension, and rales.

Treatment

Medical management for patients with RCM is similar to that for DCM and includes diuretics, sodium and water restriction, anticoagulation, and treatment of dysrhythmias. Eventually, patients may require treatment to augment SV such as an intraaortic balloon pump or LV assist device. A heart transplant may eventually be necessary.

Anesthetic Considerations

Maintenance of normal sinus rhythm, adequate preload, and minimization of myocardial depression are essential to anesthetic management. As with DCM, an anesthetic technique that minimizes myocardial depression that is accomplished using higher doses of narcotic compared with inhalation agent may be prudent. Results from studies are often conflicting related to the degree of myocardial depressant effects of modern inhalation agents (isoflurane, sevoflurane, desflurane) in relation to cardiomyopathy and impaired systolic ejection and diastolic relaxation. Patients with moderate to severe cardiomyopathy depend on SNS activity to augment myocardial performance. Despite the minimal direct myocardial depressant effects of narcotics, their inhibition of the SNS has an indirect depressant effect on the heart. Thus, titration of narcotics and assessment of the patient's hemodynamic status are important.

ARRHYTHMOGENIC RIGHT VENTRICULAR CARDIOMYOPATHY

Definition

Also known as arrhythmogenic right ventricular (RV) dysplasia, this cardiomyopathy is an autosomal dominant genetically inherited disorder. Diagnosis is frequently made postmortem in patients with arrhythmogenic right ventricular cardiomyopathy (ARVC) because sudden cardiac death occurs frequently. Signs and symptoms can also occur during childhood but more often manifest during adolescence. During sports-related exercise, severe intolerance caused by increasing myocardial oxygen demand can result in lightheadedness, syncope, or sudden death.

Etiology

ARVC is a genetic cardiac muscle disorder that has only been differentiated from other cardiomyopathies within the past 20 years. It has been determined that ARVC is caused by an autosomal dominant inheritance. The RyR2 cardiac receptor dysfunction is thought to be partially responsible for the arrhythmogenic nature of this disease state that may cause lethal ventricular dysrhythmias.

Pathophysiology

Fibrofatty infiltrates invade the RV myocardium and cause myocyte dysfunction and death. As a result, RV cardiac output (CO) is decreased. The LV undergoes this type of pathologic change in approximately half of patients with ARVC, and CHF is a sign of disease progression. Ventricular dysrhythmias are common and range from premature ventricular contractions to ventricular fibrillation. Patients with ARVC may be exquisitely sensitive to increased catecholamine levels, which may further provoke these dysrhythmias.

Treatment

The medical management for patients with ARVC includes avoiding extreme physical activity, antiarrhythmic drugs, internal cardiac defibrillator placement, and finally cardiac transplantation.

Anesthetic Considerations

Anesthetic management for patients with ARVC should focus on identification and treatment of fatal dysrhythmias. Many events increase SNS predominance; examples include hypoxia, hypotension, hypercarbia, and surgical stimulation. Excessive catecholamine release can induce fatal dysrhythmias. Signs and symptoms associated with ARVC include tachycardia, ventricular dysrhythmias (ventricular tachycardia, ventricular fibrillation), T-wave inversion (leads V_1 and V_3), bundle branch block, hypokinetic RV, decreased RV ejection, jugular venous distention, syncope, and peripheral edema. Amiodarone has been used successfully to treat dysrhythmias in these patients. Prophylactic preoperative administration of antiarrhythmic agents has not shown to be effective at suppressing ventricular dysrhythmias intraoperatively.

HYPERTROPHIC CARDIOMYOPATHY

Definition

Hypertrophic cardiomyopathy is a genetically transmitted disorder that is a form of myocardial dysfunction, which can cause CAD, valvular dysfunction, ventricular remodeling, and hypertension. The incidence in the adult population is approximately one in 500 persons. Obstructive hypertrophic cardiomyopathy has previously been referred to as *idiopathic hypertrophic subaortic stenosis*. Currently, the preferred term is *hypertrophic cardiomyopathy with or without left ventricular outflow obstruction*. This disease is an autosomal dominant hereditary condition. The peak incidence is in patients 50 to 70 years of age. Most elderly patients diagnosed with this condition are women.

Etiology

The myocardial defect that is associated with hypertrophic cardiomyopathy is related to the contractile mechanism. An increase in the density of calcium channels appears to lead to myocardial hypertrophy. Asymmetric hypertrophy of the interventricular septum of the LV occurs. The asymmetric hypertrophy of the intraventricular septum causes a left outflow tract obstruction, and therefore the hemodynamic consequences are similar to those that are characteristic of aortic stenosis (AS). Hypertrophic cardiomyopathy is the most common cause of sudden death in the pediatric and young adult populations.

Myocardial hypertrophy is the pathophysiologic abnormality that precipitates the hemodynamic derangements associated with hypertrophic cardiomyopathy and is caused by LV outflow obstruction.

Pathophysiology

The pathophysiologic abnormalities related to hypertrophic cardiomyopathy include the presence of systolic and diastolic dysfunction. A loss of diastolic compliance results in an abnormally elevated LV end-diastolic pressure (LVEDP) in the presence of low-normal end-diastolic volume. Loss of LV diastolic compliance requires a greater contribution of volume from atrial contraction. As a result, CHF may ensue as left atrial (LA) pressures continue to increase.

Hypertrophic cardiomyopathy with obstruction is characterized by its dynamic nature. Three basic hemodynamic parameters can affect the degree of outflow obstruction. Manipulation of these parameters can exacerbate or ameliorate the hemodynamic consequences of outflow obstruction. These three parameters are preload, afterload, and contractility. Increasing myocardial contractility in patients with DCM exacerbates the obstruction by increasing septal wall contraction and decreasing CO. Increased blood flow velocity causes a greater degree of systolic anterior motion of the mitral valve's anterior leaflet, creating further obstruction. Decreased preload changes LV geometry and thereby brings the anterior leaflet of the mitral valve into closer proximity of the hypertrophic septum. Increases in LV contractility cause the LV to empty more completely and increase the degree of septal contractility, which results in a greater degree of obstruction.

In hypertrophic cardiomyopathy with obstruction, conditions that impair ventricular function under normal physiologic conditions improve cardiac function. This implies that factors that normally impair contractility, such as myocardial depression, increased end-diastolic volume, and increased SVR, improve forward flow and diminish the degree of obstruction.

Hemodynamic Goals for Management of Hypertrophic Cardiomyopathy

Preload	Increase
Afterload	Increase
Contractility	Decrease
Heart rate	Maintain
Heart rhythm	Normal sinus rhythm

Treatment

The goal of treatment in these patients is to relieve the LV outflow tract obstruction. This is often achieved with β-blockers to lower the heart rate and decrease contractility. Calcium channel antagonists may also help. Caution should be taken to prevent drug-induced hypotension and negative inotropic effects; therefore, nitroglycerin should be avoided in these patients who present with angina. If CHF also exists, treatment becomes more difficult. Diuretics can lead to hypovolemia, and digoxin can increase cardiac contractility, both of which may worsen the obstruction. Cardioversion may be necessary to maintain normal sinus rhythm. Patients with atrial fibrillation require anticoagulant treatment to prevent embolization. These patients are at risk for infective endocarditis and should receive prophylactic antibiotic treatment for dental and surgical procedures. Myotomy or myomectomy under cardiac bypass may be needed in 10% to 15% of patients. Mitral valve replacement may also be needed.

Anesthetic Considerations

Anesthetic management should focus on strategies that alleviate and do not increase LV outflow obstruction. It is imperative that adequate or slightly elevated LV volume be maintained. Measures that decrease venous return and interfere with adequate ventricular preload should be avoided. Factors that increase myocardial contractility should be avoided. Inadequate depth of anesthesia that causes SNS stimulation may be detrimental. In the event that hypotension occurs, adequate perfusion pressure should be maintained by increasing preload with fluid administration and increasing SVR with phenylephrine. Pharmacologic therapy used to treat hypertrophic cardiomyopathy (including β-blockers and calcium channel blockers) should be continued until the time of surgery.

Anesthetic management must focus on increasing LV preload, decreasing myocardial contractility, controlling the heart rate, and maintaining or increasing afterload. Regional anesthesia is not contraindicated in patients with DCM. Decreases in blood pressure must be treated immediately. Hypovolemia must be avoided and expeditiously treated if it occurs. Deep general anesthesia with a volatile agent is preferred in patients with hypertrophic cardiomyopathy and obstruction.

The potential for hemodynamic deterioration because of increasing subaortic obstruction along with secondary MR necessitates aggressive hemodynamic monitoring. Invasive monitoring via a PA catheter allows for maintenance of adequate LV end-diastolic volume (LVEDV). Because of reduced diastolic compliance associated with hypertrophic cardiomyopathy, pulmonary capillary wedge pressure (PCWP) does not correlate directly with LVEDV. The PCWP should be maintained at approximately 18 to 25 mmHg. If hemodynamic status deteriorates and exacerbation of outflow obstruction is suspected, β-blocking drugs (propranolol or esmolol) should be administered. In addition, vasoconstrictors such as phenylephrine should be used to increase SVR.

B. CORONARY ARTERY DISEASE

Definition

Coronary artery disease (CAD) is a complex disease state that involves narrowing of the coronary arteries.

Incidence

Coronary heart disease caused about one of every six deaths in the United States in 2008. Coronary heart disease's mortality in 2008 was 405,309. Each year, an estimated 785,000 Americans will have a new coronary attack, and about 470,000 will have a recurrent attack. It is estimated that an additional 195,000 silent first myocardial infarctions (MIs) occur each year. Approximately every 25 seconds, an American will have a coronary event, and approximately every minute, someone will die of one.

Pathophysiology

The pathogenesis of CAD is not definitively clear, but several theories have been proposed. Scientists believe the endothelium or innermost layer of the artery becomes injured. Over time, cholesterol agents such as low-density lipoproteins and macrophages adhere to the endothelium and form plaques. The plaques continue to build and decrease the vessels' ability to distend. Because coronary oxygen extraction is maximal at rest, the only way to increase oxygen delivery to the tissues is to increase coronary flow. In normal coronaries, flow can increase three to five times over baseline when demand increases. However, this increase in flow, known as coronary reserve, is limited in patients with CAD. Thus, when patients with CAD increase demand by exercise or stress, they develop *demand ischemia*, which can then be symptomatically experienced as predictable stable angina.

Acute coronary syndromes (ACS) and perioperative ischemia are usually caused by *supply ischemia*. Ischemia occurs when a piece of the plaque ruptures causing a thrombus to form that significantly or totally occludes a segment of a coronary artery, leading to ischemia, dysrhythmias, or MI. The problem can be exacerbated by spasm, which can develop even in normal adjacent vessels.

Treatment

Great strides have been made in the nonsurgical treatment of patients with CAD and ACS in the past 2 decades. The development and evolution of coronary stents have revolutionized care. Most patients presenting for coronary artery bypass graft (CABG) surgery with CAD or ACS will have been referred for some type of percutaneous coronary intervention (PCI). Surgeons and anesthesia providers must take this into consideration when planning care. Much research has been done comparing the risk-to-benefit ratio of surgical intervention to optimal medical management. The American College of Cardiology/American Heart Association (ACC/AHA) guidelines state that surgical intervention is indicated for patients with stenosis of greater than 50% in the left main trunk or triple vessel disease. Additionally, patients who have failed PCI or who have coronary lesions not amenable to PCI benefit from surgery. In these situations, CABG has been found to have a lower mortality risk of major cardiovascular complications or cerebral events than optimal medical management.

Anesthetic Considerations

Cardiac Evaluation

A complete history and physical examination, chest radiography, and electrocardiography (ECG) should be performed in the patient with known or suspected CAD. If the initial evaluation suggests CAD, stress testing may be indicated. An exercise ECG with or without concomitant administration of intravenous radionuclide (i.e., thallium) or pharmacologic echocardiography is usually performed. If the stress test is suggestive of CAD, cardiac catheterization may then be indicated. In addition, dobutamine stress echocardiography is also available to further evaluate overall cardiac function.

Evaluation of Left Ventricular Function

Poor Function	Good Function
1. History	1. History
a. Multiple MIs	a. Angina
b. Symptoms of CHF	b. Hypertension and obesity
2. Cardiac catheterization	c. No symptoms of CHF
a. EF <40%	2. Cardiac catheterization
b. LVEDP >18 mmHg	a. EF >50%
c. Multiple areas of ventricular dyskinesia	b. LVEDP <12 mmHg
d. Decreased CO	c. No areas of ventricular dyskinesia
e. Ventricular septal defect	d. Normal CO
f. MI in progress	
g. Extreme age	

CHF, Congestive heart failure; *CO,* cardiac output; *EF,* ejection fraction; *LVEDP,* left ventricular end-diastolic pressure; *MI,* myocardial infarction.

History

The clinician should elicit the severity and functional limitations imposed by CAD. Evaluation of symptoms as they relate to exercise tolerance, dyspnea, angina, and peripheral edema will give a qualitative estimate of the degree of impairment. Symptoms in some patients may not be present at rest, so the patient's response to physical activity should be elicited through careful, appropriate questioning (e.g., Can the patient climb a flight of stairs?). One must be able to identify borderline CHF because the stress of anesthesia and surgery may elicit overt heart failure perioperatively.

Preoperative

The goal is to decrease anxiety and thus sympathetic stimulation, which may otherwise increase myocardial oxygen demand, causing ischemia. Benzodiazepines (e.g., midazolam) or narcotics may be administered for preoperative sedation and amnesia. Nitroglycerin may also be administered prophylactically to optimize coronary blood flow. Guidelines are included in the box below based on whether the patient has good or poor LV function.

Preoperative Medication and Left Ventricular Function

Poor Function	Good Function
Light premedication	Heavy premedication
IV sedation for line insertion	IV sedation for line insertion
Slow narcotic and relaxant induction	Narcotic, relaxant, and thiopental induction
	Inhalation agent may be used

IV, Intravenous.

Intraoperative

Intraoperative events that adversely affect the balance between myocardial oxygen supply and demand should be prevented. Factors that can *decrease oxygen supply* and *increase oxygen demand* are listed in the following box. The goal is to maintain heart rate and blood pressure within 20% of normal, although it is generally accepted that a heart rate higher than 100 beats/min is more likely to cause ischemia. Current recommendations state that the ideal target heart rate is 70 beats/min or less.

Factors Influencing Oxygen Supply and Demand

Decrease Oxygen Supply	Increase Oxygen Demand
Decreased cerebral blood flow	Sympathetic stimulation
Tachycardia	Tachycardia
Increased diastolic pressure	Increased systolic blood pressure
Increased $Paco_2$	Increased myocardial contractility
Coronary artery spasm	Increased afterload
Decreased Cao_2, anemia, Pao_2	Increased preload
Increased preload	

Induction of Anesthesia

Induction drugs (with the exception of ketamine) are acceptable, provided they are administered judiciously. Laryngoscopy and intubation time should be kept at a minimum (<15 seconds) to decrease sympathetic stimulation and its deleterious effects. If hypertension exists in the patient before anesthesia, the following drugs can be used to facilitate a smooth, stress-free induction:

- Lidocaine: 1 to 2 mg/kg intravenously 90 seconds before laryngoscopy
- Nitroprusside: 1 to 2 mcg/kg intravenously 15 seconds before laryngoscopy
- Esmolol: 100 to 300 mcg/kg intravenously before induction
- Fentanyl: 1 to 3 mcg/kg intravenously during induction

Maintenance of Anesthesia

It is imperative to identify whether the patient has normal or poor LV function. In patients with normal LV function, it is important to avoid tachycardia and hypertension during periods of intense stimulation (laryngoscopy and surgical incision). Volatile anesthetics minimize increases in sympathetic activity and oxygen demand. Inclusion of nitrous oxide with an inhalational agent or alone as part of a nitrous oxide–opioid technique is also acceptable. A high-dose narcotic technique with the addition of a volatile anesthetic to treat undesired increases in blood pressure is effective. In patients with poor LV function, agents that precipitate myocardial depression are not advocated. Opioids are the agents of choice, with low-dose volatile anesthetics, nitrous oxide, and benzodiazepines added as needed.

Muscle Relaxation

Any of several nondepolarizing muscle relaxants may be used. Intermediate-acting relaxants (vecuronium, cisatracurium) have been used successfully, as have longer acting relaxants (pancuronium). Choice of relaxant may be determined by its potential effect on heart rate, length of procedure, plan for emergence (i.e., Will the patient be mechanically ventilated postoperatively, or is "fast tracking" to be considered?), and cost. Pancuronium can cause a dose-dependent increase in heart rate (which could potentially lead to myocardial ischemia); however, it can also be used to offset the bradycardia that ensues when high-dose narcotics are used.

Reversal Agents

Anticholinesterase drugs (pyridostigmine, neostigmine) and anticholinergics (atropine, glycopyrrolate, and scopolamine) are considered safe. Many clinicians prefer glycopyrrolate because of its tendency to preserve a somewhat "normal" heart rate when used in combination with an anticholinesterase. The reversal medications should be titrated in incremental doses to decrease the potential for tachycardia.

Emergence

The same considerations apply here as for induction of anesthesia (i.e., prevent increases in myocardial oxygen demand and decreases in supply). Patients with severe CAD may need treatment for hypertensive episodes during emergence from anesthesia and into the postoperative period.

Postoperative Implications

Maintenance of normal cardiac dynamics (blood pressure and heart rate), normal arterial oxygen and carbon dioxide pressure, and adequate pain relief are essential to prevent sympathetic stimulation and its deleterious effects on myocardial oxygen supply and demand.

C. HEART FAILURE

Definition

Heart failure is a complex pathophysiologic process that causes a clinical syndrome characterized by pulmonary congestion caused by the heart's inability to fill with or eject blood in a sufficient quantity to meet tissue requirements

Etiology

Heart failure is caused by an insult that alters perfusion and leads to a state of neurohumoral imbalance. Activation of the sympathetic nervous system (SNS) and the renin–angiotensin–aldosterone system (RAAS) induces a host of pathologic responses.

Pathophysiology

In the face of sympathetic activation coupled with alterations in perfusion, pressure, and volume, the heart changes its size, shape, and function; that is, it "*remodels*" itself in an attempt to maintain CO. Whereas *supply* ischemia causes an increase in ventricular compliance (dilation) and a decrease in contractility, *demand* ischemia reduces compliance (stiffening) without initially impacting contractility. The primary characteristics of remodeling are hypertrophy or dilation, myocyte death, and increased interstitial fibrosis. The clinical impact manifests as a change in systolic and diastolic function.

Systolic Dysfunction

Supply ischemia resulting in MI or chronic volume overload of the LV causes *eccentric* hypertrophy or dilation. The chamber size increases in an attempt to preserve SV. In the dilated state, the heart loses its normal elliptical football shape and becomes more spherical, resembling a basketball. In this shape, the heart is unable to contract effectively (systolic dysfunction), and the mitral apparatus is stretched potentially to a point that results in MR. About 35% to 50% of patients with heart failure experience MR. The degree of systolic dysfunction is commonly expressed as ejection fraction (EF). The EF is calculated as SV divided by end-diastolic volume. According to the American Society of Echocardiography's guidelines, normal EF is 55% or greater, and dysfunction is graded as mild (45%–54%), moderate

(30%–44%), and severe (<30%). When SV is reduced, the body compensates by activating the SNS to raise the resting heart rate in an effort to maintain CO. Systolic heart failure (SHF) is caused by CAD, DCM, chronic volume overload (regurgitant valves, high output failure), and the later stages of chronic pressure overload (AS and chronic hypertension). MI causes regional defects that can eventually encompass the entire myocardium; other causes of heart failure typically reduce global function from the onset.

Diastolic Dysfunction

Diastolic dysfunction is a more difficult concept that is equally important. Pulmonary congestion and all of the symptoms of heart failure can indeed develop with a normal EF. In fact, diastolic failure is often called heart failure with preserved (>40%) EF. *Demand ischemia,* caused by chronic pressure loads from stenotic heart valves, obstructive cardiomyopathy, chronic hypertension, or obesity causes the myocardium to thicken (*concentric hypertrophy*) and compliance to decrease. Pulmonary congestion develops because the fibrosed, nondistensible LV, with an increased LVEDP, is unable to fill adequately despite near normal systolic function. Diastolic failure is graded class I to IV based on echocardiographic examination findings. The hypertrophied LV is prone to ischemia; therefore, maintenance of a high mean arterial pressure (MAP) and slow normal heart rate is crucial. Hypotension should be treated promptly, usually with phenylephrine to avoid rapid decompensation that can potentially lead to cardiac arrest. In a hypertrophied heart, chest compressions rarely generate enough pressure to perfuse the noncompliant LV. The mortality and hospitalization rates are similar in both systolic and diastolic failure. Often, as diastolic heart failure (DHF) progresses, SHF will develop, and the two will coexist.

The characteristics of patients with SHF and DHF are listed below.

Characteristics of Patients with Diastolic and Systolic Heart Failure

Characteristic	Diastolic HF	Systolic HF
Age	Frequently elderly	Usually 50–70 years
Gender	Frequently female	Most often male
EF	Preserved, >40%	Depressed, <40%
LV cavity size	Normal with concentric LVH	Dilated with eccentric LVH
Chest radiography findings	Congestion and cardiomegaly	Congestion and cardiomegaly
HTN	+++	++
DM	+++	++
Previous MI	+	+++
Obesity	+++	+
COPD	++	0
Sleep apnea	++	++
Dialysis	++	0
Atrial fibrillation	+ Usually paroxysmal	+ Usually persistent
Gallop rhythm	S_4	S_3

+, Occasionally associated with; ++, often associated with; +++, usually associated with; *0,* no association; *COPD,* chronic obstructive pulmonary disease; *DM,* diabetes mellitus; *EF,* ejection fraction; *HTN,* hypertension; *LV,* left ventricle; *LVH,* left ventricular hypertrophy; *MI,* myocardial infarction
Adapted from Popescue WM. Heart failure and cardiomyopathies. In Hines RA, Marschall KE, eds. *Stoelting's Anesthesia and Co-Existing Disease.* 6th ed. Philadelphia: Saunders; 2012:122.

Anesthetic Considerations

The anesthetic management strategies for systolic and diastolic dysfunction are listed in the following table.

Anesthetic Considerations for Systolic and Diastolic Dysfunction

	Systolic Dysfunction	Diastolic Dysfunction
Preload	• Already ↑; avoid overload, especially coming off pump. • NTG helps reduce preload and ↑ subendocardial perfusion	• Volume will be needed to stretch noncompliant LV • Evaluate with echocardiography because LVEDP is falsely ↑
Contractility	• Reduced→ Avoid agents that cause further reductions • May need inotropic support	• Usually good but use caution with agents that suppress function • *Does not* tolerate hypotension
Afterload	• Reductions will enhance forward flow as long as coronary perfusion pressure maintained • SNP works well if volume is adequate	• Already ↑ • Higher MAP needed to perfuse thick myocardium • Treat hypotension aggressively with phenylephrine
Heart Rate	• Usually high normal because of sympathetic activation	• Slow normal to maximize diastolic time for coronary perfusion and ↓MvO_2 • Prone to ischemia • Maintain SR→ Cardiovert early
CPB	• Expect large pump volumes • Consider ultrafiltration, diuretic	• Pump volume normal

↓, Decreased; ↑, increased; →, therefore; *CPB,* cardiopulmonary bypass; *LVEDP,* left ventricular end-diastolic pressure; *MAP,* mean arterial pressure; MvO_2, myocardial venous oxygen; *N,* nitroglycerin; *SNP,* sodium nitroprusside; *SR,* sinus rhythm

Treatment

Treatment is tailored to the patient's age, current disease state, and concurrent disorders. Multimodal drug therapy is used to treat heart failure and is aimed at interrupting the response and slowing disease progression. Drug therapy may include digitalis, diuretics, β-blockers, angiotensin-converting enzyme (ACE) inhibitors, and aldosterone antagonists.

D. HYPERTENSION

Definition

The AHA defines hypertension as blood pressure of 140/90 mmHg or higher.

Incidence

Hypertension affects approximately 60 million people in the United States, and the frequency at which it occurs increases with age. Nearly two-thirds of people older than the age of 65 years have hypertension.

Etiology

Hypertension is classified on the basis of its causes. Essential (primary) hypertension, which has no identifiable cause, accounts for 95% of all cases of the disease, and its diagnosis is determined on the basis of exclusion. The relationship between an individual's genetic predisposition and environmental factors most probably influences the potential development and severity of essential hypertension. Theoretical physiologic causes of essential hypertension include SNS hyperactivity or increased activity of the RAAS. Remedial (secondary) hypertension has an identifiable and potentially curable cause. Examples of pathophysiologic conditions that cause remedial hypertension include pheochromocytoma, coarctation of the aorta, renal artery stenosis, primary renal diseases (e.g., pyelonephritis, glomerulonephritis), primary aldosteronism (Conn's disease), and hyperadrenocorticism (Cushing's disease).

The classification of hypertension is listed below.

Classification of Blood Pressure for Adults Age 18 Years and Older

Category	Systolic (mmHg)		Diastolic (mmHg)
Normal	<120	And	<80
Prehypertension	120–139	Or	80–89
Hypertension, stage 1	140–159	Or	90–99
Hypertension, stage 2	≥160	Or	≥100

DBP, Diastolic blood pressure; *SBP,* systolic blood pressure;.
From U.S. Department of Health and Human Services, National Heart Lung and Blood Institute. *Seventh Report of the Joint National Committee on Prevention, Detection, Evaluation, and Treatment of High Blood Pressure.* Bethesda, MD: NIH publication No. 04-5230; 2004. Available at www.nhlbi.nih.gov/guidelines/hypertension/jnc7full.pdf.

The risk of cardiovascular disease doubles with each increment of 20/10 mmHg above 115/75 mmHg. It is estimated that the implementation of antihypertensive therapy is associated with a 25% decrease in cardiovascular complications and a 38% decrease in stroke.

Pathophysiology

Systemic blood pressure is regulated by interactive feedback mechanisms involving the sympathoadrenal axis and baroreceptors in the heart and great vessels. It is accepted that some degree of sympathetic dysfunction is responsible for essential hypertension. Dysfunction of the SNS leads to a state of chronic vasoconstriction. In an attempt to maintain normal intravascular volume, the renal juxtaglomerular apparatus secretes renin. All of the vascular and hormonal effects of renin are caused by its conversion of angiotensin I to angiotensin II. Angiotensin II is the major stimulus for the secretion of aldosterone by the adrenal cortex.

Deposition of collagen and metalloproteinases within the intima of arteries leads to vascular stiffness, and this occurs normally as part of the aging process. Narrowing of the vascular lumen and endothelial dysfunction causing inability of complete vasodilation decreases blood flow, especially within the microvasculature. Furthermore, vascular stiffness increases afterload and myocardial oxygen demand and can cause LV hypertrophy, myocardial ischemia or infarction, and CHF.

Treatment

When the diastolic blood pressure (DBP) is greater than 90 mmHg, drug treatment is usually used, although isolated systolic hypertension may respond to diet modification and weight loss. Patients with borderline hypertension can decrease their blood pressure with exercise and weight loss. If the DBP exceeds 105 mmHg, aggressive treatment is needed to decrease morbidity and mortality from MI, CHF, cerebrovascular accident, and renal failure.

Drugs used to treat patients with hypertension include diuretics, ACE inhibitors, calcium antagonists, β-blockers, and vasodilators. A combination of two antihypertensives is often used to minimize the undesirable physiologic responses to any one particular drug (e.g., a compensatory increase in renin activity). Serum potassium levels should be monitored because hypokalemia or hyperkalemia may be a side effect.

Anesthetic Considerations

Preoperative

The most important issues to be addressed in the preoperative evaluation are the identification and the adequacy of treatment. If the perioperative DBP is maintained below 110 mmHg, the risk of perioperative cardiac morbidity does not increase significantly. Reviewing the patient's medication and determining adequacy of blood pressure control are essential.

An individualized anesthetic plan must be created by taking into account the type and extent of cardiac pathophysiology, other disease states, and the surgical procedure. To maintain a stable intraoperative course, administration of antihypertensive medications should be continued on schedule until the time of surgery. Tachycardia, hypertension, angina, and MI can result from interruption of therapy with β-blockers and calcium channel–blocking agents. These drugs should be discontinued with caution and only after utmost discretionary review of the patient's physiologic status.

Determining whether to proceed with elective surgery in a patient in whom hypertension is untreated or poorly controlled remains controversial. Patients who have DBPs greater than 110 mmHg have a significantly increased risk of perioperative cardiac morbidity. This caveat may be modified in patients with hypertension in whom DBPs greater than 110 mmHg occur frequently despite aggressive antihypertensive drug therapy (e.g., patients with end-stage renal disease).

Preoperative sedation may be indicated for patients with hypertension to attenuate sympathetic responsiveness. Establishing control of the blood pressure before induction should result in a more stable hemodynamic course during the induction, maintenance, and emergence from anesthesia. A fluid bolus and incremental titration of anesthetic induction agents may help to decrease the degree and duration of hypotension.

Induction of Anesthesia

- Patients with hypertension react in an exaggerated manner to induction agents and the stimulation associated with laryngoscopy and tracheal intubation. This response is highly variable and may result in hypertension or hypotension.
- Hypertensive patients are hypovolemic as a result of renal-compensatory mechanisms, extreme vasoconstriction, or pharmacologic therapy (diuretics). Increased vasoconstriction as a consequence of hypertension results in volume contraction and a greater susceptibility to hypotension from the vasodilating and cardiac depressant effects of anesthetic agents.

- Etomidate, propofol, and dexmedetomidine agents can be used in patients with hypertension.
- The stimulation associated with laryngoscopy and tracheal intubation can result in an exaggerated hypertensive response despite postinduction hypotension. Administration of adjunct medications before induction such as β-blockers or arterial dilators can reduce the hyperdynamic sympathetic response to tracheal intubation.
- Hypotensive episodes can be treated with fluid administration, a decrease in anesthetic depth, and administration of vasoconstrictors. The pressor response to laryngoscopy and intubation can be significantly reduced by laryngotracheal or intravenous administration of lidocaine, reducing the duration of airway manipulation to 15 seconds or less, and the administration of a β-blocker before induction. Administration of fentanyl (2–3 mcg/kg) just before induction also attenuates the pressor response.
- The maintenance of an adequate depth of anesthesia at induction that produces extreme hypotension may be more detrimental to both coronary and cerebral perfusion than the hypertensive response it was intended to prevent. Because the hypertensive patient is frequently hypovolemic compared with the normotensive patient, adequate hydration before induction may help to prevent postinduction hypotension.

Maintenance of Anesthesia

The goal of anesthetic management of patients with hypertension undergoing general anesthesia is to maintain blood pressure stability within 20% of the normal mean pressure. Intraoperative events that cause wide fluctuations in blood pressure should be anticipated and treated immediately.

The most common event precipitating intraoperative hypertension is the painful stimulus of surgery. This induces increased sympathetic tone via a neurohormonal reflex and represents the stress-induced response of surgical stimulation. Volatile and opioid anesthetic agents given alone and in combination have the ability to attenuate this response.

The adjunct use of drugs such as β-antagonists, nitroprusside, ACE inhibitors (e.g., enalapril), α_2-agonists (e.g., clonidine), calcium channel blockers (e.g., nifedipine), and α_1-blockers (e.g., droperidol) may be necessary for achieving normotension.

The onset of profound hypotension during anesthesia maintenance should be immediately recognized, diagnosed, and treated. Treatment of hypotension may require reduction of the amount of volatile agent used and infusion of adequate volume. If these measures prove inadequate or untimely, a rapid-acting vasopressor such as phenylephrine or ephedrine may be administered as a temporizing measure until the cause of the hypotension can be diagnosed. It is important to realize that hypertensive patients may have exaggerated responses to vasopressor agents.

Postoperative Implications

- Termination of anesthesia results in hyperdynamic, hypertensive responses, even in patients with well-controlled hypertension. Intraoperative control of blood pressure should continue into the immediate postoperative period.
- Initiation of adjunct administration of antihypertensive medications should be anticipated early in the postoperative period. Adequate control of pain represents a primary antihypertensive consideration. Patients with

hypertension are more susceptible to perioperative cardiac morbidity than normotensive patients during the postoperative period. Adequate control of blood pressure and postprocedural pain in the postoperative period reduces the incidence of cardiovascular complications.

E. MYOCARDIAL INFARCTION

Definition

Myocardial infarction or myocardial cell death occurs when a portion of heart muscle is deprived of its blood supply as a result of blockage, acute thrombosis, or spasm of a coronary artery. MI is considered part of a spectrum referred to as ACS. The ACS continuum representing ongoing myocardial ischemia or injury consists of unstable angina, non–ST-segment elevation MI (NSTEMI), and ST-segment elevation MI (STEMI). Patients with ischemic discomfort may or may not have ST-segment or T-wave changes denoted on the ECG.

Pathophysiology

When myocardial oxygen supply (i.e., coronary blood flow) does not meet demand (myocardial oxygen consumption), ischemia or MI may occur. The risk for perioperative MI increases when a patient who has had a previous MI undergoes anesthesia and operation.

ST-segment elevations seen on the ECG reflect active and ongoing transmural myocardial injury. Without immediate reperfusion therapy, most persons with STEMI develop Q waves, reflecting a dead zone of myocardium that has undergone irreversible damage and death. Those without ST elevations are diagnosed either with unstable angina or NSTEMI—differentiated by the presence of cardiac enzymes. Both of these conditions may or may not have changes on the surface ECG, including ST-segment depression or T-wave morphologic changes. MI may lead to impairment of systolic or diastolic function and to increased predisposition to arrhythmias and other long-term complications.

Treatment

As a general rule, initial therapy for acute MI is directed toward restoration of perfusion as soon as possible to salvage as much of the jeopardized myocardium as possible. This may be accomplished through medical or mechanical means, such as PCI or CABG.

Further treatment is based on the following:

- Restoration of the balance between the oxygen supply and demand to prevent further ischemia
- Pain relief
- Prevention and treatment of any complications that may arise

Coronary thrombolysis and mechanical revascularization have revolutionized the primary treatment of patients with acute MI, largely because they allow salvage of the myocardium when implemented early after the onset of ischemia. The modest prognostic benefit of an opened infarct-related artery may be realized even when recanalization is induced only 6 hours or more after the onset of symptoms, that is, when the salvaging of substantial amounts of jeopardized ischemic myocardium is no longer likely. The opening of an infarct-related artery may improve ventricular function, collateral blood flow, and ventricular remodeling, and it may decrease infarct expansion, ventricular aneurysm formation, LV dilatation, late arrhythmia associated with ventricular aneurysms, and mortality

Evidence suggests a benefit from the use of β-blockers, ACE inhibitors, angiotensin II receptor blockers, and statins.

Anesthetic Considerations

Anesthesia care begins with a thorough history and physical examination. The history reveals risk factors for ischemic heart disease, activity tolerance, determination of angina (stable or unstable), and use of coronary vasodilators (e.g., nitroglycerin). The physical examination may reveal extra heart sounds (i.e., S_3 or S_4), rales or rhonchi, jugular venous distention, peripheral edema, or other findings consistent with underlying cardiac disease. The anesthetist should communicate any findings with the primary physician and surgeon to weigh the risks and benefits of the proposed surgical procedure. The importance of minimizing stress (demand) and optimizing myocardial perfusion (supply) intraoperatively cannot be overemphasized. Reduction of stress begins in the preoperative area with the use of individualized sedation. Any increase in metabolic work during the perioperative period increases myocardial oxygen demand, which may result in myocardial ischemia or MI. Myocardial oxygen supply and demand must be balanced for an optimal outcome.

Four questions must therefore be answered before the patient proceeds to anesthesia and operation. The answers to these questions are often determined by careful history taking. The first three questions to be addressed are: What is the extent of CAD? Is additional therapy indicated (e.g., cardiac catheterization, angioplasty, or CABG)? What is the extent of ventricular compromise? How the clinician determines the answers to these questions will inevitably affect the administration and titration of anesthetics. Finally, the fourth question to be asked is: Will the patient tolerate surgery?

Standard monitoring should always be considered in these patients. In addition, ECG monitoring of lead II (inferior ischemia) and lead V_5 (anterior ischemia), ST-segment trend analysis, esophageal ECG (to identify P waves, posterior ischemia), or transesophageal echocardiography can be used perioperatively. Invasive intravascular lines, such as a central venous pressure (CVP) line, a PA catheter (to evaluate right- and left-sided heart pressures, PCWP, pulmonary and systemic vascular resistances, and CO or cardiac index), and an arterial line for beat-to-beat evaluation of blood pressure and frequent blood specimen analyses may need to be considered. These measures should be used to optimize anesthetic care when the patient is at risk because of the clinical history or the surgical procedure.

Recognition and aggressive treatment of ischemia are vital. Careful, vigilant monitoring perioperatively will allow rapid intervention in the patient at risk for cardiac complications. Likewise, interpretation of data and prompt initiation of treatment have been shown to improve outcome.

Fluid management in these patients should be individualized to the length and type of operation and the degree of LV compromise. A CVP or PA catheter can offer useful information in these high-risk patients. Intraoperative overhydration (i.e., fluid overload) may lead to postoperative hypertension and CHF.

Urine output should be closely monitored in cardiac patients (0.5–1.0 mL/kg/hr). It is believed to be a reflection of renal perfusion and thus

CO, provided renal function is normal. Urine output may also be an indicator of overall patient volume status.

Choice of anesthetic in these patients should be individualized to the patient and the proposed procedure. General, regional, and local anesthetic techniques have all been used successfully. It is important for the clinician to understand that patient outcome is based on how the agents are administered rather than the specific technique used.

General anesthesia and spinal anesthesia are similar when the risk of perioperative MI and death is considered. A combined general–epidural technique for vascular surgery has been suggested to lower cardiac complications. The incidence and risk of CHF are higher with general anesthesia in patients with severe CAD.

Emergence from anesthesia should be smooth and stress free, with special efforts made to maintain cardiac hemodynamics (myocardial oxygen supply and demand). The time of extubation may need to be delayed until cardiovascular stability is established.

Ongoing postoperative observation of high-risk patients is essential to identify and aggressively treat cardiac complications. Shivering, fever, pain, wide swings in blood pressure, tachycardia, arrhythmias, and CHF may alter cardiac dynamics, leading to ischemia (and MI). Careful fluid management may also minimize the potential for postoperative ischemic events and may improve outcome.

Recognizing the importance of complications and mortality related to anesthesia and surgery is the first step toward prevention. Patients at risk for perioperative cardiac complications can be risk stratified, and the information can be used to plan the safest anesthetic and intraoperative monitoring.

F. PERICARDIAL DISEASE

This section focuses on the pathophysiology, clinical presentation, and anesthetic implications of three primary pericardial disease processes: acute pericarditis, constrictive pericarditis, and cardiac tamponade.

The pericardium surrounds the heart and anchors it to its anatomic position, concomitantly reducing contact between it and surrounding structures. It consists of an inner visceral layer, which envelops the surface of the heart, and an outer parietal layer. The pericardial space between these layers usually contains 20 to 25 mL of clear fluid, which under normal circumstances can accommodate gradual volume fluctuations. Rapid accumulation of pericardial fluid in the pericardial space can result in cardiac tamponade and cardiovascular collapse.

ACUTE PERICARDITIS

Etiology

Acute inflammation of the pericardium is caused by a number of disorders. The most common cause of acute pericarditis is viral infection. Post-MI syndrome (Dressler syndrome), postcardiotomy, metastatic disease, irradiation, tuberculosis, and rheumatoid arthritis represent the remaining primary predisposing conditions that contribute to the development of this process.

Pathophysiology

It is common for a serofibrinous inflammatory reaction associated with a small intrapericardial exudative effusion to evolve. This may result in adherence of the two layers of the pericardium. The sequelae are largely dependent on the severity of the reaction as well as on the specific cause. Most often when the condition is left untreated or undiagnosed, complete resolution is the end result. Infrequently, however, extended organization of fibrinous exudate within the pericardial sac may lead to encasement of the heart by dense fibrous connective tissue (chronic constrictive pericarditis) or to the accumulation of a large amount of pericardial fluid and consequent cardiac tamponade, usually when fluid levels exceed 1 L. Constrictive pericarditis and cardiac tamponade result in impaired diastolic filling and subsequent diminution of CO.

Anesthetic Considerations

Acute pericarditis in the absence of an associated pericardial effusion or scarring does not alter cardiac function. Specific considerations for anesthetic management are directed toward the underlying illness.

CHRONIC CONSTRICTIVE PERICARDITIS

Etiology

Chronic constrictive pericarditis results from pericardial thickening and fibrosis. In the past, tuberculosis was the most common cause of pericardial constriction. Currently, the most common causes are idiopathic in nature and include complications after cardiac surgery, neoplasia, uremia, radiation therapy, and rheumatoid arthritis.

Pathophysiology

The fundamental hemodynamic abnormality in chronic constrictive pericarditis is abnormal diastolic filling. The reduced myocardial compliance impairs filling of both ventricles. Consequently, filling pressures increase, and as a result, pulmonary and peripheral congestion occurs. SV and CO can also be decreased. Equilibration of PA diastolic pressure, PCWP, and RA pressure commonly occurs. Initially, ventricular systolic function is normal. However, over time, the underlying myocardial tissue may atrophy, and systolic function may decrease.

Treatment

The treatment used for patients with hemodynamically significant constrictive pericarditis is pericardiectomy. Unfortunately, the surgical removal of adherent pericardium may precipitate malignant cardiac dysrhythmias and massive bleeding. Consequently, pericardiectomy is associated with relatively high perioperative morbidity and mortality rates, ranging from 6% to 19%.

Anesthetic Considerations

Large-bore intravenous lines must be established preoperatively because of the potential for sudden, rapid hemorrhage. A cardiopulmonary bypass circuit should be readily available. Invasive hemodynamic monitoring is essential. Arterial catheterization allows beat-to-beat blood pressure monitoring and assists in the evaluation of significant cardiac dysrhythmia. A PA catheter is useful because it permits measurement of filling pressures on both the right and left sides of the heart as well as determination of CO.

The anesthetic agents chosen for management of patients with constrictive pericarditis should preserve myocardial contractility, heart rate, preload, and afterload. Among these parameters, heart rate is of greatest concern.

CO is dependent on heart rate in patients with constrictive pericarditis. As a consequence of limited ventricular diastolic filling, bradycardia is poorly tolerated and reflects a decrease in SV that can lead to hypotension. Using anesthetic medications that preserve the heart rate and myocardial contractility, such as pancuronium or ketamine, is hemodynamically advantageous. Inhalation agents that cause myocardial depression should be used with caution. The use of opioids and etomidate, benzodiazepines, and nitrous oxide for the induction and maintenance of anesthesia is suitable in this setting. The clinician should be aware that vigorous positive-pressure ventilation may cause a decrease in venous return to the heart and result in a further decrease in CO.

Postoperative Implications

Immediate hemodynamic improvement may not occur after removal of the constricting tissue. Consistently low CO after pericardiectomy may be secondary to diffuse atrophy of myocardial muscle fibers or myocardial damage from the underlying disease. Intensive postoperative care with inotropic support and awareness of the potential for dysrhythmia or bleeding are integral components of the anesthetic management plan.

G. PERIPHERAL VASCULAR DISEASE

Definition

Peripheral vascular disease (PVD) is an inflammatory disease of the peripheral vasculature. As the lumen of the vessel decreases in diameter, increases in resistance to blood flow occur. As a result of this process, perfusion to peripheral or central tissue is decreased, which can lead to ischemia and cellular necrosis.

Etiology

Peripheral vascular disease may manifest as systemic vasculitis or arterial occlusive disease. There are several types of PVD.

TAKAYASU'S ARTERITIS

Takayasu arteritis is a chronic inflammation of the aorta and its major branches. It causes multiple organ dysfunction.

Anesthetic Considerations

Corticosteroid supplementation may be necessary for patients already treated with these drugs. These patients also may be taking anticoagulants; therefore, regional anesthesia may be controversial. Blood pressure may be difficult to measure noninvasively in the upper extremities, so an arterial line may be necessary. Preoperatively, it is wise to evaluate range of motion of the cervical spine because hyperextension of the head during laryngoscopy may compromise cerebral blood flow (the carotid arteries are shortened as a result of the vascular inflammatory process). Finally, a major anesthetic goal intraoperatively is maintenance of adequate perfusion pressure.

THROMBOANGIITIS OBLITERANS

Definition

Thromboangiitis obliterans is an inflammatory process of the wall and connective tissue surrounding the arteries and veins, especially in the extremities.

It is often associated with the thrombosis and occlusion that commonly result in gangrene. Jewish men between the ages of 20 and 40 years seem to have a higher incidence of this disease.

Anesthetic Considerations

Prevention of cold-induced vasospasm is a major concern. Increasing the ambient room temperature and using convective warming devices (e.g., warming blankets, fluid warmers) help maintain body temperature. Noninvasive blood pressure monitoring is preferable to invasive (arterial) monitoring in this patient population. Regional anesthesia is acceptable; however, the concomitant use of vasoconstrictors (i.e., epinephrine) should be avoided.

CHRONIC PERIPHERAL ARTERIO-OCCLUSIVE DISEASE

Definition

Chronic peripheral arterio-occlusive disease is typically the result of peripheral atherosclerosis and often occurs in association with coronary or cerebral atherosclerosis.

Etiology and Clinical Manifestations

Occlusion of the distal abdominal aorta or the iliac arteries frequently presents as claudication of the hips and buttocks. Elderly patients often develop occlusion of the common femoral or superficial femoral arteries. This produces a syndrome of claudication from the calf area of the lower extremity.

Treatment

Treatment includes revascularization, such as femoral–femoral bypass or any of several different femoral-to-distal bypass procedures.

Anesthetic Considerations

The major risk for operative revascularization is associated ischemic heart disease. Although these procedures can be performed while the patient is under general anesthesia, regional (i.e., epidural) anesthesia before anticoagulant therapy has not been associated with untoward events. Infrarenal cross-clamping of the distal aorta in the patient with PVD is associated with minimal hemodynamic derangements. Typically, monitoring of right-sided heart pressures (i.e., central venous pressure) is sufficient unless left-sided heart disease requires the use of a PA catheter. Thromboembolic complications, particularly in the kidneys, usually reflect dislodgement of atherosclerotic debris. Spinal cord damage is unlikely, and special monitoring is not mandatory.

SUBCLAVIAN STEAL SYNDROME

Occlusion of the right subclavian or innominate artery by an atherosclerotic plaque proximal to the origin of the vertebral artery may result in reversal of blood flow from the brain, leading to syncopal episodes. The pulse in the ipsilateral arm is usually absent or diminished (10 mmHg lower).

CORONARY–SUBCLAVIAN STEAL SYNDROME

This syndrome occurs when incomplete stenosis of the left subclavian artery leads to reversal of blood flow. The patient typically presents with angina and decreased systolic blood pressure (SBP) (at least 20 mmHg lower) in the ipsilateral arm. Bilateral brachial artery blood pressure measurement is helpful in the differential diagnosis and may be useful in the preoperative assessment in patients with an internal mammary–to–coronary artery bypass.

ANEURYSMS OF THE THORACIC AND ABDOMINAL AORTA

Definition

Diseases of the aorta are frequently aneurysmal, but occlusive disease is most likely to affect the peripheral arteries.

Etiology

The primary event in aortic dissection is a tear in the intimal wall through which blood surges and creates a false lumen. The adventitia then separates up or down (or both) the aorta for various distances. Associated conditions include hypertension (which is present in 80% of these patients), Marfan syndrome, blunt chest trauma, pregnancy, and iatrogenic surgical injury (e.g., resulting from aortic cannulation during cardiopulmonary bypass). Aortic dissections involving the ascending aorta are considered type A. Surgical repair is through a median sternotomy using profound hypothermia. Aortic dissections involving the descending aorta (i.e., beyond the origin of the left subclavian artery) are considered type B. Aneurysms can also be classified as saccular, fusiform, or dissecting.

Treatment

Early, short-term treatment includes the use of β-blockers or other cardioactive agents that decrease SBP (to 100 mmHg) and aid in decreasing myocardial contractility and vascular resistance. Ultimately, surgical intervention is often necessary using aortic stent grafts or an open approach.

H. SHOCK

HEMORRHAGIC SHOCK

Definition

Hemorrhagic shock is a complication that arises from acute blood loss, also referred to as hemodynamic or vascular collapse. There is a decreased intravascular fluid volume that leads to a decreased venous return and CO and subsequently leads to inadequate organ and tissue perfusion.

Etiology

Hemorrhagic shock is a result of acute blood loss, frequently owing to trauma. Along with a decrease in intravascular fluid volume, SNS activity is increased, redirecting blood flow to the brain and heart. If this condition persists, a detrimental decrease in renal and hepatic blood flow occurs. Anaerobic metabolism is increased (lactate production), and metabolic (lactic) acidosis is manifested.

Treatment

Blood replacement therapy typically includes administration of whole blood or packed red blood cells. Crystalloids (balanced salt solutions) are also used because fluid shifts accompany hemorrhage, but controversy exists whether colloids (albumin, dextran, hetastarch) provide a better resuscitative fluid medium. Invasive monitoring, including arterial blood pressure, central venous pressure, and urinary drainage system to guide volume replacement, may become necessary. A PA catheter is helpful to determine CO, filling pressures, systemic and pulmonary vascular resistances, and oxygen extraction and delivery to the tissues. Dopamine may be useful in some cases, especially if the goals are a mild inotropic effect and an increase in renal blood flow. Vasopressors may be necessary as well to preserve cerebral and cardiac perfusion until intravascular fluid volume can be replaced. Other blood component therapy may need to be considered as more banked blood is given (e.g., fresh-frozen plasma and platelets).

Anesthetic Considerations

- Induction (if possible) and maintenance typically require invasive monitoring of blood pressure.
- Ketamine is used to induce anesthesia because it stimulates the SNS. Additional anesthetic agents must be carefully titrated to the patient's hemodynamic status.
- Treatment of hemorrhagic shock includes control of bleeding and replacement of intravascular volume (with whole blood, packed red blood cells, or both) while maintaining adequate perfusion pressures to the vital organs.

SEPTIC SHOCK

Definition

Septic shock is shock resulting from the presence of pathogenic organisms or their toxins in the blood. Bacterial endotoxins cause severe systemic vasodilation, resulting in hypotension and decreased organ perfusion.

Etiology

Early Phase

The early phase is characterized by hypotension resulting from a decrease in SVR. An increase in CO, elevated temperature, and hyperventilation also manifest themselves. Vasodilation is probably caused by endotoxins from bacterial cell walls that release vasoactive substances (i.e., histamine) and can last up to 24 hours.

Late Phase

Cardiac output may also be increased in this phase. Dilation of peripheral vessels gives over to the shunting of blood away from vital organs, and lactic acidosis develops as a result of impaired tissue oxygenation. Intravascular fluid volume may fall because of damaged muscle. Oliguria is often present. Coagulation defects are common.

Treatment

Treatment includes intravenous antibiotics and restoration of intravascular fluid volume. Antibiotics should be started immediately. Typically, two antibiotics are used to cover both gram-positive bacteria (clindamycin) and gram-negative bacteria (gentamicin). Fluid replacement should be guided by PA catheter measurements of cardiac filling pressures and urine output. Intravenous dopamine is effective when supportive function is needed.

Anesthetic Considerations

No specific anesthetic drug has been proven ideal in the presence of septic shock. The anesthetic management should be individualized to each patient.

NEUROGENIC SHOCK

Definition

Neurogenic shock is caused by a disruption of SNS innervation to the heart and arterial and venous vasculature. The SNS and parasympathetic nervous system work in tandem to balance the physiologic cardiovascular effects. The cardiovascular centers in the brain send efferent sympathetic impulses via the spinal cord to the heart and the vasculature. The efferent parasympathetic impulses also originate in the brain but are transmitted to the cardiovascular system via the vagus nerve (cranial nerve X) directly to the heart and vasculature. When sympathetic outflow is inhibited such as in a spinal cord injury, parasympathetic predominance occurs, resulting in vasodilation and bradycardia. The extent of the cardiovascular and respiratory signs and symptoms depends on the level of spinal cord injury and the patient's comorbidities.

Etiology

Neurogenic shock is most often associated with blunt or penetrating trauma. Patients who have sustained a head injury are at risk for having a neck injury. If spinal cord transaction has occurred, then the patient's deficits will be permanent. However, the potential for limited or complete recovery is possible if partial dysfunction resulting in edema or decreased blood flow to the spinal cord can occur. Cellular damage and chemical mediator release include calcium accumulation intracellularly, potassium accumulation extracellularly, catecholamine infiltration, inflammatory mediator creation and release (phospholipase A2, arachidonic acid metabolites, free oxygen radicals, excitatory amino-acids [glutamate, aspartate], and eicosanoid production).

Diagnosis

Phrenic nerve function allowing for innervation to the diaphragm for breathing originates at C3–C5. As a result, the inability to breathe occurs with high-level spinal cord injuries, those extending into the highest level cervical vertebrae. The cardioaccelerator fibers originate from T1–T4. Innervation to a large amount of vasculature is mediated via T5–L1. The higher the spinal cord injury, the more severe the physical signs and symptoms. Hypotension, bradycardia, and vasodilation also resulting in hypothermia are cardinal signs associated with neurogenic shock. Diagnosis can be confirmed after a physical examination and radiologic evidence, including radiography, computed tomography, or magnetic resonance imaging. The classic presentation includes assessing paralysis, pain, position, paresthesias, ptosis, and priapism. Other signs associated with neurogenic shock are present.

Treatment

Initial intervention should always focus on airway, breathing, and circulation. If breathing is inadequate or the potential for aspiration is severe, endotracheal intubation is warranted. If hypotension occurs, fluid administration and, if necessary, vasopressors should be administered. Atropine is the drug of choice if symptomatic bradycardia occurs. Because of the unopposed vasodilation, the patient is at significant risk for developing hypothermia. All measures to ensure that the patient remains normothermic are necessary.

Lastly, prompt diagnosis and if possible surgical treatment are necessary.

Anesthetic Considerations

Spinal cord perfusion pressure is calculated as MAP-extrinsic pressure exerted on the spinal cord. Therefore, MAP is the major factor contributing to spinal cord perfusion. Spinal cord autoregulation is presumed to occur between a MAP of 60 and 150 mmHg. When trauma occurs, autoregulatory pressures are higher, necessitating greater pressures to ensure adequate spinal cord blood flow. Anesthesia can be achieved by using a combination of agents, inhalation, narcotic, and propofol infusion. Maintaining adequate MAP is vital. Blood pressure should be supported by initiating volume replacement and with vasopressors. If somatosensory evoked potential monitoring is used, the inhalation agent should be administered at less than 1 MAC. Succinylcholine can cause life-threatening hyperkalemia if administered 24 hours after a spinal cord injury.

CARDIOGENIC SHOCK

Definition

When myocardial oxygen demand is significantly greater than myocardial oxygen supply, myocardial performance decreases. As a result, decreased perfusion to the heart and peripheral tissues can lead to MI, stroke, and end-organ ischemia. Decreased cardiac contractility occurs, and LV SV is limited despite adequate ventricular volume. Untreated cardiogenic shock results in increasing cellular hypoxia and acidosis, culminating in cardiac arrest and death.

Etiology

Numerous potential causes can result in cardiogenic shock. One of the most common causes is myocardial ischemia and infarction. Other conditions include blunt or penetrating trauma, valvular pathology, dysrhythmias, cardiomyopathies, medications (Adriamycin), and congenital heart defects.

Diagnosis

History and physical examination by a cardiologist are vital. A number of invasive and noninvasive diagnostic cardiac examinations can be accomplished, including ECG, Holter monitoring, stress test, cardiac ultrasonography, cardiac nuclear imaging, and cardiac catheterization.

Hemodynamic signs associated with cardiogenic shock are listed in the table on pg. 29. Other characteristic signs and symptoms resulting from inadequate SV and decreased peripheral perfusion include jugular vein distention; anxiety and restlessness; pulmonary edema; oliguria; and cool, mottled skin.

Treatment

Treatment for cardiogenic shock is mainly supportive, and the cause and hemodynamic factors will determine the course of treatment. Antiarrhythmic medications (e.g., amiodarone, adenosine) are used to treat dysrhythmias. Intravenous fluid and vasopressors are used to increase blood pressure and increase myocardial contractility. An intraaortic balloon pump and the LV assist device are interventions used to increase SV and improve perfusion. Cardiac transplantation is necessary.

Anesthetic Considerations

If emergency surgery is necessary or cardiogenic shock occurs intraoperatively, minimizing myocardial depression is desirable. Induction using etomidate may be most desirable and using greater amounts of narcotics compared with inhalation agents will provide analgesia without directly affecting SV. Invasive monitoring with an arterial line and central venous pressure monitoring is warranted. Infusion of antiarrhythmics, vasopressors, and inotropes may be necessary to maintain CO. The ability to perform advanced cardiac life support procedures may be needed.

ANAPHYLACTIC SHOCK

Definition

The overall incidence of anaphylaxis is estimated at approximately five per 100,000 persons per year. Anaphylaxis is a type 1 hypersensitivity reaction caused by the degranulation of sensitized mast cells and basophils after exposure to an antigen. Mast cells are located in the perivascular spaces of the skin, lung, and intestine, and basophils are located in the blood. Upon initial exposure to an antigen, immunoglobulin E (IgE) is produced and binds to the surface of the effector cell. With subsequent exposure, the antigen binds to the IgE antibodies, releasing physiologically active mediators that include histamine, tryptase, chemotactic factors, and platelet-activating factor. This results in a series of potentially life-threatening symptoms occurring most notably in the respiratory, cardiovascular, and integumentary systems.

Etiology

The most common triggers that cause anaphylaxis to occur are foods, insect or animal venom, and medications. Antibiotics such as penicillin are among the most common medications resulting in an allergic reaction, occurring in approximately once in every 2000 to 10,000 patients. Iodine-containing contrast dye, nonsteroidal anti-inflammatory drugs, and aspirin also increase the risk of hypersensitivity reactions. Among anesthetic drugs, neuromuscular blocking medications are implicated most often with causing anaphylaxis.

Diagnosis

Anaphylaxis is diagnosed based on physical signs and symptoms. Three criteria that can be used to help confirm the diagnosis are (1) involvement of the skin or mucosa (redness, swelling, petechiae) (2) difficulty in breathing or hypotension, and (3) hypotension associated with ingestion or administration of a known allergen.

Treatment

Emergency management of anaphylaxis includes maintenance of the airway, breathing, and circulation. Epinephrine is the drug of choice for treatment of anaphylaxis because it not only helps to treat hypotension but also decreases degranulation of mast cells. Other vasopressors are listed in the table on pg. 27. Histamine receptor antagonists help to decrease tissue responsiveness to histamine. Corticosteroids help to decrease inflammation and stabilize lysosomal membranes but are not effective in treating acute episodes of anaphylaxis.

Anesthetic Considerations

Avoiding administering allergens to patients who are known to have allergies to medications and latex is vital. Presently, most anesthesia equipment is latex free, but it is essential for anesthesia providers to confirm that the products that are used at a specific facility are safe. For patients who have had or are at risk for developing latex anaphylaxis, the surgical team must

Vasopressor Agents Used During Shock States

Agent	Dose Range	Peripheral Vasculature		Cardiac Effects			Typical Use
		Vasoconstriction	Vasodilation	Heart Rate	Contractility	Dysrhythmias	
Dopamine	1–4 mcg/kg/min	0	1+	1+	1+	1+	"Renal dose" does not improve renal function; may be used with bradycardia and hypotension
	5–10 mcg/kg/min	1–2+	1+	2+	2+	2+	
	11–20 mcg/kg/min	2–3+	1+	2+	2+	3+	Vasopressor range
Vasopressin	0.04–0.1 unit/min	3–4+	0	0	0	1+	Septic shock, post–cardiopulmonary bypass shock state, no outcome benefit in sepsis
Phenylephrine	20–200 mcg/min	4+	0	0	0	1+	Vasodilatory shock, best for supraventricular tachycardia
Norepinephrine	1–20 mcg/min	4+	0	2+	2+	2+	First-line vasopressor for septic shock, vasodilatory shock
Epinephrine	1–20 mcg/min	4+	0	4+	4+	4+	Refractory shock, shock with bradycardia, anaphylactic shock
Dobutamine	1–20 mcg/kg/min	1+	2+	1–2+	3+	3+	Cardiogenic shock, septic shock
Milrinone	37.5–75 mcg/kg bolus followed by 0.375–0.75 mcg/min	0	2+	1+	3+	2+	Cardiogenic shock, right heart failure, dilates pulmonary artery; use caution in renal failure

ensure that gloves and surgical attire are latex free. If anaphylaxis is diagnosed intraoperatively, notifying the surgeon to complete surgery; decreasing anesthetic depth; and administering 100% oxygen, intravenous fluids, epinephrine, and histamine receptor antagonists are warranted.

CARDIAC TAMPONADE

Definition

Cardiac tamponade is a syndrome caused by the impairment of diastolic filling of the heart because of continuous increases in intrapericardial pressure. Slow accumulation of fluid in the pericardial space can cause minute increases in intrapericardial pressure. This occurs as a result of the pericardium's ability to stretch to accommodate this increase in volume. If the pericardial fluid accumulates rapidly, the presence of a few hundred milliliters may cause a significant increase in intrapericardial pressure that may result in cardiovascular collapse, and this process is known as cardiac compressive shock. Cardiac tamponade is the cause of cardiac compressive shock that can result in inadequate peripheral perfusion, acidosis, and death.

Classification of the causes of cardiac tamponade includes: (1) trauma, including sharp or blunt trauma to the chest and dissecting aortic aneurysms; (2) causes associated with cardiac surgery; (3) malignancy within the mediastinum; and (4) expansion of pericardial effusions after any form of pericarditis.

Pathophysiology

Normal intrapericardial pressure is subatmospheric. Accumulation of pericardial fluid leads to an increase in intrapericardial pressure. As a result, diastolic expansion of the ventricles decreases. As in constrictive pericarditis, poor ventricular filling leads to peripheral congestion and a decrease in SV and CO. The decrease in SV stimulates compensatory mechanisms for maintaining CO (tachycardia, vasoconstriction, and an increase in venous pressure). If these mechanisms fail, cardiac collapse can occur. The LV pressure volume loop associated with cardiac tamponade represents decreased LV volume and decreased SV caused by compression.

Clinical Manifestations

In addition to severe hypotension, tachydysrhythmias, and pulmonary edema, specific signs of cardiac tamponade include the Beck triad of hypotension; jugular venous distention; and distant, muffled heart sounds. Another common finding is pulsus paradoxus, an exaggerated (i.e., >10 mmHg) decrease in SBP that normally occurs with inspiration. Jugular venous distention that occurs because of decreased forward blood flow through the heart may also be present.

In cardiac tamponade, chest radiography may show enlargement of the cardiac silhouette. The ECG usually demonstrates a decrease in voltage across all leads or electrical alterations of either the P wave or the QRS complex. Echocardiography is the most sensitive, noninvasive method for detection of pericardial effusion and exclusion of tamponade. Use of a PA catheter may reveal equilibration of right and LA pressures and RV end-diastolic filling pressures at approximately 20 mmHg.

Treatment

The definitive treatment for cardiac tamponade is pericardiocentesis, performed either percutaneously by needle decompression through a subxiphoid incision or via video-assisted thorascopic surgery and creation of a pericardial

Signs Associated with Various Shock States

	Cardiogenic Shock	Cardiac Compressive Shock	Severe Hypovolemic Shock	Low-Output Septic Shock	High-Output Septic Shock	Anaphylactic Shock	Neurogenic Shock
Skin perfusion	Pale	Pale	Pale	Pale	Pale	Pale	Pale
Urine output	Low	Low	Low	Low	Low	Low	Low
Pulse rate	High	High	High	High	High	High	Low
Blood pressure	Low	Low	Low	Low	Low	Low	Low
Neck veins	Distended	Distended	Flat	Flat	Flat	Flat	Flat
Cardiac filling pressures	High	High	Low	Low	Low	Low	Low
Systemic vascular resistance	High	High	High	High	Low	Low	Low

window. In contrast to patients with constrictive pericarditis, for patients with cardiac tamponade, immediate hemodynamic improvement occurs when the pericardium is opened. However, despite this fact, pulmonary edema, acute right and LV dysfunction, and circulatory collapse can occur.

Anesthetic Considerations

Preoperatively the patient's clinical status should be optimized. This includes expansion of intravascular fluid volume, use of positive inotropic agents, and correction of acidosis. The degree to which these measures are instituted depends on the hemodynamic state of the patient. Severely compromised patients require immediate medical therapy, and therefore emergency pericardiocentesis is indicated. Invasive hemodynamic monitoring should be established before the procedure. Intraarterial and central venous pressure catheters are required for frequent sampling of blood, continuous blood pressure monitoring, and assessment of intravascular fluid status.

Local infiltration anesthesia is the technique of choice for operative correction of cardiac tamponade. The potential for decompensation that is associated with the use of general anesthetics is attributed to direct myocardial depression and vasodilation in patients with established impairment of cardiac filling. The use of positive-pressure ventilation in such patients may result in decrease venous return to the heart and can further decrease CO. After percutaneous pericardiocentesis and the improvement of hemodynamic status, induction of general anesthesia and initiation of positive-pressure ventilation are sufficient for further surgical exploration.

When it is not possible to relieve intrapericardial pressure that causes cardiac tamponade before the induction of anesthesia, the same anesthetic principles that are applied to the anesthetic management of patients with constrictive pericarditis should be used, including the use of anesthetic agents that preserve myocardial contractility, heart rate, preload, and afterload. Because of the sympathomimetic effects of ketamine, this drug has been advocated for the induction and maintenance of anesthesia. However, many combinations of anesthetic agents that preserve the previously mentioned determinants of CO have been used safely.

Postoperative Implications

Postoperative continuous blood pressure monitoring, central venous pressure, and chest tube drainage are necessary. Possible complications after pericardiocentesis include the reaccumulation of pericardial fluid, coronary laceration, cardiac puncture, and pneumothorax.

I. VALVULAR HEART DISEASE

Definition

Valvular disease is classified according to the type of lesion that exists—stenosis, insufficiency, or mixed lesions. Valvular stenosis is a stenotic narrowing of the valvular orifice, which restricts flow through the orifice when the valve is open. This situation creates an increase in flow resistance and increases turbulent blood flow. Valvular insufficiency results in regurgitation secondary to incomplete or partial valve closure, which allows blood to flow back through the valve into the previous chamber. In patients with mixed lesions (stenosis with insufficiency or insufficiency with stenosis), one type of dysfunction is considered dominant over the other on the basis of the severity of clinical symptoms.

Valvular dysfunction is classified as either primary or secondary. In primary valvular dysfunction, the valve leaflets or the anchoring and supporting structures are damaged or do not function properly. In secondary valvular dysfunction, the valve is not directly damaged. However, normal valve function is altered secondary to another pathophysiologic entity. Causes of this type of manifestation include ventricular dilation, which produces mitral insufficiency; retrograde aortic dissection, which creates aortic insufficiency (AI); and papillary muscle infarction, which causes mitral insufficiency.

Evaluation of the Patient

Evaluation of the patient with valvular heart disease should focus on the pathophysiologic derangements and their effects on cardiac function. The systematic evaluation of primary valvular dysfunction should include the following:

1. Category of valvular dysfunction
   - Stenosis (progressive narrowing of the valve orifice)
   - Insufficiency (incomplete valve closure that causes backflow through the valve)
   - Mixed (regurgitant and stenotic dysfunction)
2. Status of LV loading
   - LV overload from mitral or aortic regurgitation (AR)
   - Pressure overloading from AS
   - Volume underloading from mitral stenosis (MS)
3. Acute versus chronic evolution of the dysfunction
   - Acute lesions have severe and precipitous hemodynamic consequences
4. Cardiac rhythm and its effects on ventricular diastolic filling time
5. LV function
   - Poor LV function places the patient at a higher risk for perioperative cardiac morbidity
6. Secondary effects on the pulmonary vasculature and RV function
   - Secondary pulmonary hypertension from valvular lesions can significantly affect RV function
7. Heart rate
   - Changes in heart rate (either bradycardia or tachycardia) can significantly alter the hemodynamic manifestations of a specific valvular lesion.
   - Bradycardia occurring with regurgitant lesions can result in a significant increase in the regurgitant fraction.
   - Tachycardia is detrimental in patients with stenotic lesions because it shortens the time of ejection and increases myocardial oxygen demand.
8. Perioperative anticoagulation
9. Perioperative antibiotic therapy

Clinical Symptomatology

The most frequent clinical symptoms and signs of valvular dysfunction are CHF, dysrhythmias, syncope, and angina pectoris. Symptoms commonly associated with CHF include dyspnea, orthopnea, and fatigue. The severity of LV dysfunction can be related to the patient's activity level before the onset of cardiac symptoms.

Patient Evaluation: Compensatory Mechanisms

To maintain cardiac function despite progressive valvular dysfunction, sympathetic activity increases as a compensatory mechanism. A decrease in sympathetic tone that occurs during anesthesia can cause severe myocardial dysfunction. Evaluation of the patient should include recognition of sympathetic compensatory mechanisms and management strategies to maintain hemodynamic stability. Despite maximum medical therapy, patients with severe valvular dysfunction may remain in CHF.

The evaluation should also focus on associated organ dysfunction. CO that is decreased by chronic myocardial failure can cause significant major organ dysfunction, including renal and hepatic insufficiency as well as poor cerebral perfusion, which can produce an altered level of consciousness, restlessness, agitation, and lethargy.

Diagnostic Modalities

The most valuable diagnostic modalities used to evaluate valvular heart disease include electrocardiography, chest radiography, color flow Doppler imaging, echocardiography, and cardiac catheterization of both the right and left chambers of the heart. Electrocardiography can be used for evaluation of ventricular hypertrophy; atrial enlargement; axis deviation; and, most important, determining cardiac rhythm. Chest radiography demonstrates the size of the cardiac silhouette and signs of pulmonary vascular congestion. Color-flow Doppler imaging can be used to determine the valvular area, transvalvular gradients, degree of regurgitation, and flow velocity and direction and can measure cardiac function. Cardiac catheterization can be used directly to measure transvalvular gradients, estimate the degree of regurgitation, visualize the coronary arteries, and determine intracardiac pressures.

AORTIC STENOSIS

Incidence and Prevalence

Two types of AS are commonly identified: congenital and acquired. Provided there are no other cardiac lesions, congenital AS is the most common cardiac valvular abnormality, with rheumatic disease responsible for fewer than 5% of these cases. AS can also be acquired, in which calcific disease is the most common form. Valvular AS without accompanying mitral valve disease is more common in men.

Pathophysiology

Congenital

The congenital (nonrheumatic) form of AS results from progressive calcification and tightening of a congenitally abnormal valve. These stenotic valves may have unicuspid, bicuspid, or tricuspid leaflet morphology, but the bicuspid variety is the most common (>50%). AS resulting from rheumatic fever almost always occurs in association with mitral valve disease.

Acquired

The most common form of acquired AS is calcific AS, in which degeneration of the valve apparatus increases with age. Calcium deposits build up on normal cusps and prevent them from opening and closing completely.

The anatomic obstruction to LV outflow produces an increase in LV pressure to maintain SV. A pressure gradient across the stenotic valve develops, and there is increased workload on the ventricle. Increased wall tension contributes to LV hypertrophy. CO is maintained by the hypertrophic ventricle, which may sustain a large pressure gradient across the LV outflow tract for years without evidence of clinical symptoms. Over time, diastolic function is reduced so that small changes in volume give way to large changes in LV filling pressures.

Significant AS is associated with a peak systolic transvalvular pressure gradient exceeding 50 mmHg and an aortic valve orifice area of less than 1 cm^2 (normal area, 2.6–3.5 cm^2). The atrial contribution to ventricular filling may be as high as 40% in patients with AS (≈20% normally). LVEDP is often elevated, causing symptoms of pulmonary congestion despite normal LV contractility. LVEDP values that are normal may, in fact, represent a patient who is hypovolemic.

Diagnosis

As mentioned, a long latency period exists (≈40–50 years) during which obstruction increases gradually and the pressure load on the myocardium increases while the patient remains asymptomatic. Patients with advanced AS may begin to have angina, syncope, and signs of CHF. They also have a characteristic systolic murmur, best heard in the second right intercostal space, which transmits sound to the neck. Cardiac catheterization will give vital information about intracavitary pressures, the gradient across the aortic valve, and contractility. In patients with calcific AS, echocardiography often shows thickening and calcification of the aortic valve and decreased mobility of the valve leaflets. The incidence of arrhythmias leading to severe hypoperfusion accounts for syncope and the increased incidence of sudden death in patients with AS.

Treatment

When significant symptoms develop, most patients die without surgical treatment within 2 to 5 years. Percutaneous transluminal valvuloplasty may be an alternative to surgery, but restenosis usually occurs within 6 to 12 months.

Anesthetic Considerations

The goals of anesthesia management include maintaining hemodynamic stability without causing significant alterations in compensatory mechanisms. Anesthetic management of patients with AS should focus on the following hemodynamic factors:

- Maintain normal sinus rhythm.
- Maintain heart rate of 70 to 80 beats/min.
- Ensure sufficient preload (LVEDV) to maintain CO.
- Ensure adequate coronary perfusion through maintenance of diastolic blood pressure levels.
- Avoid myocardial depression, especially with poor LV function.
- Maintain or slightly increase afterload.

General anesthesia is the preferred technique for major surgical procedures involving patients with AS because of the ability to manipulate hemodynamic parameters, especially DBP.

Central neural blockade (spinal or epidural) must be used with extreme caution because precipitous reductions in blood pressure associated with a sympathectomy decrease SVR. Epidural anesthesia offers the advantage of a slower onset of vasodilation. A high dermatome level sensory block causes greater vasodilation or hypotension and is contraindicated in those with moderate to severe AS.

Monitoring and Premedication

In addition to standard intraoperative monitoring, complete invasive monitoring may be required for patients with AS, even for routine procedures. Any significant change in basic hemodynamic variables (i.e., heart rate, heart rhythm, LVEDV, coronary perfusion pressure [CPP]) can rapidly cause irreversible myocardial deterioration. The complexity of hemodynamic monitoring modalities depends on the physical status of the patient, the severity of AS, the extent of the surgical procedure, and the ability of the anesthesia provider to use and interpret hemodynamic values.

Absolute criteria for intraoperative invasive monitoring for patients with AS are controversial. However, clinical judgment, experience, and the ability to appropriately use a PA catheter must be considered before implementation.

Maintenance of Anesthesia

Commonly used induction agents can be used as long as profound hypotension is avoided. Tracheal intubation can be performed with any of the available muscle relaxants. However, caution must be exercised to avoid histamine release because this situation can dramatically increase the heart rate. Anesthetic maintenance can be accomplished with the use of a volatile agent in conjunction with nitrous oxide, opiates, or both. The adverse cardiovascular effects of the volatile agents must be considered before these drugs are used. Higher concentrations of inhaled agent result in greater degrees of myocardial depression and vasodilation. Volatile agents must be used with extreme caution because the myocardial depressant effect can be deleterious in patients with impaired ventricular function. The use of high-dose opioid-based agents (fentanyl, 50–100 mcg/kg, or sufentanil, 5–30 mcg/kg) is an alternative anesthetic approach that may help achieve cardiovascular stability by not causing a significant amount of myocardial depression. A combination of inhaled agents and narcotics has been used safely to provide anesthesia for patients with AS. Despite the anesthetic technique that is chosen, immediate and aggressive treatment of adverse changes that occur in heart rate and rhythm, SVR, blood pressure, and LVEDV is paramount if successful anesthetic outcomes are to be achieved in patients with AS.

AORTIC INSUFFICIENCY

Incidence and Prevalence

Aortic insufficiency, also known as *AI,* can be classified as acute or chronic and as primary or secondary, depending on the cause. Primary chronic AI is caused by rheumatic valvular disease and almost always involves the mitral valve to some degree. Primary acute AI usually is caused by infective endocarditis, which is caused by direct damage to the valve cusps. Acute secondary (functional) AI results from aortic root dissection caused either by trauma or aneurysm and results in a mechanical and functional impairment of functional aortic valve closure.

Pathophysiology

The major hemodynamic aberration related to AI occurs during diastole. A portion of the blood volume that is ejected from the LV into the aorta regurgitates backward into the ventricle because of incomplete closure of the aortic valve. AI causes LV volume overload. Chronic ventricular overload causes eccentric ventricular hypertrophy and chamber dilation. The degree of regurgitation depends on three factors: the diastolic time available for regurgitation to occur, the diastolic pressure gradient between the aorta and the LV, and the degree of incompetence of the aortic valve.

Diagnosis

Most patients with chronic AI remain asymptomatic for 10 to 20 years. When symptoms develop, exertional dyspnea, orthopnea, and paroxysmal nocturnal dyspnea are the principal complaints. Diastolic murmur is often auscultated at the left sternal border. Angina is a late and ominous symptom.

In acute AI, patients develop sudden clinical manifestations of cardiovascular collapse, weakness, severe dyspnea, and hypotension. Chronic AI is recognized by its characteristic diastolic murmur (best heard in the second intercostal space, right sternal border), widened pulse pressure, decreased diastolic pressure, and bounding peripheral pulses.

Treatment

Arterial blood pressure should be decreased to reduce the diastolic gradient for regurgitation using afterload reduction via arterial vasodilators and ACE inhibitors. Early surgery is indicated for patients with acute AI because medical management is associated with a high mortality rate. Patients with chronic AI should undergo surgery before irreversible ventricular dysfunction occurs.

Anesthetic Considerations

The goals for anesthesia management are to increase forward flow and decrease the degree of regurgitation and therefore should focus on the following hemodynamic factors:

- Maintain heart rate slightly higher than normal (80–110 beats/min).
- Decrease afterload (especially diastolic pressure).
- Avoid myocardial depression.
- Maintain normal sinus rhythm.
- Maintain or increase preload.

Central neural blockade is an appropriate anesthetic choice, depending on the invasiveness of the surgical procedure. Reduction in SVR resulting from sympathetic blockade may reduce the degree of regurgitation.

Induction of general anesthesia can be accomplished with any of the available intravenous agents. Tracheal intubation can be achieved with the use of available nondepolarizing muscle relaxants. Maintenance of anesthesia can be achieved with nitrous oxide and a volatile agent. isoflurane, with its ability to increase heart rate and decrease SVR; therefore, its use is desirable. If significant ventricular dysfunction exists, an opioid-based anesthetic technique may be preferable.

Monitoring and Premedication

Unless end-stage AR or significant preoperative ventricular dysfunction exists, aggressive invasive monitoring is not warranted. However, if the surgical procedure is extensive or if vasodilators or inotropes are being used, then an arterial line and a PA catheter should be used for assessment of the results and efficacy of these therapeutic agents. Premedication should be tailored to the patient's clinical condition. In elderly or debilitated patients, a conservative amount of premedication should be titrated until effective in a monitored environment.

MITRAL STENOSIS

Incidence and Prevalence

Pure MS occurs in 25% of patients; MS and MR occur in 40% of patients.

Pathophysiology

The predominant cause of MS is rheumatic fever, which occurs about four times more frequently in women. Less common causes are congenital MS (in children) and complications associated with carcinoid syndrome, systemic lupus erythematosus, and rheumatic arthritis.

After the initial episode of acute rheumatic fever, stenosis of the mitral valve takes about 2 years to develop. Symptoms appear after 20 to 30 years, when the mitral valve orifice is reduced from its normal 4 to 6 cm^2 to less than 2 cm^2. In MS, the anterior and posterior valve cusps fuse at their edges followed by shortening of the chordae tendineae as they thicken. This produces obstruction to flow into the LV. The narrowed valvular orifice causes an increase in LA volume and pressure. LV filling and SV in the presence of mild MS are usually maintained at rest by increased LA pressure. LV SV may decrease when effective atrial contraction is lost or with tachycardia. Acute increases in LA pressure that subsequently result are transmitted to the pulmonary capillaries.

Pulmonary hypertension occurs from rearward transmission of the elevated LA pressure and irreversible increases in pulmonary vascular resistance. Chronic increases in PCWP are partially compensated by increases in pulmonary lymph flow; however, any acute increase in PCWP may result in pulmonary edema. Transudation of fluid into the pulmonary interstitial space, decreased pulmonary compliance, and increased work of breathing lead to dyspnea on exertion.

Diagnosis

About 50% of MS patients present with an acute onset of CHF that is often associated with paroxysmal attacks of atrial fibrillation (this arrhythmia occurs in 40% of patients with MS). Stasis of blood in the LA predisposes to thrombus formation. The predominant symptom of MS is dyspnea from the reduced compliance of the lungs. Rupture of pulmonary–bronchial venous communications causes hemoptysis.

Cardiac catheterization allows quantification of the mitral valve orifice and transmitral gradients. Angiography is important in those patients with angina. Two-dimensional echocardiography can also provide information about orifice size. MS is recognized during auscultation by an opening snap that occurs early in diastole and by a rumbling diastolic heart murmur best heard at the cardiac apex. The chest radiographic study may show LA enlargement and evidence of pulmonary edema.

Treatment

Medical management is primarily supportive and includes limitation of physical activity, diuretics, and sodium restriction. Digoxin is useful in patients with atrial fibrillation, and β-blockers may control the heart rate in some patients. Anticoagulation therapy is used in patients with a history of emboli and in those at high risk (i.e., those older than 40 years of age with a large atrium and chronic atrial fibrillation). Surgical correction is undertaken when significant symptoms develop. Recurrent MS after valvuloplasty is usually managed with valve replacement. Catheter-balloon valvuloplasty using a percutaneous venous introduction and a transseptal approach to the mitral valve may be used to decrease the degree of MS in selected patients.

Anesthetic Considerations

The following goals should be achieved in the anesthetic management of the patient with MS:

- Maintain sinus rhythm at a low normal heart rate.
- Ensure that LVEDV is adequate to maintain adequate CO without increasing pulmonary congestion.
- Avoid extreme decreases in myocardial contractility.
- Reduction in both RV and LV afterload may improve hemodynamics; this must be done in a controlled manner and with careful monitoring; the extent of the surgical procedure and the degree and severity of MS determine the level of monitoring that is necessary.
- Perform cardioversion for hemodynamically compromising atrial tachyarrhythmias.
- Treat hypotension with small doses of phenylephrine.

The LVEDV is normal in approximately 85% of patients with MS. An increased LVEDV in patients with MS should alert the anesthesia provider to the presence of mitral or AI or primary CAD. Most patients with moderate MS also have low to normal SV and therefore may have a normal EF. Approximately 33% of patients with MS have an EF below normal (normal, 0.67 ± 0.08). When the mitral valve is narrowed to less than 1 cm^2 (severe MS), a mean LA pressure of 25 mmHg is necessary to maintain even an adequate resting CO. Because of the abnormal transvalvular gradient, the PCWP overestimates LVEDP. On the PCWP, a prominent *a wave* and a decreased *y descent* are present in patients with MS.

Vasoconstrictors should be avoided, and early use of positive inotropes (e.g., epinephrine, dopamine, dobutamine) may be helpful.

Regional anesthesia is acceptable in the patient with MS, provided higher levels of sympathetic blockade are avoided during conduction blockade (resulting hypotension may be difficult to treat based on the pathophysiology of MS).

Prognosis

When MS produces total incapacity, 20% of patients die within 6 months without surgical correction.

MITRAL REGURGITATION AND INSUFFICIENCY

Incidence and Prevalence

Severe MR requiring surgical repair occurs in about 5% of men and in fewer than 1.5% of women.

Pathophysiology

Abnormalities of the mitral annulus, leaflets, chordae tendineae, and papillary muscles may cause MR. Chronic MR is usually the result of rheumatic fever; congenital abnormalities; or dilatation, destruction, or calcification of the mitral annulus. Acute MR is most often the result of myocardial is chemia or infarction, infective endocarditis, or chest trauma.

The mitral valve orifice lies adjacent to the aortic valve. At the onset of ventricular contraction, about half of the regurgitant volume is ejected into the LA before aortic valve opening. The total volume of regurgitant flow into the LA depends on the SVR and forward SV. Effective CO will be effectively diminished in symptomatic patients, but “total” LV output (forward and regurgitant) is usually elevated.

There is typically little enlargement of the LA cavity; however, there is a significant rise in mean atrial pressure that leads to pulmonary congestion. The degree of atrial compliance will determine the clinical manifestations. Patients with normal or reduced atrial compliance (e.g., acute MR) demonstrate pulmonary congestion and edema. Those with increased atrial compliance (i.e., chronic MR with a large, dilated atrium) demonstrate signs of decreased CO. Most patients fall between these two extremes and exhibit symptoms of both pulmonary congestion and low CO.

Diagnosis

Symptoms of MR can take up to 20 years to develop. Chronic weakness and fatigue secondary to low CO are prominent features. On auscultation, the cardinal feature of MR is a blowing pansystolic murmur, best heard at the cardiac apex and often radiating to the left axilla. The regurgitant flow is responsible for the "v" wave present on the recording of the PA occlusion pressure. The size of the v wave correlates with the magnitude of the regurgitant flow.

Treatment

Medical treatment typically includes digoxin, diuretics, and vasodilators. Reduction of afterload increases the forward SV and decreases the regurgitant volume. Surgical treatment is usually reserved for patients with moderate to severe symptoms.

Anesthetic Considerations

The following goals should be achieved in the anesthetic management of patients with MR:

- Decrease regurgitant blood flow to enhance CO by decreasing afterload.
- Maintain or increase preload.
- Maintain cardiac contractility.
- Avoid decreases in heart rate.
- Avoid significant increases in afterload.

Selection of the anesthetic technique should take into consideration the adverse effects associated with changes in heart rate and SVR. General anesthesia is the technique of choice in patients with MR. Regional anesthesia (spinal or epidural) is not contraindicated; however, the potential for profound and precipitous decreases in blood pressure via sympathetic blockade can result in severe decreases in blood pressure.

Induction of general anesthesia can be safely achieved with any of the presently available agents. Hemodynamic goals include avoiding bradycardia and significant increases in afterload. The use of muscle relaxants does not present a significant risk as long as the resulting changes in heart rate do not cause severe bradycardia. Maintenance of anesthesia can be accomplished with nitrous oxide and a volatile agent. Any changes in vascular resistance induced by nitrous oxide are frequently offset by the pulmonary vasodilatation produced by the volatile agent. Because all volatile agents induce a dose-dependent decrease in myocardial contractility, their use may be detrimental in patients with severe ventricular dysfunction. In this instance, the use of a high-dose opioid technique may provide for a more effective hemodynamic profile.

Prognosis

In most patients with MR, the clinical course and the quality of life improve after valve replacement. The original cause of MR that warranted the operation is also important to the outcome after surgical treatment. In patients in whom mitral dysfunction is secondary to ischemic heart disease, the 5-year survival rate is approximately 30%; in rheumatic MR, the 5-year survival rate is approximately 70%.

TRICUSPID REGURGITATION

Pathophysiology

Tricuspid regurgitation is commonly a result of RV enlargement secondary to pulmonary hypertension. Pulmonary hypertension may itself be indirectly the result of chronic LV failure because chronic LV failure often leads to sustained increases in pulmonary vascular pressures. This chronic increase in afterload causes the RV to dilate progressively, and excessive dilation of the tricuspid annulus eventually results in tricuspid incompetence or regurgitation. TR can also be secondary to infective endocarditis, rheumatic fever, carcinoid syndrome, chest trauma, or congenital malformations. Fortunately, the RA and vena cava are compliant and accommodate the volume overload with a minimal increase in RA pressure.

Diagnosis

Patients with isolated TR are often totally asymptomatic for many years (>20 years). Some physical signs may be present early, such as pulsatile neck veins and systolic heart murmurs heard throughout the cardiac cycle. Other symptoms include fatigue; weakness; and a feeling of fullness in the abdomen, probably from congestion in the liver (positive hepatojugular reflex). Some patients report cyanosis, which may result from blood flow from the right to the LA in those with a patent foramen ovale.

Treatment

Tricuspid regurgitation is generally well tolerated, and some degree of regurgitation has been reported in many physiologically normal persons during echocardiography. Even surgical removal of the tricuspid valve is usually well tolerated. Treatment of the underlying disease process is more important than the TR itself.

Anesthetic Considerations

Many patients with clinically significant TR who undergo surgery and anesthesia also have pulmonary hypertension and possibly mitral or aortic valve disease.

- Maintain intravascular fluid volume and central venous pressure in the high-normal range.
- Avoid increases in pulmonary vascular resistance.
- Avoid positive end-expiratory pressure and high mean airway pressures because they reduce venous return and increase RV afterload.
- Most patients tolerate spinal and epidural anesthesia well.
- Prophylactic antibiotics are recommended.

Prognosis

Excellent results have been reported with the use of tricuspid anuloplasty in patients with moderate TR. Management of severe TR entails anuloplasty or valve replacement. Durability of more than 10 years has been established with valvular prostheses.

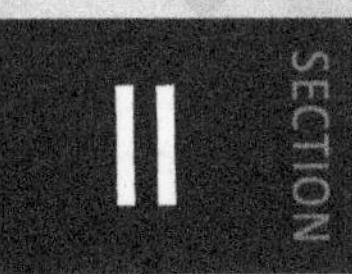

SECTION II

Central Nervous System

A. ALZHEIMER'S DISEASE AND DEMENTIA

Definition

Dementia is the clinical syndrome characterized by acquired persistent impairment of cognitive and emotional abilities severe enough to interfere with daily functioning and quality of life.

Incidence and Prevalence

Dementia occurs primarily late in life, the prevalence being about 1% at age 60 years, and it doubles every 5 years, reaching 30% to 50% by 85 years of age. Alzheimer's disease is the most common of the progressive cortical dementias, accounting for about 70% of the dementias in persons older than 55 years of age.

Pathophysiology

Alzheimer's disease is a progressive and ultimately fatal disorder in which certain types of nerve cells in particular areas of the brain degenerate and die for unknown reasons. Vulnerable brain regions include the amygdala as well as the hippocampus and areas around the hippocampus, and affected cell populations include cortical pathways involved in catecholaminergic, serotonergic, and cholinergic transmission. Advancing pathology is believed to underlie the classic clinical presentation of memory deficits followed by gradual erosion of judgment, reasoning ability, verbal fluency, and other cognitive skills.

A specific cause or pathologic process is not identified for dementia. The two "hallmark" Alzheimer's lesions observable at autopsy are amyloid plaques and neurofibrillary tangles. Plaques are extracellular deposits of abnormally processed amyloid precursor protein, and tangles are intracellular accumulations of the cytoskeletal protein tau.

Development of plaques and tangles may represent a fairly late stage in the disease process that may or may not reflect the fundamental biochemical disruptions at work in Alzheimer's disease. Although the "amyloid hypothesis," which assigns a central causative role to abnormal amyloid processing, remains the most widely embraced theory, other active areas of research include tau, inflammation, disruptions of cell-signaling pathways, and cardiovascular risk factors.

Clinical Manifestations

Multiple diseases are representative of the disorder. Cortical dementias include Alzheimer's disease, Pick's disease, and frontal lobe degeneration. Subcortical dementias are associated with Parkinson's disease, Huntington's disease, and Creutzfeldt-Jakob disease. Dementia is associated with intellectual, language, memory, and judgment impairment.

Alzheimer's disease is the most common cortical dementia and is characterized by progressive memory loss, predominantly loss of short-term memory. Language impairment manifests as difficulty in finding words for spontaneous speech. Performance of daily tasks such as meal preparation and personal hygiene becomes impaired. In addition, symptoms of mental depression and anxiety may be prominent.

Diagnosis is probable when associated with an insidious onset, progressive worsening of memory, and a normal level of consciousness. Computed tomography (CT) often displays ventricular dilation and marked cortical atrophy. A definitive diagnosis can be made only after examination of brain tissue demonstrating amyloid and fibrillar protein aggregates.

Treatment

No proven preventive therapies for dementia or Alzheimer's disease are known. Drug therapy is available to treat some symptoms but does not prevent progression of the disease. Symptomatic therapy is helpful during the early stages, especially if mental depression is prominent.

Key elements of disease management include timely diagnosis and effective use of available therapies to manage cognitive and behavioral symptoms. Other important considerations include identifying comorbid conditions and monitoring individuals for adequate nutrition, hydration, and pain management as well as signs of abuse.

Drugs currently approved specifically to treat Alzheimer's disease symptoms all act chiefly by inhibiting acetylcholinesterase, the main enzyme that breaks down acetylcholine. Anticholinesterase drugs such as tacrine and donepezil appear to have beneficial effects for some patients early in the disease.

Anesthetic Considerations

Management of this disease state is influenced by the pathophysiology of Alzheimer's disease. Preoperative challenges are related to dealing with patients who are unable to comprehend their environment. Sedatives should rarely be administered because mental confusion could result. Centrally acting anticholinergic drugs are also not recommended for inclusion in preoperative medication. Maintenance of anesthesia can be acceptably achieved with standard inhalation and intravenous agents.

Prognosis

The course of the disease is one of progressive decline, and the median survival time after the onset of dementia is 3.3 years.

B. AUTONOMIC HYPERREFLEXIA AND DYSAUTONOMIA

Definition

Autonomic dysreflexia (or autonomic hyperreflexia) is a disorder that appears after resolution of spinal shock.

Incidence and Prevalence

The incidence and prevalence depend on the level of spinal cord transection. About 85% of patients with spinal cord transection above T5 may exhibit this syndrome. Autonomic dysreflexia is unlikely to be associated with spinal cord transection below T10. The stimulation of a surgical procedure, however, is a potent trigger of autonomic dysreflexia even in patients with no previous history of this response.

Pathophysiology

Autonomic dysreflexia can be initiated by cutaneous or visceral stimulation below the level of spinal cord transection. Distention of a hollow viscus (bladder or rectum) is a common stimulus. This stimulus initiates afferent impulses that enter the spinal cord below that level. These impulses elicit reflex sympathetic activity over the splanchnic outflow tract. This outflow is isolated from inhibitory impulses such that generalized vasoconstriction persists below the level of injury. Vasoconstriction results in increased blood pressure, which is then transmitted by the carotid sinus. Subsequent activation of the carotid sinus results in decreased efferent outflow from the sympathetic nervous system. Activity from the central nervous system (CNS) is manifested as a predominance of parasympathetic nervous system activity at the heart and peripheral vasculature. This predominance cannot be produced below the level of spinal cord transection (this part of the body remains neurologically isolated). Therefore, vasoconstriction persists below the level of spinal cord transection. If spinal cord transection is above the level of splanchnic outflow (T4–T6), vasodilation in the neurologically intact portion of the body is insufficient to offset the effects of vasoconstriction (reflected by persistent hypertension).

Clinical Manifestations

The hallmark symptoms of autonomic dysreflexia are paroxysmal hypertension, bradycardia, and cardiac dysrhythmias in response to stimuli below the level of transection (e.g., bladder catheterization). Hypertension persists because vasodilation cannot occur below the level of injury. Hyperreflexia is not observed until the spinal shock phase has passed. It is therefore usually seen when patients return to surgery for such procedures as cystoscopies, which are performed later in their recovery phase. The condition is caused by stimulation below the level of the lesion. It is typically precipitated by distention of the bladder or rectum resulting from bladder fullness, defecation, childbirth, and even cutaneous stimulation. Nasal stuffiness reflects vasodilation. Other symptoms may include headache, blurred vision (from hypertension), increased operative blood loss, loss of consciousness, seizures, cardiac arrhythmias, and pulmonary edema.

Treatment

Treatment includes ganglionic blockers (trimethaphan, pentolinium), α-adrenergic antagonists (phentolamine, phenoxybenzamine), and direct-acting vasodilators (nitroprusside). General or regional anesthesia can be used. Drugs that lower blood pressure by central action alone are not predictably effective.

Anesthetic Considerations

Prevention of autonomic hyperreflexia is key in the treatment of autonomic dysreflexia. It can occur intraoperatively with local, spinal, and nitrous oxide–opioid general anesthesia. If autonomic hyperreflexia occurs, it is treated by removal of the stimulus, deepening anesthesia, and administration of direct-acting vasodilators. If left untreated, the hypertension crisis may progress to seizures, intracranial hemorrhage, or myocardial infarction. No episodes have been reported with the use of potent inhalation anesthetics. Bradycardia is treated with atropine or glycopyrrolate. Have nitroprusside and other cardioactive agents readily available to treat precipitous hypertension.

C. CEREBROVASCULAR DISEASE

Definition

Cerebral vascular disorders are characterized by sudden neurologic deficits resulting from ischemia or hemorrhagic events. Cerebrovascular disease is any of a group of disorders that affects the vasculature of the brain, the primary disorder being cerebrovascular accident (CVA or "stroke") as a result of hemorrhage and ischemia.

Incidence and Prevalence

Cerebrovascular disease is the third leading cause of death and the leading cause of disability in the United States. Women have lower stroke rates than men.

Pathophysiology

The major risk factors for the development of cerebrovascular disease are hypertension and diabetes. Other risk factors include atherosclerosis, inflammatory processes, dissecting aneurysm, disorders affecting the myocardium, congestive heart failure, polycythemia, cigarette smoking, use of oral contraceptives, and postpartum infection. The different manifestations of cerebrovascular disease can be classified as:

- Transient ischemic attack (TIA): A temporary, focal episode of neurologic dysfunction that develops suddenly and lasts a few minutes to hours but usually not more than 24 hours. Approximately 41% of these patients may eventually have a stroke.
- Reversible ischemic neurologic deficit (RIND): Neurologic symptoms that persist up to 6 to 8 weeks before resolving.
- Progressive stroke: A stroke in progress. Neurologic symptoms and deficits develop slowly and are not reversible.
- Complete stroke: Neurologic deficits are permanent.
- Amaurosis fugax: A sudden, temporary, or fleeting blindness caused by a decrease in cerebral perfusion to the retina.

Diagnostic and Laboratory Findings

Computed tomography, magnetic resonance imaging (MRI), cerebral angiography, and clinical examination are useful.

Clinical Manifestations

Clinical manifestations involve numerous neurologic deficits. See the classification of symptoms in the section on etiology.

Treatment

Treatment includes risk factor reduction through controlling hypertension, avoiding a high-fat diet, smoking cessation, and decreasing obesity.

Anesthetic Considerations

Preoperative evaluation should include a careful analysis of cardiovascular, neurologic, and pulmonary systems, as well as laboratory results and current medications. As expected, patients with cerebrovascular occlusive disease often have peripheral, renal, and cardiac occlusive disease as well. If the patient is scheduled for carotid endarterectomy, consider the benefits and risks associated with regional versus general anesthesia. Selection of anesthetic agents is based on the patient's need and the surgeon's desires. The goal is to ensure a smooth induction, maintenance, and emergence, with avoidance of wide swings in blood pressure. Moreover, an awake, extubated patient is the desired outcome so that immediate neurologic assessment can be performed. Cardioactive agents such as sodium nitroprusside, nitroglycerin, and phenylephrine (Neo-Synephrine) should be readily available.

D. GUILLAIN-BARRÉ SYNDROME

Definition

Guillain-Barré syndrome refers to acquired inflammatory peripheral neuropathies that are characterized by: (1) acute onset, (2) elevated cerebrospinal fluid (CSF) protein levels with low CSF cell counts (cyto-albumologic dissociation), and (3) a monophasic illness with at least partial recovery. Guillain-Barré syndrome is subdivided into acute inflammatory demyelinating polyneuropathy, acute motor and sensory axonal neuropathy, acute motor axonal neuropathy, and Miller Fisher syndrome.

Pathophysiology

Acute inflammatory demyelinating polyneuropathy, the demyelinating form, accounts for up to 97% of cases of Guillain-Barré syndrome in North America and Europe. It is a sporadic disorder with an incidence of 0.6 to 1.9 cases per 100,000 in North America and Europe. Men are more likely to be affected than women (2:1).

Central nervous system bulbar involvement is most frequently manifested as bilateral facial paralysis. The most common symptoms are difficulty in swallowing because of pharyngeal muscle weakness and impaired ventilation resulting from intercostal muscle paralysis. Lower motor neuron involvement gives way to flaccid paralysis, and corresponding tendon reflexes are diminished. Sensory disturbances occur as paresthesias in the distal extremities and generally precede the onset of paralysis. Pain occurs in different forms, such as headache, backache, or tenderness to deep pressure. Wide fluctuations in blood pressure (orthostatic), abnormalities on electrocardiogram (e.g., conduction disturbances, tachycardia), diaphoresis, peripheral vasoconstriction, and thromboembolism may be seen as a result of autonomic nervous system dysfunction. Complete recovery can occur within weeks when "segmental" demyelination in the CNS is the primary pathologic change. A mortality rate of 3% to 8% is the result of sepsis, respiratory distress syndrome, and pulmonary embolism.

Clinical Manifestations

Weakness, which is the most common initial symptom in both acute inflammatory demyelinating polyneuropathy and acute motor and sensory axonal neuropathy, can be mild, such as difficulty walking, or severe, such as total quadriplegia and respiratory failure. Bilateral weakness of the facial muscles (facial diplegia) occurs in about 50% of cases. The most common manifestation is leg weakness that subsequently "ascends" into the arms.

Treatment

Nonspecific therapies directed at modulating the immune system are effective in Guillain-Barré syndrome.

Diagnosis

Diagnosis is based on clinical findings of progressive bilateral weakness in the extremities. Examination of CSF by lumbar puncture reveals increased levels of protein, although cell counts remain normal. A viral origin is supported by the observation that this syndrome develops after a respiratory or gastrointestinal infection in about half of all cases.

Anesthetic Considerations

As a result of the lower motor neuron and subsequent autonomic nervous system dysfunction, these patients may have an exaggerated response to noxious stimuli during operation and anesthesia. Regurgitation or aspiration during induction of anesthesia is a very real concern; however, succinylcholine should also be avoided (i.e., use a nondepolarizing muscle relaxant). Blood pressure should be monitored invasively (arterial line) because of compensatory cardiovascular responses to changes in posture, blood loss, or positive pressure. Postoperative mechanical ventilatory support may be needed. The presence of any neurologic deficits before surgery should be documented appropriately on the preanesthetic evaluation.

Prognosis

Fifty percent of patients progress to their nadir, or maximum disability, within 2 weeks, 75% within 3 weeks, and more than 90% within 4 weeks of the onset of symptoms. With modern supportive care, acute mortality is about 2%. After a brief period of stabilization, slow, spontaneous recovery occurs over a period of weeks or months. Most patients undergo either complete recovery or are left with minor sequelae; about 20% have a persistent disability.

E. HYDROCEPHALUS

Definition

Hydrocephalus is an abnormal accumulation of CSF resulting either from an excessive production or from decreased absorption that leads to an increase in pressure in the ventricles of the brain. The rise in intraventricular pressure causes adjacent brain tissue compression and progressive enlargement of the cranium.

Incidence and Prevalence

Hydrocephalus in newborns occurs in three of every 1000 births and is usually secondary to meningomyelocele. Hydrocephalus is common after subarachnoid hemorrhage because of impaired CSF circulation through the basal cistern. It is often a complication of a ruptured brain aneurysm. Hydrocephalus may occur in neonates as a result of obstruction of CSF circulation within the brain's ventricular system or at a site of reabsorption.

Pathophysiology

Hydrocephalus can be divided into two main types, obstructive and nonobstructive. Obstructive hydrocephalus results from congenital malformation, scar tissue, fibrin deposits after intraventricular hemorrhage or infection, tumors, or cysts. There are three types of obstructive hydrocephalus: obstructive, communicating obstructive, and noncommunicating obstructive.

- Obstructive: This results from obstruction to CSF flow; depending on the site, it can be further divided into communicating or noncommunicating.
- Communicating obstructive (extraventricular hydrocephalus): This results from obstruction to CSF absorption by the arachnoid villi, usually from remote inflammatory disease or traumatic subarachnoid hemorrhage.
- Noncommunicating obstructive (extraventricular hydrocephalus): This is secondary to obstruction to CSF flow between the lateral and fourth ventricles (the ventricles dilate proximal but not distal to the obstruction).

Nonobstructive hydrocephalus results from excessive CSF production by the choroid plexus. Choroid plexus papillomas or benign tumors of the glomus of the lateral ventricles are common causes.

Diagnostic and Laboratory Findings

Hydrocephalus can be diagnosed by CT, by MRI, and by signs of increased intracranial pressure (ICP).

Clinical Manifestations

- *Early signs and symptoms:* Apnea, bradycardia, nausea and vomiting, increasing head circumference, headaches (most common), mentation changes, nystagmus, and decreased reflexes are noted.
- *Late signs and symptoms:* Bulging fontanelle, pupillary areflexia, nuchal rigidity, "setting sun" eyes, palsy of cranial nerve VI, limb spasticity, decreased level of consciousness leading to nonresponsiveness, widened pulse pressure, altered heart rate, visual changes, and hypertension are noted.

Treatment

A bypass shunt is inserted to allow CSF to flow from the lateral ventricles to the peritoneal cavity (ventriculoperitoneal shunt). This type of shunt is preferable because of the lower incidence of complications and need for revision with growth. Ventriculoatrial and ventriculopleural shunts are less popular because of the risk of infection, microemboli, and hydrothorax. The lumboperitoneal shunt (between the lumbar subarachnoid space and the peritoneal space) may be used.

Anesthetic Considerations

With hydrocephalus, ICP is elevated. Hypoventilation, hypoxia, and hypertension further increase ICP and should be avoided. Baseline neurologic status must be established, and minimal to no premedication must be administered. Intravenous induction should be rapid and smooth with cricoid pressure. After the airway is secure, hyperventilate the patient until ventricles are decompressed.

Bolus doses of propofol or thiopental are administered until ICP is reduced, and then an inhalation agent or opioid can be added. Sudden removal of large CSF volumes may lead to bradycardia and hypotension that can be prevented by rapid replacement with saline or gradual removal of CSF. Although heat is lost by surgical exposure, some degree of hypothermia may be appropriate in these patients. Narcotics are given in small amounts (or not given at all) to enable rapid neurologic assessment on awakening from anesthesia.

F. INTRACRANIAL HYPERTENSION

Definition and Etiology

Intracranial hypertension occurs with a sustained increase in ICP above 15 to 20 mmHg. Intracranial hypertension develops with expanding tissue or fluid mass, interference with normal CSF absorption, excessive cerebral blood flow (CBF), or systemic disturbances promoting brain edema. Often, multiple factors are responsible for the development of intracranial hypertension. Head injury, stroke, intracranial hemorrhage, infection, tumor formation, postischemic or posthypoxic states, hydrocephalus, osmolar imbalances, and pulmonary disease can all cause increases in ICP.

Diagnostic and Laboratory Findings

Magnetic resonance imaging and CT are the two most prominent tests to evaluate tumors, hemorrhage, stroke, and areas of ischemia. Lumbar puncture is used to diagnose infections and hydrocephalus.

Clinical Manifestations

Symptoms of increased ICP include headache, nausea, vomiting, papilledema, focal neurologic deficits, altered ventilatory function, decreasing consciousness, seizures, and coma. When ICP exceeds 30 mmHg, CBF progressively decreases, and a vicious cycle is established: ischemia produces brain edema, which in turn increases ICP and further precipitates ischemia. Cushing's triad is associated with excessively high ICP and includes hypertension, bradycardia, and irregular respirations. If this cycle remains unchecked, progressive neurologic damage or catastrophic herniation may result.

Treatment

The major methods for the treatment of elevated ICP are listed in the box below.

Methods for the Treatment of Elevated Intracranial Pressure

- Apply hyperventilation on demand ($Paco_2$ 30–35 mmHg).
- Administer diuretics (osmotic mannitol 0.25–1 g/kg IV) or furosemide.
- Perform CSF drainage (if available).
- Avoid overhydration; target normovolemia.
- Elevate patient's head; position to improve cerebral venous return; avoid neck vein compression.
- Insert ICP monitor; Sjo_2, $AVDo_2$, and CBF monitoring recommended.
- Optimize hemodynamics: mean arterial pressure, central venous pressure, pulmonary capillary wedge pressure, heart rate, and cerebral perfusion pressure; consider antihypertensive therapy as needed.
- Administer corticosteroids (dexamethasone).
- Surgical decompression; consider decompressive craniectomy if hematoma is present.
- Cerebral vasoconstriction (propofol, dexmedetomidine).
- Consider mild hypothermia.

$AVDo_2$, Arteriovenous difference in oxygen content; *CBF,* cerebral blood flow; *IV,* intravenous; *Sjo_2,* jugular bulboxyhemoglobin saturation.

Selective application of these methods often results in ICP reduction accompanied by clinical improvement. A patent airway, adequate oxygenation, and hyperventilation provide the foundation for neuroresuscitative care in acute intracranial hypertensive states. Frequently, overlap occurs among causes of increased ICP, and this may necessitate simultaneous application of a number of different therapeutic methods.

Anesthetic Considerations

Cerebral blood volume can be manipulated in various ways. Endotracheal intubation will allow prompt management of conditions related to hypoxemia and hypercarbia that could increase CBF and consequently increase ICP. Neuromuscular blockade often prevents increases in cerebral venous volume (and ICP) that result from coughing, straining, or actively exhaling. Cerebral venous drainage is facilitated by elevating the head of the bed; however, this maneuver may also decrease venous return and cardiac output (i.e., mean arterial blood pressure), thereby reducing cerebral perfusion pressure (CPP). Appropriate analgesia and sedation prevent increases in the cerebral metabolic rate for oxygen ($CMRO_2$) and any increases in CBF. Hyperventilation acutely reduces CBF, although CBF usually returns to its original level even with prolonged hyperventilation. Propofol in sufficient doses suppress both the $CMRO_2$ and CBF in association with profound electroencephalographic suppression. Caution should be used when propofol is administered of concomitant vasodilation and myocardial depression. Brain tissue volume is usually reduced by diuresis. Osmotic diuresis with mannitol reduces brain water. Mannitol can be used as a continuous infusion or as treatment for acute episodes of increased ICP. Maximum reduction of ICP is accomplished with large doses of mannitol administered rapidly, then followed by furosemide. When a patient emerges from anesthesia, increased ICP caused by any coughing or bucking (especially on the endotracheal tube) must be considered. Extubation while the patient is still anesthetized and the concomitant use of intravenous lidocaine are possible ways to ameliorate these potential problems.

G. MENTAL DISORDERS

MENTAL DEPRESSION

Definition

Mental depression is a psychiatric disorder distinguished from normal sadness and grief by severity and duration of the mood disturbances and by the presence of fatigue, loss of appetite, and insomnia.

Incidence and Prevalence

Depression is the most common psychiatric disorder, affecting 2% to 4% of the population.

Pathophysiology

Pathophysiologic causes of major mental depression are unknown, although abnormalities of amine neurotransmitter pathways are the most likely etiologic factors. Cortisol hypersecretion is present in many of these patients.

Clinical Manifestations

Diagnosis of major mental depression is based on the persistent presence of at least five characteristics and the exclusion of organic causes or a normal emotional reaction. Alcoholism and major depression often occur together, and it is presumed that toxic effects of alcohol on the brain are responsible. As stated earlier, this disease is characterized by mood disturbances and by the presence of fatigue, loss of appetite, and insomnia.

Treatment

Treatment of mental depression can be initiated using with antidepressant drugs, electroconvulsive therapy (ECT), or both. Common drug therapies include selective serotonin reuptake inhibitors, tricyclic antidepressants, and monoamine oxidase inhibitors (MAOIs). ECT is indicated for treating severe mental depression in patients who are unresponsive to drugs or who become acutely suicidal. Increased ICP is a contraindication to ECT.

Anesthetic Considerations

Treatment with tricyclic antidepressants need not be discontinued before administration of anesthesia for elective operations. Increased availability of neurotransmitters in the patient's CNS can result in increased anesthetic requirements. An increased level of norepinephrine at postsynaptic receptors in the peripheral sympathetic nervous system can be responsible for exaggerated systemic blood pressure responses after administration of indirect-acting vasopressors. Long-term treatment with tricyclic antidepressants may alter the responses to pancuronium, and the combination has been associated with tachyarrhythmias.

Anesthesia can be safely conducted despite earlier recommendation that these drugs be discontinued 14 to 21 days before elective operations. Careful consideration is needed when selecting drugs and administering doses.

During anesthesia and surgery, it is important to avoid stimulating the sympathetic nervous system, so as to decrease the incidence of systemic hypertension and cardiac dysrhythmias.

Although uncommon, adverse interactions between MAOIs and opioids have been observed. Systemic hypertension, hypotension, hyperthermia, depression of ventilation, seizures, and coma may follow administration of opioids with these agents. Meperidine has been the opioid most often incriminated, but the same syndrome can occur with other opioids.

SCHIZOPHRENIA

Definition

Schizophrenia is a psychotic disorder characterized most often with delusions and hallucinations.

Incidence and Prevalence

Schizophrenia is the most common psychotic disorder. It accounts for about 20% of all patients treated for mental illness.

Clinical Manifestations

Features of the illness include an array of symptoms, such as delusions, hallucinations, flattened affect, and social or occupational dysfunction, including withdrawal and changes in appearance and hygiene. Some patients experience exacerbations and remissions.

Treatment

Treatment of schizophrenia is with antipsychotic drugs, which most likely exert their effects by inhibiting dopamine binding at postsynaptic dopamine receptors. These agents have an array of adverse effects; their therapeutic index is high, and side effects are rarely serious or irreversible.

Anesthetic Considerations

Neuroleptic malignant syndrome is a rare, potentially fatal complication of antipsychotic drug therapy that is presumed to reflect drug-induced interference with dopamine's role in central thermoregulation. This syndrome usually manifests during the first few weeks of treatment or after an increased drug dose. Clinical manifestations usually develop over a 24- to 72-hour period and include high fever, severe skeletal muscle rigidity, autonomic nervous system instability, altered consciousness, and increased serum creatine kinase concentrations reflecting skeletal muscle damage. Treatment is with immediate cessation of antipsychotic drug therapy, administration of bromocriptine (5 mg orally every 6 hours) or dantrolene (up to 6 mg/kg daily as a continuous intravenous infusion) in an attempt to decrease skeletal muscle rigidity, and supportive therapy. These patients are vulnerable to developing malignant hyperthermia secondary to similarities between the pathophysiologies of the syndromes. This correlation is an important factor when planning for general anesthesia.

ANXIETY DISORDERS

Anxiety disorders can be responses to exogenous stimuli or endogenous stimuli. Anxiety resulting from identifiable stresses is usually self-limited and rarely requires pharmacologic treatment.

Panic disorders appear to be inherited and are characterized as discrete periods of intense fear that are not triggered by severe anxiogenic stimuli. This disorder is often accompanied by dyspnea, tachycardia, diaphoresis, paresthesias, nausea, chest pain, and fear of dying. An unexplained observation is that infusion of lactate may provoke panic attacks in susceptible persons. Tricyclic antidepressants and MAOIs are effective for treating panic attacks. Delayed recovery from anesthesia has been attributed to coexisting hysteria.

H. MULTIPLE SCLEROSIS

Definition

Multiple sclerosis (MS) is a demyelinating acquired disease of the CNS characterized by random and multiple sites of demyelination of the corticospinal tract neurons in the brain and spinal cord.

Incidence and Prevalence

There seems to be an increased risk of developing MS in persons living in northern temperate zones such as North America, Europe, and southern portions of New Zealand and Australia. The incidence is greater among inner city dwellers and affluent socioeconomic groups. Evidence for a genetic factor is demonstrated by a 12- to 15-fold increase among first-degree relatives. MS is a disease of young adults. It occurs 2 to 2.5 times more frequently in women than in men. The development of symptoms usually occurs in the third to fourth decade of life.

Pathophysiology

Although the exact cause is unknown, evidence suggests that the disease progresses from an immune-mediated attack on myelin with secondary disruption of axons leading to progressive disability.

Diagnostic and Laboratory Findings

Visual, brainstem, auditory, and somatosensory evoked potentials can be used to elicit the slow nerve conduction that occurs as a result of demyelination in specific areas. CT and MRI may demonstrate demyelinative plaques.

Clinical Manifestations

Clinical manifestations reflect the site of demyelination in the CNS and spinal cord. "Ascending" spastic paresis of skeletal muscle is often prominent. Presenting symptoms may include unilateral vision impairment, fatigue, depression, bladder urgency, weakness, impaired balance, and impaired coordination. Symptoms develop over the course of a few days, remain stable for a few weeks, and then improve. The course of MS is characterized by exacerbations and remissions of symptoms at unpredictable intervals over a period of several years. Residual symptoms persist during remission.

Treatment

There is no cure for MS, and treatment is symptomatic. Corticosteroids are used to shorten the durations of attack, and skeletal muscle spasticity is treated with baclofen (Lioresal), dantrolene, and benzodiazepines (Valium). Immunosuppressive therapy and plasmapheresis may benefit some patients. Patients should avoid stress and fatigue.

Anesthetic Considerations

A baseline neurologic examination must first be documented. The impact of surgical stress on the natural progression of MS should also be considered. Any postoperative increase in body temperature may be more likely than drugs to be responsible for exacerbation of MS. Spinal anesthesia has been implicated in postoperative exacerbation of MS, but epidural or peripheral nerve block has not. General anesthesia is most often chosen. The use of succinylcholine should be avoided because of the possible exaggerated release of potassium. The response to nondepolarizing muscle relaxants may be prolonged because of coexisting muscle weakness and decreased muscle mass.

Prognosis

The course of MS is unpredictable. Exacerbations and remissions are common. In the late-onset type, the course is generally progressive.

I. NEUROPATHY AND MYOPATHY

Definition

Neuropathy is a general term indicating nerve disorders of any kind. *Myopathy* is defined as any disorder with structural changes or functional impairment of muscle.

Pathophysiology

Neuropathies may be caused by certain drugs, diabetes mellitus, human immunodeficiency virus, Lyme disease, leprosy, herpes zoster, Bell palsy, sarcoidosis, and Guillain-Barré syndrome, among others.

Myopathies may be caused by periodic paralyses (hypokalemic, hyperkalemic, and paramyotonia congenita), metabolic alterations of glycolysis (e.g., myophosphorylase deficiency) and fatty acid utilization (e.g., carnitine palmitoyltransferase deficiency), muscular dystrophy, polymyositis, dermatomyositis, fibromyalgia, and polymyalgia rheumatica, among others.

Diagnostic and Laboratory Findings

Electrodiagnosis is used to diagnose neuropathies. Findings include slowing of nerve conduction velocity, dispersion and reduction in amplitude of evoked action potentials, or conduction block. Nerve biopsy may also be done to determine the cause of the neuropathy.

Muscle biopsy may be used to diagnose specific myopathies. Creatine kinase, which is the preferred muscle enzyme to measure in the evaluation of myopathies, may be elevated. Aspartate aminotransferase, alanine aminotransferase, and lactic dehydrogenase, enzymes in both muscle and the liver, may also be elevated. The erythrocyte sedimentation rate may be elevated in patients with certain myopathies.

Clinical Manifestations

Manifestations of neuropathy include tingling, prickling, burning, pansensory loss, areflexia, muscle atrophy, and motor weakness in the affected nerve distribution. Specific manifestations are specific to the type of neuropathy (e.g., autonomic neuropathy, pure motor neuropathy, pure sensory neuropathy, or mixed motor and sensory) and the location of the affected nerve.

Manifestations of myopathy include intermittent or persistent muscle weakness. Fatigue is a common complaint. Muscle pain associated with involuntary muscle activity, cramps, contractures, and stiff or rigid muscles may also occur. In most myopathies, muscle tissue is replaced by fat and connective tissue, but the size of the muscle is usually not affected.

Treatment

Treatment of neuropathies depends on the cause and may include use of antidepressants, anticonvulsants, neuroleptics, or corticosteroids for pain control. Glucocorticoids may be used to relieve the pain associated with myopathies.

Anesthetic Considerations

Preoperative evaluation of the patient with neuropathy should include specific documentation of signs and symptoms. Possible effects of medications should be considered. Intraoperatively, careful positioning and padding of bony prominences to avoid further damage are imperative. Regional anesthesia is not contraindicated in patients with neuropathies. However, some practitioners choose to avoid regional anesthesia to avoid confusion if new deficits appear postoperatively. The risks and benefits of general versus regional anesthesia should be weighed in deciding a plan of care. Other anesthetic care should take into consideration the underlying disease process.

Anesthetic management of patients with myopathy should take into account the affected muscle groups. Respiratory muscle involvement may diminish pulmonary reserve. Pulmonary function testing may be helpful if significant pulmonary disease is evident. History of dysphagia, regurgitation, or recurrent pulmonary infections may signal a risk of aspiration, necessitating premedication with a histamine (H_2) antagonist and prokinetic agent and rapid sequence induction. Patients with myopathies are at an increased risk of malignant hyperthermia. Therefore, the anesthesia provider may want to avoid the use of triggering agents. The anesthetic technique should be determined by the procedure and other coexisting diseases. Muscle relaxants should be avoided, if possible, because of the possibility of increased block. If muscle relaxation is necessary, a short-acting nondepolarizing agent should be used. In addition, succinylcholine should be avoided because of the risk of an unusual response (myotonic contractions, prolonged block, or phase II block), severe hyperkalemia, or malignant hyperthermia.

J. PARKINSON'S DISEASE

Definition

Parkinsonism is a clinical syndrome that consists of four cardinal signs: tremor, rigidity, akinesia, and postural disturbances (TRAP). Parkinson's disease is a common cause of TRAP syndrome, but there are numerous other causes.

Incidence and Prevalence

Parkinson's disease, which is the second most common neurodegenerative disorder after Alzheimer's disease, occurs in approximately one in 1000 persons in the general population and in 1% of persons older than 65 years. Men are affected slightly more than women (3:2).

Pathophysiology

The cause of Parkinson's disease is believed to be a variable combination of poorly understood genetic and environmental factors. Both autosomal dominant and autosomal recessive genes can cause classic Parkinson's disease. Many of the features of Parkinson's disease are attributable to loss of dopamine in the neostriatum (especially the putamen) secondary to loss of the pigmented dopaminergic neurons in the substantia nigra pars compacta of the midbrain. Approximately 60% of these dopaminergic neurons will have degenerated before clinical features of the disease develop.

Clinical Manifestations

The classic "resting tremor" of Parkinson's disease has characteristic clinical features. The tremor has a frequency of 4 to 6 cycles per second, typically with a "pill rolling" character when it involves the hand. Other motor symptoms include rigidity, akinesia, and postural disturbances.

In addition to the motor features of Parkinson's disease, a variety of nonmotor features are extremely common and include pain and other sensory disturbances. The dysautonomic complaints, such as urinary urgency and frequency, may occur.

Treatment

Treatment of Parkinson's disease is directed at slowing the progression ("neuroprotective" or "disease-modifying" treatments); improving symptoms, typically by resorting dopaminergic tone medically or by correcting basal ganglia neurophysiology surgically ("symptomatic" therapy); or attempting to restore or regenerate the damaged neurons ("neurorestorative" or "neuroregenerative" therapy).

Anesthetic Considerations

Patients being treated with L-dopa should continue to receive their medication throughout the perioperative period, including the usual morning dose the day of operation. Because of the short elimination half-life of L-dopa and dopamine, interruption in therapy for greater than 6 to 12 hours can result in loss of therapeutic effect. Abrupt withdrawal of L-dopa may lead to skeletal muscle rigidity that interferes with ventilation. L-dopa also sensitizes the cardiovascular system and may predispose the patient to perioperative arrhythmias. Long-term L-dopa therapy can cause blood pressure fluctuations because of autonomic instability; therefore, invasive blood pressure monitoring may be necessary. L-dopa therapy causes an increase in renal blood flow and sodium excretion. It also causes a concomitant decrease in renin release, intravascular fluid volume, and systemic blood pressure during induction of anesthesia. These swings in blood pressure often require aggressive fluid administration with crystalloids, colloids, or both. Drugs that block dopamine uptake (e.g., phenothiazines, butyrophenones) or dopamine receptor antagonists (metoclopramide) may exacerbate symptoms and should therefore be avoided. Anticholinergics or antihistamines may be useful during acute exacerbations. Diphenhydramine (Benadryl) is also very useful as a sedative in these patients. Ketamine may provoke an exaggerated sympathetic nervous system response, and its use is questionable.

K. SEIZURES

Definition

Seizures are the result of abnormal electrical impulse discharges in the brain.

Incidence and Prevalence

Seizures are one of the most common neurologic disorders and may occur at any age. Seizures affect approximately 0.5% to 1% of the population in the United States. Numerous types of seizures exist, but most are generalized tonic-clonic seizures. The likelihood of a recurrent seizure after a single seizure is approximately 50% in the following 3 years, with the greatest incidence during the first 6 months.

Pathophysiology

Seizures are caused by transient, paroxysmal, and synchronous discharge of groups of neurons in the brain. Most seizures are idiopathic. Idiopathic seizure disorders usually begin in childhood. Seizure onset in adults may indicate an expanding intracranial hematoma, tumor, intracranial hemorrhage, metabolic disturbance, infection, trauma, alcohol or addictive drug withdrawal, eclampsia (in pregnant women), previous trauma causing an irritative phenomenon in the brain, or local anesthesia toxicity.

Clinical Manifestations

Clinical manifestations depend on location, number of neurons involved in the seizure, discharge, and duration of the seizure. Clinical manifestations include focal or generalized tonic-clonic seizures and an increase in the cerebral metabolic rate for oxygen. Cerebral metabolic decompensation occurs after 30 minutes of uncontrolled seizure activity. Therefore, the window for treatment is limited.

Treatment

The first priority is to protect and secure the airway, oxygenate, and ventilate. Supportive care and treatment of the underlying problem are needed.

Grand Mal Seizures

Appropriate drug therapy for grand mal seizures includes midazolam, 1 mg/min by intravenous push, until seizures stop or a total of 10 mg. Phenytoin (Dilantin), with an intravenous load of 15 mg/kg over 20 minutes, is also used. No more than 50 mg/min is infused (in an adult) followed by daily maintenance doses of 300 to 500 mg orally or intravenously for adults. The therapeutic serum level is 10 to 20 mcg/mL. Phenobarbital can also be used to control seizures with an intravenous dose of 100 mg/min up to a total of 20 mg/kg. The therapeutic serum level is 20 to 40 mcg/mL.

Eclamptic Seizures

Magnesium sulfate, a mild CNS depressant and vasodilator, is used for eclamptic seizures. An initial intravenous loading dose is 2 to 4 g administered over 15 minutes followed by a continuous infusion of 1 to 3 g/hr. The therapeutic serum level is 4 to 8 mEq/L.

Anesthetic Considerations

Electrolytes, cultures, and serum drug levels should be obtained preoperatively. All current medications should be considered, and particular attention should be paid to any anticonvulsant drugs being taken and their possible cardiopulmonary effects and interactions with anesthetics, as well as consideration of protein-bound properties. When phenytoin (Dilantin) is administered intravenously, particular care should be taken to infuse and flush with normal saline; infusion should be no faster than 50 mg/min. Arrhythmias, hypotension, and cardiac arrest can occur if administration is too rapid. The intraoperative requirement for nondepolarizing muscle relaxants (NDMRs) may be increased. Other anticonvulsant medications used are phenobarbital, primidone, carbamazepine (increases requirement for NDMRs), valproic acid, and ethosuximide. Metrizamide, a water-soluble contrast agent, can produce seizures if it is allowed to enter the intracranial compartment in a high concentration.

Patients receiving antiepileptic drugs build a resistance to the effects of neuromuscular blocking agents and opioids because of changes in the number of receptors (up-regulation), altered drug metabolism, and interaction with endogenous neurotransmitters. A "paralyzing" dose of muscle relaxant stops peripheral but not CNS manifestations of seizure activity.

Etomidate and ketamine can potentially lower the seizure threshold. Atracurium possesses a laudanosine metabolite that is a CNS stimulant. Magnesium sulfate may increase sensitivity to all muscle relaxants. Hyperventilation of the lungs decreases delivery of additional local anesthesia to the brain; respiratory alkalosis and hyperkalemia result in hyperpolarization of nerve membranes.

L. SPINAL CORD INJURY

Definition

The spinal cord is vulnerable to trauma, compression by intradural or extradural tumors, and vascular injuries.

Incidence and Prevalence

Approximately 11,000 persons each year sustain acute spinal cord injuries that result in paraplegia and quadriplegia. Two-thirds are male, and 70% to 80% are ages 11 to 30 years. The mortality rate before reaching the hospital is 30% to 40%; the mortality rate during the first year decreases to 10%.

Pathophysiology

Spinal cord injuries result from motor vehicle accidents, falls, sport injuries (especially diving), and penetrating injuries (especially gunshot wounds). The spinal cord itself is not usually severed but is injured by compression from bone, foreign body, hematoma, and edema and by ischemia.

Clinical Manifestations

Clinical manifestations include changes in cardiopulmonary responses, fluids and electrolytes, temperature control function, and abnormal responses to drugs. Injuries at levels T2 to T12 cause paraplegia but leave the upper extremities and diaphragm intact. Injuries at levels C5 to T1 cause varying degrees of upper extremity paralysis as well.

Treatment

For acute injury, the ABCs (airway, breathing, circulation) of resuscitation are used. Cervical spine protection is provided by avoiding neck motion and subsequent further spinal cord damage. Spinal cord perfusion should be maintained with volume and vasoactive drugs. If the spinal cord is compressed by bone or hematoma, decompression is necessary. High-dose corticosteroid therapy (methylprednisolone, 30 mg/kg over 1 hour followed by 5 mg/kg for 23 hours) is begun soon after injury to improve neurologic outcome but has not been conclusively determined to improve outcome.

Anesthetic Considerations

Cervical ("halo") traction sometimes necessitates fundamental changes in airway management of the patient with a cervical spine injury. Airway reflex impairment may be present. An assistant may be needed to help maintain neck immobility during laryngoscopy or intubation. Alternative techniques for securing the airway (e.g., fiberoptic intubation) are sometimes necessary. Nasal intubation is contraindicated in the presence of basilar skull fracture. Be prepared for emergency cricothyroidotomy, if necessary. Succinylcholine can be used safely within the first 24 hours after injury. Use anticholinergic agents to reduce secretions. Ventilate the patient with large tidal volumes (10–15 mL/kg) to avoid hypercarbia and atelectasis. Move the patient carefully to prevent injury to the limbs and trunk. Check pressure areas to prevent breakdown. Some cardioacceleration and vasoconstrictor tone is lost as a result of cord injuries that involve levels T1 to T4. Spinal cord shock is present. Respiratory compromise is possible, depending on the level of spinal cord injury.

Endocrine System

A. ACROMEGALY

Definition

Growth hormone (GH) hypersecretion, usually caused by a GH-secreting pituitary adenoma (99% of cases), can produce a highly distinctive syndrome in adults called *acromegaly*. Acromegaly occurs because of sustained hypersecretion of GH after adolescence. The condition occurs with equal frequency in both sexes. If hypersecretion of GH occurs before puberty—that is, before closure of the growth plates—the individual grows very tall (8–9 feet), a rare condition known as *gigantism*.

Pathophysiology

The excessive production of GH associated with acromegaly does not induce bone lengthening but rather enhances the growth of periosteal bone. The unrestrained bone growth in patients with acromegaly produces bones that are massive in size and thickness. Bones of the hands and feet (acral) become particularly large. Overgrowth of vertebrae may cause kyphoscoliosis and arthritis.

Soft tissue changes are also prominent with GH hypersecretion. The patient develops coarsened facial features (acromegalic facies), including a large, bulbous nose; a supraorbital ridge overgrowth; dental malocclusion; and a prominent prognathic mandible. The changes in appearance are insidious, and many patients do not seek treatment until the diagnosis is obvious and the disease course is advanced. Overgrowth of the internal organs is less apparent clinically but no less serious. The liver, heart, spleen, and kidneys become enlarged. Lung volumes increase, which may lead to ventilation–perfusion mismatch. Exercise tolerance may be limited because of increased body mass and skeletal muscle weakness.

Cardiomyopathy, hypertension (28% of cases), and accelerated atherosclerosis in patients with acromegaly can lead to symptomatic cardiac disease (congestive heart failure, arrhythmias). Echocardiography often shows left ventricular hypertrophy. Resting electrocardiograms (ECGs) are abnormal in 50% of patients with acromegaly. ST-segment and T-wave depression, conduction defects, and evidence of prior myocardial infarction may be present. The insulin antagonistic effect of GH produces glucose intolerance in up to 50% of patients with acromegaly and frank diabetes mellitus (DM) in 10% to 25% of patients. The insulin antagonistic effect of GH produces glucose intolerance in up to 50% of patients with acromegaly and frank DM in 10% to 25% of patients.

Clinical Manifestations

Clinical manifestations resulting from the local effects of the expanding tumor may include headaches (55%), papilledema, and visual field defects (19%), which are caused by compression of the optic nerves and chiasm. Significant increases in intracranial pressure are uncommon. Compression or destruction of normal pituitary tissue by the tumor may lead to panhypopituitarism. Common features of acromegaly are summarized in the box on pg. 58.

Common Features of Acromegaly

Skeletal overgrowth (enlarged hands and feet, prominent prognathic mandible)
Soft tissue overgrowth (enlarged lips, tongue, and epiglottis; distortion of facial features)
Visceromegaly
Osteoarthritis
Glucose intolerance
Peripheral neuropathy
Skeletal muscle weakness
Extrasellar tumor extension (headache, visual field defects)

Treatment

Treatment for acromegaly is aimed at restoring normal GH levels. The preferred initial therapy for active acromegaly is microsurgical removal of the pituitary tumor with preservation of the gland. The surgical approach to the pituitary tumor most often is via a transsphenoidal route, with the patient in a semi-sitting position. Precautions associated with monitoring of venous air embolism should be part of the anesthesia management plan. Surgical ablation is usually successful in rapidly reducing tumor size, inhibiting GH secretion, and alleviating some symptoms. Administration of octreotide (a long-acting somatostatin analog), pegvisomant (a GH receptor antagonist), and gland irradiation are treatment options for patients who are not surgical candidates.

Anesthetic Considerations

Preanesthetic assessment of patients with acromegaly should include a careful examination of the airway. Facial deformities and the large nose may hamper adequate fitting of an anesthesia mask. Endotracheal intubation may be a challenge because these patients have large and thick tongues (macroglossia), enlargement of the thyroid, obstructive teeth, hypertrophy of the epiglottis, and general soft tissue overgrowth in the upper airway. Subglottic narrowing and vocal cord enlargement may dictate the use of a smaller diameter endotracheal tube. Nasotracheal intubation should be approached cautiously because of possible turbinate enlargement.

Preoperative dyspnea, stridor, or hoarseness should alert the anesthetist to airway involvement. Indirect laryngoscopy and neck radiography may be performed for thorough assessment. If difficulties in maintaining an adequate airway are anticipated, a fiberoptic-guided intubation in an awake patient is of proven value. The endotracheal tube should remain in place until the patient is fully awake and has total return of reflexes. The predisposition to airway obstruction in these patients makes assiduous postoperative monitoring of the patient's respiratory status a wise precaution.

The frequent occurrence of cardiac arrhythmias, coronary artery disease, and hypertension in patients with acromegaly warrants a thorough preanesthetic cardiac evaluation. The increased risk of DM in these patients mandates careful perioperative monitoring of blood glucose and electrolyte levels.

If preoperative assessment reveals impairment of the adrenal or thyroid axis, stress-level glucocorticoid therapy and thyroid replacement should be implemented in the perioperative period.

Entrapment neuropathies, such as carpal tunnel syndrome, are common in patients with acromegaly. An Allen test should be performed before placement of a radial artery catheter because hypertrophy of the carpal ligament may cause inadequate ulnar artery flow.

B. ADRENOCORTICAL INSUFFICIENCY

Definition

Primary adrenal insufficiency (Addison's disease) reflects the absence of cortisol and aldosterone owing to the destruction of the adrenal cortex. In 1855, an English physician, Dr. Thomas Addison, first described a relatively rare clinical syndrome characterized by wasting and skin hyperpigmentation and identified its cause as destruction of the adrenal glands. *Primary adrenocortical insufficiency Addison's disease)* becomes apparent when 90% of the gland is destroyed. Tuberculosis is a common cause of primary adrenocortical insufficiency worldwide, but in the United States, most cases are the result of autoimmune dysfunction. Primary adrenocortical insufficiency may also be associated with other autoimmune disorders, such as type 1 diabetes and Hashimoto thyroiditis. Less commonly, primary adrenal insufficiency is congenital or caused by sarcoidosis, human immunodeficiency virus infection, adrenal hemorrhage, malignancy, or trauma.

Clinical Manifestations

Clinical symptoms of Addison's disease reflect destruction of all cortical zones, resulting in adrenal androgen, glucocorticoid, and mineralocorticoid hormone deficiency (see box below).

Clinical Features of Primary Adrenocortical Insufficiency

Asthenia	Nausea
Weakness	Vomiting
Anorexia	Abdominal pain
Hypoglycemia	Mucosal and skin pigmentation
Hypotension	Weight loss
Hyponatremia	Hyperkalemia

Weakness and fatigue are cardinal features. Reduced appetite with weight loss, vomiting, abdominal pain, and diarrhea are frequently reported. Hypoglycemia is often present. Volume depletion is a common feature of the disease and may be manifested by orthostatic hypotension. Hyponatremia and hyperkalemia are commonly revealed by laboratory screening.

The adrenal–pituitary axis is intact in primary adrenal insufficiency, and adrenocorticotropic hormone (ACTH) concentrations are elevated as a result of the reduced production of cortisol. Increased melanin formation in the skin and hyperpigmentation of the knuckles of the fingers, toes, knees, elbows, lips, and buccal mucosa may be evident.

Treatment

Treatment for adrenal insufficiency aims to replace both glucocorticoid and mineralocorticoid deficiency. Normal adults secrete 15 to 30 mg of cortisol (hydrocortisone) and 50 to 250 mcg of aldosterone per day. Corticosteroids used for therapy have varying degrees of mineralocorticoid and glucocorticoid effects.

Comparative Pharmacology of Endogenous and Synthetic Corticosteroids

	Common Name	Glucocorticoid Effect*	Mineralocorticoid Effect*	Equivalent Dose (mg)	Duration of Action (hr)
Cortisol	Hydrocortisone	1	1	20	8–12
Cortisone	Cortone	0.8	0.8	25	8–36
Prednisolone	Prelone	4	0.8	5	12–36
Prednisone	Deltasone	4	0.8	5	18–36
Methylprednisolone	Medrol, Solu-Medrol	5	0.5	4	12–36
Betamethasone	Diprosone, Celestone	25	0	0.75	36–54
Dexamethasone	Decadron	25	0	0.75	36–54
Triamcinolone	Aristocort, Kenacort	5	0	4	12–36
Fludrocortisone	Florinef	10	250	2	24

*Relative to cortisol.

Data from Stoelting RK, Hillier SC. *Pharmacology and Physiology in Anesthetic Practice.* 4th ed. Philadelphia: Lippincott Williams & Wilkins; 2006:462.

A typical oral replacement dose for Addison's disease may consist of prednisone, 5 mg in the morning and 2.5 mg in the evening, or hydrocortisone, 20 mg in the morning and 10 mg in the evening. If indicated, mineralocorticoid replacement may consist of 0.05 to 0.2 mg/day of fludrocortisone. Standard glucocorticoid doses should be supplemented during periods of surgical stress.

Anesthetic Considerations

Anesthetic management for patients with primary adrenal insufficiency should provide for exogenous corticosteroid supplementation. Etomidate should be avoided because it transiently inhibits synthesis of cortisol in physiologically normal patients. Doses of anesthetic drugs should be minimized because these patients may be sensitive to drug-induced myocardial depression. Invasive monitoring (arterial line and pulmonary artery catheter) is indicated. Because of skeletal muscle weakness, the initial dose of muscle relaxant should be reduced, and further doses should be governed by peripheral nerve stimulator response. Plasma concentrations of glucose and electrolytes should be measured frequently during surgery.

SECONDARY ADRENOCORTICAL INSUFFICIENCY

Definition

Secondary adrenocortical insufficiency is caused by ACTH deficiency from two primary etiologies: (1) hypothalamic–pituitary–adrenal (HPA) axis suppression after exogenous glucocorticoid therapy and (2) ACTH deficiency secondary to hypothalamic or pituitary gland dysfunction (tumor, infection, surgical or radiologic ablation). Long-term treatment with glucocorticoids, for any cause, results in negative feedback to the hypothalamus and pituitary gland, decreased ACTH output, and eventual adrenal cortex atrophy. The longer the duration of glucocorticoid administration, the greater the likelihood of suppression, but the precise dose or duration of therapy that produces adrenal suppression is unknown. Sustained and clinically important adrenal suppression usually does not occur with treatment periods less than 14 days. Treatment periods long enough to provoke signs of Cushing syndrome are usually associated with adrenal suppression of clinically significant.

Clinical Manifestations

Clinical manifestations of secondary adrenal insufficiency resemble the primary disease except secondary insufficiency is less likely to be associated with severe hypovolemia, hyperkalemia, or hyponatremia because mineralocorticoid secretion is usually preserved. Hyperpigmentation is absent because ACTH levels are low.

ACUTE ADRENAL CRISIS

Definition

Acute adrenal crisis is a sudden exacerbation or onset of severe adrenal insufficiency. It is a rare event associated with high morbidity and mortality if allowed to progress unrecognized. A patient with chronic adrenal insufficiency may deteriorate rapidly into an acute insufficiency state as a result of some superimposed stress, such as infection, acute illness, or sepsis. The stress of surgery or trauma in the patient with inadequate adrenal reserves can precipitate acute adrenal crisis in the perioperative period.

Clinical Manifestations

Symptoms of adrenal crisis reflect acute deficiency of corticosteroids and include severe weakness, nausea, hypotension, fever, and decreasing mental status. In the surgical setting, hemodynamic instability or cardiovascular collapse may herald adrenal crisis. The index of suspicion for adrenal crisis should be particularly high if the patient has hyperpigmentation, hyponatremia, or hyperkalemia; a history of autoimmune disease (hypothyroidism, diabetes); or recent prior use of exogenous steroids. The anesthetist should be mindful of the adrenal suppressive effects of etomidate. Even a single dose of etomidate for induction of anesthesia can cause acute adrenocortical insufficiency for up to 24 hours and should be avoided in patients susceptible to adrenal insufficiency.

Treatment

Acute adrenal crisis is a medical emergency requiring aggressive treatment of the steroid insufficiency and associated hypoglycemia, electrolyte imbalance, and volume depletion. Early recognition and intervention are crucial steps in altering the course of acute adrenal insufficiency. Initial therapy begins with rapid intravenous (IV) administration of a glucose-containing isotonic crystalloid solution. If the patient is hemodynamically unstable, advanced hemodynamic monitoring and inotropic support may be necessary. Steroid replacement therapy begins with hydrocortisone, 100 mg IV, followed by hydrocortisone, 100 to 200 mg IV over 24 hours. Mineralocorticoid administration is unnecessary with large doses of steroids (hydrocortisone 100–200 mg) because mineralocorticoid effects are present at these doses.

C. CUSHING'S DISEASE

Definition

Cushing's syndrome results in diverse complex symptoms, signs, and biochemical abnormalities caused by excess glucocorticoid hormone.

Pathophysiology

The most common cause of Cushing's syndrome today is the administration of supraphysiologic doses of glucocorticoids for conditions such as arthritis, asthma, various autoimmune disorders, allergies, and a myriad of other diseases.

Endogenous Cushing's syndrome is most often the result of one of three distinct pathogenic disorders: pituitary tumor (Cushing's disease), adrenal tumor, or ectopic hormone production.

Cushing's disease specifically denotes an anterior pituitary tumor cause of the syndrome. The pituitary tumor produces excessive amounts of ACTH and is associated with bilateral adrenal hyperplasia. Patients often develop skin pigmentation as a result of excess ACTH. Cushing's disease is the most common cause of endogenous Cushing's syndrome.

Adrenal Cushing's syndrome is caused by autonomous corticosteroid production (ACTH independent) by an adrenal tumor, usually unilateral. This form of hyperadrenalism accounts for 20% to 25% of patients with Cushing's syndrome and is usually associated with suppressed plasma ACTH levels. Adrenal tumors that are malignant are usually large by the time Cushing's syndrome becomes manifest.

Ectopic Cushing's syndrome results from autonomous ACTH or corticotropin-releasing hormone (CRH) production by extrapituitary malignancies, producing markedly elevated plasma levels of ACTH. Bronchogenic carcinoma accounts for most of these cases. Carcinoid tumors and malignant tumors of the kidney, ovary, and pancreas also can cause ectopic production of ACTH.

Clinical Manifestations

Clinical features reflect cortisol excess, either from overproduction of the adrenal cortex or exogenously administered glucocorticoid. The clinical picture includes central obesity with thin extremities, hypertension, glucose intolerance, plethoric facies, purple striae, muscle weakness, bruising, and osteoporosis. Mineralocorticoid effects include fluid retention and hypokalemic alkalosis. Women manifest a degree of masculinization (hirsutism, hair thinning, acne, amenorrhea), and men manifest a degree of feminization (gynecomastia, impotence) because of the androgenic effects of glucocorticoid excess. The catabolic effects of cortisol result in skin that is thin and atrophic and unable to withstand the stresses of normal activity. Patients with Cushing's syndrome typically gain weight and develop a characteristic redistribution of fat.

Diagnosis

A widely used test for diagnosis of hyperadrenocorticism is measurement of the plasma cortisol concentration in the morning after a dose of dexamethasone. Dexamethasone suppresses plasma cortisol secretion in normal patients but not in those with endogenous hyperadrenocorticism. Diagnosis of Cushing's syndrome is also based on elevated levels of plasma and urinary cortisol, plasma ACTH, and urinary 17-hydroxycorticosteroids.

Treatment

Treatment for Cushing's syndrome depends on the cause. Transsphenoidal hypophysectomy is a primary treatment option for Cushing's disease. Complications occur in fewer than 5% of patients and include DI (usually transient), cerebrospinal fluid rhinorrhea, and hemorrhage.

Adrenal Cushing's syndrome may be treated by surgical removal of the adrenal adenoma. Because the contralateral adrenal gland is preoperatively suppressed, glucocorticoid replacement may be necessary for several months after surgery until adrenal function returns. Bilateral adrenalectomy in the patient with Cushing's syndrome is associated with a high incidence of complications and permanent corticosteroid deficiency.

The treatment of choice for an ectopic ACTH-secreting tumor is surgical removal, but this may not always be feasible because of the nature of the underlying process (e.g., metastatic carcinoma). Metyrapone, an 11-β-hydroxylase inhibitor, and mitotane, an agent that blocks steroidogenesis at several levels, may be used to help normalize cortisol levels.

Anesthetic Considerations

Important perioperative considerations for the patient with Cushing's syndrome include normalizing blood pressure, blood glucose levels, intravascular fluid volume, and electrolyte concentrations. The aldosterone antagonist spironolactone effectively decreases extracellular fluid volume and corrects hypokalemia under these conditions.

Osteopenia is an important consideration in positioning the patient for the operative procedure. Special attention must be given to the patient's skin, which can easily be abraded by tape or minor trauma. Glucocorticoids are lympholytic and immunosuppressive, placing the patient at increased risk for infection and mandating particular enforcement of aseptic techniques as indicated.

The choice of drugs for induction and maintenance of anesthesia is not specifically influenced by the presence of hyperadrenocorticism. Muscle relaxants may have an exaggerated effect in patients with preexisting myopathy, and a conservative approach to dosing is warranted when significant skeletal muscle weakness is present.

If adrenal resection is planned, glucocorticoids may be indicated after resection and administered at doses equivalent to adrenal output for maximum stress. Hydrocortisone, 100 mg IV, followed by 100 to 200 mg IV over 24 hours can be administered and then reduced over 3 to 6 days postoperatively until a maintenance dose is reached.

D. DIABETES INSIPIDUS

Definition

Diabetes insipidus (DI) reflects the absence of antidiuretic hormone (ADH) owing to the destruction of the posterior pituitary gland (neurogenic DI) or failure of the renal tubules to respond to ADH (nephrogenic DI).

Pathophysiology

Common causes of neurogenic DI include severe head trauma, neurosurgical procedures (trauma to the median eminence, pituitary surgery), infiltrating pituitary lesions, and brain tumors. DI that develops after pituitary surgery is usually transient and often resolves in 5 to 7 days.

Nephrogenic DI may occur in association with an X-linked genetic mutation, hypercalcemia, hypokalemia, and medication-induced nephrotoxicity. Ethanol, demeclocycline, phenytoin, chlorpromazine, and lithium all inhibit the action of ADH or its release.

Clinical Manifestations

The hallmark of DI is polyuria. The inability to produce concentrated urine results in dehydration and hypernatremia. The syndrome is characterized by a urine osmolarity less than 300 mOsm/L, urine specific gravity less than 1.010, and urine volumes greater than 30 mL/kg each day. The tremendous urinary water loss produces serum osmolarities greater than 290 mOsm/L and serum sodium concentrations greater than 145 mEq/L. Neurologic symptoms of hypernatremia and neuronal dehydration may be present and include hyperreflexia, weakness, lethargy, seizures, and coma.

The thirst mechanism assumes a primary role in maintaining water balance in awake patients with DI. Ingestion of large volumes of water prevents hyperosmolarity and life-threatening dehydration.

Treatment

Treatment protocols for DI depend on the degree of ADH deficiency. Most patients have incomplete DI and retain some capacity to concentrate their urine and conserve water. Mild cases (incomplete DI) may be treated with medications that either augment the release of ADH or increase the receptor response to ADH. These drugs may include chlorpropamide (sulfonylurea hypoglycemic agent), carbamazepine (anticonvulsant), and clofibrate (hypolipidemic agent).

Significant deficiency (plasma osmolarity levels >290 mOsm/L) may be treated with various ADH preparations. Aqueous vasopressin is commonly used for short-term therapy, and desmopressin is useful for long-term control. Caution is advised when administering these drugs to patients with coronary artery disease or hypertension because of the arterial constrictive action of ADH. Desmopressin (5 to 10 mcg/day intranasally, or 0.5 to 1 mcg twice daily subcutaneously) is often a preferred agent because it has less pressor activity, a prolonged duration of action (6–24 hours), and enhanced antidiuretic properties.

Anesthetic Considerations

Preoperative assessment of the patient with DI includes careful appraisal of plasma electrolytes (especially serum sodium), renal function, and plasma osmolarity. Dehydration makes these patients especially sensitive to the hypotensive effects of anesthesia agents. Intravascular volume should slowly be restored preoperatively over a period of at least 24 to 48 hours.

Perioperative administration of vasopressin is usually not necessary in the patient with partial DI because the stress of surgery causes enhanced ADH release. A surgical patient with a total lack of ADH (complete DI) may be managed with desmopressin (1 mcg subcutaneously) or aqueous vasopressin (an IV bolus of 0.1 units followed by a continuous IV infusion of vasopressin at 0.1–0.2 units/hr). Plasma osmolarity, urine output, and serum sodium concentration should be measured hourly during surgery and in the immediate postoperative period. The surgical patient with DI receiving ADH replacement therapy should be monitored for ECG changes indicative of myocardial ischemia.

Isotonic fluids can generally be administered safely during the intraoperative period. If, however, the plasma osmolarity rises above 290 mOsm/L, hypotonic fluids should be considered and the vasopressin infusion increased above 0.2 units/h.

E. DIABETES MELLITUS

Definition

Diabetes mellitus is a complex metabolic derangement caused by relative or absolute insulin deficiency. Diabetes has been called "starvation in a sea of food." Glucose is present in abundance, but because of lack of insulin or insulin resistance, it is unable to reach cells for energy provision. Guidelines for diagnosing diabetes include a fasting plasma glucose (FPG) level of 126 mg/dL or greater or a random glucose level greater than 200 mg/dL. The FPG diagnostic level was reduced from a previous value of 140 mg/dL based on findings that patients with an FPG of 126 mg/dL are at risk for diabetes-related complications.

Pathophysiology

The incidence of diabetes has increased dramatically over the past 40 years. Today, it affects nearly 21 million people in the United States (almost 7% of our population). The rise can be attributed to a combination of three factors: (1) an overweight population, (2) more sedentary lifestyles, and

(3) a rise in the number of elderly persons. As more of our population advances in age into the decades in which most cases of diabetes occur, the impact of the disease will become even more alarming.

TYPE 1 DIABETES MELLITUS

About 5% to 10% of people with DM have *type 1 DM*. This type of DM was formerly known as *insulin-dependent diabetes* or *juvenile-onset diabetes*.

Individuals with type 1 DM have an absolute deficiency of insulin and are therefore entirely dependent on exogenous insulin therapy. In the absence of sufficient exogenous insulin, the disease course may be complicated by periods of ketosis and acidosis.

In most cases, type 1 DM is caused by an unusually vigorous autoimmune destruction of the β cells of the pancreatic islets. Environmental factors, such as infection or exposure to specific antigenic proteins, are cited as possible initiators of the immune assault. Patients with type 1 DM are also more likely to have other autoimmune diseases, such as thyroid disease or Addison's disease. A genetic predisposition for development of the disease also is involved. Type 1 DM usually develops before the age of 30 years, but it can develop at any age. The classic symptoms of type 1 DM appear only when at least 80% of the β cells are destroyed. The remaining β cells usually are eliminated inexorably over 2 or 3 years. In patients with type 1 DM, daily exogenous insulin therapy is essential for life. Some type 1 DM patients may be candidates for pancreatic transplant. The transplantation of isolated pancreatic islets has been plagued by graft survival and islet isolation setbacks, but it holds out promise for a future cure.

TYPE 2 DIABETES MELLITUS

About 90% to 95% of patients with diabetes have *type 2 DM*. Type 2 DM is characterized by impaired insulin secretion, peripheral insulin resistance (a decreased number of insulin receptors or an insulin receptor or postreceptor defect), and excessive hepatic glucose production. This form of diabetes was formerly known as *non–insulin-dependent diabetes* or *maturity-onset diabetes*.

Type 2 DM occurs in patients who have some degree of endogenous insulin production but who produce quantities insufficient for sustaining normal carbohydrate homeostasis. Insulin levels may be low, normal, or even elevated, but a *relative* insulin deficiency exists. The ultimate expression is a hyperglycemic state.

Typically, type 2 DM occurs in patients who are older than 30 years of age, obese (80%), and with a family history of the disease. Type 2 DM has an insidious onset; indeed, it is estimated that half of people who have type 2 DM are not even aware of it. The disease course is rarely associated with ketosis or acidosis, but it may be complicated by a nonketotic, hyperosmolar, hyperglycemic state.

Treatment for this class of diabetes consists primarily of oral hypoglycemic agents, exercise, and diet therapy. Weight reduction in the obese diabetic patient improves tissue responsiveness to endogenous insulin and often restores normoglycemia.

The distinction between *insulin-treated* DM and *insulin-dependent* DM is important. Some people with type 2 DM may benefit from exogenously administered insulin, especially during times of illness or stress. Those with type 1 DM, on the other hand, are insulin dependent and require exogenous insulin daily to live.

DIABETES ASSOCIATED WITH OTHER CONDITIONS

Diabetes may result from other conditions such as pancreatectomy, cystic fibrosis, or severe pancreatitis. Certain endocrine conditions, including Cushing's syndrome, glucagonoma, pheochromocytoma, and acromegaly, may also be associated with a diabetic condition. Steroid-induced diabetes may occur in the patient taking supraphysiologic doses of glucocorticoids. Gestational diabetes occurs in approximately 4% of the pregnancies in the United States. Women who have had gestational DM have a 20% to 50% chance of developing type 2 DM 5 to 10 years postpartum.

Long-Term Diabetic Complications

Diabetics are subject to long-term complications that confer substantial morbidity and premature mortality. These complications include extensive arterial disease, cataracts, sensory and motor neuropathy, infection, and autonomic nervous system dysfunction.

Arterial thrombotic lesions in the diabetic population are widely distributed in the extremities, kidneys, eyes, skeletal muscle, myocardium, and nervous system. As a result of these diffuse lesions, diabetes carries a serious risk for the development of microvascular (nephropathy, retinopathy, neuropathy) and macrovascular (atherosclerosis, stroke, coronary artery disease) complications.

Treatment

Treatment includes a diabetic diet, oral hypoglycemic drugs, and exogenous insulin. Non–insulin-dependent diabetes mellitus (NIDDM) is prevented primarily by avoidance or treatment of obesity. Transplantation of pancreatic tissue may be considered in selected patients.

Anesthetic Considerations

Diabetes mellitus is the most common endocrine disorder encountered in surgical patients. Long-standing DM predisposes patients to many diseases that require surgical intervention. Cataract extraction, kidney transplantation, ulcer débridement, and vascular repair are some of the operations frequently performed on patients with DM.

Patients with DM have higher morbidity and mortality rates in the perioperative period compared with nondiabetic patients of similar age. Increased complications are not caused by the disease itself but primarily because of organ damage associated with long-term disease. Ischemic heart disease is the most common cause of perioperative mortality in the patients with DM.

For patients with DM, operations should be scheduled early in the day if possible to minimize disruptions in treatment and nutrition regimens. Day stay for minor surgery may be used for patients with well-controlled DM who are knowledgeable about their disease and treatment and who have proper home support.

Preoperative Considerations

Patients with DM may come to the operating room with a spectrum of metabolic aberrations and end-organ complications that warrant careful preanesthetic assessment.

Cardiovascular complications account for most of the surgical deaths in patients with DM. The presence of hypertension, coronary artery disease, or autonomic nervous system dysfunctions can result in a labile cardiovascular course during anesthesia. It is essential that the cardiovascular and volume status of the patient be thoroughly evaluated before surgery.

Preoperative ECG is necessary for all adult patients with DM because of the high incidence of cardiac disease.

Autonomic nervous system dysfunction may result in delayed gastric emptying. It is estimated that gastroparesis occurs in 20% to 30% of all patients with DM. These patients are prone to aspiration, nausea and vomiting, and abdominal distention. Many authorities recommend routine preoperative aspiration prophylaxis with histamine (H_2) receptor blockers, metoclopramide, or preinduction antacids for patients with DM. Intubation during general anesthesia is a logical choice for patients with gastroparesis.

Patients with significant autonomic neuropathy may have an impaired respiratory response to hypoxia. These patients are especially sensitive to the respiratory-depressant effects of sedatives and anesthetics and require particular vigilance in the perioperative period.

Peripheral neuropathies (paresthesias, numbness in the hands and feet) should be adequately documented in the preanesthetic evaluation. Their presence may affect the decision to use regional anesthesia.

An estimated 30% to 40% of patients with insulin-dependent diabetes mellitus (IDDM) demonstrate restricted joint mobility. Limited motion of the atlanto-occipital joint can make endotracheal intubation difficult. Demonstration of the "prayer sign," an inability to approximate the palms of the hands and fingers, may help identify patients with tissue protein glycosylation and potentially difficult airways.

Evidence of kidney disease should be sought, and basic tests of renal function (urinalysis, serum creatinine, blood urea nitrogen) should be performed preoperatively. The presence of renal impairment may influence the choice and dosage of anesthetic agents. The use of potentially nephrotoxic drugs should be avoided.

The anesthetist should examine the patient's history of glycemic control to ensure preoperative optimization of the patient's metabolic state. A recommended target blood glucose range for the perioperative period is 80 to 180 mg/dL.

Sustained hyperglycemia, which causes osmotic diuresis, should alert the anesthetist to possible fluid deficits and electrolyte depletion. Preoperative levels of electrolytes should be determined for all patients with DM, and adequate hydration and a good urine output should be maintained. Lactate-containing solutions are generally avoided because lactate conversion to glucose may contribute to hyperglycemia. An important part of the preoperative evaluation is a review of oral hypoglycemic and insulin regimens.

Oral Hypoglycemic Agents

Oral Glucose-Lowering Agents

Oral glucose-lowering agents and insulin are used as adjuncts to diet therapy and exercise for treating patients with type 2 DM. Currently available oral hypoglycemic agents fall into the following classifications: (1) sulfonylureas, (2) α-glucosidase inhibitors, (3) thiazolidinediones, (4) biguanides, (5) nonsulfonylurea secretagogues, and (6) others. Often, patients take a combination of therapeutic agents. The commonly used medications used to treat type 2 diabetes are listed in the following table.

Oral Agents Available for Treatment of Diabetes Mellitus

Agent	Examples	Mechanism	Action	↓ Hemoglobin A_{1c} (%)	Advantages	Disadvantages	Cost
Sulfonylureas	*First generation:* Chlorpropamide Tolazamide Tolbutamide *Second generation:* Glyburide Glipizide Glimepiride	Closes K_{ATP} channels	↑ Pancreatic insulin secretion	1–2	↓ Microvascular risk Convenience	Hypoglycemia Weight gain May blunt myocardial ischemic preconditioning ? β-cell "exhaustion"	$
Glinides	Repaglinide Nateglinide	Closes K_{ATP} channels	↑ Pancreatic insulin secretion	1–1.5	More physiologic ↓ Postprandial glucose	Hypoglycemia, weight gain May blunt myocardial ischemic preconditioning ? β-cell "exhaustion" Dosing frequency	$$$
Biguanides	Metformin	Activates AMPK	↓ Hepatic glucose production	1–2	Weight loss or weight neutrality No hypoglycemia ↓ CVD	Diarrhea, abdominal cramping Lactic acidosis risk (rare) Vitamin B_{12} deficiency Multiple contraindications to consider (e.g., CKD)	$

?, could happen.

Continued

Oral Agents Available for Treatment of Diabetes Mellitus—cont'd

Agent	Examples	Mechanism	Action	↓ In Hemoglobin A_{1c} (%)	Advantages	Disadvantages	Cost
Thiazolidinediones	Rosiglitazone Pioglitazone	Activates PPAR-γ	↑ Peripheral insulin sensitivity	0.5–1.5	No hypoglycemia βcell preservation ↑ HDL-C ↓ Triglycerides ? ↓ CVD (pioglitazone)	Weight gain Edema/heart failure ↑ Bone fractures (women) ↑ LDL-C ? ↑ CVD (rosiglitazone)	$$$
α-Glucosidase inhibitors	Acarbose Miglitol	Block SB α-glucosidase	↓ Intestinal carbohydrate absorption	0.5–1	? ↓ CVD Nonsystemic medication ↓ Postprandial glucose	Gas, abdominal bloating Dosing frequency	$$
GLP-1 receptor agonists	Exenatide Liraglutide	Activates GLP-1 receptors	↑ Insulin secretion ↓ Glucagon secretion Slows gastric emptying ↑ Satiety	1	Weight loss ? β-cell preservation ? Cardiovascular benefits	Nausea/vomiting ? Pancreatitis ? C-cell hyperplasia or tumors Injectable	$$$
Amylin mimetics	Pramlintide	Activates amylin receptors	↓ Glucagon secretion Slows gastric emptying ↑ Satiety	0.5	Weight loss ↓ Postprandial glucose	Nausea or vomiting Dosing frequency Injectable	$$$

DPP-4 inhibitors	Sitagliptin Saxagliptin	Inhibits DPP-4, ↑ endogenous incretins	↑ Insulin secretion ↓ Glucagon secretion	0.5–0.8	No hypoglycemia	? Urticaria or angioedema ? Pancreatitis	$$$
Bile acid sequestrants	Colesevelam	Binds bile acid cholesterol	Unknown	0.5	No hypoglycemia ↓ LDL-C	Constipation ↑ Triglycerides	$$$
D2 agonists	Bromocriptine	Activates dopaminergic receptors	Alters hypothalamic regulation of metabolism ↑ Insulin sensitivity	0.5	No hypoglycemia	Dizziness or syncope Nausea Fatigue Rhinitis	?

AMPK, Adenosine monophosphate–activated protein kinase; *ATP,* adenosine triphosphate; *CKD,* chronic kidney disease; *CVD,* cardiovascular disease; *D2,* dopamine-2; *DPP,* dipeptidyl peptidase; *GLP,* glucagon-like peptide; *HDL-C,* high-density lipoprotein cholesterol; *LDL-C,* low-density lipoprotein cholesterol; *PPAR,* peroxisome proliferator–activated receptor; *SB,* small bowel.

From Inzucchi SE, Sherwin RS. Type 2 diabetes mellitus. In Goldman L, Schafer AI, et al, eds. *Goldman's Cecil Medicine.* 24th ed. Philadelphia: Saunders; 2012:1496.

Insulin Preparations

Insulin preparations are generated today by DNA recombinant technology, mimicking the amino acid sequence of human insulin. All insulin formulations in the United States, except for inhaled insulin, are prepared as Unit-100 (100 units/mL).

Insulin preparations differ in onset and duration after subcutaneous administration. In addition to subcutaneous injections, insulin delivery devices (implantable pumps, mechanical syringes) are used to facilitate exogenous administration. The greatest risk with all forms of insulin is hypoglycemia. The major classes of exogenous insulin (regular, rapid acting, inhaled, intermediate acting, and long acting) are listed in the following table.

Pharmacokinetics of Insulin Preparations

Insulin Type	Onset of Action	Peak Activity	Duration	Route
Regular insulin	30–60 min	1.5–2 hr	5–12 hr	IV, Subcut, IM
Humalin R, Novolin R				
Rapid acting	10–30 min	30–60 min	3–5 hr	Subcut
Aspart (Novolog)				
Lispro (Humalog)				
Glulisine (Apidra)				
Exubera (inhaled insulin)	10–20 min	30–90 min	6 hr	Inhalation
Intermediate acting	1–2 hr	4–8 hr	10–20 hr	Subcut
NPH (Humalin N, Novolin N)				
Lente (Humalin L)				
Long acting				
Ultralente	2–4 hr	8-20 hr	16–24 hr	Subcut
Glargine (Lantus)	1–2 hr	No peak	24 hr	Subcut
Detemir (Levemir)	1 hr	No peak	20 hr	Subcut

IM, Intramuscular; *IV,* intravenous; *NPH,* neutral protamine Hagedorn. *Subcut,* subcutaneous. Time course is based on subcutaneous administration.

It is imperative to know the surgical patient's normal insulin dosage regimen and treatment compliance. Some patients are on a fixed regimen that consists of a mixture of rapid- and intermediate-acting insulins taken before breakfast and again at the evening meal. Other patients are on multiple injection regimens designed to provide more physiologic glycemic control. To determine the effectiveness and compliance of antidiabetic therapy, hemoglobin A_{1c} (HbA_{1c} glycated hemoglobin) values provide information about the plasma glucose concentration over time. An HbA_{1c} value of 6.5% or greater is indicative of DM.

Intraoperative Management

In patients with DM, operations should be scheduled early in the day, if possible, to minimize disruptions in treatment and nutrition regimens. Surgery produces a catabolic stress response and elevates stress-induced counterregulatory hormones. The hyperglycemic, ketogenic, and lipolytic effects of the counterregulatory hormones in patients with DM compound the state of insulin deficiency. For this reason, perioperative hyperglycemia and other metabolic aberrations are common in the surgical patients with DM.

No specific anesthetic technique is superior overall for patients with DM. Both general anesthesia and regional anesthesia have been used safely. General anesthesia, however, has been shown to induce hormonal changes that accentuate glycogenolysis and gluconeogenesis, compounding the patient's hyperglycemic state. Regional anesthesia may produce less deleterious changes in glucose homeostasis.

The Certified Registered Nurse Anesthetist (CRNA) must be especially careful in positioning and padding patients with DM on the operating table. Decreased tissue perfusion and peripheral sympathetic neuropathy may contribute to the development of skin breakdown and ulceration.

Patients with DM represent a heterogeneous group requiring individualized perioperative care. The specific approach to metabolic management depends on the type of diabetes (type 1 or 2), the history of glycemic control, and the type of surgery being performed. Frequent blood glucose determinations are an integral part of any diabetic management technique. A glucose meter or other accurate and rapid means of monitoring blood glucose levels should be available. At least hourly intraoperative blood glucose measurement is the prudent course for brittle patients with DM, during long surgical procedures, and for major surgery.

Strict control of even short-term elevations in blood glucose improves perioperative morbidity. Persistent hyperglycemia has been shown to impair wound healing and wound strength. In addition, reports suggest that postoperative infection is more prevalent in patients with DM who have uncontrolled blood sugar levels. Studies also provide evidence that hyperglycemia worsens the neurologic outcome after ischemic brain injury. Avoiding perioperative hyperglycemia is advisable, especially in patients at risk for acute neurologic insult (carotid endarterectomy, intracranial surgery, cardiopulmonary bypass).

Various regimens have been tendered on how to best manage the metabolic changes that occur in surgical patients who have DM. Experts differ on optimal protocols for case management and precisely defined target glucose levels. Current debate centers on the risk-to-benefit ratio of intensive or "tight" blood glucose control versus "nontight" control during surgery. The universal goal with all techniques is to avoid hypoglycemia and to minimize metabolic derangements. Patients under anesthesia are generally maintained with a mild transient hyperglycemia to avoid the potentially catastrophic effects of hypoglycemia. Frequent blood glucose determinations during surgery and in the immediate postoperative period are central to safe practice.

Three different approaches to the metabolic management of adult surgical patients with DM are described below; however, readers should note that there are numerous variations.

Intermediate-Acting Insulin Use

This is a traditional method of managing surgical patients with DM and involves less intensive control of plasma glucose but aims to avoid marked hyperglycemia and dangerous hypoglycemia. Variations of this technique are used for stable patients with DM undergoing elective operative procedures. An example of this regimen follows:

1. On the morning of surgery, fasting blood sugar level is measured.
2. An IV infusion containing 5% dextrose is started at 100 to150 mL/hr.
3. After the IV infusion is started, half of the patient's normal morning intermediate or long-acting insulin dose is administered subcutaneously.

4. The glucose-containing IV infusion is continued throughout surgery. Additional fluid requirements are met with the administration of a second, glucose-free infusate.
5. Blood glucose levels are checked every 1 to 2 hours during surgery.
6. If the blood glucose level exceeds an established maximum level, commonly 180 mg/dL, regular insulin is administered according to an established "sliding scale." Insulin sensitivity varies markedly from one patient to the next, but on the average, 1 unit of regular insulin can be expected to decrease the blood glucose level 40 to 50 mg/dL.

This time-tested regimen is easy to implement, and it is usually successful in preventing significant hypo- and hyperglycemia.

The disadvantages of nontight control are as follows:

1. Absorption of preoperatively administered subcutaneous insulin is unpredictable and erratic in surgical patients because of blood pressure, blood flow, and temperature variations that occur with anesthesia.
2. The onset and the peak effect of the preoperative intermediate-acting insulin may not correspond to the time of surgical stress, especially if the operation is delayed or prolonged.
3. The half-life of regular insulin is short, and a "rollercoaster" glucose profile may occur. Plasma glucose levels will vary considerably.

Insulin Infusion

An insulin infusion management technique may be used to maintain the blood glucose concentration within relatively narrow boundaries. Intensive perioperative regulation of blood glucose prevents hyperglycemia, but it carries the risk of hypoglycemia and therefore necessitates more frequent blood glucose assays. Regular insulin infusion may range from 0.5 to 5 units/hr depending on the clinical situation and insulin resistance.

Intraoperative insulin infusion may be considered for patients with type 1 DM having major or prolonged surgery, the poorly controlled DM patients, pregnant DM patients, DM patients undergoing coronary artery bypass grafting, and DM patients with serious concurrent illness. An example of this regimen follows:

1. On the morning of surgery, a fasting blood glucose level is measured.
2. An infusion of 5% dextrose is started at a rate of 100 to 150 mL/hr.
3. A regular insulin infusion is begun, piggybacked to the glucose infusion. The insulin infusion rate is set at: insulin (units/hr) = last plasma glucose (mg/dL) ÷ 150. (If the patient is obese, has an infection, or is taking corticosteroids, the divisor is changed to 100.)
4. Blood glucose levels are measured every hour during insulin infusion, and potassium levels are checked after the first hour of the infusion.
5. Additional fluid requirements are met with the administration of a second, glucose-free infusate.

Blood glucose levels less than 80 mg/dL may be treated with $D_{50}W$ and remeasured in 30 minutes. In a 70-kg patient, 15 mL of $D_{50}W$ can be expected to raise the blood glucose concentration by about 30 mg/dL. Surgical patients undergoing renal transplantation or coronary artery bypass graft procedures, obese and septic patients, and patients on steroid therapy usually have higher insulin infusion requirements.

The advantages of tight glucose management in the perioperative period are as follows:

1. The insulin infusion can be finely regulated to correspond to hourly variations in blood glucose levels.

2. Periods of hyperglycemia are less likely. The deleterious effects of hyperglycemia (hyperosmolarity, osmotic diuresis, impaired wound healing, infection) may be prevented.
3. The insulin–glucose infusion can be continued into the postoperative period until the patient is ready to eat, at which time subcutaneous insulin or an oral hypoglycemic agent can be reinstated.

Type 2 Diabetes and Oral Hypoglycemic Agents

Patients treated with oral hypoglycemic agents demand the same individualized perioperative management as those with type 1 DM. The duration of action of the patient's oral agent must be noted. Discontinuing long-acting agents 2 to 3 days before surgery and converting to shorter acting agents or insulin affords better perioperative glucose control. Metformin should be discontinued 2 to 7 days or more before surgery because the surgical risks of hypotension and renal hypoperfusion place patients on this drug at increased risk for lactic acidosis. It is also discontinued before computed tomography (CT) scanning when contrast dye is administered.

For well-controlled surgical patients with type 2 DM who are scheduled for minor to moderate surgery, the patient's oral hypoglycemic agent may be continued until the evening before surgery. Glucose-containing fluids may be administered intraoperatively to protect against possible residual effects of oral hypoglycemic agents. Other experts adhere to a "no glucose, no insulin" technique for well-controlled type 2 DM patients. Regardless of the technique chosen, plasma glucose should be measured regularly throughout the procedure, and hyperglycemia should be treated with insulin on a "sliding scale."

ACUTE DERANGEMENTS IN GLUCOSE HOMEOSTASIS

Hypoglycemia

Hypoglycemia is encountered more frequently in patients with DM than in healthy adults, and it can develop insidiously during the perioperative period. Medications (insulin, sulfonylureas, β-adrenergic receptor blocking agents) and toxins (ethanol) are common causes of hypoglycemia. Severe liver disease (impaired hepatic glucose output), the altered physiology associated with gastric bypass surgery, sepsis, or an insulin-secreting tumor of the islets of Langerhans (an insulinoma) are conditions that are often complicated by hypoglycemia.

The blood glucose concentration at which signs and symptoms of hypoglycemia appear varies widely from one person to the next, but blood glucose levels in the range of 45 to 50 mg/dL commonly produce mild symptoms in otherwise healthy patients. Because the brain is the predominant organ of glucose consumption, it is most sensitive to glucose deprivation. Manifestations of impaired cerebral function (confusion, dizziness, headache, weakness) are associated with lack of glucose. As the blood sugar level declines below 50 mg/dL, aberrant behavior, seizures, and loss of consciousness may occur. Other signs of hypoglycemia (tachycardia, diaphoresis, anxiety, tremors, piloerection, pupillary dilation, and vasoconstriction) reflect sympathetic-adrenal hyperactivity. Acute treatment for hypoglycemic surgical patients is the IV administration of 25 to 50 mL of 50% dextrose followed by a continuous infusion of 5% dextrose. Unless prompt glucose therapy is provided, irreversible brain damage may result.

Hypoglycemia is potentially catastrophic during surgery because most of the neural indications of glucose lack are masked by general anesthesia. Signs of sympathetic adrenal discharge may also be blunted by general anesthesia or severe diabetic autonomic neuropathy, making the diagnosis of hypoglycemia extremely difficult. β-Adrenergic receptor blocking agents can reduce the hyperglycemic effects of epinephrine in addition to diminishing the symptomatic warning signs of hypoglycemia. Frequent blood glucose determinations, maintenance of mild hyperglycemia, and diligent monitoring help to avoid this serious complication during anesthesia.

Diabetic Ketoacidosis

Diabetic ketoacidosis (DKA) is a medical emergency triggered by a hyperglycemic event, usually in a patient with type 1 DM. Treatment errors, critical illnesses (myocardial infarction, trauma, cerebrovascular accident, burns), and infections are common precipitants of DKA.

Stressful events stimulate the release of hyperglycemic counterregulatory hormones (glucagon, GH, epinephrine, cortisol). People with IDDM are unable to secrete insulin to counterbalance the serum elevations of glucose, free fatty acids, and ketone bodies produced by these stress-induced hormones. Unless exogenous insulin is provided, the glycemic event may progress to severe ketoacidosis, dehydration, and acute metabolic decompensation.

Diabetic ketoacidosis usually develops over 24 hours. Major signs and symptoms include hyperglycemia, volume depletion (average fluid deficit, 5 L), tachycardia, metabolic acidosis, a calculated anion gap greater than 10, electrolyte depletion, hyperosmolarity (>300 mOsm/L), nausea and vomiting, abdominal pain, and lethargy. Blood levels of ketone bodies are elevated, and the patient's breath may have a fruity odor from excess acetone production. The respiratory center is typically stimulated by the low plasma pH, resulting in rapid, deep breathing (*Kussmaul respiration*). Acidosis, hyperosmolarity, and dehydration may depress consciousness to the point of coma.

Gangrene and infection of an ischemic lower extremity are common surgical conditions associated with DKA. Preoperative management of surgical patients with DKA requires an aggressive approach to restore intravascular volume, correct electrolyte abnormalities, improve acid–base balance, and reduce blood glucose levels with IV insulin. The airway must be protected in the obtunded patient. After the surgical problem that initiated DKA has resolved, medical management often is more effective.

Hyperglycemic Hyperosmolar State

Hyperglycemic hyperosmolar state (HHS) is a life-threatening hyperosmolar condition triggered by a hyperglycemic event. This syndrome commonly occurs in elderly patients with type 2 DM, but it also develops in patients with no history of DM. Patients generally have some endogenous insulin secretion, but the hyperglycemic episode overwhelms the pancreas and produces severe hyperglycemia and glucosuria. The amount of insulin secreted is usually sufficient to prevent lipolysis and ketone production. Therefore, unlike DKA, this syndrome usually is not associated with acidosis or significant ketogenesis. The common features of DKA and HHS can be found on page 77.

Features of Diabetic Ketoacidosis and Hyperglycemic Hyperosmolar Syndrome

	Diabetic Ketoacidosis	Hyperglycemic Hyperosmolar Syndrome
Plasma glucose (mg/dL)	>250	>600
pH	<7.3	>7.3
Serum bicarbonate (mmol/L)	<18	>15
Serum osmolarity	+	++
Ketonemia	++	Normal or slight +
Mental obtundation	Variable	Present
Hypovolemia	Present	Present

+, Increase; ++, large increase.

Common precipitating factors of HHS include infection, sepsis, pneumonia, stroke, and myocardial infarction. A spectrum of symptoms is associated with HHS, culminating in mental confusion, lethargy, and coma. Profound dehydration is present, resulting in hypotension and tachycardia. Laboratory evaluation may reveal a biochemical profile of marked hyperglycemia, normal arterial pH, absent or minimal ketonemia, and hyperosmolarity (>330 mOsm/L). Despite depleted total body potassium stores, the serum potassium levels at presentation may be normal or elevated because of acidosis and insulin lack.

Even with appropriate treatment, the mortality figures for HHS are substantially higher (15%) than those for DKA (<5%), partly because HHS commonly affects an older population group often with accompanying comorbidities.

Treatment goals are similar to those for DKA and include identification and management of the precipitating problem, vigorous isotonic rehydration (average total body water deficit, 9 L), correction of hyperglycemia, and electrolyte replacement. The hazards inherent in aggressive fluid administration in elderly patients dictate central hemodynamic monitoring during treatment.

F. HYPERALDOSTERONISM

Definition

Conn's syndrome, the most common form of *primary aldosteronism,* results from hypersecretion of aldosterone from an adrenal adenoma independent of stimulus.

Pathophysiology

Primary aldosteronism may also be caused by adrenocortical hyperplasia or rarely carcinoma. An increase in the plasma concentration of aldosterone and an increase in the urinary excretion of potassium with coexisting hypokalemia are pathognomonic of hyperaldosteronism.

Manifestations of the syndrome reflect the exaggerated effects of aldosterone. Diastolic hypertension and hypernatremia are usually present. Aldosterone's action of promoting renal excretion of K^+ (or H^+) in exchange for Na^+ results in hypokalemic metabolic alkalosis. Hypertension associated with Conn's syndrome results from aldosterone-induced sodium retention and subsequent increase in extracellular fluid volume. Primary aldosteronism accounts for approximately 1% of all cases of hypertension.

Primary aldosteronism is associated with low renin levels, a result of the elevated blood pressure's negative feedback to the juxtaglomerular cells. With *secondary hyperaldosteronism,* the stimulus of excess aldosterone resides outside of the adrenal gland and is often associated with an increase in circulating renin levels.

Diagnostic and Laboratory Findings

Diagnosis of hyperaldosteronism is confirmed by increased plasma concentration of aldosterone and increased urinary potassium excretion (>30 mEq/L) despite coexisting hypokalemia. Measurement of plasma renin activity permits classification of the disease as primary (low renin activity) or secondary (increased renin activity).

Treatment

Treatment of primary aldosteronism involves surgical removal of the adenoma or medical management. Surgical intervention is more successful for primary aldosteronism caused by adrenocortical adenoma than for gland hyperplasia because adenomas are almost always unilateral. When the affected adrenal gland is removed, the patient is cured in most cases. For patients with adrenal hyperplasia, medical management has been used successfully to treat primary aldosteronism.

Anesthetic Considerations

Preoperative management of the patient with Conn's syndrome includes correcting electrolyte and blood glucose levels and managing hypertension. Potassium should be replaced slowly to allow for equilibration of intracellular and extracellular potassium stores. Hypokalemia may alter nondepolarizing muscle relaxant responses, making peripheral nerve stimulation monitoring especially valuable. ECG signs of potassium depletion include prominent U waves and arrhythmias. Plasma electrolyte concentrations and acid–base status should be checked often during the perioperative period. Inadvertent hyperventilation may further decrease plasma potassium concentration.

Hypertension may be controlled preoperatively with sodium restriction and aldosterone antagonists such as spironolactone. Spironolactone, 25 to 100 mg every 8 hours, slowly increases potassium levels by inhibiting the action of aldosterone on the distal convoluted tubule. Patients with primary aldosteronism have a higher incidence of left ventricular hypertrophy, albuminuria, and stroke than patients with essential hypertension. Measurement of cardiac filling pressures may be needed to assess fluid volume status in the perioperative period.

Laparoscopic adrenalectomy is currently advocated as the operation of choice for surgically remediable mineralocorticoid excess. Compared with open laparotomy, patients who undergo laparoscopic adrenalectomy have similar improvement in blood pressure control and correction of hypokalemia.

G. HYPOALDOSTERONISM

Definition

Hypoaldosteronism causes hyperkalemia in the absence of renal insufficiency. Isolated deficiency of aldosterone secretion may reflect congenital deficiency of aldosterone synthetase or hyporeninemia resulting from a defect in the juxtaglomerular apparatus or treatment with an angiotensin-converting enzyme inhibitor, leading to loss of angiotensin stimulation.

Pathophysiology

Hyporeninemic hypoaldosteronism typically occurs in patients older than 45 years with chronic renal disease, DM, or both. Indomethacin-induced prostaglandin deficiency is a reversible cause of this syndrome.

Clinical Manifestations

Symptoms include heart block secondary to hyperkalemia and postural hypotension with or without hyponatremia. Hyperchloremic metabolic acidosis is common.

Treatment

Treatment of hypoaldosteronism includes liberal sodium intake and daily administration of hydrocortisone.

Anesthetic Considerations

Begin anesthetic management with preoperative monitoring of the serum potassium level, which should be less than 5.5 mEq/L before elective surgery. ECG monitoring for effects of hyperkalemia (tall, tentlike T waves; heart block) is recommended. Hypoventilation should be avoided to prevent an additional increase in serum potassium. Succinylcholine should be avoided when possible to prevent potassium release. IV fluids should be free of potassium. If hypovolemia is suspected, fluid replacement should be initiated, possibly governed by invasive (i.e., central venous pressure) monitoring.

H. HYPERPARATHYROIDISM

Definition and Incidence

Primary hyperparathyroidism is characterized and diagnosed by the presence of elevated serum parathyroid hormone (PTH) levels despite high serum calcium levels. The incidence of primary hyperparathyroidism in the United States is approximately 0.1% to 0.5%, with a higher occurrence in females and elderly adults. Stimulation of the parathyroid gland during pregnancy or lactation, prior neck irradiation, and a family history of parathyroid disease are predisposing etiologic factors.

Pathophysiology

Primary hyperparathyroidism may result from a parathyroid adenoma, gland hyperplasia, or parathyroid cancer. In approximately 80% of cases, primary hyperparathyroidism is caused by hypersecretion of a single parathyroid adenoma. Hyperplasia of one or more parathyroid glands accounts for about 15% of the cases. Carcinoma of the parathyroid gland is found in fewer than 1% of patients and is associated with particularly high serum calcium levels. Hereditary hyperparathyroidism may exist as part of a multiple endocrine neoplasia (MEN type 1, MEN type 2A).

Clinical Manifestations

Sustained overactivity of the parathyroid glands is characterized by high serum calcium levels. Most patients remain asymptomatic until the total serum calcium level rises above 11.5 to 12 mg/dL. Severe hypercalcemia (>14 to 16 mg/dL) may be life threatening and demands immediate attention.

With the development of sensitive laboratory assays for calcium, more than half of patients today with hyperparathyroidism are asymptomatic at diagnosis. Sustained and high levels of PTH over time lead to exaggerated osteoclast activity in bone, resulting in diffuse osteopenia, subperiosteal erosions, and elevated extracellular calcium levels. As osteoblasts attempt to reconstruct the ravaged bone, they secrete large amounts of the enzyme *alkaline phosphatase.* A heightened serum alkaline phosphatase level, therefore, is a significant diagnostic feature of hyperparathyroidism. Despite an increased mobilization of phosphorus from bone, the serum phosphate concentration usually remains normal or low as a result of increased urinary excretion. The effect of hyperparathyroidism on bone becomes clinically apparent when osteoclastic absorption of bone overwhelms osteoblastic deposition. With severe and protracted disease, the weakened bones become filled with decalcified cavities, making them painful and susceptible to fracture. Because of early diagnosis, the destructive bone disease associated with hyperparathyroidism, *osteitis fibrosa cystica,* is rare today.

Many of the nonskeletal manifestations of primary hyperparathyroidism are related to the accompanying hypercalcemia. Sustained hypercalcemia may produce calcifications and other deleterious effects in the pancreas (pancreatitis), kidneys (nephrolithiasis, nephrocalcinosis, polyuria), blood vessels (hypertension), heart (shortened ventricular refractory period, bradyarrhythmias, bundle branch block, heart block), and acid-producing areas of the stomach (peptic ulcer). The mnemonic "stones, bones, and groans" summarizes the renal, skeletal, and gastrointestinal features of advanced hyperparathyroidism. Profound muscle weakness, confusion, nausea, vomiting, and lethargy are additional features of the disorder.

Secondary hyperparathyroidism develops in patients with chronically low levels of serum calcium, such as those with chronic renal failure and gastrointestinal malabsorption. A compensatory parathyroid response develops in response to the hypocalcemia. Their clinical course is marked by the same PTH-mediated skeletal assault seen in the primary form of the disorder, but because it is an adaptive response, secondary hyperparathyroidism is seldom associated with hypercalcemia.

Anesthetic Considerations

The usual treatment for symptomatic primary hyperparathyroidism is surgical removal of abnormal parathyroid tissue. Surgical treatment for asymptomatic hyperparathyroidism is more controversial. Parathyroidectomy may be performed with the patient under general anesthesia, although minimally invasive neck surgery using cervical plexus block anesthesia is increasingly utilized, especially for excision of a single adenoma.

Parathyroid tissue resembles brown fat, and this can occasionally make it difficult for the surgeon to locate. Furthermore, parathyroid tissue is sometimes footloose and can be found in such ectopic places as the deep recesses of the mediastinum, the carotid sheath, or the thymus gland. Some surgeons use periodic intraoperative determinations of serum PTH and ionized calcium levels to help guide surgical resection.

Blood loss from parathyroid surgery is usually minimal, and advanced monitoring is not required based on the surgical procedure. Serum calcium, magnesium, and phosphorous levels should be monitored in the postoperative period until stable. In most cases, serum calcium levels start to decline within 24 hours and return to normal within 3 to 4 days after successful surgery.

With current methods of detection, most patients with hyperparathyroidism are asymptomatic; however, erosive effects of elevated PTH on bone and the systemic effects of chronic hypercalcemia should be considered in the anesthetic plan for patients with severe untreated disease.

Severe or symptomatic hypercalcemia (>14–16 mg/dL) is treated aggressively. Isotonic saline hydration and loop diuretics (Lasix, 40–80 mg) can rapidly decrease serum calcium levels by hemodilution, increased glomerular filtration, and enhanced excretion. Less frequently, corticosteroids or drugs that inhibit osteoclastic bone resorption (bisphosphonates, pamidronate, plicamycin, calcitonin) are used.

Patients with hypercalcemia may be dehydrated because of anorexia, vomiting, and the impaired ability of the kidneys to concentrate urine. In these patients, hydration with non–calcium-containing solutions should be maintained throughout the perioperative period to dilute serum calcium, maintain adequate glomerular filtration and calcium clearance, and ensure adequate intravascular volume. Vigorous hydration dictates the use of bladder catheterization, central venous pressure monitoring, and frequent determinations of serum electrolytes. Elevated calcium levels may depress the central and peripheral nervous systems. The use of preoperative sedatives in patients with hypercalcemia who appear lethargic or confused should be avoided. General anesthetic requirements may be decreased as well.

Careful review of the patient's renal status is especially crucial in patients with secondary hyperparathyroidism. Associated complications of renal impairment (volume overload, anemia, electrolyte derangements) may affect anesthetic medication dosages and selection.

Cardiac conduction disturbances such as a shortened QT interval and a prolonged PR interval are observed with hypercalcemia. Dysrhythmias and hypertension may respond to calcium channel antagonists (e.g., verapamil, 5–10 mg IV).

Awareness of the effects of pH on the ionized portion of plasma calcium is important. Alkalosis shifts the ionized calcium to the protein-bound form and decreases serum levels. The response to neuromuscular blockade may be unpredictable. Muscle weakness, hypotonia, and muscle atrophy may increase the patient's sensitivity to nondepolarizing skeletal muscle relaxants. Careful titration of muscle relaxants with use of a peripheral nerve stimulator is prudent.

Patients with clinically significant bone disease are susceptible to fractures, and care must be exercised in positioning and padding. These patients are prone to postoperative nausea and vomiting; therefore, prophylactic antiemetic medications are advisable.

I. HYPOPARATHYROIDISM

Definition

Hypoparathyroidism is a disorder characterized by inadequate secretion of PTH or a peripheral resistance to its effect. Patients with hypoparathyroidism typically have low serum calcium levels. The blood phosphate concentration may be elevated because of the decreased renal excretion of phosphate.

Pathophysiology

Inadvertent removal of parathyroid tissue, parathyroid gland injury from irradiation or autoimmune destruction, and chronic severe magnesium deficiency (alcohol abuse, poor nutrition, malabsorption) are possible causes of hypoparathyroidism.

Clinical Manifestations

Clinical signs of hypoparathyroidism reflect the degree of hypocalcemia and the rapidity of calcium decline. A sudden drop in ionized calcium usually produces more severe symptoms than a slow decline. Treatment of chronic hypoparathyroidism includes vitamin D and calcium supplementation.

The decreased serum calcium ion concentration accompanying hypoparathyroidism produces hyperexcitability of nerve and muscle cells by lowering the threshold potential of excitable membranes. Cardinal features of the neuromuscular excitability are muscle spasms and hypocalcemic tetany. Symptoms vary in severity and may take the form of muscle cramps, perioral paresthesias, numbness in the feet and toes, or hyperactive deep tendon reflexes. The patient may feel restless or hyperirritable. Life-threatening laryngeal muscle spasm may occur, producing stridor, labored respirations, and asphyxia.

Two classic manifestations of latent hypocalcemic tetany are the *Chvostek's sign* and *Trousseau's sign.* The Chvostek's sign is a contracture or twitching of ipsilateral facial muscles produced when the facial nerve is tapped at the angle of the jaw. The Trousseau's sign is elicited by the inflation of a blood pressure cuff slightly above the systolic level for a few minutes. The resultant ischemia enhances the muscle irritability in hypocalcemic states and causes flexion of the wrist and thumb with extension of the fingers (*carpopedal spasm*).

Anesthetic Considerations

Temporary hypocalcemia often is observed after successful parathyroid surgery for hyperparathyroidism. This may occur within a few hours to a few days after surgery. The transient postoperative hypocalcemia is the result of parathyroid gland suppression (by preoperative hypercalcemia) and rapid bone uptake of calcium ("hungry bone syndrome"). Inadvertent removal of all parathyroid gland tissue induces a substantial decline in the serum calcium concentration, from a normal level to 6 to 7 mg/dL. Even a small amount of remaining parathyroid tissue usually is capable of sufficient hypertrophy to preserve normal calcium–phosphate balance.

Meticulous observation for signs of musculoskeletal irritability and serial measurement of serum calcium, inorganic phosphate, magnesium, and PTH levels should be performed after parathyroid surgery. The threshold for the development of signs of hypocalcemia is variable; however, manifestations of neuromuscular compromise often are observed at serum calcium levels of 6 to 7 mg/dL.

Laryngeal muscles are especially sensitive to tetanic spasm, and laryngospasm may cause life-threatening airway compromise in patients with hypocalcemia. Respiratory distress after parathyroid surgery may be secondary to laryngeal muscle spasm, edema or bleeding in the neck, or bilateral recurrent laryngeal nerve injury. Unilateral recurrent laryngeal nerve injury produces hoarseness and usually requires only close observation. Bilateral recurrent laryngeal nerve injury causes aphonia and requires immediate airway support and intubation.

Hypocalcemia may be apparent on ECG tracings as a prolonged QT interval, reflecting delayed ventricular repolarization. The cardiac rhythm usually remains normal. Decreased cardiac contractility and hypotension may occur, and congestive heart failure, although rare, is a danger.

In addition to parathyroid surgery, circulating levels of ionized calcium can decline from other causes in the perioperative period. Precipitous increases in the circulating levels of anions such as bicarbonate, phosphate, and citrate lower ionized calcium levels. Hyperventilation, the rapid transfusion of citrated blood, or the rapid administration of bicarbonate may induce overt tetany in a previously asymptomatic patient with hypocalcemia. Vigorous diuresis can also augment calcium loss.

Patients with confirmed, symptomatic hypocalcemia require prompt therapy. Those with acute hypocalcemia may be treated with an initial IV bolus of 10 to 20 mL of 10% calcium gluconate administered over 10 minutes followed by 10 mL of 10% calcium gluconate in 500 mL solution over 6 hours. Calcium, magnesium, phosphate, potassium, and creatinine levels should be monitored diligently during calcium replacement. Chronic magnesium deficiency impairs the secretion of PTH and should be corrected.

Common clinical manifestations of hyperparathyroidism and hypoparathyroidism are listed in the table below.

Clinical Features of Hyperparathyroidism and Hypoparathyroidism

System	Hyperparathyroidism	Hypoparathyroidism
Cardiovascular	Hypertension, cardiac conduction disturbances, shortened QT interval	Prolonged QT interval, hypotension, decreased cardiac contractility
Musculoskeletal	Bone pain, pathologic fractures, muscle weakness, muscle atrophy	Neuromuscular excitability
Neurologic	Somnolence, cognitive impairment, depression, hypotonia	Tetany, paresthesias, numbness in fingers and toes, seizures
Gastrointestinal	Anorexia, nausea, vomiting, constipation, abdominal pain, pancreatitis, peptic ulcer	None significant
Renal	Tubular absorption defects, diminished renal function, kidney stones, polyuria	None significant

J. HYPERTHYROIDISM

Definition

Hyperthyroidism is defined as thyroid gland hyperactivity. *Thyrotoxicosis* is more specifically defined as a state of thyroid hormone excess. The most common cause of thyrotoxicosis in the United States is *Graves' disease*. Graves' disease is an autoimmune disease in which thyroid-stimulating hormone (TSH) receptor antibodies bind to and stimulate the thyroid gland, causing excessive production and secretion of thyroxine (T_4) and triiodothyronine (T_3). The immunoglobulin G (IgG) autoantibodies mimic the action of TSH, but their effects are longer, lasting up to 12 hours compared with 1 hour for normal TSH.

The aberrant immunologic response associated with Graves' disease targets primarily the thyroid gland but also other tissues, including extraocular muscles and skin. There is a familial tendency and a higher incidence of other autoimmune disorders in patients with Graves' disease. The disease occurs most often in women (prevalence, 1%–3% in women; 0.1% in men) and between 20 and 50 years of age. Graves' disease has an unpredictable course marked by relapses and exacerbations.

Pathophysiology

Thyrotoxicosis can also be caused by benign follicular adenomas, which are not believed to have an autoimmune etiology. Exogenous iodine excess (radiocontrast agents or angiography dye) or the administration of thyroid hormones may induce iatrogenic thyrotoxicosis. The antiarrhythmic agent amiodarone is iodine rich and may cause either hypothyroidism or hyperthyroidism. Toxic multinodular goiter, subacute viral thyroiditis, postpartum thyroiditis, TSH-secreting pituitary tumors, and thyroid cancer are less common causes of thyrotoxicosis.

Clinical Manifestations

Clinical manifestations associated with thyrotoxicosis reflect the widespread hypermetabolic effects of excess thyroid hormones. Physical signs include tachycardia, tremor, goiter, and muscle weakness. Sleep is often difficult. Weight loss despite increased food consumption, anxiety, fatigue, and heat intolerance are symptoms of thyrotoxicosis.

Signs of ophthalmopathy and dermopathy are associated with Graves' disease. Thyroid-associated ophthalmopathy may cause proptosis, eye redness, and a gritty sensation in early stages, with diplopia, ocular pain, and (rarely) loss of visual acuity in more advanced stages. Graves' ophthalmopathy results from cytokine-mediated inflammation and swelling of the periorbital connective tissue and extraocular muscles.

The blood volume increases slightly under the influence of excess thyroid hormone, a result of vasodilation. Mean arterial pressure usually remains unchanged, but the pulse pressure increases. The systolic blood pressure is typically elevated 10 to 15 mmHg, and the diastolic blood pressure is reduced. Blood flow to the skin increases because of the increased need for heat elimination.

The effects of thyrotoxicosis on the heart are pronounced. Palpitations, tachycardia, and cardiac dysrhythmias affect most patients. The cardiac output increases, sometimes to 60% or more above normal. About 10% of thyrotoxic patients have atrial fibrillation. Mitral valve prolapse is more common in patients with Graves' disease than in the general population. With protracted high thyroid hormone levels, the heart muscle strength may become depressed as a result of protein catabolism. Diagnosis of thyrotoxicosis is more difficult in elderly adults because many of the hyperkinetic manifestations of hyperthyroidism are absent. Elderly patients may initially present with myocardial failure. Hyperthyroid patients may feel a constant fatigue from the exhausting effect of thyroid hormone on the musculature and on the central nervous system.

Diagnosis

The diagnosis of primary disease is biochemically established in most cases by the combined findings of an abnormally high total and unbound serum T_3 and T_4 assay and depressed TSH levels. With Graves' disease, the diagnosis may be supported by the presence of stimulatory TSH receptor autoantibodies. An elevated uptake of radioactive iodine by the thyroid gland may be used to confirm gland hyperactivity. Serum alkaline phosphatase and calcium concentrations are mildly elevated in approximately 20% of patients with Graves' disease.

Other autoimmune diseases such as myasthenia gravis, rheumatoid arthritis, systemic lupus erythematosus, and DM are more common in patients with Graves' disease.

Treatment

A variety of treatment options are available for patients with Graves' disease. The three primary treatment options for thyrotoxicosis are radioactive gland ablation, surgery, and antithyroid drug therapy.

Radioactive Iodine

A common therapy for Graves' disease is ablation of the thyroid gland with radioactive iodine. A total of 2 to 4 months is needed to reverse the effects of hyperthyroidism. Hypothyroidism is common after treatment, and it is contraindicated in pregnancy.

Subtotal Thyroidectomy

Surgery for treatment of Graves' disease is an option when antithyroid drugs are ineffective, if radioiodine treatment is refused, in children or pregnant women, or if the thyroid goiter is exceptionally large. Patients should be treated preoperatively with antithyroid medication and rendered euthyroid before surgery. Complications associated with thyroid surgery occur in less than 1% of cases and include damage to the recurrent laryngeal nerve, hypoparathyroidism, and neck hematoma.

Antithyroid Drugs and β-Adrenergic Receptor Blockade

The main class of antithyroid medications are the *thionamides,* which include propylthiouracil (PTU), methimazole, and carbimazole. All thionamides inhibit thyroid hormone synthesis by interfering with the incorporation of iodine into tyrosine residues of thyroglobulin. PTU also inhibits conversion of T_4 to T_3. A euthyroid state is usually obtained in 6 to 7 weeks. Hepatitis and agranulocytosis are the most serious side effects of these drugs.

About 10 days before surgery, oral potassium iodide (SSKI, Lugol's solution) is added to the course of therapy to decrease gland vascularity and to block hormone synthesis and release. Propranolol is added to the antithyroid regimen to reduce cardiovascular symptoms and to inhibit the peripheral conversion of T_4 to T_3.

Anesthetic Considerations

Preoperative

The key to successful preoperative preparation of the hyperthyroid surgical patient is a careful assessment of the extent of thyrotoxicosis and the severity of end-organ manifestations. Thyrotoxicosis is associated with increased operative risk, and elective surgery should not proceed until the patient has been rendered euthyroid by medical management. Antithyroid medications should be continued through the morning of surgery.

Hyperthyroid patients have increased blood volume, decreased peripheral resistance, and a wide pulse pressure. The cardiac output, heart rate, and systolic blood pressure may be increased. Appropriate corrections of the patient's fluid volume and electrolyte status should be accomplished before surgery.

A careful preoperative evaluation of the airway is mandatory in all hyperthyroid patients undergoing surgery. Thyroid gland enlargement can cause tracheal deviation and tracheoesophageal compression. Hoarseness, sore throat, a feeling of pressure in the neck, coughing, or dyspnea suggests tracheal compression that can be caused by thyromegaly. Chest and airway radiographs and CT scans are useful to detect tracheal deviation and compression.

A patient with a large goiter and an obstructed airway poses the same challenge as any other patient in whom airway management is problematic. An awake fiberoptic intubation with topical anesthesia is of proven value under these conditions. Tracheomalacia weakens thyroid cartilage from chronic pressure, and its presence may necessitate a more prolonged intubation and vigilant observation after surgery.

Only life-threatening emergency surgery should be performed in an untreated symptomatic hyperthyroid patient. In an emergency situation, the otherwise healthy patient can be expeditiously prepared for surgery with the oral administration of potassium iodide (3–5 drops every 6 hours) and carefully titrated IV propranolol (1–10 mg) or esmolol (50–300 mcg/kg). Elderly patients who require emergency surgery and have rapid ventricular rates require central pressure monitoring to guide therapy.

Intraoperative

A major goal of perioperative management of hyperthyroid patients is prevention of sympathetic nervous system stimulation. This is accomplished by providing sufficient anesthetic depth and avoiding medications that stimulate the sympathetic nervous system.

A preoperative anxiolytic medication is generally warranted. Atropine should be avoided as an antisialagogue because of its vagolytic effects and its ability to impair sweating.

Induction of anesthesia may be achieved with a number of IV medications. Ketamine should be avoided because it can stimulate the sympathetic nervous system. If the airway is not compromised by an enlarged goiter, administration of a muscle relaxant can facilitate intubation of the trachea. Pancuronium should be avoided because it has the potential to increase the heart rate. Because of the increased incidence of myasthenia gravis and skeletal muscle weakness in hyperthyroid patients, precaution dictates careful titration of muscle relaxant doses with use of a peripheral nerve stimulator.

Isoflurane and sevoflurane are attractive choices for inhalation anesthetics because of their ability to offset sympathetic nervous system responses to surgical stimulation and because they do not sensitize the myocardium to catecholamines. Hyperthyroid patients do not generally require a higher minimum alveolar concentration (MAC) for inhalational anesthesia. The increased cardiac output accompanying hyperthyroidism may accelerate the uptake of an inhaled anesthetic, resulting in the need to increase the delivered concentration, and this may be perceived clinically as an increased anesthetic requirement.

Monitoring of the hyperthyroid patient should focus on early recognition of increased thyroid gland activity, suggesting the onset of thyroid storm. Core body temperature should be monitored closely. The ECG should be assessed for tachycardia or dysrhythmias. Hypotension occurring during surgery is better treated with direct-acting vasopressors than with indirect-acting vasoactive drugs that stimulate the release of catecholamines. Hypercarbia and hypoxia should be stringently avoided because they stimulate the sympathoadrenal axis.

Meticulous care of the eyes is required. The patient with proptosis is at risk for corneal exposure and damage, so special care should be taken to lubricate and protect the eyes perioperatively. The key anesthesia implications for patients with hyperthyroidism are listed below.

Anesthesia Implications for Patients with Hyperthyroidism

Ensure a euthyroid state before surgery.
Determine the extent of thyrotoxicosis and end-organ complications.
Evaluate the airway closely.
Avoid sympathetic nervous system activation and sympathomimetic drugs.
Titrate muscle relaxants carefully, considering possible myopathy and myasthenia gravis.
Position carefully (decreased bone density and predisposition to osteoporosis).
Monitor closely for early signs of thyroid storm.
Pad and protect the eyes.

THYROID STORM

A feared complication in hyperthyroid patients is *thyroid storm* or *thyrotoxic crisis*. Thyroid storm is a rare event that is caused by acute stress in the previously undiagnosed or incompletely treated hyperthyroid patient. Precipitating events may include trauma, surgery (especially thyroid surgery), the peripartum period, radioiodine treatment, acute illness, and infection.

Thyroid storm is a life-threatening medical emergency that represents a severe exacerbation of hyperthyroid signs and symptoms. The clinical manifestations may include marked tachycardia, hyperthermia, hypertension, atrial fibrillation, sweating, tremor, vomiting, weakness, agitation, shock, and congestive heart failure (see box below). Metabolic acidosis may be present secondary to increased lactate production from the overactive metabolism.

Clinical Manifestation of Thyroid Storm

Fever >38.5°C	Nausea and vomiting
Tachycardia	Hypertension
Confusion and agitation	Congestive heart failure
Dysrhythmias	Abnormal liver function test results

Similarities exist between the clinical features of thyroid storm and those of pheochromocytoma, neuroleptic malignant syndrome, light anesthesia, and malignant hyperthermia, making clinical diagnosis challenging in some cases.

Thyroid storm associated with surgery may occur anytime in the perioperative period but is more likely to occur 6 to 18 hours after surgery. Treatment must be initiated as soon as the diagnosis is made to prevent substantial morbidity and mortality. Mortality rates are as high as 30% even with early diagnosis and management. The high mortality rate associated with thyroid storm underscores the importance of achieving a euthyroid state before surgery.

Management of perioperative thyroid storm includes identifying and treating the precipitating cause, administering antithyroid medications, and providing hemodynamic support. Carefully titrated β-adrenergic receptor blockers, potassium iodide, and antithyroid drugs (PTU or methimazole) block thyroid hormone synthesis and adrenergic manifestations. Supplemental glucocorticoids should be administered because the turnover of endogenous steroids is accelerated by the hypermetabolism of thyrotoxicosis.

Supportive measures include IV hydration with glucose-containing crystalloid solutions, correction of electrolyte and acid base imbalances, and management of hyperthermia. Salicylates may displace T_4 from its carrier protein; therefore, acetaminophen is the recommended antipyretic for lowering body temperature. Adequate oxygenation is of paramount importance during thyroid storm. Vasoactive medications and advanced hemodynamic monitoring may be necessary to help manage the labile cardiovascular course.

Management of Thyroid Storm

Administer propylthiouracil, 200–400 mg PO or NGT every 4–6 hr.
Administer IV fluids.
Administer hydrocortisone100 mg IV every 8 hr.
Administer propranolol 10–80 mg PO every 6 hr or esmolol IV infusion.
Use cooling blankets and acetaminophen for hyperthermia.
Use digoxin for heart failure in the presence of atrial fibrillation with a rapid ventricular response.

IV, Intravenous; *NGT, nasogastic tube*; *PO,* oral.

K. HYPOTHYROIDISM

Definition and Incidence

Hypothyroidism is a state of thyroid gland hypofunction resulting in decreased circulating concentrations of thyroid hormones. Laboratory findings show decreased plasma T_3 and T_4 concentrations and increased TSH levels in patients with primary hypothyroid disease. The clinical spectrum of thyroid hormone deficiency can range from the asymptomatic patient with no overt physical findings to the classic myxedematous patient with profound symptoms. Hypothyroidism is the most common disorder of thyroid function, occurring in 5% to 10% of women and 0.5% to 2% of men.

Pathophysiology

Primary hypothyroidism accounts for 95% of all cases of hypothyroidism. An autoimmune-mediated destruction of the thyroid gland, known as *Hashimoto's thyroiditis,* is the most common form of hypothyroidism in the

United States. The disorder most often occurs in women of middle age and is associated with other autoimmune disorders such as myasthenia gravis and adrenal insufficiency.

Primary hypothyroidism may also be the result of severe iodine deficiency, previous thyroid surgery, neck irradiation, or treatment for hyperthyroidism (radioiodine therapy). The antiarrhythmic agent amiodarone is associated with hyper- and hypothyroidism. Lithium inhibits the release of thyroid hormone and causes hypothyroidism in some patients.

Rarely, secondary hypothyroidism is the result of pituitary or hypothalamic disorders. Secondary hypothyroidism is associated with decreased concentrations of both thyroid hormones and TSH. Regardless of the etiology, the clinical manifestations of hypothyroidism are similar.

Clinical Manifestations

Most cases of hypothyroidism are subclinical, with laboratory findings of increased plasma TSH but no overt signs. Patients with more significant disease develop signs and symptoms that reflect a slowed metabolism and impaired cellular functions. The thyroid gland usually is enlarged, nontender, and firm. Patients may have dry skin, cold intolerance, paresthesias, slow mental functioning, ataxia, a puffy face, and constipation. Lack of thyroid hormones causes the muscles to become sluggish. Patients with severe hypothyroidism may be hypersomnolent with a decreased ventilatory response to hypoxia and hypercarbia. The hair and nails frequently are brittle.

The accumulation of proteinaceous fluid in serous body cavities is a well-recognized feature of hypothyroidism. The most common sites of effusions associated with hypothyroidism are the pleural, pericardial, and peritoneal cavities. Inappropriate ADH secretion and impaired free water clearance can lead to hyponatremia. Accumulation of mucopolysaccharides and fluid imparts the characteristic edematous appearance, called *myxedema*.

Cardiovascular complications include sinus bradycardia, dysrhythmias, cardiomegaly, impaired contractility, congestive heart failure, and labile blood pressure. Symptoms of low exercise tolerance and shortness of breath with exertion may be partially the result of decreased cardiac function. Chronic vasoconstriction produces diastolic hypertension and decreases the intravascular fluid volume. The autonomic nervous system response is blunted, and there is a decrease in the sensitivity and number of β-receptors.

Overt hypothyroidism is associated with a number of abnormalities in lipid metabolism that may predispose patients to accelerated coronary artery disease. Hypothyroidism is associated with anemia and decreased erythrocyte production of 2,3-diphosphoglycerate, leading to a leftward shift of the oxyhemoglobin dissociation curve and decreased oxygen delivery to the tissues.

These "classic" clinical features of hypothyroidism are often lacking in elderly hypothyroid patients. In older patients, thyroid status may not always be predicted from clinical signs and symptoms, and diagnosing hypothyroidism is more difficult.

Treatment

Treatment of hypothyroidism requires replacement with thyroid hormone. The agent of choice is synthetic *levothyroxine sodium* (T_4) because of its long half-life (7 days) and its ability to attain physiologic levels of T_3. Replacement dosages range from 75 to 150 mcg/day, depending on the underlying autonomous thyroid function.

An area of particular concern during thyroid hormone replacement is the effect on the cardiovascular system. Initiation of thyroid hormone replacement in a patient with coexisting angina pectoris or underlying risk factors for coronary artery disease is potentially hazardous and requires careful monitoring of both cardiovascular and thyroid status. Myocardial oxygen consumption is augmented by thyroid hormone, and a hypothyroid patient with deficient coronary artery circulation may not tolerate full replacement doses.

Anesthetic Considerations

Patients with subclinical disease have an overall low risk of complications when undergoing anesthesia and surgery. These patients should receive a careful preoperative evaluation and preoperative continuation of levothyroxine therapy. Patients with severe hypothyroidism are predisposed to multiple complications with anesthesia. Depression of myocardial function, abnormal baroreceptor function, and reduction in plasma volume may be present. Slowed hepatic metabolism and renal clearance of injected drugs may prolong their effects, but MAC is not decreased significantly. Elective surgical procedures should be postponed in the presence of severe or symptomatic hypothyroidism to restore normal thyroid status.

All patients with hypothyroidism should undergo careful preoperative evaluation of the airway. A large goiter may cause airway compromise in the form of tracheal deviation or compression. In some patients with severe hypothyroidism, adequate air exchange may be compromised by an enlarged tongue and myxedematous infiltration of the vocal cords. Depression of the ventilatory responses to hypoxia and hypercarbia must be considered. Preoperative sedation should be avoided in patients with macroglossia or preexisting hypoventilation. The risk of pulmonary aspiration is increased because of associated somatic obesity and delayed gastric emptying.

Patients with hypothyroidism may respond to opioids with increased central nervous system and respiratory depression and to volatile agents with increased hypotension and myocardial depression. Although ketamine has been proposed as the ideal induction agent, even ketamine can produce cardiovascular depression in the absence of a robust sympathetic nervous system.

Intubation of the trachea may be facilitated by the administration of succinylcholine or a nondepolarizing muscle relaxant; however, hypothyroid patients may be more sensitive to standard doses of nondepolarizing muscle relaxants because of coexisting muscle weakness and decreased hepatic metabolism and renal elimination of these drugs. Maintaining muscle paralysis with minimal doses of muscle relaxants is an appropriate goal.

Supplemental perioperative cortisol should be considered in patients with symptomatic disease as a potential for adrenal insufficiency when stress exists. In hypothyroidism, the number of β-receptors is diminished, and responses to inotropic drugs and sympathetic stimulation may be influenced by the altered β-receptor pool.

Body temperature should be monitored closely in hypothyroid patients, and mechanisms for warming the patient should be used during surgery. The box on pg. 91 summarizes the anesthesia implications of hypothyroidism.

Anesthesia Implications for Patients with Hypothyroidism

Delay elective surgery for patients with severe symptomatic disease.
Evaluate the airway closely.
Monitor for exaggerated central nervous system depression with anesthetic agents.
Titrate muscle relaxants carefully considering possible coexisting muscle weakness.
Consider decreased hepatic metabolism and renal elimination when dosing medications.
Maintain normothermia.
Monitor ventilation closely considering blunted ventilatory response to hypercarbia and hypoxia.

MYXEDEMA COMA

Myxedema coma is a rare syndrome that reflects the end stage of untreated hypothyroidism. The presence of coma is a marker of the patient's clinical deterioration rather than a primary effect of hypothyroidism. A critical insult (infection, surgery, cerebrovascular accident, pneumonia, gastrointestinal bleeding, cold exposure) can precipitate myxedema coma in a patient with hypothyroidism.

Generally, the patient is elderly; has severe clinical features of hypothyroidism; and is hypothermic, hypoventilating, and hyponatremic. The response to hypoxia and hypercapnia is measurably decreased, and mechanical ventilation may be required. The patient is typically lethargic or stuporous. The skin often is pale as a result of cutaneous vasoconstriction. Myxedema coma is a medical emergency. Vigorous therapeutic attention should be paid to body temperature, shock, and ventilatory failure. Treatment consists of hemodynamic and ventilatory support and the IV administration of levothyroxine (300–500 mcg) with continuous ECG monitoring for myocardial ischemia. Supplemental cortisol is appropriate because myxedematous patients may have adrenal atrophy and decreased adrenal reserve. Because these patients may be vulnerable to water intoxication and hyponatremia, meticulous fluid replacement is important. Only lifesaving surgery should proceed in a patient with myxedema coma.

L. PHEOCHROMOCYTOMA

Definition

Pheochromocytomas are catecholamine-secreting tumors derived most commonly from adrenomedullary chromaffin cells. The tumors synthesize, store, and secrete catecholamines, mostly norepinephrine and epinephrine. Unlike a normal adrenal medulla, norepinephrine is the predominant catecholamine secreted by most of these tumors. In the majority of cases, however, it is impossible to predict the degree of catecholamine secretion from the clinical features. The tumors are not innervated, and neural stimulation does not stimulate hormone release.

The tumors are sometimes broadly defined as following the "rule of 10s." Pheochromocytomas involve both adrenal glands in 10% of adult patients with the tumor. Approximately 10% of the tumors arise from extraadrenal chromaffin cells. Approximately 10% of the tumors are in children. Malignant spread of pheochromocytomas occurs in fewer than 10% of cases. Malignant pheochromocytomas are more often extraadrenal and often secrete norepinephrine exclusively. Malignant pheochromocytoma metastasis usually proceeds via venous and lymphatic channels to the liver. See the tables below for the locations of pheochromocytomas.

Locations of Pheochromocytomas

	Percentage		
Location	**Total**	**Familial**	**Children**
Solitary adrenal	80	<50	50
Extraadrenal	10	<10	25
Bilateral adrenal	10	>50	25

From Landsberg L, Young JB. Catecholamines and the adrenal medulla. In Wilson JD, Foster DW, eds. *Williams Textbook of Endocrinology.* 9th ed. Philadelphia: Saunders; 1998:707.

Locations of Extraadrenal Pheochromocytomas

Location	%
Cervical	2
Thoracic	10–20
Intraabdominal	70–80
Upper abdomen	40
Organ of Zuckerkandl	30
Bladder	15

From Landsberg L, Young JB. Catecholamines and the adrenal medulla. In Wilson JD, Foster DW, eds. *Williams Textbook of Endocrinology.* 9th ed. Philadelphia: Saunders; 1998:707.

Diagnostic tests for determining the presence of a catecholamine tumor include measurements of urinary or plasma catecholamines and their metabolites, vanillylmandelic acid, and metanephrines. Free norepinephrine measurement in a 24-hour urine sample is a sensitive index of pheochromocytoma (see the table below). Other methods that can be used to assess for the presence of a pheochromocytoma include a clonidine suppression test, CT scan, and metaiodobenzylguanidine (MIBG) scintigraphy.

Values for Catecholamines and Catecholamine Metabolites

Hormone or Metabolite	Reference Range
Vanillylmandelic acid, urine	2.0–7.0 mg/24 hr
Metanephrines, urine	<1.3 mg/24 hr
Norepinephrine, urine	<100 mcg/24 hr
Norepinephrine, plasma	150–450 pg/mL
Epinephrine, plasma	<35 pg/mL
Catecholamines, free urinary	<110 mcg/24 hr

Incidence and Prevalence

Pheochromocytomas are rare, occurring in approximately 0.1% of hypertensive patients. These tumors may be associated with neurocutaneous syndromes such as von Hippel-Lindau disease, tuberous sclerosis, and Sturge-Weber syndrome. The tumors may also be a component of MEN type 2A or 2B (see the table below). Patients with a family history of MEN syndrome should be regularly screened for pheochromocytoma. Twenty-five percent of pheochromocytomas occur as part of an inherited autosomal dominant trait.

Manifestations of Multiple Endocrine Neoplasia

Syndrome	Manifestations
MEN type 1 (Wermer's syndrome)	Hyperparathyroidism, pituitary adenomas, pancreatic islet cell tumors
MEN type 2A (Sipple's syndrome)	Medullary thyroid cancer, hyperparathyroidism, pheochromocytoma
MEN type 2B (mucosal neuroma syndrome)	Medullary thyroid tumor, pheochromocytoma, neuromas of the oral mucosa, marfanoid habitus

MEN, Multiple endocrine neoplasia.

Pheochromocytomas can occur at any age but usually occur within the third to the fifth decades of life, with equal frequency in both sexes in adults.

Clinical Manifestations

Manifestations of a pheochromocytoma reflect massive catecholamine release and include hypertension, diaphoresis, headache, tremors, and palpitations. Hypertension may be paroxysmal or sustained. The combination of paroxysmal diaphoresis, tachycardia, and headache in hypertensive patients is a recognized triad of symptoms for pheochromocytoma.

A catecholamine-mediated paroxysm typically consists of a sudden and alarming increase in blood pressure, a severe throbbing headache, profuse sweating, palpitations, tachycardia, a sense of doom, anxiety, pallor (rarely flushing), and nausea. Orthostatic hypotension may result from plasma volume deficit or a lack of tone in the postural reflexes that defend upright blood pressure caused by the sustained excesses of catecholamines. Paroxysmal symptoms may last several minutes to days and are often followed by physical exhaustion. The frequencies of clinical symptoms associated with pheochromocytoma are outlined in the table below.

Frequency of Symptoms in 100 Patients with Pheochromocytoma

Symptom	%
Headache	80
Excessive perspiration	71
Palpitation (with or without tachycardia)	64
Pallor	42
Nausea (with or without vomiting)	42
Tremor or trembling	31
Weakness or exhaustion	28

Continued

Frequency of Symptoms in 100 Patients with Pheochromocytoma—cont'd

Symptom	%
Nervousness or anxiety	22
Epigastric pain	22
Chest pain	19
Dyspnea	19
Flushing or warmth	18
Numbness or paresthesia	11
Blurring of vision	11
Tightness of throat	8
Dizziness or faintness	8
Convulsions	5
Neck or shoulder pain	5
Extremity pain	4
Flank pain	4

From Landsberg L, Young JB. Catecholamines and the adrenal medulla. In Wilson JD, Foster DW, eds. *Williams Textbook of Endocrinology.* 9th ed. Philadelphia: Saunders; 1998:706.

Multiple endocrine neoplasia is a group of rare diseases caused by genetic defects that lead to hyperplasia and hyperfunction of two or more components of the endocrine system.

A paroxysm may be triggered by abdominal palpation, defecation, or any event that provokes pressure on the tumor. Micturition may trigger symptoms if the pheochromocytoma is present in the urinary bladder wall. In some patients, no clearly defined precipitating factor can be found. Mental or psychological stress does not usually initiate a crisis.

Because of the predominance of norepinephrine secretion, the symptoms associated with a pheochromocytoma reflect α-adrenergic activity over β-adrenergic effects. As a result of α-adrenergic inhibition of insulin and enhanced hepatic glucose output, hyperglycemia may be present. The cardiac output and heart rate may be significantly increased. An overall increase in metabolism accelerates oxygen consumption and can cause hyperthermia. Vasoconstriction in the extremities may produce pain, paresthesias, intermittent claudication, or ischemia.

Hypertension is the most common symptom, occurring in more than 90% of patients. Severe paroxysmal hypertension is present in approximately 40% of patients and is a distinctive manifestation of the disease. Sustained hypertension is often resistant to conventional treatment. When pheochromocytomas are predominantly epinephrine secreting, hypertension can alternate with periods of hypotension associated with syncope. Hypotension reflects surges of epinephrine, causing disproportionate β-adrenergic stimulation with vasodilation in the presence of a contracted vascular space.

A catecholamine-induced increase in myocardial oxygen consumption, hypertension, and coronary artery spasm can precipitate myocardial infarction or congestive heart failure even in the absence of coronary artery disease. ECG changes are common. Nonspecific ST-segment and T-wave changes and prominent U waves may be seen. Sinus tachycardia, supraventricular tachycardias, and premature ventricular contractions are commonly noted. Right and left bundle branch blocks and ventricular strain sometimes occur. Ventricular tachycardia has also been reported.

Treatment and Anesthetic Considerations

Preoperative Management

The pharmacologic effects of released catecholamines present major anesthetic challenges. Medical management before tumor excision aims to reverse the effects of excessive adrenergic stimulation. Preoperative antihypertensive therapy and volume replacement has helped to decrease the surgical mortality rate from about 50% to the current 1% to 3%. The preoperative use of α-adrenergic antagonists in concert with reexpansion of the intravascular fluid compartment greatly improves cardiovascular stability intraoperatively. Myocardial infarction, congestive heart failure, cardiac dysrhythmias, and cerebral hemorrhage decrease in frequency when the patient has been treated preoperatively with α-adrenergic receptor antagonists. The drugs used in the management of pheochromocytoma are listed in the following table on pg. 96.

α-Adrenergic Receptor Blockade

Phenoxybenzamine (Dibenzyline) is the drug of choice for preoperative α-adrenergic blockade and blood pressure stabilization. It is a noncompetitive presynaptic (α_2) and postsynaptic (α_1) adrenergic receptor antagonist of long duration (24–48 hours). Most patients with a pheochromocytoma require an oral dose between 60 and 250 mg/day. Postural hypotension is a common side effect of treatment.

Typically, patients require 10 to 14 days of α-adrenergic antagonist therapy to stabilize blood pressure, restore fluid volume, and decrease symptoms. Establishment of normotension facilitates reexpansion of the intravascular fluid compartment. Satisfactory α-adrenergic blockade is implied if the hematocrit decreases by 5% during treatment. Half to two-thirds of the normal oral phenoxybenzamine dose may be given the morning of surgery. α-Blockade must be initiated before β-blockade to avoid the potential for a hypertensive crisis.

Prazosin (Minipress), a specific postsynaptic α_1-adrenergic receptor antagonist, has also been used successfully to treat the hypertension of pheochromocytoma preoperatively. Labetalol (Trandate, Normodyne), a mixed α- and β-receptor antagonist, has not been as effective as a first-line drug in controlling the blood pressure response, but it may be used as an adjunctive agent.

β-Adrenergic Receptor Blockade

A β-adrenergic receptor antagonist is usually introduced in the preoperative period for control of tachycardia, hypertension, and catecholamine-induced supraventricular dysrhythmias. An important caveat is that β-adrenergic receptor antagonists should not be administered until after α-adrenergic blockade is established. Blocking β-receptor–mediated vasodilation in skeletal muscle without prior α-adrenergic blockade can increase the blood pressure even further in patients with pheochromocytoma.

Other Treatment Regimens

Calcium channel blockers and magnesium sulfate infusion have been used with variable success as monotherapy for the perioperative management of pheochromocytoma. Some regimens use these agents in conjunction with adrenergic blocking drugs.

α-Methyl tyrosine (Demser) is used for patients requiring long-term therapy such as in patients for whom surgery is contraindicated. The drug competitively inhibits catecholamine formation by blocking tyrosine hydroxylase, the rate-limiting enzyme in catecholamine synthesis.

Drugs Used in the Management of Pheochromocytoma

Drug	Action	Pressor Crisis	Preoperative Blood Pressure Control	Comments
Phentolamine	α-Blocker	IV: 2–5 mg	—	Rapid onset, short acting; bolus every 5 min or infuse initially 1 mg/min
Phenoxybenzamine	α-Blocker	—	PO: 30 mg/day, increasing daily dosage by 30 mg	Long half-life; may accumulate; administer two or three times daily
Prazosin	α-Blocker	—	PO: 1.0 mg single dose, increasing to tid regimen	First-dose phenomenon; may cause syncope; start with low dose before bedtime
Propranolol	β-Blocker	IV: 1.0 mg bolus to total of 10 mg	PO: 40 mg bid; increase to 480 mg/day	Should not be administered without first creating α-blockade
Atenolol	β-Blocker	—	PO: 50 mg/day initially; may increase to 100 mg/day	Long-acting, selective β1-antagonist eliminated unchanged by kidney
Esmolol	β-Blocker	IV 500 mcg/kg min loading followed by maintenance infusion	—	Ultrashort-acting selective β1-antagonist; may be used during anesthesia
Labetalol	α- and β-blocker	IV 10 mg bolus to 150 mg	PO: 200 mg tid	A much weaker α-blocker than β-blocker; may cause pressor response in pheochromocytoma
Nitroprusside	Vasodilator	IV infusion: initially 0.5–1.5 mcg/kg min	—	Powerful vasodilator; short acting; may be used during anesthesia
Magnesium sulfate	Vasodilator	IV: 40–60 mg/kg bolus followed by 2 g/hr and additional 20 mg/kg boluses as needed	—	May potentiate neuromuscular blockade
Diltiazem	Calcium channel blocker	IV 3–10 mcg/kg/min	—	May also directly block release of catecholamines
Nicardipine	Calcium channel blocker	IV 2–6 mcg/kg/min	—	Better vasodilator than diltiazem
α-Methyl-tyrosine	Inhibitor of biosynthesis of catecholamines	—	PO: 1–4 g/day	Suitable for patients not amenable to surgery; may be nephrotoxic

bid, Twice a day; *IV,* intravenous; *PO,* oral; *tid,* three times a day.

Adapted from Schwartz JJ, Rosenbaum S, Graf GJ. Anesthesia and the endocrine system. In Barash PG, Cullen BF, Stoelting RK, eds. *Clinical Anesthesia.* 4th ed. Philadelphia: Lippincott; 2001:1132.

The following criteria are proposed as end points for the patient awaiting surgery for pheochromocytoma resection:

1. No in-hospital blood pressure reading higher than 160/90 mmHg 24 hours before surgery
2. No blood pressure on standing lower than 80/45 mmHg
3. No ST-segment or T-wave abnormality on the ECG that cannot be attributed to a permanent defect
4. No marked symptoms of catecholamine excess; no more than 1 premature ventricular contraction every 5 minutes

Anesthetic Considerations

Effective anesthetic management is based on selecting drugs that do not stimulate catecholamine release and implementing monitoring techniques that facilitate early and appropriate intervention when catecholamine-induced changes in cardiovascular function occur.

Pheochromocytomas are excised by open laparotomy or laparoscopy. Postoperative morbidity is similar with both approaches. During pneumoperitoneum for laparoscopy, significant catecholamine release has been reported.

A number of drugs and conditions can precipitate hypertension in surgical patients with pheochromocytoma. Dopamine antagonists (metoclopramide, droperidol), radiographic contrast media, indirect-acting amines (ephedrine, methyldopa), drugs that block neuronal catecholamine reuptake (tricyclic antidepressants, cocaine), histamine, and glucagon may enhance the physiologic effect of tumor product.

Pheochromocytomas are vascular tumors. Large-bore IV lines and a peripheral arterial catheter should be established preoperatively. A central venous pressure or pulmonary artery catheter should be placed to help guide fluid management and intervention with inotropes or vasoactive drugs. Arterial blood gases, electrolyte concentrations, and blood glucose levels should be assessed regularly during the anesthetic.

Critical intraoperative junctures are: (1) during induction and intubation of the trachea (possible hypertension), (2) during surgical manipulation of the tumor (possible hypertension), and (3) after ligation of the tumor's venous drainage (possible hypotension).

Anesthesia induction may be accomplished with barbiturates, etomidate, or propofol. Anesthetic depth can be enhanced by mask ventilation of the lungs with a volatile anesthetic prior to laryngoscopy and intubation. Lidocaine (1–2 mg/kg IV) administered 1 minute before intubation may help attenuate the hemodynamic response to laryngoscopy. Rapid-acting vasodilating drugs such as nitroprusside should be readily available to treat hypertension. Short-acting opioids, such as fentanyl or remifentanil, administered before intubation may also help blunt the blood pressure responses to intubation. Morphine sulfate should be avoided because of its propensity for histamine release.

Sevoflurane and short-acting opioids, such as remifentanil, provide cardiovascular stability and possess the ability to rapidly change anesthetic depth, attractive features in the anesthetic management of patients with pheochromocytoma. The tachycardia associated with desflurane makes it a less desirable choice for these cases.

The use of succinylcholine has been questioned because compression of an abdominal tumor by drug-induced skeletal muscle fasciculations may provoke catecholamine release. However, a predictable adverse effect of succinylcholine has not been supported clinically when administered to patients with pheochromocytoma. Skeletal muscle paralysis with a nondepolarizing muscle relaxant devoid of vagolytic or histamine-releasing effects is desirable. Pancuronium should be avoided because of its known chronotropic effect.

The anesthetist should anticipate a labile cardiovascular course during surgery. Hypertension can be treated by increasing the anesthetic depth and administering nitroprusside if necessary. Propranolol, lidocaine, labetalol, or esmolol may be given IV to decrease tachydysrhythmias. β-Adrenergic antagonists must be used cautiously in patients with catecholamine-induced cardiomyopathy because even minimal β-adrenergic blockade can accentuate left ventricular dysfunction. The short half-life of esmolol makes it an advantageous choice for β-adrenergic blockade. Dysrhythmias associated with hypertension may be resolved by lowering an abnormally high blood pressure. Indirect-acting sympathomimetics have an unpredictable pressor effect in these patients and should be avoided.

After surgical ligation of the veins that drain a pheochromocytoma, the rapid decrease in circulating catecholamines and the associated down-regulation of adrenergic receptors may precipitate a decrease in blood pressure. During this juncture, close communication with the surgical team is important. Decreasing the inhaled anesthetic agent concentration and increasing the administration of IV crystalloid or colloid solution should adequately increase blood pressure. IV administration of phenylephrine hydrochloride (Neo-Synephrine) or dopamine may be needed until the peripheral vasculature can adapt to the decreased level of endogenous α-stimulation.

Hyperglycemia is common before excision of the pheochromocytoma. With tumor removal, the sudden withdraw of catecholamine stimulation can result in hypoglycemia. Furthermore, β-adrenergic blockade impairs hepatic glucose production. β-Adrenergic blockers may also mask hypoglycemic signs by preventing tachycardia and tremor. Blood glucose levels should be monitored at frequent intervals intraoperatively and postoperatively.

Some pheochromocytomas may first present as a hypermetabolic state during anesthesia for unrelated surgery. The hypertension, tachycardia, hyperthermia, and respiratory acidosis of a pheochromocytoma may mimic light anesthesia, thyroid crisis, malignant hyperthermia, or sepsis.

Postoperative Implications

Fluid shifts, pain, hypoxia, hypercapnia, autonomic instability, urinary retention, or residual tumor are all potential causes of postoperative hypertension. Invasive monitoring is indicated during the initial postoperative period to assess blood pressure changes and cardiac status. Fifty percent of patients remain hypertensive during the immediate postanesthesia recovery period despite removal of the pheochromocytoma. Transient hypertension postoperatively usually reflects fluid shifts and autonomic instability. Postoperative catecholamine levels decrease to normal over several days. In 75% of patients, normal blood pressure returns within 14 days after surgery. Relief of postoperative pain can be accomplished with neuraxial opioids and may contribute to early tracheal extubation in otherwise healthy patients.

A. CARCINOID TUMORS AND CARCINOID SYNDROME

Definition

Carcinoid tumors consist of slow-growing malignancies composed of enterochromaffin cells usually found in the gastrointestinal tract. They may also occur in the lung, pancreas, thymus, and liver. Carcinoid tumors have a low incidence rate of 1.9 per 100,000.

Pathophysiology

Speculation is that the advent and increasing use of proton pump inhibitors is a major contributory factor to the development of carcinoid tumors. A delay of several years frequently occurs before a diagnosis of carcinoid tumor is made. The gastrointestinal tract accounts for about two-thirds of carcinoids. Within the gastrointestinal tract, most tumors occur in the small intestine (41.8%), rectum (27.4%), and stomach (8.7%). Distant metastases may be evident at the time of diagnosis in 12.9% of patients, but better diagnostic techniques have contributed to improved survival rates.

The tumors can secrete several biologically active substances, including serotonin (5-hydroxytryptamine), kallikrein, histamine, prostaglandins, adrenocorticotropic hormone, gastrin, calcitonin, and growth hormone, among others. Approximately 5% to 10% of patients with carcinoid tumors develop carcinoid syndrome.

Clinical Manifestations

The manifestations of carcinoid syndrome are in the table on pg. 100 and as follows:

- Episodic cutaneous flushing (kinins, histamine)
- Diarrhea (serotonin, prostaglandins E and F)
- Heart disease
- Tricuspid regurgitation, pulmonic stenosis
- Supraventricular tachydysrhythmias (serotonin)
- Bronchoconstriction (serotonin, bradykinin, substance P)
- Hypotension (kinins, histamine)
- Hypertension (serotonin)
- Abdominal pain (small bowel obstruction)
- Hepatomegaly (metastases)
- Hyperglycemia
- Hypoalbuminemia (pellagra-like skin lesions resulting from niacin deficiency)

Vasoactive peptides released from carcinoid tumors located in the bronchi and ovaries exert a faster effect because of their direct drainage into the portal vein. Carcinoid tumors are also functionally autonomous. Two factors that enhance release of carcinoid hormones are direct physical manipulation of the tumor and β-adrenergic stimulation.

Principal Mediators of Carcinoid Syndrome and Their Clinical Manifestations

Mediator	Clinical Manifestations
Serotonin	Vasoconstriction (coronary artery spasm, hypertension), increased intestinal tone water and electrolyte imbalance (diarrhea), tryptophan deficiency (hypoproteinemia, pellagra)
Kallikrein	Vasodilation (hypotension, flushing), bronchoconstriction
Histamine	Vasodilation (hypotension, flushing), arrhythmias, bronchoconstriction

Treatment

Patients with carcinoid syndrome may undergo primary resection of the carcinoid tumor. Examples of other procedures that these patients often undergo include cardiac valve replacement and hepatic resection (e.g., lobectomy) for excision of metastases.

Anesthetic Considerations

Many anesthetic techniques have been used successfully in the treatment of patients with carcinoid syndrome (see the following section). Preoperative preparation of the patient requires correction of deficiencies in circulating volume and electrolyte levels. Use of histamine-releasing agents, such as morphine, and atracurium should be avoided. Fasciculations may induce release of carcinoid hormones and are therefore prevented by avoidance of succinylcholine, although it has been used successfully many times, especially for rapid sequence induction.

Anesthetic Considerations in Carcinoid Syndrome

- The most common clinical signs are flushing, wheezing, blood pressure and heart rate changes, and diarrhea.
- Preoperative assessment should include complete blood count, measurement of electrolytes, liver function tests, measurement of blood glucose, electrocardiogram (echocardiogram if indicated), and determination of urine 5-HIAA levels.
- Optimize fluid and electrolyte status and pretreat with octreotide as noted. Continue octreotide throughout the postoperative period. Interferon-α has shown success in controlling some symptoms.
- Both histamine-1 and -2 receptor blockers must be used to fully counteract histamine effects.
- Avoid histamine-releasing agents such as morphine, thiopental, and atracurium.
- Avoid sympathomimetic agents such as ketamine and ephedrine.
- Treat hypotension with an α-receptor agonist such as phenylephrine.
- General anesthesia is preferred over regional anesthesia. Patients with high serotonin levels may exhibit prolonged recovery; therefore, desflurane and sevoflurane, which have rapid recovery profiles, may be beneficial.
- Aggressively maintain normothermia to avoid catecholamine-induced vasoactive mediator release.
- Monitor intraoperative plasma glucose because these patients are prone to hyperglycemia. Treat with insulin as is customary.

Octreotide, a somatostatin analog, is used to blunt the vasoactive and bronchoconstrictive effects of carcinoid tumor products. Octreotide mimics the inhibitory action of somatostatin on the release of several gastrointestinal hormones, as well as those derived from carcinoid tumors. Treatment for 2 weeks preoperatively with a dose of 100 mcg subcutaneously three times a day is standard. If prior therapy was not used, a dose of 50 to 150 mcg subcutaneously is given preoperatively. Intraoperative infusion may be continued at 100 mcg/hr. Bolus doses of 100 to 200 mcg given intravenously may be used for intraoperative carcinoid crises. Lantrotide (which is administered every two weeks) and octreotide LAR (which can be given monthly) are long-acting formulations that are superior in terms of patient acceptance and cost effectiveness.

Patients with hypotension should be treated with an α-adrenergic agonist (e.g., phenylephrine infusion) to avoid hormone release by β-adrenergic stimulation. Bronchospasm resulting from histamine or bradykinin release has been shown to be resistant to ketamine and inhalation anesthetics. Low-dose β_2-agonists are effective in bronchodilation and have relatively little influence on carcinoid hormone release. In the presence of high levels of serotonin in carcinoid syndrome, adjustments in anesthetic selection and dosage must be considered if further compromise of cardiovascular function is to be prevented.

B. GALLSTONES AND GALLBLADDER DISEASE

CHOLECYSTITIS

Definition

Obstruction of the cystic duct by gallstones results in acute, severe midepigastric pain, typically radiating to the right abdomen. Inspiratory effort usually accentuates the pain (Murphy's sign).

Clinical Manifestations

Increases in plasma bilirubin, alkaline phosphatase, and amylase levels frequently occur. Ileus and localized tenderness may indicate perforation with peritonitis. Leukocytosis and fever are often present. The presence of jaundice indicates complete obstruction of the cystic duct. Symptoms are frequently confused with those of myocardial infarction. Differential diagnosis is accomplished through serial electrocardiogram (ECG) evaluations and laboratory analysis of serum enzymes that are specific to cardiac muscle. Cholescintigraphy (a contrast study that evaluates gallbladder excretion of a radiographically labeled substance) and ultrasonography are often used for clinical confirmation of the diagnosis.

Anesthetic Considerations

Patients with symptoms indicative of acute cholecystitis are often volume depleted as a result of intolerance of oral intake, vomiting, and possible preoperative nasogastric evacuation of gastric contents. Dehydration warrants preoperative intravenous fluid replacement. Gastric suction may be warranted in the presence of ileus. The presence of free abdominal air, as determined by abdominal radiography or symptoms of an acute abdomen (fever, ileus, rigid and painful abdomen, vomiting, dehydration), suggests the presence of a ruptured viscus, possibly including perforation of the gallbladder. Under these circumstances, emergency exploratory laparotomy is undertaken.

CHOLELITHIASIS AND CHOLEDOCHOLITHIASIS

Acute obstruction of the common bile duct often produces symptoms similar to those seen in patients with cholecystitis. Recurrent bouts of acute cholecystitis induce the development of fibrotic changes in gallbladder structure, thereby impeding the ability of the gallbladder to adequately expel bile. The presence of Charcot's triad (fever and chills, jaundice, upper quadrant pain) aids in establishing the differential diagnosis in acute ductal obstruction. Weight loss, anorexia, and fatigue complete the symptomatology. Diagnostic modalities include radiography, transhepatic cholangiography, ultrasonography, cholescintigraphy, and computed tomography (CT) scan. A dilated common bile duct and biliary tree are typically observed in these studies.

Anesthetic Considerations

Removal of gallstones is undertaken not only for relief of symptoms but also for prevention of further sequelae, including cholecystitis, cholangitis, jaundice, pancreatitis, and peritonitis, all of which may result from stasis or impediment to bile flow.

C. HIATAL HERNIA AND GASTRIC REFLUX

Definitions

Hiatal Hernia

A hiatal hernia consists of a defect in the diaphragm that allows a portion of the stomach to migrate upward into the thoracic cavity. Two types of esophageal hiatal hernias are the sliding type (type I), which is formed by the movement of the upper stomach through an enlarged hiatus, and the paraesophageal type (type II), in which the esophagogastric junction remains in normal position but all or part of the stomach moves into the thorax and assumes a paraesophageal position. A third type of hiatal hernia (type III) has been identified that combines the features of a sliding and a paraesophageal hernia. A fourth type of hiatal hernia (type IV) occurs when other organs, such as the colon or small bowel, are contained in the hernia sac that is formed by a large paraesophageal hernia. Hiatal hernia and peptic esophagitis often exist concurrently, although one does not cause the other.

Gastric Reflux

Gastric reflux relates to a reduced lower esophageal sphincter tone, which can increase the risk for regurgitation and aspiration. Reflux can occur without the presence of hiatal hernia. The lower sphincter is a physiologic sphincter with no specialized musculature. Tone is 15 to 35 mmHg.

Incidence and Prevalence

Types I to IV hiatal hernias are present in 10% of the population, usually without symptoms. Only 5% of the population has reflux symptoms along with a hiatal hernia.

Pathophysiology

In most cases, the cause is unknown, whether the condition is congenital, traumatic, or iatrogenic.

Clinical Manifestations

The major symptom is retrosternal pain of a burning quality that commonly occurs after meals. It is assumed that patients with a hiatal hernia are predisposed to developing peptic esophagitis, thereby providing a rationale for surgical correction of this condition. Most patients with hiatal hernia do not have symptoms of reflux esophagitis, however, and do not require H_2-agonist and oral antacid therapy. Nevertheless, implementation of aspiration precautions on induction of general anesthesia and emergence is still strongly recommended.

Treatment

The primary goal in the surgical correction of hiatal hernia consists of reestablishment of gastroesophageal competence. This usually entails repair of the sliding hernia, reduction by 2 cm or more of the tubular distal esophagus below the diaphragm, and valvuloplasty. An abdominal, thoracic, or thoracoabdominal surgical approach may be selected. Common procedures for correction of hiatal hernia include the Nissen, Belsey, and Hill operations. Laparoscopically assisted fundoplication techniques are also more commonly being used. A gastroplasty may be performed (the Collis procedure) in association with repair of the hiatal hernia when indicated, usually in patients with a shortened esophagus. If a thoracic approach is selected, the patient must be assessed for ability to tolerate one-lung anesthesia.

Anesthetic Considerations

Symptomatic patients require pretreatment with a nonparticulate antacid and an H_2-blocker. For induction of anesthesia, elevation of the head of the bed or stretcher and rapid-sequence induction to prevent aspiration should be considered. If the hernia is large, one-lung anesthesia may be used to improve surgical access during repair. Communication with the surgical team is imperative when the thoracoabdominal approach is being considered.

D. INFLAMMATORY BOWEL DISEASE

Definition

In the United States, between 200,000 and 300,000 individuals have inflammatory bowel disease, and approximately 30,000 new cases are diagnosed each year. The two major types of inflammatory bowel disease are Crohn's disease and ulcerative colitis. Ulcerative colitis is an inflammatory disease, primarily of the mucosa of the rectum and distal colon. It is a chronic disease that is fraught with remissions and exacerbations.

Incidence and Prevalence

Ulcerative colitis affects female patients more frequently than male patients and has a bimodal age distribution that shows a first peak incidence between ages 15 and 20 years and a second, smaller, peak between ages 55 and 60 years. The disorder is speculated to have a strong familial genetic predisposition, but psychological factors have also been implicated in its cause. Crohn's disease most commonly occurs at about 30 years of age.

CROHN'S DISEASE

Pathophysiology

Crohn's disease involves primarily the distal ileum and large colon in approximately 50% of patients. The remainder of patients experience disease that is localized to either the colon or portions of the small intestine (regional enteritis). The deeper layers of the intestinal mucosa are typically involved, a situation that leads to derangements in colonic absorption.

Clinical Manifestations

Owing to the loss of functional absorptive surfaces in the large colon, patients with Crohn's disease are often deficient in magnesium, phosphorus, zinc, and potassium. They also have deficiencies secondary to the loss of absorptive capability in portions of the small intestine. Protein-losing enteropathy is often encountered, as is anemia resulting from occult blood loss and deficiencies in vitamin B_{12} and folic acid. Iron deficiency secondary to insufficient intestinal absorption also contributes to development of an anemic state. Involvement of the distal ileum in the disease process results in deficiencies in vitamin B_{12} and in nutrients that are dependent on bile acids for absorption. Disturbance in the enterohepatic circulation of bile in the terminal ileum is reflected in complex nutrient deficiencies, including proteins, zinc, magnesium, phosphorus, fat-soluble vitamins, and vitamin B_{12}. This state is typical of patients with chronic Crohn's disease. Folate deficiency may also be present in patients with Crohn's disease who receive sulfasalazine preparations.

Fistulas often develop between inflamed portions of the intestine and adjacent abdominal structures. Abdominal and pelvic abscesses, rectocutaneous fistulas, and perirectal abscesses have a high incidence in these patients. Increased calcium oxalate absorption in the terminal ileum frequently occurs, resulting in a high rate of renal calculi and cholelithiasis.

Treatment

Medical therapy for Crohn's disease includes a variety of drugs and is given in the box below.

Agents Used to Treat Crohn's Disease

5-Aminosalicylates (5-ASAs)
Sulfasalazine
Sulfa free (mesalamine, olsalazine, balsalazide)

Antibiotics
Metronidazole
Ciprofloxacin
Glucocorticoids
Classic
Novel (controlled ileal-release budesonide)

Agents Used to Treat Crohn's Disease—cont'd

Immunomodulators
6-Mercaptopurine, azathioprine
Methotrexate
Cyclosporine
Biologic Response Modifiers
Infliximab

From Sands BE. Crohn's disease. In Feldman M, Friedman LS, Brandt LJ. *Sleisenger and Fordtran's Gastrointestinal and Liver Disease.* 9th ed. Philadelphia: Saunders; 2010:1962.

Surgery is warranted when medical treatment fails or when complications supervene. Although effective in the relief of complications, surgical resection of the diseased colon and ileum does not alter the progression of the disease. The primary principle of surgical management is to limit the operation to the correction of the presenting complication, which could include bowel obstruction, fistulas, abscesses, and symptoms that indicate widespread symptomatic disease (for which total colectomy and ileal resection may be warranted).

Most patients with Crohn's disease undergo surgery, and a large number require repeat or continued procedures. The recurrence rate at 10 years after surgery is 50%. A high likelihood of repeat surgery involves areas of the remaining bowel proximal to the area of a previous anastomosis. Patients with a history of Crohn's disease are also shown to have a higher prevalence of bowel carcinoma.

ULCERATIVE COLITIS

Clinical Manifestations

Symptoms usually include abdominal pain, fever, and bloody diarrhea. Ulcerative colitis is typically chronic, with relatively low-grade symptoms, such as bloody stools, malaise, diarrhea, and pain. In approximately 15% of patients, however, ulcerative colitis that has acute, fulminating characteristics may occur. Under this circumstance, severe abdominal pain, profuse rectal hemorrhage, and high fever are seen. Associated symptoms include nausea and vomiting, anorexia, and profound weakness. Physical signs usually include pallor and weight loss.

Associated with an acute onset of fulminating ulcerative colitis is toxic megacolon, which is characterized by severe colonic distention that causes shock. In patients with this condition, the distended bowel lumen provides an environment that is conducive to bacterial overgrowth. This condition, coupled with erosive intestinal inflammation and perforation, allows for the systemic release of bacteria-produced toxins. Clinical signs and symptoms of toxic megacolon include fever, tachycardia, abdominal distention, pain, ileus, and dehydration. Electrolyte derangements, anemia, and hypoalbuminemia are also commonly present.

An increased incidence of large joint arthritis is seen in patients when the disease is clinically active. Concomitant liver disease, as evidenced by fatty infiltrates and pericholangitis, may also complicate the clinical picture. Other extracolonic manifestations of ulcerative colitis include iritis, erythema nodosum, and ankylosing spondylitis.

Treatment

Therapy for ulcerative colitis is initially medical. As with Crohn's disease, sulfasalazine preparations, antidiarrheal agents, and corticosteroids are the cornerstones of medical therapy. Both Crohn's disease and ulcerative colitis result in systemic disorders, such as anemia and nutritional deficiencies, which are handled in the same supportive manner. In both diseases, surgical resection is reserved for patients with intractable complications. Whereas surgery for Crohn's disease is nondefinitive and complication oriented, proctocolectomy with ileostomy is generally curative for ulcerative colitis.

Anesthetic Considerations

Anesthetic management of patients with inflammatory bowel disease begins with a thorough, systematic patient history, and particular attention is paid to the patient's fluid and electrolyte status. Possible extracolonic complications (e.g., sepsis, liver disease, anemia, arthritis, hypoalbuminemia, and other metabolic derangements) must also be considered during planning and perioperative management. Efforts to optimize the medical condition of such patients before elective surgery are strongly recommended.

Prophylactic steroid coverage is likely to be indicated, particularly in patients receiving long-term steroid therapy. Inclusion of nitrous oxide in anesthesia delivery should be reconsidered with the possibility of bowel distention associated with its prolonged intraoperative use. Awareness of complications from parenteral nutritional therapy (e.g., hyperglycemia or hypoglycemia, increased carbon dioxide production, renal or hepatic dysfunction, nonketotic hyperosmolar hyperglycemic coma, and hyperchloremic metabolic acidosis) is also necessary for patients receiving total or partial parenteral nutritional support. Administration of a preexistent parenteral nutritional support infusion should be maintained throughout the perioperative period at the ordered infusion rate. Periodic laboratory assessment of metabolic status (i.e., serum glucose and electrolytes) should be performed and guide corrective interventions for detected derangements. The severity of extracolonic influence on the function of other organ systems dictates appropriate technique and drug selection, as well as the extent to which invasive monitoring is used. Correction of fluid, electrolyte, and hematologic derangements may be necessary before surgery. Increased intraluminal pressure caused by the administration of anticholinesterases for reversal of neuromuscular blockade has been shown to have no effect on colonic suture lines. No particular anesthetic technique is mandated; however, the use of a combined technique (epidural and general anesthesia) is attractive for both intraoperative use and postoperative analgesia needs.

E. PANCREATITIS

ACUTE PANCREATITIS

Pathophysiology

The cause of pancreatitis is multifactorial. Common causes include alcohol abuse, direct or indirect trauma to the pancreas, ulcerative penetration from adjacent structures (e.g., the duodenum), infectious processes, biliary tract disease, metabolic disorders (e.g., hyperlipidemia and hypercalcemia), and certain drugs (e.g., corticosteroids, furosemide, estrogens, and thiazide diuretics). Patients who have undergone extensive surgery involving mobilization of the abdominal viscera are at risk for development of postoperative pancreatitis, as are patients who have undergone procedures involving cardiopulmonary bypass.

Clinical Manifestations

Acute pancreatitis is characterized as a severe chemical burn of the peritoneal cavity. Enzymes implicated as major culprits in the syndrome of pancreatitis are those activated by trypsin, enterokinase, and bile acids. Cardiovascular complications of acute pancreatitis can lead to pericardial effusions, alterations in cardiac rhythmicity, and signs and symptoms mimicking acute myocardial infarction, thrombophlebitis, and cardiac depression. Acute pancreatitis also predisposes patients to the development of acute respiratory distress syndrome and disseminated intravascular coagulopathy.

Pain is the foremost symptom of acute pancreatitis and may be variable in quality (i.e., localized or radiating, dull and tolerable, or severe and unremitting). Pancreatic pain may radiate from the midepigastric to the periumbilical region and may be more intense when the patient is in the supine position.

Abdominal distention is often seen and is largely attributable to the accumulation of intraperitoneal fluid and paralytic ileus. Nausea and vomiting and fever are common symptoms. Hypotension is seen in 40% to 50% of patients and is attributable to hypovolemia secondary to the loss of plasma proteins into the retroperitoneal space. Acute renal failure secondary to dehydration and hypotension may occur.

Hypocalcemia frequently develops in patients with acute pancreatitis, and this condition obviates monitoring the ECG for cardiac rhythm disorders (e.g., lengthened QT interval with possible reentry dysrhythmias). The clinician must also be observant for signs of tetany. Clinical shock may develop that is largely secondary to the effects of vasoactive kinin peptides (e.g., bradykinin) released during the inflammatory process; these peptides enhance vasodilation, vascular permeability, and leukocyte migration.

Elevated serum amylase levels are often present but do not necessarily indicate primary pancreatic disease; other intraabdominal disease processes result in such elevations, including biliary tract disease, tubo-ovarian disease, peptic ulcer disease, and acute bowel disease, including obstruction, inflammation, and ischemia. Elevated serum lipase levels may also be observed. Compressive obstruction of the common bile duct by an edematous head of the pancreas contributes to elevations in serum bilirubin and alkaline phosphatase levels.

Radiographic and ultrasonographic findings aid in the differential diagnosis of pancreatic disease. Evidence of free intraperitoneal air by radiography suggests the presence of a perforated viscus. CT is highly effective in the diagnosis of an enlarged, edematous pancreatic head, which is typically seen in patients with pancreatitis.

Treatment

Supportive therapy is initially undertaken in acute pancreatitis. This regimen usually includes intensive care unit admission and may involve implementation of invasive monitoring, fluid and hemodynamic resuscitation, and interventions necessary for the preservation of perfusion and function of the abdominal viscera. Severely ill, malnourished patients are often given parenteral nutritional support.

If the cause of pancreatitis is obstructive biliary disease caused by the presence of a stone in the common bile duct or by inflammation of the gallbladder, cholecystectomy and possibly common bile duct exploration are indicated.

Anesthetic Considerations

The choice of anesthetic technique and the extent to which monitoring modalities are used are based on an assessment of the patient's history, the acuity of disease, and the degree of preexisting physical compensation. Special attention is directed toward the correction of significant intravascular volume deficits. The presence of labile hemodynamics and alterations in hepatic function must also be discerned, and appropriate accommodating modifications must be made to the anesthetic plan, for example, ensuring stable arterial pressure, using anesthetic agents and adjuvants that require minimal hepatic biotransformation, ensuring adequate oxygenation, and replacing electrolytes and blood volume.

CHRONIC PANCREATITIS

Pathophysiology

Chronic alcoholism is a common etiologic factor in chronic pancreatitis. This condition is strongly suggested by the classic diagnostic triad of steatorrhea, pancreatic calcification (evidenced radiographically), and diabetes mellitus. Individuals with chronic pancreatitis are often malnourished and emaciated. They are more often male than female. Other conditions besides chronic alcohol abuse that are associated with the development of chronic pancreatitis include significant and usually chronic biliary tract disease and the effects of pancreatic injury sustained at an earlier age.

Formation of a pseudocyst occurs in up to 8% of alcoholic patients after resolution of a bout of acute pancreatitis. Pancreatic abscess occurs in 3% to 5% of patients with acute pancreatitis but is present in 90% of patients dying as a result of acute pancreatitis.

Clinical Manifestations

The clinical picture may also include hepatic disease, as evidenced by jaundice, ascites, esophageal varices, derangements in coagulation factors, serum albumin, and transferase enzymes. Perturbation in pancreatic exocrine function with consequent enzymatic insufficiency results in malabsorption of fats and proteins in the intestine. Patients with chronic pancreatitis also have a predisposition for the development of pericardial and pleural effusions.

Pancreatic abscesses develop from infected peripancreatic collections of fluid. Abscesses are usually secondary manifestations of chronic pancreatitis and warrant surgical drainage to prevent spread of the infectious contents to the subphrenic and pericolic spaces. Fistula formation is possible, particularly into the transverse colon. Severe intraabdominal hemorrhage is also possible as a result of erosion into major proximal arteries.

Treatment

Surgical drainage of a pancreatic pseudocyst is usually undertaken after a period of maturation of the cyst (usually 6 weeks). The procedure consists of formation of a cystogastrostomy, cystojejunostomy, cystoduodenostomy, or possibly distal pancreatectomy. The location of the pseudocyst dictates the extent and type of procedure used for the provision of drainage of cystic contents into the gastrointestinal tract. Percutaneous external drainage, guided by CT, is reserved for cases in which the pseudocyst is particularly friable. Spontaneous resolution of pseudocysts may be expected in 20% or more of patients who have undergone surgical drainage.

Anesthetic Considerations

The patient undergoing surgical treatment of pancreatic disease exhibits a variable clinical picture: the patient may be jaundiced and stable with a painless pancreatic mass or may be severely ill with multiorgan system involvement. Patients may have severe, acute abdominal pain with possible intestinal obstruction or ileus. Aspiration precautions should be in effect during induction of anesthesia and emergence from anesthesia. Perioperative assessment of serum glucose level and institution of appropriate control measures are warranted because these patients are likely to have diabetes (secondary to β-cell dysfunction) or hypoglycemia (as in the case of insulinoma). Derangements in fluid and electrolyte balance must also be anticipated. Rigorous blood product and crystalloid resuscitation may be necessary throughout the perioperative period and likely will necessitate the placement of invasive hemodynamic lines in order to guide therapy and to monitor central pressures.

Potential electrolyte disorders include hypocalcemia, hypomagnesemia, hypokalemia, and possibly hypochloremic metabolic alkalosis. The serum hematocrit value may be falsely increased secondary to hemoconcentration, or it may be decreased secondary to the presence of a bleeding diathesis. Coagulation parameters, including platelet count, prothrombin time, activated partial thromboplastin time, and fibrinogen level, should be assessed at regular intervals perioperatively. Preservation of renal function mandates the preoperative assessment of blood urea nitrogen, serum creatinine, and 24-hour creatinine clearance (if possible); urinalysis should also be performed. Intraoperatively a urine output of at least 0.5 to 1 mL/kg/hr should be maintained.

A significant incidence of postoperative respiratory morbidity associated with upper abdominal surgery, as well as the possible preexisting debilitated state of the patient, mandates a thorough assessment of preexisting pulmonary status. This assessment includes arterial blood gas analysis; chest radiography; and, when appropriate, pulmonary function tests. The pulmonary assessment assumes added importance because of the high incidence of pleural effusion secondary to pancreatic disease and secondary to the potential history of heavy tobacco use.

Cardiovascular assessment should assimilate related findings from the assessment of other organ systems so that the degree to which functional hemodynamic impairment may need to be corrected is fully appreciated. Correction of preexisting hemodynamic disturbances entails restitution of plasma volume and the oxygen-carrying capacity of the blood. Ischemic changes noted on the ECG must be treated promptly. ECG changes mimicking myocardial ischemia are often seen in pancreatitis.

General endotracheal anesthesia is the technique of choice. Preoperative placement of an epidural catheter allows greater flexibility in the intraoperative management of pain and in the provision of postoperative pain control. Patients undergoing extensive pancreatic surgery often require postoperative ventilatory support and intensive care unit monitoring because of the magnitude and the length of the procedure, as well as their preexisting cardiopulmonary status.

Laboratory results should be reviewed, and the patient should be evaluated for shock, hemorrhage, and pain relief (meperidine is the drug of choice). Fluid and electrolyte status is of concern because the patient should receive nothing by mouth. The patient will have a nasogastric tube, and H_2 blockers will be given. In addition, the patient should undergo typing and crossmatching for possible transfusion. Plasma expanders, crystalloids, and invasive monitoring may be used.

F. SPLENIC DISORDERS

Definition

A palpable spleen is the major physical sign produced by diseases affecting the spleen and suggests enlargement of the organ. The normal spleen is said to weigh less than 250 g, decreases in size with age, normally lies entirely within the rib cage, has a maximum cephalocaudal diameter of 13 cm by ultrasonography or maximum length of 12 cm or width of 7 cm by radionuclide scan, and is usually not palpable.

Incidence and Prevalence

A palpable spleen was found in 3% of 2200 asymptomatic male freshman college students. Follow-up at 3 years revealed that 30% of those students still had a palpable spleen without any increase in disease prevalence. Ten-year follow-up found no evidence for lymphoid malignancies. Furthermore, in some tropical countries (e.g., New Guinea), the incidence of splenomegaly may reach 60%. Thus, the presence of a palpable spleen does not always equate with the presence of disease.

Pathophysiology

Hyperplasia or hypertrophy is related to a particular splenic function such as reticuloendothelial hyperplasia (work hypertrophy) in diseases such as hereditary spherocytosis or thalassemia syndromes that require removal of large numbers of defective red blood cells and to immune hyperplasia in response to systemic infection (infectious mononucleosis, subacute bacterial endocarditis) or to immunologic diseases (immune thrombocytopenia, systemic lupus erythematosus, Felty's syndrome). Passive congestion results from decreased blood flow from the spleen in conditions that produce portal hypertension (cirrhosis, Budd-Chiari syndrome, congestive heart failure). Infiltrative diseases of the spleen include lymphomas, metastatic cancer, amyloidosis, Gaucher's disease, and myeloproliferative disorders with extramedullary hematopoiesis.

The differential diagnostic possibilities are fewer when the spleen is "massively enlarged," that is, it is palpable more than 8 cm below the left costal margin or its drained weight is 1000 g or more. Most such patients have non-Hodgkin's lymphoma, chronic lymphocytic leukemia, hairy cell leukemia, chronic myelogenous leukemia, myelofibrosis with myeloid metaplasia, or polycythemia vera.

Laboratory Results

The major laboratory abnormalities accompanying splenomegaly are determined by the underlying systemic illness. A complete blood count is the diagnostic examination needed with any patient presenting with splenic disorders. It is vital for a differential diagnosis. A complete blood count also identifies platelet or white blood cell dysfunction.

Clinical Manifestations

The most common symptoms produced by diseases involving the spleen are pain and a heavy sensation in the left upper quadrant. Massive splenomegaly may cause early satiety. Pain may result from acute swelling of the spleen with stretching of the capsule, infarction, or inflammation of the capsule. Symptoms of hypersplenism include fatigue, malaise, recurrent infection, and easy or prolonged bleeding. These symptoms occur from a hyperfunctional spleen that removes and destroys normal blood cells. In portal hypertension, transmitted backpressure results in hypersplenism, which leads to congestive failure of splenic function.

Vascular occlusion with infarction and pain is commonly seen in children with sickle cell crises. Rupture of the spleen, either from trauma or infiltrative disease that breaks the capsule, may result in intraperitoneal bleeding, shock, and death. The rupture itself may be painless.

Treatment

Correction or amelioration of certain hematologic and immunologic disorders may be attempted through splenectomy. Commonly accepted medical disease processes for which splenectomy is considered include idiopathic thrombocytopenic purpura, thrombotic thrombocytopenic purpura, Hodgkin's disease, lymphoma, certain leukemias, hereditary spherocytosis, hereditary hemolytic anemia, idiopathic autoimmune hemolytic anemia, and hypersplenism. Splenectomy may also be performed in the treatment of patients with thalassemia and sickle cell disease when these diseases are refractory to medical management and when hypersplenism supervenes. The development of primary (with no identifiable underlying cause) or secondary (from a known cause) hypersplenism may warrant splenectomy. Treatment of the primary disease process usually provides relief of symptoms. Splenectomy, however, is often a necessary part of therapy, particularly in long-standing disorders.

V SECTION

Hematologic System

A. AIDS/HIV INFECTION

Definition

Human immunodeficiency virus (HIV) is the most significant etiology of secondary immunosuppression that can result from infection that causes depletion of immune cells. The virus exists as two main types, HIV-1 and HIV-2. Of the two, HIV-1 is more prevalent and more pathogenic. The primary targets of HIV infection are $CD4^+$ lymphocytes. A glycoprotein on the viral envelope binds to the CD4 antigen to allow the virus to enter the T cell. HIV is a retrovirus, that is, its genome contains 2 strands of single-stranded RNA. After the virus enters the host cell, its RNA undergoes reverse transcription to produce complementary DNA that is incorporated into the host cell DNA. Synthesis of new viral RNA then occurs in the host cell followed by formation of new virus particles and their release to infect other $CD4^+$ cells. Infection with HIV alters T-cell function and causes cytotoxicity, leading to the characteristic decline in $CD4^+$ cells. Exactly how HIV infection kills T cells, though, is not known and may involve several mechanisms. Ultimately, with a sufficient fall in $CD4^+$ cells, individuals become susceptible to life-threatening opportunistic infections.

Pathophysiology

The epidemiologic basis for HIV infection begins with transmission of the virus through certain body fluids. Infection with HIV can progress to acquired immune deficiency syndrome (AIDS) and fatal disease. Although more than 25 million individuals have died as a result of AIDS complications since the first description of the disease, early detection, evaluation, and pharmacologic intervention have become very successful in controlling HIV infection in many individuals while preserving immune system integrity.

The potential sources of transmission of HIV are blood contact, sexual transmission, and perinatal exposure (see box below).

Routes of HIV Transmission

Absolute
Blood
Body fluids containing blood

Possible
Cerebrospinal fluid
Pericardial fluids
Amniotic fluids
Semen, vaginal secretions
Synovial fluid
Pleural fluid

Remote
Feces
Saliva
Sputum
Sweat
Tears
Urine
Wound drainage
Nasal secretions

Not Implicated in Health Care Settings
Human breast milk

Human immunodeficiency virus is transmitted through mucous membranes during anal, vaginal, and oral intercourse. Transmission of HIV also occurs through sharing injection equipment and needles. Vertical transmission occurs from mother to child. Blood, semen, vaginal fluid, breast milk, cerebrospinal fluid (CSF), amniotic fluid, and serosanguineous fluid can transmit HIV; saliva, tears, and sweat do not. The virus cannot survive outside the host, and 90% to 99% of infective HIV on dry surfaces is eliminated within hours. Insect bites and casual contact carry no risk.

As epidemic and scientific approaches to HIV infection evolved, the focus shifted from "risk groups" to "risky behaviors." This distinction is important because risk groups can give a false sense of security by implying that certain groups of individuals are less vulnerable to infection. *Risky behaviors* is a more useful term, falling along a spectrum of "no risk" (e.g., complete sexual abstinence), "very low risk" (e.g., 100% use of latex condoms), to "very high risk" (e.g., unprotected receptive anal intercourse with ejaculation), with other behaviors in midspectrum. The physician serves as a source of accurate information to be provided in simple, nonjudgmental terms because ultimately the patient will decide the acceptable degree of risk.

Acute infection with HIV is characterized by a mononucleosis-like illness, in which release of inflammatory mediators, including interleukin-1 (IL-1) and tumor necrosis factor α (TNF-α), causes symptoms such as malaise, fever, myalgias, and rash. At the same time, a transient decline in circulating $CD4^+$ cells occurs. Over several weeks after the primary infection, antibodies directed against virus envelope proteins are produced, and cytotoxic T lymphocytes (CTLs) begin to kill infected T cells that display HIV peptides. These immune responses permit resolution of the symptoms of acute infection; however, anti-HIV antibodies and CTLs become overwhelmed by viral replication and mutation, and progression of HIV infection occurs.

Spontaneous resolution of the acute symptoms of HIV infection is followed by a variable period of asymptomatic infection. If the infection is not treated, a gradual, progressive fall in $CD4^+$ cells occurs in conjunction with a gradual increase in the plasma viral load. Progression to AIDS in untreated individuals occurs in an average time of 10 years, although in some individuals, progression may occur much more rapidly or perhaps not at all. With respect to the latter possibility, there are reports of individuals who have not developed AIDS despite multiple exposures to HIV, suggesting that the adaptive immune system in some individuals may provide chronic protection by an as yet undefined mechanism. Clinically, AIDS is defined as a $CD4^+$ cell count less than 200 cells/μL or by the presence of an AIDS-indicator condition.

About 33 million people worldwide are living with HIV/AIDS in 2007. Of these, 2.7 million have been newly infected, and 2 million people have died of HIV/AIDS. Developing countries account for more than 95% of these infections (UN AIDS, 2007). From 2004 to 2007, there has been an increase of 15% in the incidence of HIV/AIDS cases in the United States. This increase occurred mainly in persons age 40 to 44 years, who accounted for 15% of all HIV/AIDS cases, likely caused by both changes in reporting systems and increased HIV testing.

A disproportionate number of minorities and women are affected by HIV. Blacks constituted 45% of newly diagnosed cases in 2006, with a rate of infection of 83.7 per 100,000. Of these, 60% are women. Blacks living with HIV/AIDS constituted about 60% of the adult HIV-positive population in 2007, with a rate of 76.7 per 100,000. Similarly, Hispanics, although constituting 12% of the population, reflected 17% of persons newly infected with HIV in 2006 and 20% of those living with HIV/AIDS in 2007, with rates of 29.3 and 20 per 100,000, respectively. Year-end prevalence rates in 2007 were 185.1 per 100,000 population, with a range between 2.2 in Samoa and 1750 per 100,000 in the District of Columbia.

Acquired immunodeficiency syndrome was diagnosed within 12 months of diagnosis of HIV infection for a larger percentage of Hispanics and male intravenous drug users (IVDUs) and men with high-risk heterosexual contact. Survival after AIDS diagnosis has increased in those who were diagnosed between 1998 and 2000, among men who have sex with men, and those who have acquired HIV perinatally. More whites survive 48 months after a diagnosis of AIDS than minorities. Survival has declined in IVDUs and with each year of age at diagnosis after age 35 (HIV/AIDS Surveillance Report, 2007).

The three main modes of transmission of HIV are as follows:

1. Through the mucous membranes during anal, vaginal, or oral sexual intercourse with an HIV-infected person. The average risk of transmission in heterosexual exposure is one in 1000 and increases with commercial sex workers to about five to 10 in 100. Whereas co-infection with other sexually transmitted diseases (STDs), rough sex, and higher viral load increase risk, condom use and male circumcision reduce risk. Uncircumcised men a run risk similar to a woman, and circumcised men may transmit the virus to female partners four times as efficiently as uncircumcised men. Postmenopausal women are more susceptible because of thinning of the vaginal mucosa. Risk of infection per act has been suggested from cohort studies, so physicians should avoid discussing risks in numeric terms.
2. Through the veins while sharing needles or injection paraphernalia with an HIV-infected person
3. Vertically from an HIV-infected mother to an infant during pregnancy, delivery, or through breastfeeding. High viral load, prolonged time after rupture of membranes, and chorioamnionitis increase risk of transmission, and peripartum prophylactic antiretroviral therapy decreases risk. The overall risk of transmission by breastfeeding is about 15% to 25% in 18- to 24-month-old infants.

Occupational exposure occurs by needlestick injuries (risk, 3:1000), infected blood or fluid splashing into the mouth or nose, or exposure to infected blood through a cut or an open wound. Mucous membrane exposure carries a risk of infection of about nine in 10,000. Transmission of HIV through infected blood is extremely rare after routine screening of the blood supply was initiated in 1985. With risk of transmission as low as two per million, 16 annual infections are accounted for by infectious donations. Neither insect bites nor casual contact carry any risk.

Human immunodeficiency virus can be transmitted by blood, semen, vaginal fluid, breast milk, and serosanguineous body fluids. Contact with CSF, amniotic fluid, and synovial fluid can be a risk factor for HIV transmission. Importantly, although HIV can be present in small quantities in saliva, sweat and tears, contact with these fluids does not transmit HIV. The virus cannot survive outside the host, and the amount of infective virus dried on surfaces is reduced by 90% to 99% in a few hours.

The two classification systems currently in use to monitor the severity of HIV illness and assist with its management have been developed by the Centers for Disease Control and Prevention (CDC) (see table on pg. 115) and the World Health Organization (WHO) (see box below). The CDC classification, last modified in 1993, uses $CD4^+$ counts and specific HIV-related conditions, but the WHO classification, developed in 1990 and revised in 2007, is guided by clinical observations and can be used in settings where access to $CD4^+$ tests is unavailable. The CDC lists AIDS categories as A3, B3, C1, C2, and C3, with 23 AIDS-defining conditions. The WHO includes primary HIV infection and four clinical stages.

Centers for Disease Control and Prevention Classification System of HIV/AIDS

CD4 Cell Count	Clinical Categories		
	A Asymptomatic Acute HIV or PGL	**B Symptomatic Conditions, not A or C**	**C AIDS Indicator Conditions**
>500 cells/mm^3	A1	B1	C1
200–499 cells/mm^3	A2	B2	C2
<200 cells/mm^3	A3	B3	C3

PGL, Persistent generalized lymphadenopathy.
Data from US Centers for Disease Control and Prevention. 1993 Revised classification system for HIV infection and expanded surveillance case definition for AIDS among adolescents and adults. *MMWR* 1992;41(RR-17):1-19.

World Health Organization Clinical Staging of HIV/AIDS

Primary HIV infection
Asymptomatic
Acute retroviral syndrome

Clinical Stage 1
Asymptomatic
Persistent generalized lymphadenopathy

Clinical Stage 2
Moderate unexplained weight loss (<10% body weight)
Recurrent respiratory infections (sinusitis, tonsillitis, otitis media, pharyngitis)
Herpes zoster
Angular cheilitis
Recurrent oral ulceration
Papular pruritic eruptions
Seborrheic dermatitis
Fungal nail infections

Clinical Stage 3
Severe, unexplained weight loss (>10% body weight)
Unexplained diarrhea lasting >1 month
Unexplained, persistent, constant or intermittent fever >1 month (>37.6° C)
Persistent oral candidiasis
Oral hairy leukoplakia
Pulmonary tuberculosis
Severe presumed bacterial infections (pneumonia, empyema, pyomyositis, bone and joint infections, meningitis, bacteremia)
Acute necrotizing gingivitis, stomatitis, periodontitis

Continued

World Health Organization Clinical Staging of HIV/AIDS—cont'd

Unexplained anemia (hemoglobin <8 g/dL)
Neutropenia (<500 cells/mm^3)
Chronic thrombocytopenia (<50,000 cells/mm^3)

Clinical Stage 4
All of the AIDS indicator conditions as defined by the CDC classification *and*
Atypical disseminated leishmaniasis
Symptomatic HIV-associated nephropathy
Symptomatic HIV-associated cardiomyopathy
Reactivation of American trypanosomiasis (meningoencephalitis or myocarditis)

CDC, Centers for Disease Control and Prevention.
Modified from World Health Organization. Case definitions of HIV for surveillance and revised clinical staging and immunological classification of HIV related disease in adults and children. Geneva, WHO, 2007. www.who.int/hiv/pub/guidelines/HIVstaging150307.pdf.

Category B: Symptomatic Conditions

These conditions must indicate defective cell-mediated immunity caused by HIV infection, or their clinical course and management must be complicated by HIV. Category B conditions include the following:

- Constitutional symptoms (fever >38.5° C or diarrhea) lasting more than 1 month
- Candidiasis: oropharyngeal or persistent or recurrent vulvovaginal
- Pelvic inflammatory disease
- Moderate or severe cervical dysplasia or carcinoma in situ
- Oral hairy leukoplakia
- Idiopathic thrombocytopenic purpura
- Peripheral neuropathy
- More than two episodes of multidermatomal herpes zoster
- Bacillary angiomatosis

Category C: AIDS-Defining Illnesses

Including bacterial, viral, fungal infections, parasitic infestations, and some cancers

Bacterial

- *Mycobacterium tuberculosis* infection at any site, pulmonary or extrapulmonary
- *Mycobacterium avium* complex disease; infection with *Mycobacterium kansasii* or other species, disseminated or extrapulmonary
- *Mycobacterium,* any species disseminated or extrapulmonary
- Bacterial pneumonia, recurrent (>2 episodes in 12 months)
- Nontyphoid *Salmonella* septicemia, recurrent

Viral

- Cytomegalovirus disease (other than liver, spleen, or nodes) and retinitis with vision loss
- Herpes simplex virus (chronic ulcer persisting >1 month, bronchitis, pneumonitis, esophagitis)
- Progressive multifocal leukoencephalopathy

Fungal

- Candidiasis of the esophagus, bronchi, trachea, or lungs
- Coccidioidomycosis, disseminated or extrapulmonary
- Cryptococcosis, extrapulmonary
- Histoplasmosis, disseminated or extrapulmonary
- Isosporiasis, chronic intestinal (persisting for >1 month)
- Pneumonia, recurrent (*Pneumocystis jiroveci*)

Parasitic

- Cryptosporidiosis, chronic intestinal (persisting for >1 month)
- Toxoplasmosis of brain
- Isosporiasis, chronic intestinal (persisting for >1 month)

HIV-Related Conditions

- Encephalopathy, HIV related
- Wasting syndrome, HIV related (weight loss >10% body weight with either chronic diarrhea of >2 stools/day for 1 month or chronic weakness and documented fever >1 month)

Cancers

- Cervical cancer, invasive
- Kaposi sarcoma
- Lymphoma (Burkitt, immunoblastic, or primary lymphoma of the brain)
- Cancers and chronic renal failure associated with AIDS and lipodystrophy, insulin resistance, osteoporosis, and cardiovascular complications of HAART are being increasingly recognized and addressed.

The best defense is a good offense, and there is no substitute for strict adherence to universal precautions. If despite these efforts you or a coworker are exposed to HIV, postexposure prophylaxis is available. Because most occupational exposures do not result in HIV transmission, the guidelines for postexposure prophylaxis weigh the relative risk of infection against the potential toxicity of treatment. The relative risk of infection depends on both the type and amount of blood exposure. The risk of transmission is increased by (1) percutaneous exposure, (2) devices contaminated with visible blood, (3) hollow-bore needles, and (4) high viral titer (i.e., a patient late in the course of the disease). The three classes of antiretroviral agents recommended for prophylactic treatment include nucleoside reverse transcriptase inhibitors, non-nucleoside reverse transcriptase inhibitors, and protease inhibitors. All are associated with a number of toxicities. A basic two-drug regimen is most often recommended, with an expanded three-drug regimen reserved for high-risk exposure (see table on pg. 118). The U.S. Public Health Service guidelines recommend that clinicians consider known drug resistance in their area or documented drug resistance in the source patient, or both, when selecting a prophylactic protocol. The duration of treatment is 4 weeks.

Anesthetic Considerations

HIV-infected patients may require a variety of surgical interventions. Although several studies have evaluated the effects of surgery and anesthesia in HIV-infected patients, to date there is no conclusive evidence to support any particular set of recommendations. Most alterations caused by various anesthetic agents and techniques are transient and have not been shown to contribute to any adverse outcome.

Recommended HIV Postexposure Prophylaxis (PEP) for Percutaneous Injuries

	Infection Status of Source				
Exposure Type	**HIV Positive Class 1***	**HIV Positive Class 2***	**Source of Unknown HIV Status†**	**Unknown Source‡**	**HIV Negative**
Less severe§	Recommend basic two-drug PEP	Recommend expanded three-drug PEP	Generally, no PEP warranted; however, consider basic two-drug PEP‖ for source with HIV risk factors¶	Generally, no PEP warranted; however, consider basic two-drug PEP‖ in settings where exposure to HIV-infected persons is likely	No PEP warranted
More severe**	Recommend expanded three-drug PEP	Recommend expanded three-drug PEP	Generally, no PEP warranted; however, consider basic two-drug PEP‖ for source with HIV risk factors¶	Generally, no PEP warranted; however, consider basic two-drug PEP‖ in settings where exposure to HIV-infected persons is likely	No PEP warranted

From U.S. Public Health Service: Updated U.S. Public Health Service guidelines for the management of occupational exposures to HBV, HCV, and HIV and recommendations for postexposure prophylaxis. *MMWR Recomm Rep* 50(RR-11):1-42, 2001.

*HIV positive, class 1—asymptomatic HIV infection or known low viral load (e.g., $<$1500 RNA copies/mL). HIV positive, class 2— symptomatic HIV infection, AIDS, acute seroconversion, or known high viral load. If drug resistance is a concern, obtain expert consultation. Initiation of PEP should not be delayed pending expert consultation, and because expert consultation alone cannot substitute for face-to-face counseling, resources should be available to provide immediate evaluation and follow-up care for all exposures.

†Source of unknown HIV status (e.g., deceased source person with no samples available for HIV testing).

‡Unknown source (e.g., a needle from a sharps disposal container).

§Less severe (e.g., solid needle and superficial injury).

‖The designation "consider PEP" indicates that PEP is optional and should be based on an individualized decision between the exposed person and the treating clinician.

¶If PEP is offered and taken and the source is later determined to be HIV negative, PEP should be discontinued.

**More severe (e.g., large-bore hollow needle, deep puncture, blood visible on device, or needle used in a patient's artery or vein).

Antiretroviral Medicines

Generic (Brand)	Abbreviation
Nucleoside/Nucleotide Reverse Transcriptase Inhibitors	
Abacavir (Ziagen)	ABC
Emtricitabine (Emtriva)	FTC
Didanosine (Videx)	ddI
Lamivudine (Epivir)	3TC
Stavudine (Zerit)	d4T
Tenofovir (Viread)	TDF
Zalcitabine (Hivid)	ddC
Zidovudine (Retrovir)	ZDV
Abacavir and lamivudine (Epzicom)	ABC + 3TC
Emtricitabine and tenofovir (Truvada)	FTC + TDF
Lamivudine and zidovudine (Combivir)	3TC + ZDV
Non-nucleoside Reverse Transcriptase Inhibitors (NNRTIs)	
Delavirdine mesylate (Rescriptor)	DLV
Efavirenz (EFV)	EFV
Etravirine (Intelence)	TMC-125
Nevirapine (Viramune)	NVP
Efavirenz, emtricitabine, and tenofovir (Atripla)	EFV + FTC + TDF
Protease Inhibitors	
Atazanavir (Reyataz)	ATZ
Darunavir (Prezista)	TMC-114
Fosamprenavir calcium (Lexiva)	FPV
Indinavir sulfate (Crixivan)	IDV
Lopinavir and ritonavir (Kaletra)	LPV/r
Nelfinavir mesylate (Viracept)	NFV
Ritonavir (Norvir)	RTV
Saquinavir mesylate (Invirase)	SQV
Tipranavir (Aptivus)	TPV
Fusion Inhibitor	
Enfuvirtide (Fuzeon)	T-20
CCR5 Inhibitor	
Maraviroc (Selzentry)	
Integrase Strand Transfer Inhibitor	
Raltegravir (Isentress)	

It is important to understand the patient's status both in response to and the application of antiretroviral therapy and other treatments when an operative procedure is planned. Appreciation of both recent and past therapeutic efforts and the patient's response is important in preparing the HIV-infected patient for anesthesia and related care. Consultation with and participation of the patient's primary care provider in the planning process can be beneficial.

When anesthesia care is planned, attention should focus on possible end-organ and systemic dysfunction. Clinically significant alterations occur in many organ systems, particularly in the advanced disease stages of HIV infection, when vigilant monitoring and, at times, intensive intervention may be necessary. The patient (or his or her legal representative or caregiver)

Antiretroviral Regimens for Treatment-Naïve Patients

Preferred Regimens: Level 1
Ritonavir-boosted darunavir + tenofovir + emtricitabine
Ritonavir-boosted atazanavir + tenofovir + emtricitabine
Efavirenz + tenofovir + emtricitabine
Raltegravir + tenofovir + emtricitabine

Alternative Regimens: Level 2
Efavirenz + (abacavir *or* zidovudine)/lamivudine
Nevirapine + zidovudine/lamivudine
Atazanavir/ritonavir + (abacavir *or* zidovudine)/lamivudine
FPV/r* (once or twice daily) + *either* [(abacavir *or* zidovudine)/lamivudine] *or* tenofovir/emtricitabine
LPV/r† (once or twice daily) + *either* [(abacavir *or* zidovudine)/lamivudine] *or* tenofovir/emtricitabine
Saquinavir/ritonavir + tenofovir/emtricitabine

*Fosamprenavir calcium and ritonavir.
† Lopinavir and ritonavir (Kaletra).
From Rakel RE, Rakel DP. *Textbook of Family Medicine.* 8th ed. St. Louis: Saunders; 2011.

should be included in the planning and evaluation of potential care options. Informed consent may be the responsibility of a legal guardian or durable power of attorney designee for the patient who may be mentally incompetent.

The immunocompromised patient may have combined deficiencies that predispose to significant or fatal outcomes. It is important to remember that microorganisms that are not routinely pathogenic can cause the demise of these patients. Meticulous implementation of infection control measures throughout the perioperative period should be a primary focus in the care of these vulnerable patients. Respiratory isolation should be used when it is either known or suspected that airborne pathogens may be transmitted. Examples of such pathogens include the causative agents of tuberculosis and varicella. The immune system compromise resulting from HIV infection markedly increases the susceptibility to tuberculosis, and recurrent or newly acquired tuberculosis is frequently the cause of death for persons infected with HIV. A striking clinical feature of tuberculosis in HIV-infected patients is a high incidence of extrapulmonary involvement, usually with concomitant pulmonary presentation.

Although equipment preparedness is important for every patient to whom anesthesia is administered, it is of particular significance for immunocompromised patients. Meticulous attention to behaviors and adherence to strict aseptic technique in providing care to these most vulnerable patients are paramount to safe practice and quality patient care. The anesthesia machine and its multitude of components should be adequately maintained, cleaned, and disinfected, and appropriate sterile components should be changed between each use in accordance with both approved infection control practices and manufacturers' recommendations.

A multitude of clinical presentations have the potential to affect anesthesia management in patients infected with HIV. Oxygenation and metabolic functions are frequently impaired during progressive HIV infection. Pulmonary infections can alter both gas exchange and lung perfusion and create ventilation–perfusion mismatch. Dehydration and hypovolemia secondary to gastrointestinal disturbances can further complicate the patient's clinical course. A thorough preoperative assessment, including current physical examination, laboratory results, and radiographic examination, combined with other studies as indicated by patient presentation and current disease state, is critical before anesthesia.

Complications from HIV

Wasting syndrome may be seen in HIV-infected patients and results from disturbances in food absorption and metabolism. This syndrome is defined as profound, involuntary weight loss greater than 10% of baseline body weight. Chronic diarrhea frequently contributes to this scenario. Parenteral nutrition and appetite stimulation are usually required when this syndrome is persistent. Preoperative assessment should include evaluation of volume status and related physiologic studies to plan appropriate management.

Neurologic evaluation is essential for HIV-infected patients. Both the central and peripheral nervous systems can be impaired because of direct disease effects, concomitant opportunistic infections, or adverse effects of therapeutic agents used to combat viral insult. Peripheral neuropathies may result in considerable discomfort or physical limitations, and autonomic neuropathy may result in some degree of cardiovascular instability requiring immediate or continuous intervention. AIDS-related dementia can influence both motor and cognitive states, particularly in advanced disease states.

Non-Hodgkin's lymphoma, manifesting as a space-occupying lesion within the central nervous system, may require surgical or chemotherapeutic intervention. Kaposi's sarcoma, a cancer that invades endothelial tissues, can attack both skin and internal organs. Women infected with HIV may develop cervical dysplasia and cancers.

As HIV infection progresses to AIDS, advanced disease combinations emerge that would otherwise be resisted in the immunocompetent host. These opportunistic disease processes increase in both manifestation and severity as the immune system fails. Both acute and chronic bacterial infections tend to plague HIV-infected individuals. *Mycobacterium avium-intracellulare* (MAI) infection is characterized by intractable diarrhea and resultant wasting states. Splenic and pulmonary infections with MAI lead to severe thrombocytopenia and tuberculosis. MAI attacks the immunosuppressed host easily and is transmittable.

Several viral infections can occur or recur from previously dormant states as HIV disease progresses. Herpes simplex and varicella infections can invade oral and esophageal tissues and the central nervous system. Cytomegalovirus can affect the gastrointestinal and pulmonary systems, resulting in colitis and pneumonia. Retinal invasion may lead to marked visual disturbances and blindness. Ganciclovir is used to treat cytomegalovirus infection.

Opportunistic protozoal infections can develop in persons with advanced HIV infection. *Pneumocystis carinii* pneumonia is responsible for the majority of deaths secondary to opportunistic infection in HIV-infected persons. Fever and impaired gas exchange frequently result in hypoxemia, and pneumothorax is not uncommon. Toxoplasmosis encephalitis can affect both central nervous system function and the sensorium. Cryptosporidiosis can trigger considerable diarrhea, resulting in significant dehydration and related electrolyte imbalance. Volume status must be judiciously evaluated and monitored.

Fungal infection is responsible for histoplasmosis and aspergillosis pneumonia in HIV-infected patients. Such insults can result in significant febrile and hypoxic states, with impairment of gas exchange and overall sensorium. Disseminated candidiasis infections are responsible for oropharyngeal and esophageal pathology that includes stomatitis, dysphagia, and esophagitis. Patients with cryptococcal meningitis can experience increased intracranial pressure.

Childbearing women constitute a significant portion of reported cases of HIV and AIDS. This is of considerable significance because perinatal transmission accounts for greater than 80% of all pediatric AIDS cases that have been reported in the United States. Pregnant patients with HIV present unique challenges for health maintenance. In advanced stages of HIV infection, anemia can be particularly significant, frequently necessitating transfusion therapy. Elective cesarean section in HIV-positive parturients appears to reduce the risk of HIV transmission from mother to neonate. However, complications of cesarean section, including blood loss and wound infection, may be exaggerated in HIV-infected parturients as a result of immunosuppression.

Because many physical manifestations of HIV-related illness involve neuromuscular disorders, pain management can be a difficult challenge in patients with advanced HIV infection. Both routine analgesic modalities and analgesic agents combined with the use of various chemotherapies, nerve blocks, and complementary therapies have been beneficial in treating acute postoperative and obstetric pain in HIV-infected patients.

Managing HIV Infection

Occupational Safety

The primary emphasis in managing HIV infection during anesthesia and other aspects of patient care is an effective prevention program. Because the routes of HIV transmission are well known, an appropriate infection control program with consistent application of proven blood and body substance precautions can prevent disease transmission. Universal precautions were developed after known modes of transmission of both HIV and hepatitis B virus (both bloodborne pathogens) were clarified. More recent efforts to apply this practice throughout all patient care areas have resulted in the consistent application of standard precautions during patient care. The basic premise on which these guidelines is based is the prevention of parenteral, mucous membrane, and nonintact skin exposure to blood and certain body fluids from all patients. Guidelines include the following:

1. Gloves must be worn when contact with body substances is suspected or possible.
2. A plastic gown or apron must be worn when soiling with body substances is likely.
3. Protective masks and eyewear must be worn in the presence of airborne disease or for preventing splash or aerosolization of body substances to eyes or mucous membranes.
4. Hands must be thoroughly washed before and after body substances or articles possibly covered with body substances have been handled and after gloves have been removed at the completion of each task or procedure.
5. Uncapped needles and syringes must be discarded in puncture-resistant receptacles placed as close to their point of use as is practical.

6. Trash and linens must be discarded in impervious, sealed plastic bags that are labeled as infectious and transported according to standard precautions.

Self-protection against HIV and all other infectious bloodborne pathogens such as hepatitis B and C viruses is an essential element of safe practice. The Occupational Safety and Health Administration (OSHA) Act, which became effective in 1992, mandates that employers minimize occupational exposure to all bloodborne pathogens in workplaces where a potential for such exposures exists. Known or suspected exposure to bloodborne pathogens should be responded to immediately with appropriate action, as recommended by OSHA and institutional infection control standards.

B. ANEMIA

Definition

Anemia is a deficiency of erythrocytes caused by either too rapid a loss or too slow production of the cells. Therefore, numeric concentrations of hemoglobin are reduced, and the oxygen-carrying capacity of blood is decreased. This results in reduced oxygen delivery to peripheral tissues.

Pathophysiology

Anemia may result from acute blood loss; however, iron-deficiency anemia from persistent blood loss is the most frequent form of chronic anemia. Anemia is also associated with many chronic diseases, such as persistent infections, neoplastic processes, connective tissue disorders, and renal and hepatic disease. Other forms of anemia include aplastic anemia, which involves bone marrow depression, and megaloblastic anemias, which are related to deficiencies of vitamin B_{12} or folic acid. Finally, various anemias can result from intravascular hemolysis of erythrocytes.

Laboratory Results

Erythrocyte production can be assessed from the reticulocyte count in peripheral blood. For instance, a low reticulocyte count in the presence of a low hematocrit suggests an erythrocyte production defect, rather than blood loss or hemolysis, as a cause of anemia. A decrease in hematocrit that exceeds 1% per day is most likely related to acute blood loss or intravascular hemolysis.

Clinical Manifestations

A history of reduced exercise tolerance characterized as exertional dyspnea is a frequent clinical sign of chronic anemia. A functional heart murmur and evidence of cardiomegaly may be detected on physical examination. The decreased oxygen-carrying capacity of arterial blood is reflected in the arterial oxygen content equation (i.e., arterial oxygen content = [hemoglobin × 1.39] × oxygen saturation + [arterial oxygen tension × 0.003]). This decrease is compensated for by a rightward shift oxyhemoglobin dissociation curve and an increase in cardiac output. Decreased blood viscosity and vasodilation lower systemic vascular resistance and increase blood flow. Blood pressure and heart rate remain unchanged with increased cardiac output. The decreased exercise tolerance reflects the inability of cardiac output to increase to maintain tissue oxygenation when these patients become physically active.

Treatment

Packed erythrocytes can be transfused preoperatively to increase hemoglobin concentrations, with peak effect at 24 hours to restore intravascular fluid volume and blood viscosity. Compared with a similar volume of whole blood, erythrocytes produce about twice the increase in hemoglobin concentration. Packed red blood cells have a hematocrit of 70%, and cell saver has a hematocrit of 45% to 65%.

Anesthetic Considerations

Transfusion guidelines include assessment of the patient's cardiovascular status, age, anticipation of further blood loss, arterial oxygenation, mixed venous oxygen tension, cardiac output, and infection risk. (Minimum acceptable hemoglobin concentrations for elective surgery have changed over the years. The "old" value of 10 g/dL has been lowered to approximately 8 g/dL, depending on the patient's preoperative status, intraoperative status, operation, and institution.) The presence of neurovascular and cardiovascular disease can diminish blood flow to the brain and heart. Further decreasing oxygen delivery to these tissues caused by anemia can result in acute stroke or myocardial ischemia or infarction. If elective surgery is performed, the anesthetic regimen should be geared toward preventing changes that may interfere with tissue oxygen delivery. Adequate oxygenation can be obtained with a hemoglobin of 8 g/dL as long as the patient is normovolemic. For example, myocardial depression produced by volatile agents may reduce cardiac output and thus impair the patient's compensatory mechanisms. Likewise, leftward shifts of the oxyhemoglobin dissociation curve (as produced by hyperventilation resulting in respiratory alkalosis) can impair release of oxygen from hemoglobin to the tissues. It is also important to maintain body temperature because hypothermia will cause a leftward shift of the curve. Intraoperative blood loss should be promptly replaced and closely monitored. Finally, it is important to minimize shivering or increases in body temperature postoperatively because these changes can greatly increase total body oxygen requirements.

Rule-of-Thumb Transfusion Guidelines

- Blood loss >20%
- Hemoglobin <8 g/dL
- Hemoglobin <10 g/dL with major disease or with autologous blood
- Hemoglobin <12 g/dL when ventilator dependent

C. DISSEMINATED INTRAVASCULAR COAGULATION

Definition

Disseminated intravascular coagulation (DIC) is a coagulation disorder characterized by ongoing activation of the coagulation cascade in response to a clinical or systemic event. Organ damage and death are the result of widespread microvascular bleeding and thrombosis.

Pathophysiology

The diagnosis of DIC is usually secondary to a systemic illness or insult. Coagulation activation ranges from mild thrombocytopenia and prolongation of clotting times to acute DIC characterized by extensive bleeding and thrombosis. During overactive coagulation, the available platelets and coagulation factors are consumed. This consumption along with fibrinolysis exhausts the hemostatic balance. Rarely is the primary cause a coagulation deficiency or dysfunction.

Several factors play an important role in the pathogenesis of DIC, including the propagation of thrombin, alteration in anticoagulant activity, impaired functioning of the fibrinolytic system, and the release of cytokines. Tissue factor release is considered to play the most important role in the development of a hyperthrombinemia in DIC. Mediators such as antithrombin and tissue factor pathway inhibitor that normally inhibit coagulation are altered. Reasons for this impairment include septicemia, liver impairment, capillary leakage, and the release of endotoxins and proinflammatory cytokines. The initial increased fibrinolytic activity is followed by the release of plasminogen activator inhibitor type 1 (PAI-1), which in turn impairs fibrinolysis and leads to accelerated thrombus formation in DIC. And, lastly, activated protein C mediates the release of inflammatory cytokines such as TNF and ILs from endothelial cells. Complement activation and kinin generation increase the coagulation response, leading to subsequent vascular occlusion.

Diagnosis

A diagnosis of DIC is made by considering the patient's clinical picture in conjunction with laboratory tests (platelet count, activated partial thromboplastin time [aPTT], prothrombin time [PT], fibrin-related markers such as fibrin degradation products, D dimer, fibrinogen, and antithrombin). Additionally, a scoring system developed by the International Society of Thrombosis and Haemostasis assists with the diagnosis. Overt (acute) DIC is characterized by ecchymosis, petechiae, mucosal bleeding, depletion of platelets, clotting factors, and bleeding at puncture sites. A score of 5 or above is comparable with overt DIC. Nonovert (chronic) DIC is characterized by thromboembolism accompanied by evidence of activation of the coagulation system. A score of below 5 is suggestive for nonovert DIC.

Treatment

The management and treatment of patients with DIC always depends on the underlying cause. In obstetric catastrophes, DIC may resolve as a result of prompt delivery, and treatment of sepsis with antibiotic therapy may halt the progression of DIC. Restoration of physiologic anticoagulant pathways with activated protein C in the treatment of sepsis with overt DIC holds promise. Activated protein C inactivates factors Va and VIIIa, resulting in decreased thrombin formation. Its use in treating patients with severe sepsis in DIC has been approved by the U.S. Food and Drug Administration. For individuals requiring surgery who are bleeding or at risk for active bleeding, correction of coagulopathy with platelets ($<$50,000/mm^3), fresh-frozen plasma, and cryoprecipitate (fibrinogen $<$50 mg/dL) must be used. Continued replacement of blood products should be based on the clinical picture and reassessment of laboratory results.

The use of anticoagulants for DIC remains controversial, especially for a patient who is prone to bleeding. Also, the use of antithrombin III concentrates may prove effective in inhibiting coagulation; however, its use is yet to be conclusive.

D. HEMOPHILIA

Definition and Incidence

Hemophilia is an X-linked recessive disorder. It is a hematologic disorder of unpredictable bleeding patterns. Patients are either deficient in factor IX (hemophilia A) or factor VIII:C (hemophilia B). Hemophilia affects males, and females are carriers of the disease.

Pathophysiology

Hemophilia A is grouped into mild (bleeding surfaces after trauma or surgery), moderate (rarely have extensive unprovoked bleeding), and severe (absence of factor VIII:C in the plasma) forms. People with hemophilia exhibit spontaneous bleeding, muscle hematomas, and generalized joint pain. Continued joint bleeding often results in decreased range of motion and progressive joint arthropathy and often requires orthopedic surgical intervention throughout their lives. Hemophiliacs also exhibit excessive bleeding after trauma.

Anesthetic Considerations

For patients with hemophilia or a family history of hemophilia, a preoperative assessment of hemostasis is imperative. Preoperative laboratory tests should include a platelet count and function, a coagulation panel (PT, partial thromboplastin time [PTT], factor VIII, factor IX, and fibrinogen), as well as an inhibitor test. If the hemophiliac was given a test dose of factor VIII preoperatively, the response to the test dose should be evaluated. The patient should be typed and cross-matched because even a low-risk procedure for bleeding can be catastrophic for patients with hemophilia.

A clearly defined anesthesia plan is essential for patients with hemophilia because uncontrolled bleeding is certainly a possibility. Factor VIII concentrated can be given before surgery. Factor VII is administered intraoperatively to augment thrombin generation and deter bleeding. The dose should be precalculated and vial availability confirmed before going into the operating room. Desmopressin (0.3 mcg/kg) can also be administered to increase plasma levels of factor VIII:C and von Willebrand factor VIII for mild to moderate hemophilia. There is no risk for viral transmission when either of these drugs is administered.

E. HEPARIN-INDUCED THROMBOCYTOPENIA

Definition and Incidence

Heparin-induced thrombocytopenia (HIT) is a disorder of coagulation that is a direct consequence of heparin therapy. One of the few relative versus absolute contraindications to heparin therapy is HIT. In the United States, a yearly estimate of 600,000 new cases of HIT occur, with as many as 300,000 patients developing thrombotic complications and 90,000 patients dying.

Pathophysiology

HIT is a special case of drug-induced immune-mediated thrombocytopenia associated with arterial and venous thrombosis, rather than bleeding. It is seen in 2% to 5% of patients exposed to unfractionated heparin and in 0.7% of patients given low-molecular-weight heparin (LMWH); it almost never occurs in patients exposed only to fondaparinux. To understand this disease, one must know that platelets can secrete a protein, platelet factor 4 (PF4), that can bind to heparin. HIT is caused by an antibody that binds to this PF4–heparin complex. Large complexes of antibodies directed against heparin-bound PF4 accumulate on the surface of platelets. At times, these anti-PF4 immunoglobulins bind to the Fc receptor that is also present on the platelet surface. The interaction of platelet Fc receptors and anti-PF4 antibodies causes activation of the platelet, release of more PF4, and a cycle of events that leads to the stimulation of even more platelets. Ultimately, it also leads to activation of the coagulation cascade. The activation of platelets and the clotting cascade leads to the formation of thrombi and thrombocytopenia.

Heparin-induced thrombocytopenia typically occurs 4 to 14 days after patients are given heparin by any route (even subcutaneously or in extremely low doses by heparin flush). This lag between heparin exposure and the appearance of HIT is due to the time it takes for the immune response to generate the requisite antibodies against the heparin–PF4 complex. Some patients who have been exposed to heparin within the past several months already have preexisting antibodies, and they may develop an acute onset of HIT within the first day of reinitiating the drug.

If a patient has HIT, all heparin should be stopped immediately. This includes subcutaneous injections of "minidose" heparin, heparin flushes of intravenous lines, and LMWH; even heparin-coated intravenous catheters should be withdrawn. Alternative anticoagulation, such as a direct thrombin inhibitor such as recombinant hirudin or argatroban, should be administered, at least until the platelet count normalizes. Warfarin should not be used in cases of acute HIT because of its delayed therapeutic effect and its association with venous limb gangrene. Because patients rarely become profoundly thrombocytopenic as a result of HIT alone, platelet transfusions are typically not required. In fact, some reports suggest that platelet transfusions can actually precipitate thrombotic complications, although this remains controversial.

Laboratory Assays for Heparin-Induced Thrombocytopenia

Assay	Sensitivity (%)	Specificity (%)	Positive Predictive Value (%)	Negative Predictive Value (%)
Functional assay (e.g., serotonin release assay)	88	≈100	≈100	81
PF4/heparin enzyme immunoassay (ELISA)	95–98	86	93	95

ELISA, Enzyme-linked immunosorbent assay; *PF4,* platelet factor 4.

F. LEUKEMIA

Definition

Leukemia is the uncontrolled production of leukocytes caused by cancerous mutation of lymphogenous cells or myelogenous cells. Lymphocytic leukemias begin in lymph nodes or other lymphogenous tissues and then spread to other areas of the body. Myeloid leukemias begin as cancerous production of myelogenous cells in bone marrow, with spread to extramedullary organs. Cancerous cells usually do not resemble other leukocytes and lack the usual functional characteristics of white blood cells. Leukemia cells may infiltrate the liver, spleen, and meninges and produce signs of dysfunction at these sites.

Incidence, Pathophysiology, Laboratory Results, and Treatment

Acute lymphoblastic leukemia accounts for approximately 15% of all leukemias in adults. Central nervous system dysfunction is common. These patients are highly susceptible to life-threatening infections, including those produced by *Pneumocystis carinii (jiroveci)* and cytomegalovirus.

Chronic lymphocytic leukemia accounts for approximately 25% of all leukemias and is most common in elderly men. The diagnosis is confirmed by the presence of lymphocytosis ($>15{,}000/mm^3$) and lymphocytic infiltrates in bone marrow. There may be neutropenia with an associated increased susceptibility to bacterial infections. Treatment is with cancer chemotherapeutic drugs classified as alkylating agents.

Acute myeloid leukemia can result in death in about 3 months if untreated. Patients present with fever, weakness, bleeding, and hepatosplenomegaly. Chemotherapy produces a temporary remission in about half of patients.

Patients with chronic myeloid leukemia present with massive hepatosplenomegaly and white blood cell counts greater than $50{,}000/mm^3$. Fever and weight loss reflect hypermetabolism. Anemia may be severe. Splenectomy is routine in these patients.

Chemotherapy is the best available therapy for irradiation of cancerous cells anywhere in the body. Adverse clinical effects of these drugs include bone marrow suppression (susceptibility to infection, thrombocytopenia, and anemia), nausea, vomiting, diarrhea, ulceration of the gastrointestinal mucosa, and alopecia. Destruction of tumor cells by chemotherapy produces a uric acid load that may result in urate nephropathy and gouty arthritis. Bone marrow transplantation is also becoming an increasingly successful treatment for leukemia.

Anesthetic Considerations

Management of anesthesia for patients with leukemia requires a clear understanding of the mechanisms of action, potential interactions, and likely toxicities associated with the use of cancer chemotherapeutic drugs. Patients taking doxorubicin or daunorubicin (antibiotics) may develop cardiomyopathy leading to congestive heart failure, which is often refractory to cardiac inotropic drugs. Cardiomegaly or pleural effusions may be found on chest radiographs. Marked left ventricular dysfunction was found to persist for as long as 3 years after the drug was discontinued. Nonspecific and usually benign electrocardiographic changes have been observed in 10% of patients. Bleomycin is an antibiotic that can cause pulmonary toxicity, with dyspnea and nonproductive cough being the initial manifestations. Pulmonary function tests demonstrate "restrictive" pulmonary disease. The inspired fraction of oxygen should be maintained at less than 30% during surgery because patients are susceptible to the toxic pulmonary effects of oxygen while they are receiving bleomycin therapy.

Strict aseptic technique is important because of immunosuppression. Preoperatively, signs of central nervous system depression, autonomic nervous system dysfunction, and peripheral neuropathies should be noted. Renal or hepatic dysfunction should influence the choice of anesthesia and muscle relaxants. Volatile anesthetics may reduce myocardial contractility in patients with cardiotoxicity related to chemotherapeutic drugs (i.e. Adriamycin). Arterial blood gases should be monitored. Replacing fluid losses with colloid rather than crystalloid solutions in patients with pulmonary fibrosis may be considered. In addition, possible postoperative ventilation, depending on the length of the procedure and the degree of fibrosis, should be considered. Other considerations include:

- A risk of infection from immunosuppression exists.
- Renal function is affected by uric acid production.
- A thorough neurologic assessment related to chemotherapy treatment is indicated.
- Patients with acute lymphoblastic leukemia may develop malignant hyperthermia.
- Nitrous oxide should be avoided in bone marrow transplantation. (The use of nitrous oxide in patients donating bone marrow or undergoing bone marrow transplantation should be avoided because of the potential for drug-induced adverse effects on the bone marrow itself. Donors may be given heparin before removal of bone marrow, and anticoagulation can complicate the use of spinal or epidural anesthesia for this procedure.)

G. POLYCYTHEMIA VERA

Definition and Pathophysiology

Polycythemia vera is a myeloproliferative neoplastic disorder that generally occurs in patients between 60 and 70 years of age. Hyperactivity of myeloid progenitor cells results in increased production of erythrocytes, leukocytes, and platelets.

Laboratory Results

Hemoglobin concentrations typically exceed 18 g/dL, and platelet counts can be greater than 400,000/mm^3.

Clinical Manifestations

Clinical symptoms are the result of hyperviscosity of the blood, which leads to stasis of blood flow and an increased incidence of vascular thrombosis, particularly in the cardiovascular and central nervous systems. Erythromelalgia (burning pain) in the fingers and toes is caused by digital ischemia. Defective platelet function is the most likely mechanism for spontaneous hemorrhage, which may occur in these patients. Splenomegaly is often present.

Treatment

Treatment entails reducing the hematocrit to near-normal levels to about 40% by phlebotomy before elective surgery.

Anesthetic Considerations

Surgery in the presence of uncontrolled polycythemia vera is associated with a high incidence of perioperative hemorrhage and postoperative venous thrombosis. In emergency situations, viscosity of the blood can be reduced by intravenous infusions of crystalloid solutions or low-molecular-weight dextrans. NPO (nothing by mouth) fluid replacement should be infused early to assist in decreasing blood viscosity.

H. SICKLE CELL DISEASE

Definition

Sickle cell disease is one of the more commonly inherited hemoglobinopathies.

Pathophysiology

Sickle cell is a disorder transmitted as an autosomal recessive trait that causes an abnormality of the globin genes in hemoglobin. A person who is homozygous for hemoglobin S manifests the disorder. Individuals may have the sickle cell trait or sickle cell disease. The sickle cell trait is a heterozygous disorder seen in 10% of African Americans. Their hemoglobin S levels are normally 30% to 50%, and sickling is seen with a Po_2 of 20 to 30 mmHg. Sickle cell disease is a homozygous disorder seen in 0.5% to 1.0% of African Americans. The majority of the hemoglobin molecule is hemoglobin S, and sickling is seen with a Po_2 of 30 to 40 mmHg. A crisis may be caused by a decrease of oxygen saturation and temperature, infections, dehydration, stasis, or acidosis. These complicated scenarios translate into perioperative mortality rates of 10% and postoperative complications of 50%.

Anesthetic Considerations

Suggestions for intraoperative management of patients with sickle cell disease are listed in the following box.

Intraoperative Management of Patients with Sickle Cell Disease

- Standard monitors
- Anesthetic technique appropriate for patient and surgical procedure
- Continue hydration (usually 1.5 times maintenance depending on renal status)
- At least 50% inspired oxygen concentration
- Controlled ventilation or titration of sedation to maintain normocapnia
- Maintain oxygen saturation >95% at all times
- Transfuse if necessary to replace surgical blood loss, avoid increasing the Hb >11 g/dL
- Maintain normothermia

From Lewis MA, Goodwin SR: Sickle cell disease and acute porphyria. In Lobato EB, Gravenstein N, Kirby RR. *Complications in Anesthesiology.* Philadelphia: Lippincott Williams & Wilkins; 2008:550.

There is no universal method for caring for patients with a sickle cell disorder. It is suggested that patients with a preoperative hemoglobin A level of at least 50% and a hematocrit of at least 35% may have less risk of an intraoperative crisis as an effort is made to correct anemia. By providing preoperative transfusion supplement, there is a risk of increasing the blood's viscosity causing end-organ damage. Anesthesia management that includes adequate hydration, saturation, normothermia, normal acid–base balance, and proper positioning and analgesia may interrupt an intraoperative and postoperative crisis.

I. THALASSEMIA

Definition

Thalassemia is an inherited autosomal recessive disorder resulting in a person's inability to synthesize structurally normal hemoglobin.

Incidence and Prevalence

Thalassemia major usually affects Greek and Italian children.

Pathophysiology

Patients have a genetic inability to synthesize structurally normal hemoglobin. Thalassemia major reflects an inability to form the chains of hemoglobin. As a result, adult hemoglobin A is not formed, and anemia develops during the first year of life as fetal hemoglobin disappears. Thalassemia minor reflects a heterozygote state that results in mild anemia. Thalassemia results from the lack of production of chains of adult hemoglobin. The homozygous form of thalassemia is incompatible with life, resulting in intrauterine demise or early neonatal death.

Clinical Manifestations

Thalassemia major is associated with jaundice, hepatosplenomegaly, and susceptibility to infection. Death can result from cardiac hemochromatosis. Supraventricular cardiac dysrhythmias and congestive heart failure are common. Hemothorax and spinal cord compression may occur secondary to massive extramedullary hematopoiesis and destruction of vertebral bodies. Overgrowth of the maxillae can make visualization of the glottis difficult during direct laryngoscopy for tracheal intubation.

In thalassemia minor, a relatively normal RBC count distinguishes anemia caused by thalassemia minor from iron-deficiency anemia. Finally, the homozygous form of thalassemia is incompatible with life; the heterozygous presentation usually results in mild hypochromic and microcytic anemia.

Treatment

Treatment varies depending on variant form. Patients with β-thalassemia major can be treated with hydroxyurea. Occasionally, bone marrow transplantation may be recommended in these patients, and a splenectomy may be necessary if hypersplenism leads to pancytopenia. For α-thalassemia, blood transfusion is occasionally necessary.

Anesthetic Considerations

Check the patient's complete blood count preoperatively.

J. VON WILLEBRAND DISEASE

Definition

von Willebrand disease (vWD) has traditionally remained the most common inherited coagulation diathesis. von Willebrand factor (vWF) VIII is a heterogeneous multinumeric glycoprotein that serves two main functions: to facilitate platelet adhesion and to behave as a plasma carrier for factor VIII:C of the coagulation cascade. vWF is synthesized in the endothelial cells and in megakaryocytes. An acquired form of vWD:VIII is seen with lymphomyeloproliferative or immunologic disease states secondary to antibodies against vWF:VIII.

Clinical Manifestations

Similar to many coagulopathies, vWD:VIII has varying degrees of severity: mild, moderate, and severe. In the milder or moderate forms, regular or spontaneous bleeding is not evident, but it is likely after surgery or when trauma occurs. In the more severe form, spontaneous epistaxis and oral, gastrointestinal, and genitourinary bleeding can be relentless.

Anesthetic Considerations

Most patients with vWF:VIII exhibit a prolonged bleeding time, a deficiency in vWF:VIII, decreased vWF:VIII activity measured by a ristocetin(an antibiotic) cofactor assay, and a decreased VIII:C. The recommended treatment for vWF:VIII is to supplement with recombinant factor VIII preoperatively and to administer it during surgery to raise the level of circulating vWF:VIII. Cryoprecipitate is another means of acquiring factor VIII; however, there is a risk of viral transmission. DDAVP (synthetic vasopressin) is an excellent option for the milder forms and should not be overlooked. DDAVP helps to increase plasma levels of vWF:VIII and augment aggregation.

Hepatic System

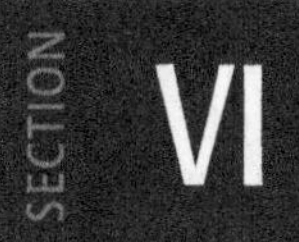

A. CIRRHOSIS AND PORTAL HYPERTENSION

Definition

Cirrhosis is a progressive and ultimately fatal syndrome of hepatic failure.

Pathophysiology

Chronic alcoholism is the most common cause of cirrhosis (Laënnec's cirrhosis) in the United States. Cirrhosis is also caused by biliary obstruction, chronic hepatitis, right-sided heart failure, α_1-antitrypsin deficiency, Wilson disease, and hemochromatosis. Anatomic alterations secondary to hepatocyte necrosis are the primary cause of the deterioration that occurs in liver function.

Over time, the liver parenchyma is replaced by fibrous and nodular tissue, which distorts, compresses, and obstructs normal portal venous blood flow. Portal hypertension develops and impairs the ability of the liver to perform various metabolic and synthetic processes. Obstructive engorgement of vessels within the portal system ultimately results in transmission of increasing backpressure within the splanchnic circulation. Therefore, splenomegaly, esophageal varices, and right-sided heart failure ensue in addition to deterioration in liver function.

The development of esophageal varices places the patient at risk for spontaneous, severe upper gastrointestinal hemorrhage. Fluid sequestration resulting from ascites causes consequent alteration in intravascular fluid dynamics and alteration in the renin–angiotensin system. Subsequent reduction in renal perfusion results in eventual renal failure in conjunction with hepatic failure (hepatorenal syndrome). Failure of the liver to clear nitrogenous compounds (ammonia) from the blood contributes to the development of progressive mental status changes (caused by encephalopathy), ultimately leading to coma.

Clinical Manifestations

The clinical manifestations of cirrhosis may not be strongly correlated with the severity of the disease process. Patients may have severe liver disease without overt jaundice and ascites. However, the eventual development of jaundice and ascites is observed in most patients as the disease process progresses. Other signs of severe liver disease include gynecomastia, spider angiomata, palmar erythema, and asterixis. Hepatic fibrosis results from the presence of other diseases; portal hypertension ensues, along with its sequelae. These diseases include Budd-Chiari syndrome (vena cava or hepatovenous obstruction), idiopathic portal fibrosis (Banti syndrome), schistosomiasis, and certain rare congenital fibrotic disorders. Venous occlusive disease secondary to metastases, primary hepatic neoplasia, or thromboembolism is also associated with portal hypertension.

Diagnostic and Laboratory Results

Laboratory changes in the presence of portal hypertension include a hematocrit of 30% to 35%; hyponatremia resulting from increased secretion of antidiuretic hormone; blood urea nitrogen greater than 20 mg/dL; and elevated plasma bilirubin, transaminases, and alkaline phosphatase concentrations.

Treatment

Treatment is supportive until liver transplantation can be undertaken. Variceal bleeding involves replacement of blood loss, vasopressin infusion (0.1–0.9 units/min intravenously), balloon tamponade (Sengstaken-Blakemore tube), endoscopic sclerosis, or the transjugular intrahepatic portosystemic shunt–stent procedure to stop the bleeding. If bleeding does not stop or recurs, emergency surgical procedures such as shunts (portocaval or splenorenal), esophageal transection, or gastric devascularization may be needed. Coagulopathies should be corrected by replacing clotting factors with fresh-frozen plasma (FFP) or cryoprecipitate. Platelet transfusions should be performed preoperatively for counts less than 100,000 mm^3. Preservation of renal function involves avoiding aggressive diuresis while correcting acute intravascular fluid deficits with colloid infusions.

Anesthetic Considerations

The dosage of muscle relaxants should be reduced, depending on hepatic elimination (e.g., pancuronium, vecuronium) because of reduced plasma clearance. Cisatracurium may be the relaxant of choice. The duration of action of succinylcholine may be prolonged as a result of reduced levels of pseudocholinesterase. Half-lives of opioids may be prolonged, leading to prolonged respiratory depression. Regional anesthesia may be used in patients without thrombocytopenia or coagulopathy if hypotension is avoided (perfusion to the liver becomes highly dependent on hepatic arterial blood flow). After removal of large amounts of ascitic fluid, colloid fluid replacement may be necessary to prevent hypotension. Whole blood may be preferable to packed red blood cells when replacing blood loss. Coagulation factors and platelet deficiencies should be corrected with FFP and platelet transfusions, respectively. Citrate toxicity can occur in these patients because of impaired metabolism of the citrate anticoagulant in blood products. Intravenous calcium should be given to reverse the negative inotropic effects of a reduction in serum ionized calcium levels. For patients with esophageal varices, placement of a nasogastric tube or esophageal can cause rupture and uncontrolled bleeding.

Therapeutic Modalities for Portal Hypertension

Pharmacologic management of patients with portal hypertension and acute variceal bleeding is considered secondary to endoscopic treatment and traditionally consists of intravenous infusion of vasopressin or somatostatin. Vasopressin is a splanchnic vasoconstrictor but may also induce undesirable systemic vasoconstriction. Infusion of vasopressin is initiated at 0.1 to 0.4 U/min. Concurrent infusion of nitroglycerin, titrated at 40 mcg/min, may be used to attenuate coronary arterial vasoconstriction and to control systolic blood pressure at 100 to 110 mmHg. In the presence of profound variceal exsanguination and hemodynamic instability, vasopressin may be used in conjunction with mechanical compression of bleeding esophageal varices provided by insertion of a triple-lumen Sengstaken-Blakemore tube. Use of this device also requires endotracheal intubation for airway support and for prevention of pulmonary aspiration.

Octreotide, a somatostatin analog, has been shown to be equally as effective as vasopressin in pharmacologic control of variceal bleeding. Infused at 50 mcg/hr, octreotide acts as a potent and reversible inhibitor of gastrointestinal peptide hormone activity, thereby decreasing gut motility and venous return to the portal circulation. Octreotide has also been shown to be equally as efficacious as sclerotherapy in acute treatment of variceal hemorrhage. Endoscopic sclerotherapy, usually performed with the patient under intravenous titrated sedation, has been recognized as the treatment of choice in definitive correction of variceal bleeding. Sclerotherapy is accomplished endoscopically by injection of a thrombosing agent either directly into the bleeding variceal or through creation of a fibrotic overlayer over the varix, accomplished by injection of the sclerosing agent proximal to the paravariceal mucosa. A course of treatments is usually necessary to reduce the incidence of rebleeding. Rebleeding, however, continues to be problematic in this subset of patients, with an incidence of up to 60%.

B. HEPATIC FAILURE

Definition

Hepatic failure occurs when massive necrosis of liver cells results in the development of a life-threatening loss of functional capacity that exceeds 80% to 90%. Hepatic failure can result from acute or chronic liver disease.

Incidence

The major causes of hepatic failure in the United States are related to the effects of viral hepatitis or drug-related liver injury. Each year, an estimated 2000 cases of hepatic failure in the United States are related to viral hepatitis. This accounts for 1% of all deaths and 6% of all liver-related deaths.

Pathophysiology

The following box is a categoric list of the potential causes of hepatic failure.

Potential Causes of Hepatic Failure

Viral
Hepatitis A, B, C, D, and E viruses
Herpes simplex virus
Cytomegalovirus
Adenovirus
Epstein-Barr virus
Varicella zoster virus
Dengue fever virus
Rift Valley fever virus

Metabolic
Wilson's disease
Acute fatty liver of pregnancy
Reye's syndrome
Sickle cell disease
Galactosemia

Toxic Damage
Isoniazid
Phenytoin
Halothane
Methyldopa
Tetracycline
Valproic acid
Nicotinic acid
Carbon tetrachloride
Phosphorus
Pesticides
Ethyl alcohol

Other
Autoimmune hepatitis
Amanita phalloides (mushroom) poisoning
Acetaminophen
Budd-Chiari syndrome
Veno-occlusive disease
Hyperthermia
Partial hepatectomy
Jejunoileal bypass

Diagnostic and Laboratory Findings

Most proteins associated with the promotion or inhibition of coagulation are synthesized in the liver. When one is reviewing laboratory data, special attention should be given to coagulation studies, liver function studies, complete blood count, electrolytes, glucose, blood urea nitrogen, and creatinine.

A 12-lead electrocardiogram (ECG) should be performed to rule out any possible cardiac arrhythmias related to acidemia, electrolyte abnormalities, or hypoxemia associated with hepatic failure. The patient with liver failure is at risk for the development of acid–base derangements. Respiratory alkalosis may result from hyperventilation related to an abnormality of central regulation. Respiratory acidosis may be caused by endotoxins, increased intracranial pressure, or pulmonary sequelae, which depress respiratory centers. Metabolic acidosis is also possible, related to substantial tissue damage and decreased clearance of lactic acid by the failing liver.

The hypoxemia associated with liver failure can be attributed to aspiration, atelectasis, infection, hypoventilation, or their combinations. Results of chest radiography should be obtained to rule out evidence of pulmonary edema or adult respiratory distress syndrome. Listed in the following table is a guide to laboratory results in liver failure.

Laboratory Results in Liver Failure

Laboratory Study	Normal	Liver Failure
White blood cell count	3.5–10.6 cells/mm^3	Decreased
Hemoglobin	11.5–15.1 g/dL	Decreased
Hematocrit	34.4%–44.2%	Decreased
Platelet count	150–450/mm^3	Decreased
Prothrombin time	11–14 sec	Increased
Partial thromboplastin time	20–37 sec	Increased
Bilirubin	Plasma: 0.3–1.1 mg/dL Indirect: 0.2–0.7 mg/dL Direct: <0.5 mg/dL	Increased; jaundice seen with plasma bilirubin levels >3 mg/dL
Serum glutamic oxaloacetic transaminase (aspartate aminotransferase)	10–40 units/L	Increased
Serum glutamic-pyruvic transaminase (alanine aminotransferase*)	5–35 units/L	Increased
Lactate dehydrogenase (LD-5*)	5.3%–13.4%	Increased
Alkaline phosphatase	87–250 units/L	Normal; used to differentiate biliary obstruction
Albumin	3.3–4.5 g/dL	Decreased; levels <2.5 g/dL are precarious
Ammonia	<50 g/dL	Increased ammonia converted to urea by the normal liver

Laboratory Results in Liver Failure—cont'd

Laboratory Study	Normal	Liver Failure
Blood urea nitrogen	7–20 mg/dL	Normal or decreased by impaired excretion of sodium and retention of water; increased in hepatorenal syndrome
Creatinine	0.6–1.3 mg/dL	Increased in hepatorenal syndrome
Sodium	135–145 mEq/L	Usually decreased; increased sodium may result after the administration of lactulose or if replacement of free water is inadequate
Potassium	3.6–5 mEq/L	Decreased; related to the secondary effects of hyperaldosteronism, vomiting, diuretic use, or inadequate replacement; increased potassium may result from the use of blood products
Magnesium	1.6–3 mEq/L	Decreased
Calcium	8.8–10.4 mg/dL	Decreased
Phosphorus	2.5–4.5 mg/dL	Decreased
Glucose	70–110 mg/dL	Decreased; related to impaired gluconeogenesis and decreased insulin clearance

*Specific for liver damage.

Clinical Manifestations

No matter the exact cause of the patient's liver failure, it inevitably affects the entire physiologic makeup. Physical examination is important for the approximation of liver and spleen size, evidence of bleeding abnormalities, identification of extravascular fluid shifts, and any other organ dysfunction. Listed in the table below are common clinical features of hepatic failure and their associated causes.

Clinical Features of Hepatic Failure and Associated Causes

Clinical Feature	Cause
Anemia	Iron, vitamin B_{12}, or folate deficiency; hypersplenism; bone marrow suppression
Ascites	Portal hypertension; hypoalbuminemia; sodium and water retention
Fetor hepaticus (pungent sour odor detected in exhaled breath)	Inability to metabolize methionine
Gynecomastia	Increased circulating estrogen

Continued

Clinical Features of Hepatic Failure and Associated Causes—cont'd

Clinical Feature	Cause
Hepatic encephalopathy (hepatic coma)	Inability to metabolize ammonia; increased cerebral sensitivity to toxins; hypoglycemia
Hepatorenal syndrome	Decreased renal blood flow, particularly to the cortex; vasoconstriction; decreased glomerular filtration rate; renal retention of sodium
Increased bleeding tendencies, nosebleeds, gingival bleeding, menstrual bleeding, easy bruising	Anemia; thrombocytopenia; decreased production of clotting factors; decreased adherence of circulating platelets
Increased risk of infection	Endotracheal intubation with impaired cough reflex; intravenous catheters; central lines; urinary catheters; leukopenia; decreased neutrophil adherence; complement deficiencies
Increased skin pigmentation	Increased activity of melanocyte-stimulating hormone
Jaundice	Increased circulating bilirubin
Leukopenia	Hypersplenism; bone marrow suppression
Palmar erythema	Increased circulating estrogen
Pectoral and axillary alopecia	Increased circulating estrogen
Peripheral edema	Hypoalbuminemia; failure of the liver to inactivate aldosterone and antidiuretic hormone, with subsequent sodium and water retention
Spider angiomas, "nevi"	Increased circulating estrogen
Testicular atrophy	Increased circulating estrogen
Thrombocytopenia	Hypersplenism; bone marrow suppression
Weight loss and muscle wasting	Nausea and vomiting; anorexia; impaired gluconeogenesis; impaired insulin functioning; hypoproteinemia

Treatment

Management of patients with liver failure should include admission to the intensive care unit. The health care team should be on constant guard for complications associated with liver failure, such as sepsis, cerebral edema, hypoglycemia, and electrolyte and bleeding abnormalities. Liver failure associated with acetaminophen poisoning or mushroom poisoning should be identified immediately because antidotes are available for both. Patients who are not responsive to conventional treatment should be considered for liver transplantation as early as possible before they are excluded by the development of infection or encephalopathic brain damage.

General treatment modalities for patients with liver failure include the following:

- Antibiotic prophylaxis
- Urinary catheter
- Central venous pulmonary catheter
- Histamine-2 (H_2) antagonist or sucralfate
- Blood glucose checks every 1 to 2 hours
- Aspiration precautions
- Periodic assessment of neurologic status (neurologic status may rapidly deteriorate because of increasing ammonia levels or increasing intracranial pressure)
- Prevention of sepsis

- Monitoring of renal function and fluid status
- Monitoring of fluid volume
- Increase in gastric pH and decrease in risk of gastrointestinal bleeding
- Prevention of hypoglycemia and guiding administration of intravenous dextrose
- Prevention of aspiration pneumonia and adult respiratory distress syndrome
- Early nutritional supplementation: prevention of nutrition-related complications

Anesthetic Considerations

Only surgery to correct life-threatening conditions should be performed on patients with liver failure. The patient's condition should be optimized before the surgical procedure. A normally "minor" procedure can become a major catastrophe in patients with liver failure.

Premedication must be considered, taking into account the severity of the patient's disease process, the presence of altered consciousness, and the liver's diminished ability to metabolize pharmacologic agents. If the patient is thought to have a full stomach, antacids and H_2 antagonists may be administered.

Monitoring should conform to the established standards of care. The size and number of intravenous catheters should be individualized. Most cases involving liver failure require the use of an arterial line, a central venous pressure or pulmonary artery catheter, and a urinary drainage catheter to monitor the patient's fluid status.

The use of local anesthesia with sedation or regional anesthesia should be considered whenever possible. Coagulopathies must first be ruled out, and the surgical procedure itself must be considered. Patients may be considered to have a full stomach, especially in the presence of ascites. In this case, a rapid-sequence induction is standard. The choice of induction agent and dosage administered should reflect the liver's diminished ability to metabolize pharmacologic agents and the patient's increased volume of distribution. Hyperammoniaemia causes central nervous system inhibition, resulting in increased sensitivity to anesthetic agents. Increased ammonia also causes myocardial depression, which can be potentiated and cause severe hypotension when inhalation agents are administered.

Both nondepolarizing and depolarizing muscle relaxants may be administered. Dosages may need to be individualized according to the patient's initial response. A peripheral nerve stimulator aids the practitioner in gauging the patient's response and adjusting subsequent doses. The breakdown of succinylcholine remains relatively normal despite advanced disease states. Muscle relaxants metabolized by the liver (e.g., vecuronium) should be avoided. Cisatracurium may be the muscle relaxant of choice because of its unique metabolic properties, which do not involve either the liver or the kidneys. If cisatracurium is unavailable, any other nondepolarizing muscle relaxant may be used, taking into account the patient's specific organ involvement and the drug's metabolic properties.

Isoflurane and desflurane are the inhalational agents of choice. Nitrous oxide may be safely instituted according to the nature of the surgical procedure and as long as a high fraction of inspired oxygen is not required.

The use of opioids must take into account a prolonged half-life and decreased clearance. Because fentanyl does not decrease hepatic blood flow, it is often the opioid of choice for the patient with liver failure.

The patient with liver failure is at risk for major blood loss with any invasive procedure. Blood products should be available, and all losses should be replaced accordingly.

Prognosis

In the United States, mortality rates from liver disease have increased since the 1960s. Overall, the mortality rate from hepatic failure is 70% to 95%. Liver transplantation should be considered when conventional medical management fails; such consideration should take place early before infection or encephalopathic brain damage renders the potential candidate ineligible for the procedure. One-year patient survival rates after liver transplantation are 63% to 78%.

C. HEPATITIS

Definition

Hepatitis is an inflammatory disease of hepatocytes that may be either acute or chronic (lasting more than 6 months) and can progress to cell necrosis and eventual hepatic failure.

ACUTE HEPATITIS

Acute hepatitis presents a variable clinical picture. Manifestations may extend from mild inflammatory increases in serum transaminase levels to fulminant hepatic failure.

Pathophysiology

The cause of this syndrome is usually exposure to an infectious virus. Other causes include exposure to hepatotoxic substances and adverse drug reactions. Viral hepatitis may be attributable to exposure to one of a number of viruses, including hepatitis viruses (A, B, C [formerly referred to as *non-A, non-B*], D [delta virus], E [enteric non-A, non-B]), Epstein-Barr virus, herpes simplex virus, cytomegalovirus, and coxsackievirus. The most common culprits are hepatitis A, hepatitis B, and hepatitis C. Hepatitis A and E are transmitted by the oral–fecal route, and hepatitis B and C are transmitted by contact with body fluids and physical contact with disrupted cutaneous barriers.

Clinical Manifestations

The common clinical course of viral hepatitis begins with a 1- to 2-week prodromal period, the signs and symptoms of which include fever, malaise, and nausea and vomiting. Progression to jaundice typically occurs, with resolution within 2 to 12 weeks. However, serum transaminase levels often remain increased for up to 4 months. If hepatitis B or C is the cause, the clinical course is often more prolonged and complicated. Cholestasis may manifest in certain cases. Fulminant hepatic necrosis in certain individuals is also possible. The major characteristics of hepatitis types A, B, C, D, and E are listed in the table on pg. 141.

Acute viral hepatitis may evolve into a chronic active syndrome, which develops in 3% to 10% of cases involving hepatitis B and in 10% to 50% of cases involving hepatitis C. Many patients become asymptomatic infectious carriers of hepatitis B and C. These patients include many who are immunosuppressed or require chronic hemodialysis.

Five Causes of Acute Viral Hepatitis

Hepatitis Virus	Size (nm)	Genome	Route of Transmission	Incubation Period (Days)	Fatality Rate (%)	Chronic Rate (%)	Antibody
A	27	RNA	Fecal-oral	15–45 (mean, 25)	1	None	Anti-HAV
B	45	DNA	Parenteral	30–180 (mean, 75)	1	2–7	Anti-HBs
			Sexual				Anti-HBc
							Anti-HBe
C	60	RNA	Parenteral	15–150 (mean, 50)	<0.1	70–85	Anti-HCV
D (delta)	40	RNA	Parenteral	30–150	2–10	2–7	Anti-HDV
			Sexual			50	
E	32	RNA	Fecal–oral	30–60	1	None	Anti-HEV

anti-HDV, Hepatitis D virus antibody; *anti-HEV,* hepatitis E virus antibody; *HAV,* hepatitis A virus; *HBc,* hepatitis B core; *HBe,* hepatitis B e antigen; *HBs,* hepatitis B surface; *HCV,* hepatitis C virus.
From Hoofnagle JH: Acute viral hepatitis. In Goldman L, Ausiello D, eds. *Cecil's Textbook of Medicine*. 23rd ed. Philadelphia: Saunders; 2008: 1101.

DRUG-INDUCED HEPATITIS

Drug-induced hepatitis results from an idiosyncratic drug reaction, from direct hepatic toxicity or from a combination of the two, as shown in the box below. Clinically, its manifestations resemble those of viral hepatitis, thereby complicating diagnosis. Alcoholic hepatitis is probably the most common form of drug-induced hepatitis and results in fatty infiltration of the liver (causing hepatomegaly), with impairment in hepatic oxidation of fatty acids, lipoprotein synthesis and secretion, and fatty acid esterification.

Drugs and Substances Associated with Hepatitis

Toxic
Alcohol
Acetaminophen
Salicylates
Tetracycline
Trichloroethylene
Vinyl chloride
Carbon tetrachloride
Yellow phosphorus
Poisonous mushrooms
Amanita
Galerina

Idiosyncratic
Volatile anesthetics
Inhalation
Phenytoin
Sulfonamides
Rifampin
Indomethacin

Toxic and Idiosyncratic
Methyldopa
Isoniazid
Sodium valproate
Amiodarone

Primarily Cholestatic
Chlorpromazine
Chlorpropamide
Oral contraceptives
Anabolic steroids
Erythromycin estolate
Methimazole

From Morgan GE, Mikhail MS. Anesthesia for patients with liver disease. In Morgan GE, Mikhail MS, eds. *Clinical Anesthesiology*. 4th ed. Norwalk, CT: Appleton & Lange: 2006: 791.

CHRONIC HEPATITIS

Pathophysiology

Chronic hepatitis occurs in 1% to 10% of acute hepatitis B infections and in 10% to 40% of hepatitis C infections. Patients are classified as having one of three distinct syndromes based on liver biopsy:

1. Chronic persistent hepatitis
2. Chronic lobular hepatitis
3. Chronic active hepatitis

Chronic persistent hepatitis is relatively benign and is confined to portal areas. Hepatocellular integrity is preserved, and progression to cirrhosis is rare. Chronic lobular hepatitis involves recurrent exacerbations of acute inflammation, but as in persistent hepatitis, progression to cirrhosis is rare. The most serious form of chronic hepatitis is chronic active hepatitis, which is progressive and results in hepatocyte destruction, cirrhosis, and ultimately hepatic failure. Death often results from related manifestations of hepatic failure, such as hemorrhage from esophageal varices, multiorgan system failure (e.g., hepatorenal syndrome), and encephalopathy. The typical etiologic agent is hepatitis B or hepatitis C virus. Autoimmune disorders (e.g., systemic lupus erythematosus) and exposure to certain drugs (e.g., methyldopa, isoniazid, and nitrofurantoin) have been implicated as etiologic factors as well.

Clinical Manifestations

Marked fatigue and jaundice are common in chronic hepatitis. Arthritis, neuropathy, myocarditis, thrombocytopenia, and glomerulonephritis may also be present. Plasma albumin levels are usually decreased, and the prothrombin time (PT) is often prolonged.

Treatment

Dehydration and electrolyte abnormalities should be corrected. Vitamin K or FFP is used to correct coagulopathies. Bacterial infections should be treated, and neomycin, lactulose, or both should be used to decrease plasma ammonia levels. Factors that may aggravate hepatic encephalopathy should be avoided. Orthotopic liver transplantation may be considered in selected patients.

Anesthetic Considerations

Increased perioperative mortality (10%) and morbidity (12%) rates have been reported with surgery, particularly laparotomy, in patients with acute viral hepatitis. Operative procedures performed in patients with alcohol intoxication are also likely to be associated with increased perioperative complications. Surgery performed in those undergoing alcohol withdrawal is associated with a mortality rate as high as 50%.

With acutely intoxicated alcoholic patients, certain anesthetic issues must be kept in mind: (1) less anesthetic is needed; (2) aspiration precautions must be implemented; (3) surgical bleeding may be increased as a result of interference with platelet aggregation; (4) the brain is less tolerant of hypoxia; and (5) the level of circulating catecholamines is increased, as evidenced by lability in vital signs and exaggerated responses to drugs and stimuli (probably indicating decreased neurotransmitter uptake).

It is recommended to postpone elective surgical procedures until liver function has been normalized. Surgery and anesthesia greatly increase the risk for further hepatic decompensation in patients with hepatitis; this risk may be compounded by the development of renal failure (hepatorenal syndrome), encephalopathy, and the decompensation of other organ systems.

If urgent or emergency surgery is necessary, as thorough a preoperative history as possible must be obtained. If serious time constraints are imposed, the preoperative evaluation should focus on signs and symptoms (e.g., encephalopathy, bleeding diatheses, jaundice, ascites, and hemodynamic findings) and on the results of laboratory studies (e.g., levels of electrolytes, blood urea nitrogen, creatinine, serum glucose, hemoglobin, hematocrit, liver enzymes, and bilirubin, as well as arterial blood gas determinations and coagulation studies). Other pertinent studies include chest radiography and ECG. If not previously ordered, blood typing and crossmatching are warranted, depending on the magnitude of the planned procedure. Any history of hospitalizations and anesthetic use also should be obtained. In general, as much pertinent information as possible should be procured and recorded.

Dehydration and electrolyte derangements should be anticipated and corrected before surgery. Metabolic alkalosis and hypokalemia are often present as a result of vomiting. The presence of hypomagnesemia predisposes to the development of perioperative dysrhythmias. Elevated enzyme (e.g., alkaline phosphatase, alanine aminotransferase [ALT], aspartate aminotransferase [AST]) and serum bilirubin levels are nonspecific with regard to the degree of hepatic necrosis. Alcoholic hepatitis and obstructive hepatitis are commonly associated with an elevation in AST. Viral hepatitis and drug-induced hepatitis often reflect elevated ALT levels. The highest measured levels of AST are seen in viral hepatitis or in fulminant hepatic failure.

The PT is the best indicator of the liver's ability to synthesize coagulation factors. Severe hepatic dysfunction results in a persistent prolongation of PT even after the administration of vitamin K. Evaluation of serum albumin level is warranted, although deficiencies in serum albumin, as well as in all proteins synthesized by the liver (i.e., coagulation factors), are manifestations of severe hepatic dysfunction and malnutrition.

Preoperative medication (e.g., sedation) may best be avoided, so that exacerbation of preexisting encephalopathy or respiratory depression is prevented. Administration of FFP, vitamin K, and packed red blood cells may be necessary for the correction of coagulopathy and red blood cell deficiency before surgery. Premedication with benzodiazepines and thiamine may be necessary for alcoholic patients in impending withdrawal. Child's classification system is useful in conjunction with other available assessment parameters for determining the degree to which liver disease influences surgical and anesthetic risk (see table below).

Child-Turcote-Pugh Score of Severity of Liver Disease

Points	1	2	3
Encephalopathy	None	1–2	3–4
Ascites	Absent	Slight	Moderate
Bilirubin (mg/dL)	<2	2–3	>3
For PBC/PSC	<4	4–10	>10
Albumin (g/dL)	<3.5	2.8–3.5	>2.8
PT (INR)	<1.7	1.7–2.3	>2.3

INR, International normalized ratio; *PBC,* primary biliary cirrhosis; *PSC,* primary sclerosing cholangitis.

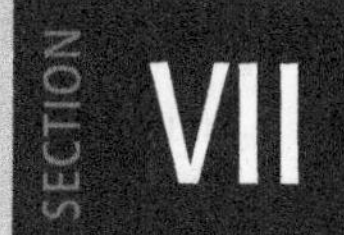

Musculoskeletal System

A. ANKYLOSING SPONDYLITIS

Definition and Incidence

Ankylosing spondylitis (AS), also known as *rheumatoid spondylitis* and *Marie-Strumpell disease*, is a chronic inflammatory disorder that primarily affects the spine and sacroiliac joints and produces fusion of the spinal vertebrae and the costovertebral joints. It is a disease of adults younger than 40 years, and it demonstrates a predilection for males (male-to-female ratio is 9:1). The disease is rare in Caucasians.

Pathophysiology

The cause of AS remains unclear. However, it is strongly associated with the histocompatibility antigen HLA-B27, the presence of which is detected in more than 90% of Caucasians with the disease.

Clinical Manifestations and Diagnosis

Ankylosing spondylitis is diagnosed on the basis of clinical criteria that include: (1) chronic low back pain with limitation of spinal motion (<4 cm as measured by the Schober test), (2) radiographic evidence of bilateral sacroiliitis, and (3) limitation of chest wall expansion (<2.5-cm increase in chest circumference measured at the fourth intercostal space). Extraskeletal manifestations of this disease include iritis, cardiovascular involvement (cardiac conduction defects, aortitis, and aortic insufficiency in 20% of individuals), peripheral arthritis, fever, anemia, fatigue, weight loss, and fibrocavitary (fibrobullous) disease of the apexes of the lungs. The most limiting factors associated with the disease are pain, stiffness, and fatigue.

Complications

Pulmonary complications are reported to occur in 2% to 70% of patients with AS. Apical fibrosis is the most commonly occurring abnormality followed by aspergilloma and pleural effusion with nonspecific pleuritis. In apical fibrosis, the pulmonary lesion begins with apical pleural thickening and patchy consolidation of one or both apexes and often progresses to dense bilateral fibrosis and air space enlargement. Patients with apical fibrosis usually have advanced AS. Impaired thoracic cage excursion caused by AS results in a greater impairment of apical ventilation, and this may be one factor in the pathogenesis of apical fibrosis.

The most common thoracic complication is fixation of the thoracic cage as a result of costovertebral ankylosis, which can lead to pulmonary dysfunction. In patients with this complication, motion of the thoracic cage is restricted because of fusion of the costovertebral joints; this restriction leads to a decrease in thoracic excursion. Respiratory function typically demonstrates a restrictive pattern with mild diminution of total lung capacity (TLC), vital capacity (VC), and carbon monoxide diffusing capacity (DLCO) and normal or slightly increased residual volume (RV) and functional residual capacity (FRC). Pulmonary compliance, diffusion capacity, and arterial blood gas (ABG) values usually are normal. Despite having abnormal pulmonary function, the majority of patients with AS are able to perform normal physical activities without pulmonary symptoms. It has been suggested that patients who exercise regularly and thus improve cardiovascular fitness could maintain a satisfactory work capacity.

Bone ankylosis may occur in the numerous joints around the thorax (the thoracic vertebrae and the costovertebral, costotransverse, sternoclavicular, and sternomanubrial joints), resulting in limitation of chest wall movement. Patients with AS rarely complain of respiratory symptoms or functional impairment unless they have coexisting cardiovascular or respiratory disease. Progressive kyphosis is equivalent to progressive rigidity of the thorax. Increased diaphragmatic function compensates for decreased thoracic motion, allowing lung function to be well preserved. Patients with advanced disease may have an entirely diaphragmatic respiration. Regional lung ventilation in patients with AS is normal unless they have preexisting apical fibrosis.

Cervical spondylosis affects levels C5 to C6 and C6 to C7 most often and less frequently C4 to C5, C7 to T1, and C3 to C4. The degenerative changes may result in nerve root entrapment by foraminal encroachment. The phrenic nerve, which innervates the diaphragm, is supplied primarily by the C4 nerve root and to a lesser extent by the C3 and C5 nerve roots.

Cricoarytenoid involvement may exist and can lead to respiratory dysfunction and upper airway obstruction. Cricoarytenoid dysfunction can manifest as a hoarse, weak voice. Respiratory failure from cricoarytenoid ankylosis has necessitated therapeutic tracheostomy. In all reported cases, laryngeal symptoms were present before cricoarytenoid arthritis caused airway compromise. A case of acute respiratory failure and cor pulmonale resulting from cricoarytenoid arthritis has also been reported in a patient with AS.

Treatment

Medical therapy for adult patients with AS is supportive and preventive. Most patients with AS are asymptomatic. Depending on the severity of disease involvement, management may consist of the use of corticosteroids and nonsteroidal anti-inflammatory drugs (NSAIDs). Patients should refrain from smoking tobacco.

Anesthetic Considerations

Patients with AS have specific anesthetic requirements. Management of the upper airway is the priority because of the potential for obstruction. Cervical spine involvement may result in limitation of movement. The ankylosed neck is more susceptible to hyperextension injury, and cervical fracture may occur. Intubation awake with or without the use of a fiberoptic bronchoscope is indicated. In rare situations, tracheostomy must be performed with the patient under local anesthesia before anesthesia can be induced. A regional anesthetic technique may not be feasible because of skeletal involvement that precludes access or because of neurologic complications such as spinal cord compression, cauda equina syndrome, focal epilepsy, vertebral basilar insufficiency, and peripheral nerve lesions. Patients with cardiovascular system involvement may require antibiotics, treatment of heart failure, or insertion of a temporary pacemaker before surgery. Restriction of chest expansion and, rarely, pulmonary fibrosis necessitate performance of a thorough preoperative assessment and immediate postoperative mechanical ventilation. Careful attention to positioning is essential.

B. KYPHOSCOLIOSIS

Definition and Incidence

Kyphosis is a deformity marked by an accentuated posterior curvature. Scoliosis is a lateral curvature of the spine. Kyphoscoliosis results when both kyphosis and scoliosis occur concomitantly, causing a lateral bending and rotation of the vertebral column. Scoliosis alone, despite its severity, does not cause sensory or motor impairment. In contrast, kyphosis and kyphoscoliosis may induce spinal cord damage because of the sharp angulation of the spine. Respiratory dysfunction is associated with scoliosis, significant kyphosis, and severe kyphoscoliosis. Scoliosis is the most common spinal deformity, with an incidence of four persons per 1000.

Scoliosis is classified in five categories: idiopathic, congenital, neuropathic (e.g., poliomyelitis, cerebral palsy, syringomyelia, and Friedreich ataxia), myopathic (e.g., muscular dystrophy and amyotonia), and traumatic. Idiopathic scoliosis is the most common deformity, accounting for 80% of all cases. On the basis of the time of onset, idiopathic scoliosis is divided into the following two categories: (1) the rare infantile form (male-to-female ratio is 6:4) and (2) the common adolescent form (male-to-female ratio is 1:9). The children in the adolescent group are born with straight spines; however, at some point during the growth period, their spines begin to bend and deform, with deformation progressively worsening until growth ends. In general, whereas curves associated with adolescent idiopathic scoliosis are convex and deviated to the right, those related to other disease may be deviated to the left. The presence of cervical scoliosis should alert anesthesia personnel to potential difficulties in airway management. Any significant curvature involving the thoracic spine may alter lung function. Unless the deformity is severe, patients with kyphosis are able to maintain normal pulmonary function; in contrast, even mild forms of scoliosis can result in impaired ventilatory function. Severe thoracic deformity may result in respiratory alterations during sleep. Several types of breathing abnormalities have been documented, including obstructive sleep apnea and hypopnea. The lowest HbO_2 saturations occurred during rapid eye movement sleep.

Pathophysiology

Diminution of pulmonary function occurs with curvatures of greater than 60 degrees, and pulmonary symptoms develop with curvatures greater than 70 degrees (as measured by the Cobb technique). Curvatures greater than 100 degrees may be associated with significant gas exchange impairment.

In general, the greater the curvature, the greater the loss of pulmonary function. Because of this, mechanical ventilation becomes inefficient; this inefficiency is the major factor causing respiratory compromise. At the time of diagnosis, it often is possible to document a reduction in lung capacity. The characteristic deformity seen in scoliosis causes one hemithorax to become relatively smaller than the other.

Skeletal chest wall deformity in kyphoscoliosis leads to a reduction in lung volumes and the pulmonary vascular bed. Ventilatory failure associated with severe kyphoscoliosis produces a lung size that is 30% to 65% of normal. As the patient ages, the chest wall becomes less compliant; this increases the work of breathing and leads to hypoventilation and respiratory muscle weakness.

The main features of lung mechanics in the patient with early-stage scoliosis are reduced lung volumes (VC, TLC, FRC, and RV) and reduced chest wall compliance; in the late stages of disease, ventilation/perfusion mismatching with hypoxemia (attributed to alveolar hypoventilation because of a decrease in tidal volume [V_T]), increased pulmonary artery pressure (PAP), hypercapnia, abnormal response to CO_2 stimulation, increased work of breathing, and cor pulmonale occur and eventually lead to cardiorespiratory failure. Reduction in VC to 60% to 80% of the predicted value is a typical finding. The ratio of forced expiratory volume in 1 second to forced vital capacity (FEV_1/FVC) is normal unless other pulmonary diseases are present. Although normocarbia prevails for most of the clinical course, an elevated $Paco_2$ signifies the onset of respiratory failure. The severity of hypercapnia most closely correlates with the patient's age and inspiratory muscle strength.

Associated Conditions

Scoliosis may be associated with several cardiovascular abnormalities, of which mitral valve prolapse is the most common. If mitral regurgitation is present, antibiotic prophylaxis is indicated before surgical manipulation. Other common changes include an increase in pulmonary vascular resistance (PVR) and ensuing pulmonary hypertension (PH), which leads to the development of right ventricular hypertrophy. Several contributing factors are thought to be responsible for the development of increased PVR. First, arterial hypoxemia results in pulmonary vasoconstriction. Second, changes in the pulmonary arterioles consequent to the increased pulmonic pressure may cause narrowing and result in irreversible PH. Third, a compressed chest wall may increase vascular resistance in affected areas. Fourth, development of scoliosis at an early age inhibits growth of the pulmonary vascular bed. Alveolar multiplication is nearly complete by 2 years of age but continues until the age of 8 years. During the first few years, lung growth occurs primarily by enlargement of existing alveoli.

Treatment

The management of scoliosis may include the following: (1) observation of the problem without active medical treatment; (2) treatment by nonoperative methods that include the use of braces or electronic stimulators; and (3) operative methods such as anterior or posterior spinal fusion and instrumentation, such as Harrington rod insertion. The mortality rate among persons with untreated scoliosis is twice that of the normal population, and the rate for those with thoracic curvatures alone was fourfold that of the normal population. Patients with congenital thoracic scoliosis are particularly at risk for cor pulmonale.

Anesthetic Considerations

Preoperative Evaluation

Before surgery, a thorough review of systems is essential. The severity of scoliosis and of any underlying conditions must be noted. Any reversible pulmonary involvement such as pneumonia should be corrected before elective surgery. Laboratory data should include complete blood count; prothrombin time; partial thromboplastin time; values for electrolytes, blood urea nitrogen, and creatinine; electrocardiography (ECG); chest radiography; and routine pulmonary function test values. ABG analysis may be indicated if the results of the pulmonary function tests reflect significant impairment or if the surgical procedure dictates its need. Because these procedures can potentially involve large blood losses, young, healthy, asymptomatic patients may donate autologous blood. Blood typing and crossmatching also are required.

When sedatives are used in the preoperative area, care must be taken to ensure that respiratory status is not depressed. The need for intraoperative monitoring is dictated by the type of surgery and the physical status of the patient. No specific anesthetic techniques have been shown to be superior in patients with scoliosis; however, N_2O may increase PVR by direct vasoconstrictive effects on the pulmonary vasculature. It has been suggested that scoliosis is associated with an increased incidence of malignant hyperthermia (MH). Ventilation should be adjusted so that adequate arterial oxygenation and normocarbia are maintained.

Patients undergoing surgery for correction of the spinal curvature should be informed preoperatively of the possible need for the "wake-up" test; when the patient is able to move both feet on request and surgical correction has been achieved, anesthesia can be quickly reinstituted. The use of somatosensory evoked potentials may require an alteration in anesthetic technique. All anesthetic agents depress somatosensory evoked potentials to a varying degree. Administration of volatile anesthetics should not exceed a minimum alveolar concentration of 1. A continuous infusion opioid technique often is preferred. Communication between the technician and anesthetist is essential.

Intraoperative Management

Considerable fluid and blood loss may occur during surgery. The surgeon may request the institution of deliberate hypotension. Deliberate hypotension can be produced with the use of one or more of the following: potent inhalation anesthetics, vasodilators (e.g., sodium nitroprusside, nitroglycerin), or β-adrenergic blocking agents (e.g., propranolol and esmolol). The risks and potential benefits should be weighed against the effects of deliberate hypotension. The mean arterial blood pressure should be maintained at no lower than 60 to 65 mmHg. Cell saver blood is often used. Interventions for prevention of hypothermia, such as use of a hot air warming blanket or heated humidifiers, should be used. Careful positioning is essential.

Postoperative Implications

The decision whether to use mechanical ventilation postoperatively is based on the severity of scoliosis and intraoperative events. Most patients with mild to moderate pulmonary dysfunction are able to undergo safe extubation in the operating room. Those with severe deformity or patients who have received massive fluid and blood replacement therapy should be weaned slowly.

C. LAMBERT-EATON MYASTHENIC SYNDROME

Incidence

Lambert-Eaton myasthenic syndrome (LEMS) is a rare autoimmune disease that classically occurs in patients with malignant disease, particularly small cell carcinoma of the bronchi. One-third to half of patients, however, have no evidence of carcinoma. Most patients with myasthenic syndrome are men between the ages of 50 and 70 years.

Pathophysiology

The basic defect associated with LEMS appears to be an autoantibody-mediated derangement in presynaptic Ca^{2+} channels leading to a reduction in Ca^{2+}-mediated exocytosis of acetylcholine (ACh) at neuromuscular and autonomic nerve terminals. The decreased release of ACh quanta from the cholinergic nerve endings produces a reduced postjunctional response. Unlike in myasthenia gravis, the number and the quality of postjunctional AChRs remain unaltered, and the end plate sensitivity is normal. The neuromuscular junction abnormality of LEMS is similar in location to that of Mg^{2+} intoxication or botulism poisoning, in which the release of presynaptic ACh is attenuated.

Clinical Manifestations

Muscle weakness, fatigue, hyporeflexia, and proximal limb muscle aches are the dominant features of LEMS. The diaphragm and other respiratory muscles are also involved. Autonomic nervous system dysfunction is often present and is manifested as impaired gastric motility, orthostatic hypotension, and urinary retention.

Patients with LEMS experience a brief increase in muscle strength with voluntary contraction, distinguishing it from myasthenia gravis. Tetanic stimulation results in a progressive augmentation in muscle strength as the frequency of the stimulation is increased. Post-tetanic potentiation is also enhanced.

Treatment

There is no cure for LEMS. Treatment is aimed at removal of the small cell carcinoma if present improving muscle strength and reversing autonomic deficits. 3,4-Diaminopyridine improves muscle strength in some patients by promoting presynaptic Ca^{2+} influx and increasing the number of ACh quanta that are liberated by a single nerve action potential. Anticholinesterase agents, plasmapheresis, corticosteroids, intravenous immunoglobulin, and immunosuppressive drugs provide improvement for some patients with LEMS.

Anesthetic Considerations

An index of suspicion for LEMS should be maintained in surgical patients with a history of muscle weakness and suspected or diagnosed carcinoma of the lung. Patients with LEMS are extremely sensitive to the relaxant effects of both depolarizing and nondepolarizing muscle relaxants. Inhalational anesthetics alone may provide adequate relaxation, but if muscle relaxants are required, their dosages should be reduced and the neuromuscular blockade closely monitored. Neuromuscular reversal with an anticholinesterase agent may be used. Prolonged ventilatory assistance may be required postoperatively.

D. MALIGNANT HYPERTHERMIA

Definition and Incidence

Malignant hyperthermia is an uncommon, life-threatening hypermetabolic disorder of skeletal muscle triggered in susceptible individuals by potent inhalation agents, including sevoflurane, desflurane, isoflurane, and halothane and the depolarizing muscle relaxant succinylcholine. About 52% of cases occur in patients younger than age 15 years, with a mean age of 18.3 years. The exact incidence of MH is unknown, but the rate of occurrence has been estimated to be one in 50,000 in adults and one in 15,000 in children.

Pathophysiology

Although the cause of MH is not yet known with certainty, it is generally agreed that MH is an inherited disorder of skeletal muscle in which a defect in calcium regulation is expressed by exposure to triggering anesthetic agents; intracellular hypercalcemia results. The ryanodine receptor is the major calcium release channel of the sarcoplasmic reticulum, and much attention has been focused on this receptor as the site of the MH defect. The defect involves skeletal muscle, and there is no evidence for a primary defect in cardiac or smooth muscle cells.

Malignant hyperthermia is initiated when specific triggering agents induce increased concentrations of calcium in the muscle cells of MH-susceptible (MHS) patients. Actomyosin cross-bridging, sustained muscle contraction, and rigidity result. Energy-dependent reuptake mechanisms attempt to remove excess calcium from the myoplasm, increasing muscle metabolism two- to threefold. The accelerated cellular processes increase oxygen consumption, augment carbon dioxide and heat production, deplete adenosine triphosphate (ATP) stores, and generate lactic acid. Acidosis, hyperthermia, and ATP depletion cause sarcolemma destruction, producing a marked regress of potassium, myoglobin, and creatine kinase (CK) to the extracellular fluid. Skeletal muscle constitutes 40% to 50% of our body mass, so relatively small changes in muscle metabolism may produce the dramatic systemic biochemical changes observed with MH.

Clinical Manifestations

Not all cases of MH are fulminant, but rather there is a spectrum or continuum of severity, ranging from an insidious onset with mild complications to an explosive response with pronounced rigidity, temperature rise, arrhythmias, and death. Although MH may present in several ways, a typical MH episode begins while the patient is under general anesthesia with a volatile anesthetic. Use of succinylcholine may or may not precede the MH episode. The onset of MH symptoms may occur immediately after induction of anesthesia or several hours into the surgery. Desflurane is a weaker MH trigger and has been associated with delayed onset of MH, as long as 6 hours after induction of anesthesia. Succinylcholine appears to accelerate the onset and increase the severity of the MH episode. The presentation of MH may follow a dose-dependent response, with lower concentrations of volatile anesthetics resulting in a more protracted onset of hypermetabolic symptoms. Rarely, MH occurs in the recovery room, usually within 1 hour after general anesthesia.

The clinical features of MH reflect increased intracellular muscle Ca^{2+} concentration and greatly increased body metabolism and are listed in the following section. Common signs of MH include tachycardia, tachypnea, skin mottling, cyanosis, and total body or jaw muscle rigidity. Muscle rigidity is clinically apparent in 75% of cases. The most sensitive indicator of MH is an unanticipated increase in end-tidal carbon dioxide ($ETCO_2$) levels out of proportion to minute ventilation. The increased $ETCO_2$ may be abrupt, or it may rise gradually over the course of the anesthetic. Hyperthermia, which may climb at a rate of 1° to 2° C every 5 minutes and exceed 43.3° C (110° F), is often a late but confirming sign of MH.

Clinical Events

- Unexplained, sudden rise in end-tidal CO_2 (>55 mmHg)
- Unexplained tachycardia, tachypnea, labile blood pressure, or arrhythmias
- Masseter muscle or generalized muscle rigidity
- Unanticipated respiratory or metabolic acidosis
- Rising patient temperature
- Cola-colored urine (myoglobinuria)
- Mottled, cyanotic skin
- Decreased Sao_2

Laboratory Results

- ABG analysis: $Paco_2$ >60 mmHg, base excess more negative than –8 mEq/L, pH <7.25
- Serum potassium >6 mEq/L
- CK >20,000 international units/L
- Serum myoglobin >–170 mcg/L
- Urine myoglobin >–60 mcg/L

The combination of acidosis, hyperkalemia, and hyperthermia leads to cardiac irritability, a labile blood pressure, and arrhythmias that can rapidly progress to cardiac arrest. Laboratory findings mirror the muscle breakdown and include myoglobinuria and increased serum potassium and CK. Serum CK levels peak 12 to 24 hours after the onset of MH. Myoglobin appears in the plasma within minutes of the hypermetabolic muscle response. Arterial and venous blood gas analysis reveals decreased oxygen tension and mixed metabolic and respiratory acidosis. Late complications may include cerebral edema, myoglobinuric renal failure, disseminated intravascular coagulopathy, hepatic dysfunction, and pulmonary edema.

The variable time course and the nonspecific clinical features and laboratory findings can make the diagnosis of MH difficult. Insufficient anesthetic depth, hypoxia, neuroleptic malignant syndrome, propofol infusion syndrome, thyrotoxicosis, pheochromocytoma, and sepsis can share several characteristics with MH, making the clinical picture ambiguous and the differential diagnosis challenging to even the most experienced practitioner. Surgical procedures performed of necessity in a darkened operating room can further compromise the practitioner's diagnostic acumen.

In addition to being a trigger of MH, succinylcholine may also induce hyperkalemic-mediated cardiac arrest in children with occult myopathies. Because of this concern, most anesthetists use nondepolarizing muscle relaxants for elective intubation in children and reserve the use of succinylcholine for treatment of laryngospasm or emergency airway management.

Preoperative Assessment and Prevention

Malignant hyperthermia–susceptible patients may be otherwise healthy and completely unaware of their risk until exposed to a triggering anesthetic. Furthermore, not everyone who has the MH gene develops an MH episode upon each exposure to triggering anesthetics. It is estimated that about 21% of MHS patients have at least one uneventful anesthetic before having an MH episode. Although MH susceptibility cannot be ruled out by history alone, every surgical patient should be questioned about the following information:

- Family or personal history of muscle disorders
- Family history of unexpected intraoperative complications or deaths

- Family or personal history of muscle rigidity or stiffness or high fever under anesthesia
- Personal history of dark or cola-colored urine after surgery

Because MH is considered an inherited disorder, all members of a family in which MH has occurred must be considered MHS unless proven otherwise. Moreover, the absence of a positive family history does not preclude MH susceptibility.

Certain disorders should alert the anesthetist to an increased possibility of MH susceptibility. A clear genetic association between MH and the inherited myopathy central core disease has been demonstrated. Case reports have also linked MH or an MH-like disorder to DMD and BMD dystrophy and forms of periodic paralysis and myotonia. MH-triggering agents should not be administered to patients with these disorders. This caveat is especially consequential in patients undergoing outpatient procedures, who may have more limited postoperative observation.

All patients given general anesthesia for more than 30 minutes should have core temperature monitoring. Stress, fever, prior exercise, and cocaine and alcohol ingestion have been implicated as causal factors of MH, but it is debated whether these factors cause, exacerbate, or have no effect on MH triggering in humans.

Treatment

Enhanced patient monitoring, earlier diagnosis and treatment, and dantrolene administration are responsible for the dramatic decrease in mortality rates from nearly 80% 20 years ago to less than 10% today.

Dantrolene is a unique muscle relaxant that works by reducing the release of calcium from skeletal muscle sarcoplasmic reticulum, counteracting the abnormal intracellular calcium levels accompanying MH. At clinical concentrations, dantrolene does not render the muscle totally flaccid and without tone, but it may cause significant muscle weakness and respiratory insufficiency, especially in patients with preexisting muscle disease. Dantrolene should not be used with calcium channel blockers because the combination may induce life-threatening myocardial depression.

The Malignant Hyperthermia Association of the United States (MHAUS) provides an "Emergency Therapy for MH" poster that should be posted in every surgical site. The following treatment sequence is recommended for an acute MH episode:

- Call for help and alert the surgeon to conclude the procedure promptly.
- Discontinue the volatile anesthetic and succinylcholine.
- Hyperventilate with 100% oxygen at high flows (at least 10 L/min) to improve tissue oxygenation and eliminate CO_2.
- Administer 2.5 mg/kg of dantrolene intravenous bolus and repeat as necessary until symptoms abate. Occasionally, a total dose greater than 10 mg/kg may be needed, but if greater than 20 mg/kg is given without reversal of symptoms, the diagnosis should be reassessed. The alkaline solution is highly irritating to vessels and should be administered into fast-running large peripheral veins or via central venous catheters.
- Dysrhythmias usually respond to treatment of acidosis or hyperkalemia. Treat persistent or life-threatening arrhythmias with standard antiarrhythmic agents (avoid calcium channel blockers).

- If fever is present, initiate cooling by lavage (orogastric, bladder, open cavities), administration of chilled intravenous normal saline, and surface cooling (hypothermia blanket; ice packs to the groins, axilla, and neck).
- Determine ABGs, serum electrolytes, and blood glucose every 15 minutes until the syndrome stabilizes. Correct severe metabolic acidosis with sodium bicarbonate. Baseline values for coagulation studies, CK, myoglobin, and liver enzymes should be established.
- Treat hyperkalemia with hyperventilation, bicarbonate, and intravenous insulin and glucose.
- Maintain urine output greater than 2 mL/kg/hr with hydration and furosemide (0.5–1.0 mg/kg).
- Large losses of intravascular volume should be anticipated. Consider central venous or pulmonary artery hemodynamic monitoring.

Each vial of dantrolene must be reconstituted with 60 mL of sterile water, and its poor water solubility makes it very time consuming to mix and administer the requisite doses. During an MH emergency, the full-time efforts of additional medical personnel should be enlisted. Warming the diluent fluid to 41° C using an intravenous fluid–warming device expedites dantrolene preparation. Documentation of an MH episode should include patient responses, personnel involved, medications, interventions, and patient outcomes.

Anesthetic Considerations

Standard intraoperative monitoring for the MHS surgical patient includes blood pressure, ECG, pulse oximetry, capnography, and continuous measurement of core body temperature. A cooling water mattress should be placed under the MHS patient at the start of the procedure. Dantrolene pretreatment for MHS surgical patients is no longer routine. Inconsistent reports of emotional stress or anxiety predisposing a patient to MH have led to recommendations that anxiolytic agents be included in the premedication.

If the surgical site permits, a regional or local anesthetic technique is preferable for MHS patients. Local anesthetics (both amide and ester) are nontriggering drugs. Nontriggering general anesthetics can also be administered safely in concert with close monitoring of appropriate vital functions. The list of "nontriggering" anesthetic agents is comprehensive enough to meet most anesthetic requirements and are listed below. All volatile inhalation anesthetics and succinylcholine are MH triggers and should not be administered to MHS patients.

Triggering and Nontriggering Agents

Triggering Agents

- All volatile inhalation anesthetics (halothane, desflurane, isoflurane, sevoflurane)
- Succinylcholine

Nontriggering Agents

- Local anesthetics
- Opioids
- Nitrous oxide
- Barbiturates, propofol, ketamine, etomidate
- Benzodiazepines

- Nondepolarizing skeletal muscle relaxants (vecuronium, atracurium, cisatracurium, pancuronium, mivacurium, rocuronium)
- Digoxin, tricyclic antidepressants, magnesium
- Anticholinesterase agents
- Anticholinergic agents

Not all drugs have been thoroughly screened as potential MH triggers, but it is clear that the vast majority of prescription and nonprescription drugs are safe, including antibiotics, antihypertensive agents, and drugs used in the treatment of gastrointestinal disorders. Keys to successful perioperative outcome for the MHS patient include the following:

- Avoidance of MH-triggering medications
- Preparation of an anesthesia machine by changing the soda lime and breathing circuits, removing or inactivating vaporizers, and flushing with oxygen or air at 10 L/min for at least 20 minutes or 10 minutes if the fresh gas hose is also replaced
- Assiduous perioperative observation for signs of MH, including continuous intraoperative monitoring of the patient's $ETCO_2$, arterial oxygen saturation, and core temperature
- A full appreciation of a preestablished treatment protocol by all perioperative medical personnel
- A machine to manufacture ice or the ready availability of ice and the ability to crush it, and a refrigerator containing at least 3000 mL of cold intravenous solution, should be available.

Ambulatory surgery can be safely performed in most MHS patients, provided that appropriate monitoring is used and an adequate supply of dantrolene is available. Patients known or suspected of having MH should be assessed well before their date of outpatient surgery, so that anesthesia records and MH testing center reports (if available) can be collected to corroborate the history.

Outpatient surgical cases for the MHS patient are best scheduled early in the day, allowing for at least 2.5 hours of postanesthesia observation time, including a minimum initial recovery period of 1 hour of monitoring vital signs every 15 minutes. Most MHS patients who experience uneventful outpatient surgery may be discharged on the day of surgery. Some experts recommend conservative management with overnight postoperative hospital admission for patients who have survived a previous fulminant or severe MH episode or when dantrolene prophylaxis is used.

All locations where general anesthesia is administered should contain a fully stocked MH cart with drugs and supplies, including 36 vials of dantrolene. Each minute is critical in an MH emergency, and therefore a dantrolene supply should not be shared with a nearby facility. Dantrolene should be kept in or very close to the operating room so that it is available immediately if MH occurs.

Diagnostic Testing

The most accurate and commonly accepted test available for determining MH susceptibility is the caffeine halothane contracture test (CHCT). This test involves taking a biopsy of skeletal muscle from the patient's thigh and measuring its contractile response to caffeine, halothane, or both. Normal muscle contracts in response to caffeine or halothane, but this is augmented in patients with MH. The test is available at eight medical centers in North America; because it must be completed within hours after muscle biopsy, the patient must travel to the testing site. Patients who have survived an unequivocal episode of MH are considered to have MHS. The CHCT is indicated for family members of an MHS patient or for patients who have had a previous suspicious but undiagnosed reaction to anesthesia. Genetic testing from a blood sample is available, but, at present, this assessment is not highly diagnostic.

Postoperative Implications

The patient who has experienced an acute MH episode should be observed in an intensive care unit for at least 24 hours. Intravenous dantrolene should be continued at approximately 1 mg/kg every 6 hours for a minimum of 24 hours after control of the episode. Recrudescence of an intraoperative episode may occur in 20% to 25% of cases. Patients who experience recrudescence are more likely to have a muscular body type and to have had greater than 150 minutes transpire from induction to MH reaction.

For the MHS patient who has undergone an uneventful surgical course, close observation and monitoring should continue into the postanesthesia care unit. MH can first manifest in the recovery room after uneventful surgery and anesthesia.

Masseter Muscle Rigidity

Masseter muscle rigidity (MMR) or trismus is a sustained and forceful contracture of the masseter muscle. The contracture may be severe enough to make opening the jaw impossible ("jaws of steel"). A mild increase in masseter muscle tone or incomplete jaw relaxation following succinylcholine is fairly common and may be a normal response. However, severe jaw tightness that interferes with intubation may portend an episode of MH. If trismus is further accompanied by generalized body rigidity, MH is highly likely.

Management of trismus in surgical patients is a contentious issue, and authorities are divided on how to proceed after MMR. Some experts recommend cautiously continuing the anesthetic with nontriggering agents after an episode of MMR while monitoring for rhabdomyolysis and signs and symptoms of MH. Others maintain that the safer course is to assume that trismus is a harbinger of MH, discontinue the anesthetic, and cancel elective surgery until results of a muscle biopsy are available.

Because of the likelihood of MH or rhabdomyolysis, the surgical patient should be admitted to the hospital and observed for at least 24 hours after marked jaw rigidity and at least 12 hours after a mild increase in jaw tension. Myoglobinuria may be apparent in the recovery room, and inducing a brisk urine output may lessen the risk of myoglobinuric renal damage. Studies indicate that after MMR, if the CK is greater than 20,000 IU and a concomitant myopathy is not present, the diagnosis of MH is likely. Patients who have experienced MMR should be counseled concerning the possibility that they are MHS and should be referred to a well-informed primary or specialty care physician or genetic counselor for further investigation.

Information Resources

The MHAUS is a nonprofit organization that provides educational and technical information to patients and health care providers. Information is available via fax-on-demand at 800-440-9990 or at http://www.mhaus.org. An MH hotline may be accessed for MH emergencies 24 hours a day at 800-MH-HYPER (800-644-9737). Health care providers are encouraged to report MH episodes to the North American MH Registry.

E. MUSCULAR DYSTROPHY

Definition

Muscular dystrophy is a heterogeneous set of diseases that includes fascioscapulohumeral dystrophy, limb-girdle dystrophy, Becker muscular dystrophy (BMD), Duchenne muscular dystrophy (DMD), and others. DMD, also known as *pseudohypertrophic muscular dystrophy,* is the most common and most severe form.

Pathophysiology

Duchenne muscular dystrophy is an inherited, sex-linked recessive disease. The disease presents in early childhood between 2 and 6 years of age. It is clinically evident in boys and has an incidence of one in 3500 live male births. Girls and women are generally unaffected but are carriers of the disorder. Mental retardation, of varying degrees, occurs in about 30% of patients with DMD. Death often occurs in late adolescence or early adulthood and is usually caused by respiratory failure.

Clinical Manifestations

Patients with DMD experience an infiltration of fibrous and fatty tissue into the muscle followed by a progressive and painless degeneration and necrosis of muscle fibers. Muscle weakness ends with muscle destruction.

Duchenne muscular dystrophy is characterized by an unremitting weakness and a steady deterioration of the proximal muscle groups of the pelvis and shoulders. The child exhibits a clumsy, waddling gait and falls frequently. Weakness of the pelvic girdle leads to the classic finding of the Gower sign, in which patients use their hands to climb up their legs to arise from the floor. A steady deterioration of muscle strength forces most of these boys to start using wheelchairs by the age of 8 to 12 years.

Skeletal muscle atrophy is usually preceded by fat and fibrous tissue infiltration, resulting in pseudohypertrophy. The infiltrative process is most apparent in the calf muscles, which become particularly enlarged.

Degeneration of respiratory muscles occurs and leads to a restrictive type of ventilatory impairment. Unopposed action by healthy, nondystrophic axial muscles predisposes these patients to kyphoscoliosis, which further decreases the pulmonary reserve. Decreasing muscle strength also results in ineffective cough, impaired swallowing, and an inability to mobilize secretions.

More progressive forms of the disease affect not only skeletal muscle but also smooth muscle of the alimentary tract and cardiac muscle. Alimentary tract involvement can lead to intestinal hypomotility, delayed gastric emptying, and gastric dilation.

Myocardial involvement occurs in almost all patients with progressive disease. Myocardial disease includes fibrotic changes localized primarily to the left ventricle. Echocardiography can effectively evaluate left ventricular function in patients with DMD. Clinical symptoms of heart failure do not usually appear unless the patient is severely stressed or until advanced stages of the disease.

Electrocardiographic changes characteristic of preclinical cardiomyopathy include a large or polyphasic R wave in lead V_1, deep Q waves in the lateral precordial leads (V_4 to V_6), premature beats (atrial and ventricular), and labile sinus or atrial tachycardia.

Although often severe, the compromised cardiac and respiratory conditions may be masked by the limited activity imposed by the patient's skeletal myopathy. Added stress, such as that produced by surgery and anesthesia, may suddenly increase cardiorespiratory demand and uncover the weakened cardiac and respiratory states.

Laboratory Results

Laboratory findings include a serum CK level that is 30 to 300 times normal, even early in the disease, reflecting skeletal muscle necrosis and the increased permeability of skeletal muscle membranes. CK concentration is elevated in approximately 70% of female carriers. Skeletal muscle biopsy early in the course of the disease may demonstrate necrosis and phagocytosis of muscle fibers.

Anesthetic Considerations

Patients with DMD are susceptible to untoward anesthesia-related complications. When possible, local or regional anesthesia should be considered.

Generalized muscle weakness, especially in the advanced stages of muscular dystrophy, makes these patients exquisitely sensitive to the respiratory depressant properties of opioids, sedatives, and general anesthetic agents. Preoperative sedation should be minimal, and the smallest possible amounts of anesthetic agents should be used.

Preoperative and postoperative respiratory therapy can help to maximize the patient's pulmonary condition. In patients with more advanced disease, ABG determinations and preoperative pulmonary function studies may elucidate the extent of respiratory involvement and the amount of respiratory reserve. An FVC of less than 35% of that predicted indicates a risk for postoperative pulmonary complications.

The effects of nondepolarizing muscle relaxants must be scrupulously monitored. There is increased muscle relaxant sensitivity, and recovery may be prolonged by three to six times in patients with DMD. Short-acting nondepolarizing muscle relaxants that are carefully titrated with the use of a nerve stimulator are recommended.

Attention to respiratory function must be continued into the postoperative period. Delayed pulmonary insufficiency, as late as 36 hours after surgery, has been reported. At least 24 hours of observation should be instituted after the patient undergoes anesthesia.

Their decreased cardiac reserve makes these patients sensitive to the myocardial depressant effects of general anesthetic agents, sedatives, and narcotics. Cardiac arrest associated with inhalation anesthetics has been reported. A carefully titrated intravenous "balanced" technique may help to provide a smoother cardiovascular course. Ketamine has been used successfully for anesthesia during diagnostic muscle biopsy in patients with DMD. Judicious administration of intravenous fluids is warranted. The sudden occurrence of tachycardia during anesthesia may indicate acute heart failure.

The potential for delayed gastric emptying, in addition to the presence of weak laryngeal reflexes, dictates that the anesthesia plan of care include measures for guarding against aspiration of stomach contents. Gastrokinetic agents and the prophylactic use of a nasogastric tube are recommended to avoid gastric dilation.

Succinylcholine and the potent inhalational agents should not be used in patients with muscular dystrophy because the altered sarcolemma can lead to rhabdomyolysis with their administration. The resultant massive breakdown of muscle fibers produces a profound hyperkalemia that requires extensive and tenacious treatment with hyperventilation, calcium chloride, sodium bicarbonate, and glucose and insulin. Several cases of ventricular fibrillation or cardiac arrest occurring during anesthetic induction have been associated with succinylcholine or potent inhalational agent administration. Additionally, DMD is included among the myopathies that may be associated with MH. The anesthetist should avoid MH-triggering agents and should vigilantly observe for signs and symptoms of MH when these children undergo surgery. Dantrolene and other treatment modalities for MH should be readily available.

F. MYASTHENIA GRAVIS

Definition

Myasthenia gravis, a chronic disease of the neuromuscular junction, is manifested by increasing skeletal muscle weakness, fatigability on effort, and at least partial restoration of function after rest.

Incidence

In the United States at least one in 7500 people have myasthenia gravis. In individuals younger than 50 years, the ratio of women to men with the disease is 3 to 2; however, in those older than 50 years, the disease is equally distributed between the sexes. Myasthenia gravis can begin spontaneously at any age, but it occurs most frequently between the ages of 30 to 40 years. The onset may be abrupt or insidious, and the course is fluctuating, marked by periods of exacerbation and remission. Spontaneous remissions that do occur sometimes persist for years.

Pathophysiology

Electron microscopic examination of the neuromuscular junction of the patient with myasthenia gravis shows a decrease in the number of functional postsynaptic ACh receptors (AChRs). The AChR lesion appears to be caused by immune-mediated destruction, blockage, or inactivation. The prejunctional ACh pool is normal.

Myasthenia gravis is a prototype autoimmune disease. Circulating antibodies react with myoneural AChR proteins, leading to varying degrees of dysfunction. Anti-AChR antibodies (immunoglobulin G [IgG]) are found in the sera of 85% to 90% of patients with myasthenia gravis, but the antibody level does not necessarily correlate with the severity of the disease. Most patients in clinical remission continue to show elevated serum levels of AChR antibodies.

The initiating stimulus for the production of anti-AChR IgG antibodies is unclear. A genetic cause or induction by microbial antigens has been postulated. The thymus gland seems to play a central role in the pathogenesis.

Pregnancy exacerbates the symptoms of myasthenia gravis in 40% of pregnant women with the disease; however, other patients with the disease experience remission or no change in symptoms during pregnancy. Anti-AChR antibodies that pass across the placenta may produce transitory symptoms of weakness in approximately 10% to 15% of infants born to mothers with myasthenia gravis. Signs of weakness (difficulty with breathing, ptosis, facial weakness) in the affected infant are usually present within the first few hours after birth. The condition lasts as long as 21 days, mirroring the half-life of the IgG antibodies.

Clinical Manifestations

The clinical hallmarks of myasthenia gravis include a generalized muscle weakness, which improves with rest, and an inability to sustain or repeat muscular contractions. Enhanced effort produces enhanced weakness. The severity of myasthenia gravis can range from mild (slight ptosis only) to severe (respiratory failure). Environmental, physical, and emotional factors seem to affect the disease process, although unpredictably.

Mouth, eyes, pharynx, proximal limb, and shoulder girdle musculature are most often affected. Visual symptoms (ptosis and diplopia) from extraocular muscle weakness occur in more than 50% of patients with myasthenia gravis. The disease is restricted to the extraocular muscles in 20% of patients. Sensation and cognition are not affected by the disease process.

Thymus gland abnormalities are detectable in about 75% of patients with myasthenia gravis. Other autoimmune disorders, such as thyroid disease, collagen vascular diseases, polymyositis, and RA, occur more frequently in patients with myasthenia gravis. Myocarditis may complicate myasthenia gravis, especially in patients with thymomas. Microscopic lesions of myasthenic cardiac muscles are similar to skeletal muscle lesions, indicating a common pathogenesis. The myocardial inflammation produces dysrhythmias, particularly atrial fibrillation and atrioventricular block.

Treatment

Therapy for patients with myasthenia gravis is directed toward improving neuromuscular transmission and includes cholinesterase inhibitors, corticosteroids and other immunosuppressants, plasmapheresis, intravenous immunoglobulin, and thymectomy.

Treatment with cholinesterase inhibitors can dramatically reduce the symptoms of myasthenia gravis by inhibiting the hydrolysis of ACh and therefore increasing the neurotransmitter's concentration at the neuromuscular junction. Increasing the synaptic concentration of ACh enhances the possibility of postsynaptic AChR occupation, which is critical for the production of a threshold-reaching end plate potential for muscle contraction. Anticholinesterase treatment is particularly successful in patients with milder disease.

The most commonly used anticholinesterase agent in the United States is oral pyridostigmine. Oral pyridostigmine, 60 mg, lasts 3 to 4 hours and is equivalent to an intramuscular or intravenous dose of pyridostigmine, 2 mg, or neostigmine, 1 mg. Titration of the anticholinesterase dose is challenging. Underdosing does not sufficiently retard the muscle weakness and can result in *myasthenic crisis*, a severe exacerbation of myasthenic symptoms.

Overmedicating with a cholinesterase inhibitor can produce a surplus of ACh at the myoneural junction, causing a depolarizing-like block and augmenting skeletal muscle weakness. This situation is called *cholinergic crisis*. Muscarinic side effects (e.g., abdominal cramping, diarrhea, salivation, bradycardia, and miosis) predominate in a cholinergic crisis.

Corticosteroid therapy produces an 80% remission rate in patients with myasthenia gravis, partly by reducing AChR antibody levels. Glucocorticoid therapy is often used in combination with other agents. Use is limited by the side effects (e.g., osteoporosis, gastrointestinal bleeding, suppression of endogenous cortisol release, cataracts, increased susceptibility to acute infections, hypertension, and glucose intolerance) observed with long-term administration.

In patients with more debilitating, widespread disease, immunosuppressive drugs such as azathioprine (Imuran) and cyclosporine may induce remission by interfering with the production of AChR antibodies. Side effects of azathioprine include severe hemopoietic depression and liver dysfunction. Cyclosporine side effects include hypertension and nephrotoxicity.

Excision of the thymus gland is recommended for adults with generalized disease and for patients with thymomas, thymus gland hyperplasia, or drug-resistant myasthenia gravis. Thymectomy effectively arrests or reverses the myasthenic process by removing a major source of antibody production. Clinical improvement of myasthenic symptoms is seen in 75% to 96% of patients within weeks to months after surgery.

Plasmapheresis (plasma exchange) arrests severe refractive myasthenia gravis by reducing the concentration of circulating antibodies. It is used primarily as a short-term treatment because the improvement that it produces in symptoms is generally short lived. Intravenous immunoglobulin may also be used for short-term control of symptoms before surgery.

Anesthetic Considerations

Several days before the operation and again immediately before surgery, the surgical candidate with myasthenia gravis should be evaluated for disease control and, if applicable, for stabilization of anticholinesterase dose.

The use of anticholinesterase medication in the immediate preoperative period is controversial. Some experts believe that an awareness of drug mechanisms can enable anticholinesterase therapy to be safely continued into the preoperative period, especially in patients who depend on this therapy for their well-being. Others recommend discontinuing or tapering anticholinesterase medication before surgery to avoid complicating the anesthetic management. Patients with mild myasthenia gravis can usually tolerate the temporary disruption in treatment.

The presence of cholinesterase inhibitors may potentiate vagal responses and complicates both the intraoperative administration of muscle relaxants and the differential diagnosis and treatment of postoperative muscle weakness. Emotional stress and surgery may precipitate or worsen skeletal muscle weakness. Pharyngeal and laryngeal muscle weakness, difficulty in eliminating oral secretions, and the risk of pulmonary aspiration should be considered in the anesthesia plan of care. Swallowing and respiratory muscle dysfunction account for much of the morbidity and potential mortality in patients with myasthenia gravis.

Regional or local anesthesia with careful monitoring are the preferred anesthetic techniques when appropriate. If general anesthesia is indicated, the respiratory depressant effects of barbiturates, sedatives, narcotics, and volatile anesthetic agents, compounded by the presence of an already weakened respiratory system, must be carefully considered.

In many patients, the relaxant effects of a volatile anesthetic in combination with the patient's preexisting skeletal muscle weakness are sufficient to facilitate intubation of the trachea. Enhanced muscle relaxation may be seen with the administration of all the potent volatile anesthetics.

Small doses of succinylcholine may be used to facilitate tracheal intubation, but the response may be unpredictable. Untreated patients with myasthenia gravis appear to be two to three times more resistant to succinylcholine. Normal dosages of succinylcholine may not effectively depolarize the end plate because of the deficiency of viable AChRs. On the other hand, patients treated with cholinesterase inhibitors exhibit a normal or prolonged response to succinylcholine. Cholinesterase inhibitors block the effects of plasma cholinesterase, as well as those of true cholinesterase; hence, succinylcholine and other medications metabolized by plasma cholinesterase (e.g., ester local anesthetics) may have a delayed hydrolysis and a prolonged duration of action. The ester hydrolysis of atracurium is independent of plasma cholinesterase activity.

The deficient number of functioning AChRs in patients with myasthenia gravis produces an extraordinary sensitivity to nondepolarizing muscle relaxants. Small doses of nondepolarizing agents can produce a profound block with a prolonged effect even in patients being treated with cholinergic drugs. Some patients require no medication at all for surgical muscle relaxation. If muscle relaxation is necessary, cisatracurium offers an advantage of being metabolized by non–organ-dependent mechanisms.

Generally, muscle relaxant requirements are widely variable in patients with myasthenia gravis, a characteristic that makes neuromuscular blockade monitoring an essential and integral part of the anesthetic management. The orbicularis oculi muscle may overestimate the degree of muscle relaxation in patients with myasthenia gravis. This site may be the most ideal site to monitor neuromuscular blockade to avoid the possibility of undetected residual muscle weakness. When needed, the use of smaller doses (half to two-thirds the normal dose) of shorter acting nondepolarizing relaxants is the prudent choice.

Reversal of neuromuscular blockade with an acetylcholinesterase inhibitor should be performed cautiously in patients with myasthenia gravis. Overtreatment with an anticholinesterase agent can precipitate a cholinergic crisis and aggravate rather than reverse the muscle weakness. In many circumstances, the neuromuscular block can be titrated to allow complete spontaneous recovery, avoiding the use of reversal.

Complete, sustained return of muscle strength must be demonstrated before extubation and resumption of spontaneous ventilation. The patient should be informed that postoperative tracheal intubation and ventilatory support may be required. Skeletal muscle strength may appear to be adequate shortly after surgery but may deteriorate a few hours later. Postoperative ventilation is recommended for patients undergoing transsternal thymectomy, who have the disease for longer than 6 years, who take a daily pyridostigmine dose greater than 750 mg, who have chronic obstructive pulmonary disease, or have a preoperative VC less than 2.9 L.

G. MYOTONIC DYSTROPHY

Definition

The myotonias are a group of hereditary degenerative muscle diseases that include myotonic dystrophy, myotonia congenita (Thomsen disease), and paramyotonia congenita. A symptom common to all myotonias is the inability of skeletal muscles to relax after chemical or physical stimulation.

Myotonic dystrophy, also known as *Steinert disease, myotonia atrophica,* or *myotonia dystrophica,* is the most common and the most severe form of the myotonias. It is characterized by skeletal muscles that are hypoplastic, dystrophic, and weak yet prone to persistent contraction. Although muscles are primarily affected, myotonic dystrophy is distinguished from nondystrophic myotonias by being a multisystem disease.

Incidence

Myotonic dystrophy is inherited as an autosomal dominant trait. In most cases, an affected person has one affected parent. The onset of symptoms can occur at any age but usually occurs in the second to third decade of life. A slow, progressive deterioration of skeletal, cardiac, and smooth muscle occurs, resulting in death by the sixth decade. An estimated one in 20,000 people worldwide have the disorder, with an equal occurrence in males and females. The severity of clinical symptoms usually increases with transmission to subsequent generations (*genetic anticipation*). Myotonic dystrophy is the most common and severe inherited muscular dystrophy of adulthood.

Pathophysiology and Treatment

Myotonic dystrophy is a disorder of muscle membrane excitability that results in self-sustaining runs of depolarization. Electrophysiologic studies show a lowered resting membrane potential in muscle cells from patients with myotonic dystrophy. Therapeutic agents used to treat the myotonic contractures include quinine, procainamide, and phenytoin. These agents delay the return of membrane excitation by blocking rapid Na^+ influx into muscle cells. Regional anesthesia and muscle relaxants do not prevent or relieve the recalcitrant contraction. Dantrolene has also been ineffective in reversing myotonia. Warming the ambient temperature or injecting local anesthetics into the involved muscles may induce relaxation. Steroids and inhalation anesthetic agents may also attenuate the contraction in some patients. No treatment is available for the muscle weakness that develops with myotonic dystrophy.

Clinical Manifestations

A wide variety of symptoms are characteristic of myotonic dystrophy. Facial weakness ("expressionless facies"), ptosis, and sternocleidomastoid muscle and distal limb weakness are prominent features of the disease. Frontal balding, cataracts, and testicular atrophy in men form a frequently recognized triad of characteristics. Endocrine abnormalities, such as diabetes mellitus and thyroid disease, occur with a greater frequency in this patient group than in the general population.

Myotonia, an inability to relax a muscle, occurs in most symptomatic patients and may be worsened by pressure, touch, cold, or shivering. Insidious muscle atrophy, particularly of the face, neck, pharynx, and distal limbs, causes severe muscle debility in the later stages of the disease. Myotonic symptoms usually precede the atrophy and weakness.

Cardiac disturbances occur in most patients with myotonic dystrophy, often manifesting as conduction defects and arrhythmias. Conduction defects were present in about 50% of the patients in one series. First-degree atrioventricular block is the most common finding, but greater degrees of heart block are also seen. Arrhythmias include sinus bradycardia, atrial flutter or fibrillation, and ventricular extrasystoles.

Weakening of the thoracic muscles, including the diaphragm, reduces the respiratory reserve and the VC, and a restrictive type of ventilatory impairment develops with progression of the disease. Central sleep apnea and hypersomnolence cause hypoventilation and decreased ventilatory response to carbon dioxide.

Anesthetic Considerations

Any drug that has the potential to depolarize skeletal muscle may produce an exaggerated contraction in patients with myotonia dystrophica. Administration of succinylcholine to patients with myotonic dystrophy should be avoided because it can produce an intense generalized myotonic contracture that makes ventilation and intubation difficult or impossible. Agents associated with myoclonus (methohexital, etomidate) have the potential to produce similar effects.

Nondepolarizing muscle relaxants may be used in these patients as long as the degree of muscle wasting and weakness is appreciated. The dose of the nondepolarizer should be reduced according to the degree of muscle impairment, and the neuromuscular block should be monitored closely with a peripheral nerve stimulator.

An abnormal swallowing mechanism resulting from palatal, pharyngeal, and esophageal muscle involvement and gastrointestinal hypomotility renders these patients vulnerable to pulmonary aspiration of gastric contents.

Reversal of neuromuscular blockade with anticholinesterase agents may theoretically precipitate skeletal muscle contraction by producing an ACh-induced depolarizing block. Shorter acting nondepolarizing muscle relaxants have the obvious advantage of being less likely to require reversal. Hypothermia and shivering should be avoided by raising the room temperature, warming inhaled gases and intravenous fluids, and providing a forced-air thermal blanket.

Underestimating the severity of respiratory compromise is not uncommon in these patients. Preoperative ABG determinations and pulmonary function results may serve as useful baselines in the patient with advanced disease. The respiratory depressant effects of barbiturates, opioids, and volatile anesthetics may compromise already weakened respiratory musculature and may lead to unexpected decompensation. Even small doses of short-acting anesthetic agents may be associated with an exaggerated and prolonged anesthetic effect.

Diligent monitoring of cardiovascular parameters should be maintained intraoperatively and postoperatively. Cardiac function that was clinically normal preoperatively may become unacceptably depressed as a result of the administration of general anesthetic agents. The patient should be questioned preoperatively about syncope, and the ECG should be examined closely for advanced conduction blocks to help ascertain the need for cardiac pacing. It may be wise to assume that even asymptomatic patients have some degree of cardiac involvement. Pregnancy may exacerbate the symptoms of myotonia. Uterine atony, postpartum hemorrhage, and retained placenta have accompanied delivery in patients with myotonic dystrophy. Increased progesterone levels are linked to the deleterious effects.

Malignant hyperthermia–triggering agents should be avoided in these patients because associations between some forms of myotonia and MH have been described.

H. PECTUS DEFORMITIES

PECTUS EXCAVATUM

Definition

Pectus excavatum, also referred to as *funnel chest,* is the most common chest wall deformity, occurring in one in 400 children.

Pathophysiology

Pectus excavatum is a congenital abnormality characterized by depression of the sternum (usually above the xiphisternal junction) and symmetric or asymmetric prominence of the ribs on either side. Its origin is unknown; however, it is thought that excessive diaphragmatic traction on the lower sternum or displacement of the heart into the left hemithorax is largely responsible. Family history of some type of anterior thoracic deformity is present in 37% of patients. If uncorrected, the disease usually worsens at adolescence. Self-limiting deformities are either gone or vastly improved by the age of 3 years.

Clinical Manifestations

Clinically, the majority of patients are asymptomatic unless pectus excavatum is extreme. Patients with pectus excavatum have reduced chest cavities and TLC. Pulmonary function often is normal except in severe cases, in which VC, TLC, and maximum breathing capacity may be diminished.

Treatment

The indications for repair of pectus excavatum are the subject of controversy. Conflicting data have been presented regarding whether the repair of pectus excavatum is performed only for cosmetic purposes or whether it actually improves cardiorespiratory function and exercise tolerance. Some clinicians suggest that pectus excavatum should be corrected in childhood—ideally, when patients are between the ages of 4 and 6 years—to relieve the structural compromise of the chest, allow normal growth of the thorax, prevent pulmonary and cardiac dysfunction in teens and adults, and improve cosmetic appearance. Others have found that surgery does not significantly improve pulmonary function and that exercise tolerance and cardiorespiratory function during exercise do not benefit significantly from surgical correction. Patients with Marfan syndrome have a high incidence of chest wall deformities; they usually are seen in their most severe form, often accompanied by scoliosis. Congenital heart disease, mitral valve prolapse, and asthma also occur more frequently in patients with pectus excavatum. Electrocardiographic abnormalities are common and attributable to the abnormal chest wall configuration and to the displacement and rotation of the heart into the left thoracic cavity. A systolic ejection murmur of grades II to III or IV frequently is identified.

PECTUS CARINATUM

Definition and Incidence

Pectus carinatum is characterized by a longitudinal protrusion of the sternum. It is the second most common chest deformity, occurring in one or two persons per 1000. A familial tendency exists, and the disorder is more frequent in males than in females (4:1 ratio).

Pathophysiology

The pathogenesis is unclear, and the disorder may be congenital or acquired. The development of pectus carinatum is thought to result from the overgrowth of the costal cartilages, which results in displacement of the sternum.

Clinical Manifestations

The development of pectus carinatum has also been associated with severe childhood asthma and rickets. The physiologic effects are probably related to the restriction of thoracic excursion. Patients with pectus carinatum have an increased incidence of congenital heart disease, including ventricular septal defect, patent ductus arteriosus, atrial septal defects, and mitral valve abnormalities.

Three classifications of pectus carinatum exist. Type I, pigeon breast or keel chest, consists of symmetric protrusion of the sternum and costal cartilages. Type II, pouter pigeon breast or Currarino-Silverman syndrome, is characterized by protrusion of the manubrium of the first two sternal cartilages, backward arching of the sternal body, and anterior displacement of the xiphoid process. Type III, lateral pectus carinatum, is manifested by unilateral protrusion of the anterior chest wall.

Treatment

Surgery is the only effective treatment for pectus carinatum and is performed to alleviate possible cardiopulmonary dysfunction and to prevent progressive postural deformities, as well as for cosmetic reasons.

I. RHEUMATOID ARTHRITIS

Definition

Rheumatoid arthritis (RA) is a chronic inflammatory polyarthropathy with myriad degrees of systemic involvement. The disease is multifactorial, and the clinical picture varies widely in severity, extent of involvement, and symptoms. The capricious course of the disease may be persistent and debilitating or relapsing and remitting. With each successive exacerbation, new joints may become involved.

Incidence

Rheumatoid arthritis is the most common form of inflammatory arthritis, affecting approximately 0.8% of the U.S. population. The onset of RA can occur at any age, but most cases are diagnosed in patients between the ages of 35 and 50 years. RA is two to three times more likely to develop in women than in men. Patients with RA have a reduced life expectancy ranging from 3 to 7 years.

Pathophysiology

The exact cause of RA remains elusive, but heredity plays some role in increasing a person's susceptibility. Impaired immunity, stress, and other environmental factors may precipitate or aggravate the disease.

A viral or a bacterial infection that alters the immune system in a genetically susceptible host may play a role in the etiology. The invading microbe may produce a protein similar to those in the body's own tissue, particularly joint tissue (*molecular mimicry*). To destroy the antigen, the immune system may mount an autoimmune response and mistakenly direct its attack against its own tissue. Circulating autoantibodies called *rheumatoid factors* are detectable in 70% to 80% of patients with RA.

Clinical Manifestations

Joint Involvement

Inflammation and destruction of synovial tissues are responsible for most of the symptoms and chronic disability associated with RA. Joint involvement progresses in three main stages: (1) inflammation of the joint synovial membrane and infiltration by polymorphonuclear leukocytes; (2) rapid division and growth of cells in the joint (synovial proliferation and pannus formation); and (3) liberation of osteolytic enzymes, proteases, and collagenases, which damage small blood vessels, cartilage, ligaments, tendons, and bones. Collapse of normal cortical and medullary architecture leads to erosion and dislocation of bone that is contiguous with the inflammatory cell mass.

The onset of symptoms is most often insidious, evolving over a period of weeks to months. The most common sites of onset are the hands, wrists, and feet. There is often symmetric joint involvement. Swelling, warmth, and pain in the affected joints are caused by the inflammatory process. Morning stiffness, weight loss, and fatigue are noted early in the disease course.

Dissolution of bone and disuse atrophy of bone (osteoporosis) are found in all seriously affected areas. Pain, inflammation, and erosion of bone and tissue may permanently limit the joint's full range of motion. Later stages of the disease are characterized by severe pain, joint instability, and crippling deformities. Nerve entrapment may occur at any site where peripheral nerves pass near the inflamed joint. Carpal tunnel syndrome is a common peripheral neuropathy.

Synovitis in the temporomandibular joint may limit jaw motion. An estimated 30% to 70% of patients with RA have involvement of the temporomandibular joint. As the disease progresses, flexion contractures and soft tissue swelling may lead to a marked limitation in the patient's ability to open the jaw.

Although the thoracic and lumbar spine are usually spared, involvement of the cervical spine may be extensive and can lead to limited movement or deformity of the neck and to severe laryngeal deviation.

The most common site of cervical spine synovitis is C1 to C2. Atlantoaxial (C1–C2) instability results from erosion and collapse of bone and from destruction of supporting cervical ligaments. Symptoms occur when excessive motion between C1 and C2 exerts pressure on the spinal cord. Additionally, separation of the atlanto-odontoid articulation may allow the odontoid process of the axis to impinge on the spinal cord, leading to neurologic damage. The atlantoaxial subluxation may also exert pressure and impair blood flow through the vertebral arteries.

Arthritis extends to the cricoarytenoid joint of the larynx in 40% of patients with severe RA. The joint may become swollen, inflamed, and fixed in a position that obstructs air flow. Vocal cord nodules and polyps may also be present. Symptoms of cricoarytenoid arthritis include tenderness over the larynx, hoarseness, pain on swallowing with radiation to the ear, and dyspnea or stridor. Patients with no overt clinical symptoms may also have significant laryngeal disease.

Systemic Involvement

Although the effects of RA are most clearly seen in joints, the disease is systemic. The immune-mediated destructive process affects a wide variety of organs, including the heart, lungs, muscle, vasculature, and eyes. The occurrence of extraarticular manifestations is usually associated with more active, erosive articular disease.

Firm, painless subcutaneous nodules occur in approximately 20% to 30% of patients with RA. The nodules usually occur over pressure points, such as the occiput, sacrum, ulna, or Achilles tendon and may be associated with pressure ulcerations. Rheumatoid nodules can also occur in most visceral organs, including the lungs and the heart. Dural nodules can cause spinal cord compression and neurologic complications.

Pericarditis and pericardial effusion may accompany severe progressive RA and impair cardiac performance. Although rare, rheumatoid nodules have been isolated from the cardiac conduction system and may be associated with conduction defects.

Pulmonary involvement manifests as pleural effusion, pneumonitis, pulmonary nodules, or interstitial fibrosis. Decreased lung volume, diffusion capacity, and VC may result from the lung alterations.

Rheumatoid myositis, which is characterized by muscle weakness and eventual muscle necrosis and atrophy, may accompany RA. Inflamed, painful, and underused joints contribute to the skeletal muscle atrophy. Lacrimal duct and salivary gland destruction may result in dryness of the eyes and the mouth (Sjögren syndrome) in about 15% of patients with RA.

Treatment

There is no cure for RA, and all treatment interventions are palliative. Medical therapy is directed toward relief of pain, nonspecific suppression of the inflammatory process, immunosuppression, prevention and correction of deformity, and control of systemic involvement. Most patients, including those with mild to moderate disease, obtain some relief of symptoms with rest, joint immobilization, and use of NSAIDs. NSAIDs relieve joint pain, stiffness, heat, and swelling, partly by blocking cyclooxygenase and inhibiting prostaglandin, thromboxane, and prostacyclin synthesis. Despite their potent antiinflammatory properties, they do not alter the underlying disease process.

Corticosteroids are potent anti-inflammatory drugs that suppress many symptoms of RA. Long-term side effects (osteoporosis, predisposition to infection, suppression of endogenous cortisol release, cataracts, gastrointestinal bleeding, hypertension, and hyperglycemia), however, limit their use to isolated flares of the disease or to adjunctive, rather than primary treatment.

Disease-modifying antirheumatic drugs (DMARDs) can slow the progressive damage and arrest the underlying disease process. Agents such as the anticytokines etanercept (Enbrel), adalimumab (Humira), and infliximab (Remicade) work by interfering with the proinflammatory cytokine, tumor necrosis factor. Notably, these drugs increase the risk of developing serious infection. Biologic agents such as interleukin-1 receptor antagonists offer the potential for more effective treatment of RA. Leflunomide (Arava) is a DMARD that inhibits the proliferation of T lymphocytes and slows disease progression. The major side effect of leflunomide is liver enzyme elevation and liver disease.

The antimetabolite methotrexate (Rheumatrex) is widely used as an effective DMARD for patients with aggressive RA. Bone marrow suppression, oral ulcerations, pneumonitis, and hepatic damage are potential side effects of methotrexate. Gold salts, sulfasalazine, antimalarial drugs, and D-penicillamine are effective DMARDs used when more conservative measures fail to retard symptoms. Immunosuppressive drugs such as cyclophosphamide (Cytoxan) and cyclosporine (Sandimmune) and antimetabolites such as azathioprine (Imuran) are effective agents, generally reserved for more refractory cases. Surgical interventions for relief of pain or for correction or prevention of deformities include total joint replacement, synovectomy, and tenolysis.

Anesthetic Considerations

Overall, no individual anesthetic agent or mode of anesthesia is substantially safer than another for patients with RA. Preoperative examination of an individual patient's disease course and medication history are likely to reveal specific features that affect the anesthesia or surgical course.

NSAID ingestion may result in platelet dysfunction. Mild anemia, a common finding in patients with RA, may be secondary to the disease process or to drug therapy. Long-term NSAID therapy may exert harmful effects on the liver or kidney, exacerbate allergic rhinitis or asthma; and cause gastrointestinal bleeding; these effects may influence the choice of anesthesia.

Patients receiving long-term corticosteroid therapy may develop hypophyseal–pituitary axis suppression, which may require perioperative steroid supplementation. Long-term administration of corticosteroids may increase the patient's susceptibility to infection by inhibiting normal host defense mechanisms. The newer tumor necrosis factor inhibitors are also associated with serious infections, mandating close attention to sterile techniques.

A thorough preoperative assessment of the airway is essential. Particular attention should be directed to the temporomandibular joints (TMJs), the cervical spine, and the cricoarytenoid joints. Range of motion of the TMJ must be assessed before anesthesia is induced. Patients with severe TMJ involvement may be able to open their mouths only 1 to 2 cm. In such cases, the use of the flexible fiberoptic bronchoscope for tracheal intubation is of proven value.

A thorough neurologic assessment and a radiographic evaluation of the cervical spine should be performed, especially for patients with advanced disease. Some patients with significant radiographic evidence of atlantoaxial or subaxial instability may be entirely asymptomatic. Neck pain is an early symptom of cervical spine instability. Paresthesias that extend into the shoulders and arms, muscle weakness, paresis, and bowel or bladder dysfunction are some of the clinical manifestations of spinal cord compression secondary to atlantoaxial or subaxial subluxation. Compression on the vertebral arteries, with interruption of vertebral artery blood flow, may lead to symptoms such as nausea, vomiting, dysarthria, dysphagia, blurred vision, or transient loss of consciousness.

Altered cervical spine anatomy or laryngeal deviation can make intubation of the trachea an extreme challenge. Deviation of the larynx can frequently be detected preoperatively by palpating the location of the larynx in relation to the sternal notch. Flexion, extension, and rotation of the neck must be avoided in the presence of cervical instability. Such circumstances dictate fiberoptic-guided intubation of the trachea in an awake patient.

Hoarseness in a patient with RA should alert the anesthetist to possible cricoarytenoid joint involvement. A smaller endotracheal tube may be necessary because of narrowing of the glottic opening. Laryngoscopy can assess normal cord motion and glottic patency. The patient should be observed closely for signs of airway obstruction after extubation.

Generalized demineralization of bone may increase the risk of fractures in patients with RA. Glucocorticoid therapy may aggravate the osteopenia. Proper patient positioning and padding of pressure points prevent nerve palsies, skin ulcerations, and further structural damage to the joints.

Renal System

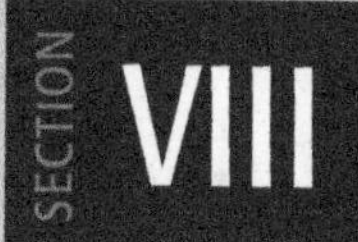

A. ACUTE RENAL FAILURE

Definition

Acute renal failure (acute tubular necrosis, vasomotor neuropathy, lower nephron necrosis) is defined as the sudden inability of the kidneys to vary urine volume and content appropriately in response to homeostatic needs.

Pathophysiology

Acute renal failure is classified according to its predominant cause or on the basis of urine flow rates. The cause of acute renal failure has prerenal, renal, or postrenal origins. Prerenal failure results from hemodynamic or endocrine factors that impair renal perfusion, renal failure results from tissue damage, and postrenal failure results from urinary tract obstruction. Prerenal or postrenal failure is reversed with attention to hemodynamics or relief of obstruction. Acute renal failure caused by parenchymal disease or damage is more serious and often requires hemodialysis. Common causes are listed below.

Common Causes of Acute Renal Failure

- Hypovolemia
- Impaired renal perfusion
- Sepsis
- Drugs
  - Radiocontrast media
  - Antimicrobials
- Hepatic dysfunction
- Vascular occlusion
- Obstruction of collecting system

PRIMARY RENAL DISEASE

Failure classified according to urine flow rates is known as *oliguric, non-oliguric,* or *polyuric* failure. Oliguria is defined as a urinary flow rate less than 0.5 mL/kg/hr in a patient subjected to acute stress. This rate is higher than that seen in unstressed patients because acutely stressed patients cannot maximally concentrate urine. Polyuric failure is associated with elevations of blood urea, nitrogen, and serum creatinine levels and is characterized by urine flow rates that exceed 2.5 L/day.

Conditions that lead to prerenal oliguria include acute reductions in glomerular filtration rate (GFR), excessive reabsorption of salt or water, or both. Increases in circulating levels of catecholamines, antidiuretic hormone (ADH), or aldosterone are physiologic factors that can decrease urinary output. Hypotension may or may not be present in the initiation of acute renal failure. If not reversed, prerenal oliguria may progress to parenchymal damage and tubular necrosis.

Acute Tubular Necrosis

Acute tubular necrosis may be produced by a variety of factors that interfere with glomerular filtration or tubular reabsorption. The pathogenesis of acute tubular necrosis may be divided into an initiation period, a maintenance period, and a recovery period. Renal hypoperfusion or a nephrotoxic insult may initiate renal failure. Surgical patients with external and internal fluid losses or sepsis may have renal hypoperfusion. The initiating insult culminates in the development of one or more maintenance factors, such as decreased tubular function, tubular obstruction, and sustained reductions in renal blood flow and glomerular filtration. Urine flow and solute excretion are reduced. When the maintenance period has begun, pharmacologic interventions to improve renal blood flow do not reverse the failure.

Prerenal Oliguria

Prerenal oliguria is associated with physiologic mechanisms that conserve salt and water. In this case, urine has low sodium levels and high osmolality. Urine sodium levels are high, and osmolality is low. Renal damage is also associated with a progressive rise in serum urea, creatinine, uric acid, and polypeptide levels. Serum potassium levels may increase by 0.3 to 3 mEq/L/day, and a decrease occurs in the serum levels of sodium, calcium, and proteins such as albumin. The creatinine clearance remains the single most helpful test in defining renal status and predicting the prognosis in cases of severe renal dysfunction.

Risk Factors

A number of conditions may place patients at high risk for acute renal failure and are listed in the following section. Renal reserve decreases progressively with age. For each year after 50 years of age, creatinine clearance decreases by 1.5 mL and renal plasma flow by 8 mL. Older patients are less able to cope with fluid and electrolyte imbalance and are more prone to renal damage. Overall mortality rates associated with acute renal failure increase from 50% for those younger than age 40 years to 80% for those older than age 60 years.

Classification of Acute Renal Failure

- I. **Prerenal failure**
  - A. Hypoperfusion or hypovolemia
    1. Skin losses
    2. Fluid losses
    3. Hemorrhage
    4. Sequestration
  - B. Cardiovascular failure
    1. Myocardial failure
    2. Vascular pooling
    3. Vascular occlusion
       - a. Thromboembolic phenomena
       - b. Aortic or renal artery clamping
- II. **Renal or acute tubular necrosis**
  - A. Prolonged renal ischemia
  - B. Nephrotoxic injury
    1. Hemepigments
    2. Some anesthetics
    3. Antibiotics
    4. Radiocontrast dyes
    5. Chemotherapeutic agents

   C. Miscellaneous
      1. Cellular debris
      2. Acute interstitial nephritis
      3. Hypersensitivity reactions
      4. Acute glomerulonephritis

III. Postrenal failure
   A. Obstruction
      1. Calculi
      2. Blood clots
      3. Neoplasm
   B. Surgical ligation
   C. Edema

Prevention and Management

Prevention of renal failure can be based on the following generalizations:

- The most common cause of failure is prolonged renal hypoperfusion.
- Prophylaxis reduces mortality more effectively than dialytic therapy.
- The duration and magnitude of the initiating renal insult are critical in determining the severity of failure.

A key strategy in reducing the incidence of renal failure is limiting the magnitude and duration of renal ischemia. Although a number of preventive strategies have been described, none apart from maintenance of normovolemia appears to be effective.

Anesthetic Considerations

Preoperative

In the preoperative preparation of surgical patients, high-risk patients and procedures should be identified. Reversible renal dysfunction should be sought, and fluid losses and hypovolemia should be corrected by intravenous fluids. Perioperative ADH and renin–angiotensin–aldosterone secretion can be minimized with adequate hydration before anesthetic induction. Administration of saline rather than solutions low in sodium is helpful in prevention of aldosterone secretion, hyponatremia, and oliguria.

Oliguria often signals inadequate systemic perfusion, and prevention of acute renal failure requires its rapid recognition through adequate monitoring. In addition to standard monitors and a urinary catheter, monitors for patients with questionable cardiac and pulmonary function should include a direct arterial line for blood pressure monitoring and a central venous pressure (CVP) or Swan-Ganz catheter, when appropriate, for assessment of cardiac function and volume status.

Perioperative

Use of a urinary catheter is the only means of monitoring renal function in the operating room. A fluid challenge is necessary if hourly urinary output decreases to below acceptable levels.

The use of diuretics in the face of inadequate urinary output must be carefully evaluated. Although diuretics may not be effective during the initiation of failure, large doses of furosemide may convert oliguric renal failure into nonoliguric failure, which is easier to manage. In the maintenance phase, doses of furosemide in excess of 1 g may be required to convert oliguric failure to nonoliguric failure. Diuretic therapy must be associated with aggressive monitoring and intravascular volume expansion.

Although the mechanism is unknown, prophylactic administration of mannitol in well-hydrated patients protects renal function. Loop diuretics may also prevent acute renal failure. Mechanisms for protection include the inhibition of sodium reabsorption and the prevention of tubular obstruction through the maintenance of high flow and pressure within the tubules and the reversal of intrinsic renal vasoconstriction. Prophylactic use of diuretics may be of benefit in the case of jaundice in surgical patients, excessive exposure to contrast media, hyperuricemia, or the presence of pigment in the urine. Fenoldopam, a dopamine receptor agonist, also may be helpful.

Fenoldopam mesylate (Corlopam) is a selective DA_1 receptor agonist. It causes both systemic and renal arteriolar vasodilation and has no impact on DA_2, α-adrenergic, or β-adrenergic receptors. Unlike dopamine, which causes renal vasoconstriction at higher doses, fenoldopam at high dose produces even greater renal vasodilation. Fenoldopam is more than six times as potent as dopamine in increasing renal blood flow.

Management of Acute Renal Failure

If acute renal failure develops, it progresses through four distinct phases: onset, the oliguric phase, the diuretic phase, and the recovery phase. Onset, or the initiation phase, precedes actual necrotic injury and correlates with a major alteration in renal hemodynamics. The oliguric phase reflects four pathophysiologic processes:

1. Obstruction of tubules by cellular debris, tubular casts, or tissue swelling
2. Total reabsorption or backleak of urine filtrate through damaged tubular epithelium and into the circulation
3. Tubular cell damage with leakage of adenosine triphosphate (ATP) and potassium and edema
4. Continuation of renal vasoconstriction

The diuretic phase signifies that tubular function is returning. It is marked by a large daily urinary output (more than 3 L) secondary to the osmotic diuretic effect produced by an elevated blood urea nitrogen (BUN) and impaired ability of tubules to conserve sodium and water. The recovery phase is characterized by gradual improvement of renal function over 3 months to 1 year.

After renal failure is established, the primary consideration in management is the maintenance of fluid and electrolyte balance. The early use of hemodialysis for the prevention of severe fluid and electrolyte imbalance is necessary during the oliguric and diuretic phases. The clinical management of oliguria is discussed in the following section.

Algorithm for Clinical Management of Perioperative Oliguria

- Oliguria is less than 0.5 mL/kg but may be 1 to 2 mL/kg in a patient who has received mannitol.
- Assume oliguria is prerenal until proven otherwise.
- Do not give a diuretic to "make urine" in the face of intravascular hypovolemia or hypotension.
- Do not give diuretics if there are signs of fluid overload or if oliguria persists despite fluid challenges and stabilized hemodynamics or if there is pigment nephropathy.
- If improvement is not noted with fluid challenge or diuretics, institute invasive hemodynamic monitoring.

- Maximize renal blood flow by enhancing cardiac function: normalize preload, heart rate, rhythm, consider afterload reduction with vasodilators or inodilator agents.
- Prophylactic pharmacologic agents may be used when renal risk is high, but there is little evidence to suggest that they are better at maintaining GFR than volume.
- Diuretic resistance may be related to:
  - Acute tolerance induced by hypovolemia
  - Chronic tolerance
  - Refractory states

B. CHRONIC RENAL FAILURE

Definition

Chronic renal failure is a slow, progressive, irreversible condition characterized by diminished functioning of nephrons and a decrease in renal blood flow, GFR, tubular function, and reabsorptive capacity.

Pathophysiology

Although many conditions may lead to renal failure, primary causes include glomerulonephritis, pyelonephritis, diabetes mellitus, vascular or hypertensive insults, and congenital defects. The systemic effects of chronic renal failure are shown in the following box.

Systemic Effects of Renal Disease

System	Effects
Cardiovascular	Hypertension Congestive heart failure Peripheral and pulmonary edema Pericarditis Coronary artery disease
Hematologic	Normochromic, normocytic anemia Platelet dysfunction Leukocyte, immunologic dysfunction
Neurologic	Encephalopathy Peripheral and autonomic neuropathy
Endocrine	Hyperparathyroidism Adrenal insufficiency
Respiratory	Pneumonitis Pulmonary edema
Gastrointestinal	Bleeding Nausea, vomiting Delayed gastric emptying
Metabolic	Acidosis Electrolyte imbalance

The general course of progressive renal failure may be divided into three stages: decreased renal reserve, renal insufficiency, and end-stage renal failure or uremia. As the number of functioning nephrons declines, the signs, symptoms, and biochemical abnormalities become more severe.

Clinical signs or laboratory evidence of renal disease are absent until fewer than 40% of normal-functioning nephrons remain. Loss of nephron function without symptoms is known as a *decrease in renal reserve.* Renal insufficiency occurs when only 10% to 40% of nephrons are functioning adequately. Nocturia occurs secondary to a decrease in concentrating ability. Although affected patients seem well compensated when excretory capacity is unstressed, little renal reserve is present. Elimination of a large protein load or excretion of certain drugs is impaired, and preservation of remaining nephron function is a major goal. Toxic substances such as aminoglycosides potentiate existing damage, and aminoglycoside toxicity is enhanced in the presence of either volume depletion or arterial hypotension. Radiocontrast exposure in patients with chronic renal insufficiency often causes further reversible decreases in renal function in those with either myocardial failure or diabetes mellitus.

As renal function deteriorates further, end-stage renal disease (ESRD) develops. During this stage, concentrating and diluting properties of the kidney are severely compromised, and electrolyte, hematologic, and acid–base disturbances are common. The loss of 95% of functioning nephrons culminates in uremia, which is associated with volume overload and congestive heart failure. Uremia, which can be viewed as urine in the blood, adversely affects almost every organ system. Death occurs unless dialysis is performed.

Treatment

Dialytic Therapy

Approximately 250,000 people in the United States today require chronic dialysis with an estimated 8% increase each year.

Dialysis Techniques

Dialysis is a general term used to describe therapy in which solute moves from blood through a semipermeable membrane into a chemically prescribed solution. The movement of solute, which is called *diffusive transport,* depends on differences in molecular concentration between the blood compartment and the dialysate. *Ultrafiltration* is a technique in which a hydraulic pressure difference across a semipermeable membrane causes the bulk removal of fluid and solute by convective transport.

Major types of dialysis include hemodialysis and peritoneal dialysis. In hemodialysis, blood moves through a device that exposes it to an individually prescribed dialysate solution across a semipermeable membrane. Hemodialysis requires systemic or regional anticoagulation. In peritoneal dialysis, the blood compartment is the peritoneal microvasculature, and the semipermeable membrane is the peritoneal lining. The dialysate is infused into and withdrawn from the abdominal cavity. Movement of water occurs down an osmotic gradient from blood to dialysate and may be increased with an increase in the glucose concentration of the dialysate. Diffusive transport is influenced by the solute concentration within the dialysate.

Anesthetic Considerations

Preoperative

Preoperative preparation of patients with advanced renal disease should include an evaluation of recent laboratory measurements, coexisting diseases, and current medications. Patients with ESRD should undergo determination of BUN and serum creatinine levels, complete blood count, bleeding time measurement, and electrolyte studies preoperatively. Special attention should be given to serum potassium, the type of and schedule for dialysis, and volume status.

Discussions regarding premedication should take into consideration unexpected sensitivity to central nervous system depressants and delayed gastric emptying. Benzodiazepines are useful as premedicants because of their oral route of administration and hepatic metabolism. Midazolam has virtually no active metabolites, and its half-life is only slightly prolonged in renal failure. Although this drug is useful when it is carefully titrated, patients with renal disease may be more susceptible to the sedative-hypnotic effects of this benzodiazepine than those without renal dysfunction. Reduced protein binding may be responsible for increased sensitivity to these drugs in these patients.

Gastric hyperacidity and gastrointestinal bleeding are common in patients with renal failure. H_2 blockers and magnesium-free antacids should be considered. Cimetidine has been used, but renal elimination accounts for 80% of total elimination, and elimination is impaired with reduced renal function. Although newer H_2 antagonists are now available, all H_2-receptor blockers are very dependent on renal excretion. Metoclopramide is partly excreted unchanged in the urine and accumulates in patients with renal failure.

Intraoperative Monitoring

The selection of monitors for a patient with diminished or absent renal function is based on the physiologic status of the patient and the proposed surgical procedure. Frequent measurements of blood pressure and continuous recording of temperature and heart rate and rhythm are essential. Electrocardiography may allow early detection of hyperkalemia.

The decision to use invasive monitors depends on the patient's functional cardiac reserve and the severity and control of hypertension. Continuous monitoring of intraarterial blood pressure is helpful when major surgical procedures are performed. A femoral or dorsalis pedis artery is sometimes used for cannulation because vessels in the upper extremities may be needed later for vascular shunts. Vascular volume and fluid replacement can be guided by CVP or pulmonary artery catheter monitoring. A pulmonary artery catheter is useful if interpretation of the CVP is questionable or cardiac disease is present.

Vascular shunts and fistulas must be protected. Patency is easily monitored with Doppler imaging. Because of the immunocompromised state of these patients, strict aseptic technique is required during the placement of vascular catheters.

Regional Anesthesia

Regional anesthesia is tolerated by patients with advanced renal disease, provided no significant coagulation disorder is present and the mean arterial pressure is maintained. Regional techniques avoid most of the pharmacokinetic and pharmacodynamic problems associated with general anesthetics and sedative drugs. Major concerns regarding this type of anesthesia include psychological intolerance, coagulation abnormalities, the presence of peripheral neuropathies, difficulty in making intravascular volume adjustments, and risk of infection.

Arteriovenous shunts or fistulas may be surgically created with the use of local infiltration or brachial plexus block. In addition to providing analgesia, brachial blocks improve surgical conditions by providing maximum vascular vasodilation and abolishing vasospasm. The duration of brachial plexus block has been reported to be shortened by 40% in patients with chronic renal failure. A shortened duration of action would support the use of a longer acting local anesthetic, such as bupivacaine, especially if prolonged surgery is anticipated. However, data suggest a similar duration of anesthesia with brachial plexus blocks in patients with renal failure and normal renal function.

With regard to spinal or epidural anesthesia, patients with long-standing renal disease often have undergone multiple procedures and prefer general anesthetic techniques. In addition to the history, the bleeding time, platelet count, prothrombin time, partial thromboplastin time, and fibrinogen level should be evaluated before subarachnoid or epidural catheters are placed in uremic patients. An opioid or opioid and local epidural solution rather than local solution alone allows continuous monitoring of neurologic function.

Peripheral neuropathies should be discussed with the patient and documented before regional anesthesia is undertaken. The incidence of hypotension with subarachnoid or epidural blockade may be increased because of effects of chronic hypertension or hypovolemia related to recent dialysis. Correction of hypovolemia postoperatively is hazardous. Recession of the sympathetic block in patients who cannot undergo diuresis may lead to pulmonary edema. One must weigh the advantages of fluid infusion against the effects of pressor drugs with these factors in mind.

Patients with ESRD are often acidotic, and local anesthetic toxicity may be increased with acidosis. The onset and duration of blocks also have been shown to vary in these patients.

General Anesthesia

Intravenous Drugs

Intravenous anesthetics can be used in patients with advanced renal disease, but the response of these patients may be more variable than normal. Variability arises from a complex interplay among changes in volume of distribution (which is often increased), protein binding (which may be low), low pH, and dependence on renal excretion for the parent drug or metabolites.

The action of many drugs is potentiated by metabolic abnormalities associated with renal failure. Highly protein-bound drugs have more target organ effect in the presence of hypoalbuminemia. The acidemic state associated with renal failure increases the proportion of the agent that is unionized and unbound and therefore more available to target tissue. Anemia associated with renal failure increases cardiac output and enhances delivery to the brain. Uremia alters the blood–brain barrier; this also increases the sensitivity to intravenous drugs.

Uremic patients are generally anemic and may require high inspired oxygen concentrations. Because intravenous anesthesia is often supplemented with nitrous oxide, the inspired concentration of oxygen is reduced. Volatile agents are more reliable in controlling hypertension, and their action is more easily reversed. For these reasons, inhalation agents may be preferable for general anesthesia.

Volatile Anesthetic Agents

Inhalation agents offer some advantage in patients with renal failure. Although biotransformation of some agents may produce metabolites excreted by the kidneys, elimination of volatile agents does not rely on renal function. Inhalation agents potentiate neuromuscular blocking drugs, allowing administration of reduced doses. Although the potency of these agents allows them to be administered without nitrous oxide, excessive depth of anesthesia may lead to a depression of cardiac output. Reductions in cardiac output and tissue blood flow must be avoided in these patients with anemia if tissue oxygen delivery is to be maintained. A disadvantage of sevoflurane relates to its biotransformation and potential nephrotoxic effects.

Both regional and general anesthesia have been used successfully in patients with advanced renal disease. Advantages and disadvantages of both techniques are shown in the table below.

Regional versus General Anesthesia

Technique	Advantages	Disadvantages
Regional	Patient responsiveness Minimal changes in renal hemodynamics	Presence of peripheral neuropathy Tendency for bleeding Patient anxiety Prolonged procedures Hypotension with sympathetic block; may cause reluctance to expand volume
Inhalation anesthetics	Good airway control Blood pressure control Duration not dependent on urinary excretion Less neuromuscular blocking with drugs required FiO_2 can be increased because N_2O not necessary	Alterations in renal hemodynamics Decreased cardiac output Hypotension Biodegradation and potential nephrotoxicity; halothane, 15%–20%; sevoflurane, 5%; isoflurane, 0.2%; desflurane, 0.02%
Intravenous anesthetics	Hemodynamic stability	Unpredictable response Hypertension Greater need for N_2O and neuromuscular blockers

FiO_2, Fraction of inspired oxygen; *N_2O*, nitrous oxide.

Intravenous Fluid Management

Perioperative management of fluids and electrolytes in patients with renal disease is critical. The state of hydration affects renin, aldosterone, and antidiuretic levels. Dehydration and hypovolemia lead to elevations in these hormones and to a decline in urinary output.

Perioperative Renal Function

Surgical patients at high risk for acute renal failure and those with advanced disease who do not require hemodialysis present unique challenges. Preservation of renal function intraoperatively is a major goal. Preservation of renal function is dependent on the maintenance of intravascular volume and cardiovascular stability and on the avoidance of events that cause renal vasoconstriction. Preoperative hydration with 10 to 20 mL/kg of balanced salt solution may be helpful. Intraoperatively, urinary output is the only time monitor for renal function. A urinary output of 0.5 to 1 mL/kg/hr intraoperatively and postoperatively is recommended in these patients.

Decreased Renal Reserve

The goal of fluid management in patients with decreased renal reserve is the maximization of renal perfusion. Basal fluids should be replaced; 5% dextrose in water (D_5W) with 50 to 70 mEq/L of Na^+ is appropriate. Potassium should be administered as needed to sustain a normal plasma level. Deficit and intraoperative losses should be replaced as for a normal patient. Third-space losses can be replaced with balanced salt solution. Although it is better to err on the side of excess with respect to volume replacement in these patients, if the ratio of replacement crystalloid solution to lost blood exceeds 3:1, consideration should be given to the use of a colloid solution. The administration of large volumes of crystalloid solution may be associated with pulmonary edema as fluids are mobilized. This generally occurs on the second to the fourth postoperative day.

Renal Insufficiency

In patients with renal insufficiency, volume deficits should be replaced preoperatively, as in normal patients. Basal fluids must be carefully regulated because these patients cannot tolerate much deviation. Overall basal fluid requirements must be related to metabolic rate and be designed to provide an overall fluid balance that allows an isotonic urine to carry excreted electrolytes and waste products. Intraoperative losses greater than 10% to 15% of the blood volume should be replaced with colloid solution on a 1:1 basis after red blood cell losses are corrected. Smaller losses can be replaced with the usual 3:1 ratio of crystalloid infusion to blood loss. Third-space losses are ideally replaced initially with crystalloid solution without potassium or excess chloride. Initial third-space losses should be replaced with crystalloid solution at a rate of 2 to 3 mL/kg/hr. The critical goal in patients with renal insufficiency is sustaining blood volume. Monitoring of colloid osmotic pressure and hemoglobin can guide the choice between crystalloid and colloid infusions. If hemoglobin and colloid osmotic pressure are increasing, crystalloid solution is clearly indicated. If they are decreasing, crystalloid solution should be withheld in favor of colloid solution. Close monitoring of blood pressure, heart rate, CVP, pulmonary artery occlusion pressure, and cardiac output also guides fluid titration. This is especially true in patients with cardiac or respiratory compromise.

End-Stage Renal Disease

With regard to perioperative fluid management, patients with ESRD who are hemodialysis dependent require special attention. Although these patients are similar to normal patients in terms of fluid deficit, basal, and third-space requirements, they have a narrow margin of safety. The patient's ability to compensate for either fluid excess or fluid deficiency progressively declines as renal function is lost.

Fluid deficits must be replaced preoperatively in patients with ESRD. If deficits exceed 10% to 15% of the blood volume, invasive monitoring is justified. Dialysis is recommended on the day before anesthesia to allow time for equilibration of fluid and electrolyte shifts that are common with dialysis. Electrolyte levels must be checked before anesthesia.

Basal fluids in patients with ESRD should be replaced in a manner similar to that for patients with renal insufficiency. Volume restriction is recommended for intraoperative losses. Third-space losses should be replaced with a balanced salt solution that contains no potassium and small amounts of chloride. Close monitoring of hemoglobin and cardiac filling pressures is indicated for all major procedures. Patients with ESRD generally require dialysis within 24 to 36 hours after major surgery.

Uremia

Deficit replacement in patients with uremia must be guided by hemodynamic monitoring. Basal fluids should be replaced with red blood cells, fresh-frozen plasma, or colloid solutions. Third-space losses are best replaced with crystalloid solutions in association with frequent monitoring of hemoglobin and cardiac filling pressures. A moderate degree of volume overload is not a grave problem. Many uremic patients require dialysis within 24 to 36 hours for the removal of mobilized fluid and the control of hypertension.

Although volume overload is most often emphasized in patients with ESRD, complications of hypovolemia are also serious. Hypotension associated with hypovolemia increases the risk of thrombosis of the arteriovenous fistula and predisposes to cardiac and cerebral ischemia. Hemodynamic goals include the avoidance of hypotension and gross fluid overload. This can be accomplished only through careful titration with the patient well monitored.

C. UROLITHIASIS

Definition

Urolithiasis, or "kidney stones," refers to the presence of calculi, typically composed of calcium oxalate, in the urinary system. These calculi result from hypercalcemia or hyperoxaluria. Other types of stones include magnesium ammonium phosphate, calcium phosphate, and uric acid.

Pathophysiology

Causes of hypercalcemia and hypercalciuria are primarily hyperparathyroidism, vitamin D intoxication malignancies, and sarcoidosis. Small bowel bypass is associated with hyperoxaluria. Alterations in urine pH and the presence of metabolic disturbances can also result in formation of renal stones, which differ in composition from the typical oxalate variety.

Treatment

Extracorporeal shock wave lithotripsy is a noninvasive treatment of renal stones. It transmits shock waves through water and focuses them on the stone by biplanar fluoroscopy. For patients with arrhythmias, shock waves can be delivered during the heart's refractory period ($\approx$20 msec after R wave) to avoid initiating further cardiac arrhythmias. Patients with artificial cardiac pacemakers risk pacemaker dysfunction with this form of therapy. Percutaneous nephrostomy can also be performed for removal of stone, obstruction, or biopsy. A needle is passed into the renal collecting duct, a catheter can be placed over the needle, and the kidney is drained. Anesthetic options include local anesthesia with sedation, regional anesthesia, and general anesthesia.

Anesthetic Considerations

General anesthesia, intravenous sedation, or regional anesthesia, including epidural and intercostal nerve blocks with local infiltration, may be used to provide analgesia during lithotripsy. Regardless of anesthetic regimen, the patient must remain still because movement (including excessive diaphragmatic excursion) can move the stone from the wave focus. The sitting position may be associated with peripheral pooling of blood, especially with the use of regional anesthesia and resultant vasodilation. Immersion in water increases hydrostatic pressures on the abdomen and thorax, which can displace blood into the central circulation. This increase in CVP may result in acute congestive heart failure in patients with limited cardiac reserve. The hydrostatic forces on the thorax likewise result in decreases in chest wall compliance and functional residual capacity. This may produce ventilation/perfusion mismatches. Water in the immersion tub should be kept warm to avoid hypothermia. An alternative option to an immersion tank is a lithotripsy table. Extracorporeal shock wave lithotripsy is contraindicated in patients with abdominal aortic aneurysms, spinal cord tumors, or orthopedic implants in the lumbar region. Parturients, obese patients, and patients with coagulopathies also are not good candidates for this procedure.

Respiratory System

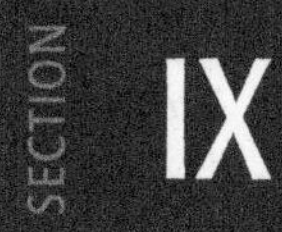

A. ADULT RESPIRATORY DISTRESS SYNDROME

Definition

The term *acute respiratory failure* is often used synonymously with *acute* (formerly *adult*) *respiratory distress syndrome* (ARDS). Although ARDS may be caused by or associated with a variety of clinical conditions, most patients with this disease demonstrate similar clinical and pathologic features regardless of the cause of lung injury. Common features include: (1) a history of a preceding noxious event that served as a trigger for the subsequent development of ARDS; (2) an interval from hours to days of relatively normal lung function after the insult; and (3) the rapid onset and progression over several hours of dyspnea, severe hypoxia, diffuse bilateral pulmonary infiltration, and stiffening and noncompliance of the lungs.

Incidence and Prevalence

Risk factors for the development of ARDS appear to be additive. The incidence of occurrence is 25% with the presence of one risk factor, 42% with the presence of two, and 85% with the presence of three. The mortality rate for ARDS remains high, ranging from 50% to 70% and often exceeds 90% when gram-negative septic shock precedes ARDS development. Events and risk factors associated with the development of ARDS include: (1) shock (septic, cardiogenic, or hypovolemic), (2) trauma, (3) pulmonary infection (e.g., with *Pneumocystis carinii* [*jiroveci*] or *Escherichia coli*), (4) disease states that result in the release of inflammatory mediators (e.g., extrapulmonary infections, disseminated intravascular coagulation, anaphylaxis, coronary bypass grafting, and transfusion reactions), (5) exposure to various agents (e.g., narcotics, barbiturates, and O_2), (6) diseases of the central nervous system (CNS), (7) aspiration (e.g., of gastric contents or as in drowning), and (8) metabolic events (e.g., pancreatitis and uremia).

Pathophysiology

The pathophysiology of ARDS is centered around severe damage and inflammation to the alveolocapillary membrane. Irrespective of the cause of acute respiratory failure, the lung's structural response to injury and subsequent repair occurs in a similar fashion. Although the exact mechanisms of this response and repair remain unclear, research has focused on the release of cytokines and membrane-bound phospholipids from the capillary endothelium and the activation of leukocytes and macrophages (via the complement system) within the lungs.

Clinical Manifestations

The clinical presentation includes patients who are dyspneic, hypoxic, and hypovolemic and require intubation and mechanical ventilation. Recovery of lung function is unpredictable. Milder cases resolve quickly, but others progress to fibrosis and death.

Treatment

Because lung infections (e.g., *P. carinii [jiroveci]* pneumonia) mimic ARDS, antibiotic therapy often is initiated before the cause of respiratory failure is known. Maintenance of tissue oxygenation and replacement of lost intravascular fluids are the main goals of therapy. Preservation of end-organ perfusion is of utmost importance. Treatment is supportive and includes correction of hypoxia, preload and afterload reduction, and inotropic support as indicated.

Anesthetic Considerations

Anesthetic preparation includes evaluation of the patient's respiratory, cardiac, and renal status. Ventilator settings should be noted and special attention devoted to peak inspiratory pressures and positive end-expiratory pressure (PEEP) levels. If the anesthesia ventilator cannot accommodate these settings, then arrangements must be made to bring the patient's ventilator into the operating room. The nature of lung sounds and amount of secretions should be noted. The presence of excess secretions should alert the anesthesia provider to the potential risk of airway obstruction. The degree of barotrauma from prolonged mechanical ventilation with high levels of PEEP can be assessed by the presence of chest tubes and subcutaneous emphysema secondary to pneumothorax. The effectiveness of therapy with bronchodilators should be assessed because the use of these drugs may be initiated preoperatively and continued intraoperatively if effective. An arterial line should be placed preoperatively and arterial blood gas (ABG) analysis performed. If possible, lactic acid values should be determined.

Volume status should be evaluated closely because patients with ARDS often are hypovolemic. Invasive monitoring via central venous lines and pulmonary artery catheters often is available, and cardiac filling pressures along with CO values should be assessed. Patients requiring inotropic support may arrive for surgery with infusions of dopamine or dobutamine. For all procedures, renal function should be monitored with a bladder catheter. Antibiotic therapy should be continued intraoperatively, and continuation of steroid preparations should be considered if patients were receiving these medications preoperatively.

Because patients with ARDS often are hemodynamically unstable, careful titration of anesthetic agents and adjunct agents is necessary. Owing to the multisystemic involvement characteristic of ARDS, drug metabolism and elimination should be carefully considered.

Transport should be carefully planned so that complications are minimized and safe arrival in the intensive care unit is ensured. Patients should undergo pulse oximetry, electrocardiography (ECG), and blood pressure transport monitoring (by arterial line or noninvasively) before departure from the operating room.

Breath sounds should be continually assessed with a precordial stethoscope. A full tank of O_2 and PEEP adapter valves should be available for transport. The potential need for emergency medications and a defibrillator should be considered. If the patient's ventilator needs to be returned to the intensive care unit, plans should be made so that it arrives there before the patient does. Finally, if possible, another member of the anesthesia team should accompany the patient during transport. Pulmonary dysfunction is the most common cause of postoperative complications after the administration of general anesthesia. To minimize pulmonary derangement, the anesthesia provider must identify patients who are at risk for the development of pulmonary impairment and must have a thorough understanding of the preexisting lung dysfunction.

B. ASPIRATION PNEUMONIA

Definition

Two entirely separate clinical aspiration disorders exist. One occurs after the aspiration of solid food and produces a picture of laryngeal or bronchial obstruction, an the other results from direct acid injury to the lung and produces an "asthma-like" syndrome. Pulmonary aspiration occurs when the gastric contents escape from the stomach into the pharynx and then enter the lungs. This results from preexisting disease, airway manipulation, and the inevitable compromise in protective reflexes accompanying the anesthetized state. Aspirates are commonly categorized as contaminated, acidic, alkaline, particulate, and nonparticulate. Fewer than half of all aspirations lead to pneumonia. Pneumonia occurs most often in patients with aspiration of infected material or who are immunocompromised.

Incidence and Prevalence

Although the incidence of regurgitation is estimated to be frequent (as high as 15%), pulmonary aspiration complicates only about one in 3000 anesthetics. This incidence is roughly doubled for cesarean section surgery and emergency surgery. Fortunately, the majority of aspiration incidents require little or no treatment.

Pathophysiology

Although vomiting and gastroesophageal reflux are common clinical events, aspiration usually occurs only when normal protective reflexes (swallowing, coughing, gagging) fail. Three broad categories of failure are (1) depression of reflex protection, (2) alteration in anatomic structures, and (3) iatrogenic disorder. Reflex responses to aspiration are automatically blunted with depression of consciousness. The most common setting for depression of reflex protection occurs during anesthesia induction and emergence.

Three aspiration syndromes have been identified: (1) chemical pneumonitis (Mendelson syndrome), (2) mechanical obstruction, and (3) bacterial infection. Because acute chemical pneumonitis poses the greatest difficulty to anesthesia providers, the pathophysiology, presentation, and anesthetic implications of Mendelson syndrome are discussed. The triphasic sequence of (1) immediate respiratory distress combined with bronchospasm, cyanosis, tachycardia, and dyspnea followed by (2) partial recovery and (3) a final phase of gradual return of function is characteristic of Mendelson syndrome. This acute chemical pneumonitis is caused by the irritative action of hydrochloric acid, alkaline aspirates, or particulate materials, which are damaging to the lungs.

The pathophysiology of aspiration pneumonitis is typically characterized by four stages: (1) The aspirated substance causes immediate damage to the lung parenchyma, resulting in tissue necrosis. (2) Atelectasis results within minutes caused by a parasympathetic response that leads to airway closure and a decrease in lung compliance. (3) One to two hours after the injury, there is an intense inflammatory reaction characterized by pulmonary edema and hemorrhage. Inflammatory cytokines play a central role in this, including interleukin-8 and tumor necrosis factor alpha (TNF-α) released by alveolar macrophages. Neutrophils also play a key role in this phase by releasing oxygen radicals and proteases. Fluid fills the alveolar capillary membrane, causing hypoxia and hypercarbia. (4) Later, secondary injuries result from fibrin deposits and necrosis of alveolar cells by 24 hours after the insult.

Clinical Manifestations and Diagnosis

Arterial hypoxemia, the hallmark sign of aspiration pneumonitis, is frequently the first sign of aspiration. Because the majority of aspiration incidents are asymptomatic or mildly symptomatic, unexplained hypoxemia occurring in otherwise healthy patients postoperatively may frequently be a vague sign of silent aspiration. Other signs to alert the anesthetist to the possibility of aspiration include tachypnea, dyspnea, tachycardia, hypertension, and cyanosis.

Anesthetic Considerations

Preoperative Management

When dealing with aspiration, "an ounce of prevention is worth a pound of cure." Avoiding the use of general anesthesia is the most effective means of preventing aspiration. However, regional and local sedation anesthesia is unrealistic for many procedures and in certain patient populations. When the use of general anesthesia is unavoidable, taking the following steps may help minimize the risk of aspiration or at least limit its consequences.

- Adhere to *nil per os* (NPO) policy.
- Use pharmacologic prophylaxis for aspiration. Agents such as gastrokinetics, histamine blockers, anticholinergics, antacids, proton pump inhibitors, and antiemetics are all used alone or in various combinations to raise gastric pH and lower volume (see the table below).
- Consider rapid sequence induction and the application of cricoid pressure.
- Other nonpharmacologic mechanisms such as elevating the patient's head may offer limited benefit.

Drug Prophylaxis for Anesthesia

Medication Type	Common Examples	Recommendation
Gastrointestinal stimulants	Metoclopramide	No routine use*
Gastric acid secretion blockers	Cimetidine	No routine use*
	Famotidine	No routine use*
	Ranitidine	No routine use*
	Omeprazole	No routine use*
	Lansoprazole	
Antacids	Sodium citrate	No routine use*
	Sodium bicarbonate	
	Magnesium trisilicate	
Antiemetics	Droperidol	No routine use*
	Ondansetron	
Anticholinergics	Atropine	No use†
	Scopolamine	
	Glycopyrrolate	
Combinations of the medications above		No routine use*

*The routine preoperative use of these medications to decrease aspiration risk in patients with no apparent increased risk is not recommended.

†The use of anticholinergics to decrease aspiration risk is not recommended.

Data from American Society of Anesthesiologists. Practice guidelines for preoperative fasting and the use of pharmacologic agents to reduce the risk of pulmonary aspiration: application to healthy patients undergoing elective procedures. *Anesthesiology* 2011;114(3):495-511.

Intraoperative Management

If intubation is not expected to be difficult, a rapid-sequence induction (rather than awake endotracheal intubation) is indicated in the patient with aspiration risk. There is little evidence that "modified" rapid sequence technique (which allows for gentle mask ventilation) would worsen aspiration incidence, and this approach may be preferable in patients at risk for rapid oxygen desaturation. Because difficult intubation itself is a risk factor for aspiration, there should be a low threshold for performing awake intubation in a patient with aspiration risk who may also pose airway challenges. Endotracheal intubation is considered the optimal approach for airway isolation; however, regurgitated material can seep around the endotracheal tube (ETT) cuff, particularly if it is not lubricated. Preventive measures in the anesthetic plan include ensuring that the patient is fully awake before extubation, that the patient is manifesting protective reflexes, minimizing any residual neuromuscular blockade, avoiding narcosis, and emptying the stomach.

If vomiting or aspiration occurs during induction, immediate treatment includes tilting of the patient's head downward or to the side, rapid suctioning of the mouth and pharynx, and intubation. There is little benefit in performing tracheal or bronchial suctioning in most cases, and bronchoscopy should be reserved for patients who are suspected of having aspirated solid material. If aspiration is severe, surgery may be postponed. ABG analysis should be performed for determination of the extent of hypoxemia. Early application of PEEP is recommended for improving pulmonary function and combating atelectasis. Oxygenation should be supported with supplemental oxygen only to the minimum extent necessary.

Treatment of Aspiration Pneumonitis

- Suction the mouth and pharynx.
- Use deeper suctioning only for particulate material.
- Administer oxygen only to the extent needed.
- Administer lidocaine to inhibit neutrophil response.
- Steroids can lead to superinfection and are generally not indicated
- Intubate as needed to support oxygenation.
- Use a bronchodilator and PEEP to support ventilation.
- Administer antibiotics only if indicated or for fever or an elevated white blood cell count lasting longer than 48 hours.

C. ASTHMA

Definition

Asthma is a chronic inflammatory disorder of the airways characterized by increased responsiveness of the tracheobronchial tree to a variety of stimuli. Many cells and cellular elements play a role, particularly mast cells, eosinophils, T lymphocytes, neutrophils, and epithelial cells. In susceptible individuals, this inflammation causes recurrent episodes of wheezing, breathlessness, chest tightness, and cough, particularly at night and in the early morning. These episodes are usually associated with widespread but variable airflow obstruction that is often reversible either spontaneously or with treatment.

Various subtypes of asthma exist. The most important consideration is the identification of exacerbating factors whenever possible. A well-known system classifies asthmas as either extrinsic or intrinsic. Although this system is conceptually helpful, its two groups are not mutually exclusive. Whereas extrinsic asthma (or allergic asthma) most commonly affects children and young adults and involves infectious, environmental, psychological, or physical factors, intrinsic asthma (or idiosyncratic asthma) usually develops in middle age without specifically identifiable attack-provoking stimuli. The term *atopy,* which refers to a hereditary, immunoglobulin E (IgE)–mediated, clinical hypersensitive state, is often used when extrinsic asthma is described.

Incidence and Prevalence

Up to 15 million persons in the United States have asthma. It is the most common chronic disease of childhood, affecting an estimated 4.8 million children. People with asthma collectively have more than 100 million days of restricted activity and 470,000 hospitalizations annually. More than 5000 people die of asthma each year.

Pathophysiology

Asthma is a heterogeneous clinical syndrome characterized by episodes in which airways are hyperresponsive, interspersed with symptom-free periods. Bronchoconstriction is a factor long associated with the asthmatic symptom complex, but asthma is much more than bronchoconstriction. Airway inflammation and a nonspecific hyperirritability of the tracheobronchial tree are now recognized as being central to the pathogenesis of even mild cases of asthma. Permanent changes in airway anatomy, referred to as *airway remodeling,* magnify the inflammatory response.

Allergic asthma (atopic or immunologic disease) is triggered by antigens that provoke a T-lymphocyte–generated, IgE-mediated immune response. It is often associated with a personal or familial history of allergic disease. Potent biochemical mediators released from proinflammatory and airway epithelial cells promote vasoconstriction, increased smooth muscle tone, enhanced mucous secretion, submucosal edema, increased vascular permeability, and inflammatory cell chemotaxis. Leukotrienes have been identified as especially potent spasmogenic and proinflammatory substances. Released molecules that are toxic to the airway epithelium cause patchy desquamation, which exposes cholinergic nerve endings and compounds the bronchoconstrictive and hyperresponsive response.

The asthmatic diathesis creates airways that are inflamed, edematous, and hypersensitive to irritant stimuli, and the degree of airway hyperresponsiveness and bronchoconstriction appears to parallel the extent of inflammation. When airway reactivity is high, asthmatic symptoms are generally more severe and unrelenting, and the amount of therapy required to control the episode is greater.

The mechanisms underlying idiosyncratic asthma (nonimmunologic disease) are less clearly defined. Nonimmunologic asthma occurs in patients with no history of allergy and normal serum IgE. These patients typically develop asthmatic symptoms in response to some provocative or noxious stimulus such as cold air, airway instrumentation or irritation, climate changes, or an upper respiratory illness. Recent upper respiratory infection may precipitate bronchospasm in any patient, but the risk is higher in patients with a history of asthma.

The mechanism of exercise-induced asthma is unknown. Regardless of the mechanism, most symptoms last less than 1 hour and are usually quickly reversed with administration of β_2-adrenergic receptor agonists. Occupational asthma develops when irritants directly stimulate vagal nerve endings in the airway epithelium. Infection-induced asthma with acute inflammation of the bronchi may be caused by viral, bacterial, or mycoplasmal infections. Aspirin-induced asthma occurs when, in some predisposed persons, cyclooxygenase promotes an increase in leukotriene levels via the arachidonic acid pathway, thereby triggering the asthma attack. This peculiar response can occur with the use of other nonsteroidal anti-inflammatory agents. The aspirin-induced asthma variant is not IgE mediated or allergic in nature; furthermore, it is clinically associated with nasal polyps. Patients with aspirin-induced asthma may be at increased risk of bronchospasm after ketorolac (Toradol) administration.

Clinical Manifestations

Key hallmarks of asthma in the awake patient include the following:

- Wheezing
- Dyspnea (may parallel the severity of expiratory airflow obstruction)
- Cough (productive or nonproductive; frequently at night or early morning)
- Labored respirations with accessory muscle use
- Tachypnea (a respiratory rate >30 breaths/min and a heart rate of 120 beats/min suggests severe bronchospasm)
- Chest tightness
- Prolonged expiratory phase of respiration
- Fatigue

Typically, attacks are short lived, lasting minutes to hours. Between attacks, the patient with asthma may be entirely symptom free; however, underlying airway remodeling is still evident. Severe obstruction persisting for days or weeks is known as *status asthmaticus*. Use of accessory muscles of respiration and the increased work of breathing associated with a protracted asthmatic episode can result in respiratory muscle fatigue and respiratory failure. During exacerbations, pulmonary function tests may reflect acute expiratory airflow obstruction (decreased forced expiratory flow $[FEF]_{25\%-75\%}$ and decreased ratio of forced expiratory volume in one second to forced vital capacity [FEV_1/FVC]). Viscid mucous secretion may compound the airway narrowing and produce airway collapse.

The asthmatic episode produces not only airflow obstruction but also gas exchange abnormalities. The resulting low ventilation/perfusion (V/Q) state produces arterial O_2 desaturation. Hypoxemia is common, but in most patients with acute bronchospasm, CO_2 elimination is relatively well preserved until V/Q abnormalities are severe. An increased arterial CO_2 tension may indicate impending respiratory failure in an acutely ill patient with asthma. Chronic asthma may eventually lead to irreversible lung destruction, loss of lung elasticity, pulmonary hypertension (PH), and lung hyperinflation.

Anesthetized Patients

In anesthetized patients, prominent manifestations of the asthmatic episode are wheezing, mucous hypersecretion, high inspiratory pressures, a blunted expiratory CO_2 waveform, and hypoxemia. Mechanical ventilation and positive airway pressure (PAP) are associated with a higher incidence of air trapping and lung hyperinflation, and the associated barotrauma can result in a pneumothorax. Additionally, alveolar overdistention may lead to decreased venous return and diminution of CO. The combination of impaired ventilation and hypoxia can precipitate increased pulmonary vascular resistance, enhanced right ventricular afterload, and finally hemodynamic collapse.

The onset of an asthmatic episode may occur abruptly in surgical patients. Airway manipulation, acute exposure to allergens, or the stress of surgery can provoke wheezing in a patient who was previously asymptomatic. Wheezing often suggests potentially reversible bronchoconstriction, but the extent or degree of wheezing is a notoriously poor indicator of the degree of airway obstruction. Care must be taken to differentiate wheezing of asthmatic origin from other causes of wheezing such as pneumothorax, ETT obstruction, endobronchial intubation, anaphylaxis, pulmonary edema, and pulmonary aspiration.

Anesthetic Considerations

Several important anesthetic considerations and risk reduction strategies have been reported (see the following box).

Risk Reduction Strategies for Anesthetization of Patients with Asthma

Preoperative

- Encourage cessation of cigarette smoking for at least 8 weeks.
- Aggressively treat airflow obstruction.
- Administer antibiotics and delay surgery if respiratory infection is present.
- Begin patient education regarding lung-expansion maneuvers.

Intraoperative

- Limit the duration of surgery to less than 3 hours.
- Use regional anesthesia when possible.
- Avoid the use of long-acting neuromuscular blocking agents.
- Use laparoscopic procedures when possible.
- Substitute a less ambitious procedure for upper abdominal or thoracic surgery when possible.

Postoperative

- Encourage deep-breathing exercises or incentive spirometry.
- Use continuous positive airway pressure.
- Perform chest percussion.
- Use intercostal nerve blocks and local anesthesia infiltration of incisional area for pain when appropriate.

Modified from Smetana GW. Current concepts: preoperative pulmonary evaluation. *N Engl J Med* 1999;340:937-944; Hurford WE. The bronchospastic patient. *Int Anesthesiol Clin* 2000;38:77-89.

D. CHRONIC OBSTRUCTIVE PULMONARY DISEASE

Definition

Chronic obstructive pulmonary disease (COPD) is a "disorder characterized by abnormal tests of expiratory flow that does not change markedly over periods of several months of observation." Asthma, chronic bronchitis, and emphysema are all common obstructive diseases characterized by decreased air flow through the tracheobronchial tree and small airways.

The terms *chronic obstructive pulmonary disease* and *chronic obstructive lung disease* are widely used as synonyms for the combination of chronic bronchitis and emphysema. Because of the prevalence of cigarette smoking, the combination of these two entities is encountered much more commonly than either of the two in its "pure" form. As a rule, the combination of chronic bronchitis and emphysema is seen in those who smoke heavily, and the disease process takes 30 years or longer to manifest. Differential diagnosis of COPD compared with other common lung disorders is described in the following table.

Differential Diagnosis of Chronic Obstructive Pulmonary Disease

Diagnosis	Suggestive Features*
COPD	Onset in midlife; symptoms slowly progressive; long-term smoking history; dyspnea during exercise; largely irreversible airflow limitation
Asthma	Onset early in life (often childhood); symptoms vary from day to day; symptoms occur at night or in early morning; allergy, rhinitis, or eczema also present; family history of asthma; largely reversible airflow limitation
Congestive heart failure	Fine basilar crackles on auscultation; chest radiograph shows dilated heart, pulmonary edema; pulmonary function tests indicate volume restriction, not airflow limitation
Bronchiectasis	Large volumes of purulent sputum; commonly associated with bacterial infection; coarse crackles or clubbing on auscultation; chest radiograph or CT scan shows bronchial dilation, bronchial wall thickening
Tuberculosis	Onset at all ages; chest radiograph shows lung infiltrate or nodular lesions; microbiologic confirmation; high local prevalence of tuberculosis
Obliterative bronchiolitis	Onset at younger age, in nonsmokers; may have history of rheumatoid arthritis or fume exposure; CT scan taken on expiration shows hypodense areas
Diffuse panbronchiolitis	Most patients are male and nonsmokers; almost all have chronic sinusitis; chest radiograph and HRCT scan show diffuse small centrilobular nodular opacities and hyperinflation

*These features tend to be characteristic of the respective diseases but do not occur in every case. For example, a person who has never smoked can develop COPD (especially in developing countries, where other risk factors may be more important than cigarette smoking); asthma can develop in adult and even elderly patients.

COPD, Chronic obstructive pulmonary disease; *CT,* computed tomography; *HRCT,* high-resolution computed tomography.

From Rable KF, Hurd S, Anzueto A, et al. Global strategy for the diagnosis, management, and prevention of chronic obstructive pulmonary disease. *Am J Respir Crit Care Med* 2007;176:532-555.

Incidence and Prevalence

COPD affects an estimated 15 to 20 million Americans and is the fifth leading cause of death in the United States, accounting for approximately 60,000 deaths each year. Chronic bronchitis and emphysema are the most common causes of COPD.

Pathophysiology

The dominant feature of the natural history of COPD is progressive air flow obstruction, as reflected by a decrease in FEV_1. Three causes of decreases in FEV_1 are as follows:

1. A decrease in the intrinsic size of bronchial lumen
2. An increase in the collapsibility of bronchial walls (this cause is the most difficult to quantify)
3. A decrease in elastic recoil of the lungs

Clinical Manifestations

The clinical presentation of COPD varies markedly, and crippling changes for one person may be a minor incapacity for another. Chronic productive cough and progressive exercise limitation are the hallmarks of COPD. The clinical and functional changes are noted in the following tables.

Clinical Hallmarks: Predominant Bronchitis versus Predominant Emphysema

	Blue Bloater, Predominant Bronchitis	Pink Puffer, Predominant Emphysema
General appearance	Overweight; dusky; warm extremities	Thin, often emaciated; pursed-lip breathing; anxious; prominent use of accessory muscles; normal-to-cool extremities
Age (years)	40–55	50–75
Onset	Cough	Dyspnea
Cyanosis	Marked	Slight to none
Cough	More evident than dyspnea	Less evident than dyspnea
Sputum	Copious	Scanty
Upper respiratory infections	Common	Occasional
Breath sounds	Moderately diminished	Markedly diminished
Cor pulmonale and right-sided heart failure	Common	Only during bouts of respiratory infection
Radiographic features	Normal diaphragm position; cardiomegaly; lungs normal or with increased bronchovascular markings	Small pendulous heart; low, flat diaphragm; areas of increased radiolucency
Course	Ambulatory but constantly on verge of right-sided heart failure and coma	Incapacitation of breathlessness punctuated by life-threatening bouts of upper respiratory infections; prolonged course culminating in right-sided heart failure and coma

Modified from Fishman AP, et al, ed. *Fishman's Pulmonary Diseases and Disorders*. 4th ed. New York: McGraw-Hill; 2008.

Functional Hallmarks: Predominant Bronchitis versus Predominant Emphysema

	Blue Bloater, Predominant Bronchitis	Pink Puffer, Predominant Emphysema
FEV_1/FC	Reduced	Reduced
FRC	Mildly increased	Markedly increased
TLC	Normal to slight increase	Considerably increased
RV	Moderately increased	Markedly increased
Lung compliance	Normal or high	Normal or low
Recoil pressure	Normal or high	Low
MVV	Moderately decreased	Markedly decreased
Airway resistance	Increased	Normal to slightly increased
DLCO	Normal or low	Low
Arterial PaO_2	Moderate to severe decrease	Mildly to moderately reduced
Arterial hypercapnia	Often present	Present during an acute respiratory infection
Hematocrit	Generally high; may reach 70%	Normal or slightly high; uncommonly exceeds 55%
Pulmonary arterial pressure	Generally increased	Normal or slightly increased

DLCO, Diffusing capacity of carbon monoxide; *FEV1*, forced expiratory volume in 1 second; *FRC*, functional residual capacity; *MVV*, maximum voluntary ventilation; *PaO_2*, partial pressure of arterial oxygen; *RV*, residual volume; *TLC*, total lung capacity.
From Fishman AP, et al, ed. *Fishman's Pulmonary Diseases and Disorders*. 4th ed. New York: McGraw-Hill; 2008.

Anesthetic Considerations

Preoperative Evaluation

The surgical site and the preoperative status of the patient are critical factors in determining the incidence of postoperative complications. Multiple factors are predictive of postoperative respiratory difficulties, but no preoperative pulmonary function test establishes absolute contraindications to surgery. The preoperative evaluation of patients with COPD should determine the severity of the disease and identify treatments for reducing inflammation, improving secretion clearance, treating underlying infection, and increasing airway caliber that can ensure the best surgical outcome. Supplemental administration of O_2 usually is recommended if the PaO_2 is less than 60 mmHg, the hematocrit is greater than 55%, or evidence of cor pulmonale is present. Bronchodilators should be used if the patient exhibits some degree of airway obstruction.

The presence of COPD does not dictate the use of specific drugs or techniques for the management of anesthesia. It is crucial to realize that COPD patients are susceptible to the development of acute respiratory failure during the postoperative period. Therefore, continued intubation of the trachea and mechanical ventilation of the lungs may be necessary, particularly after thoracic and upper abdominal surgery. Postoperative ventilation is more likely to be needed in those patients with low PaO_2 and dyspnea at rest.

Regional Anesthesia

Regional anesthesia is useful if sedation is not needed, and it may be safer than general anesthesia. Anesthesia providers must avoid complacency if they use regional rather than general anesthesia, monitoring for potential adverse side effects (e.g., pneumothorax, impaired muscle function). Regional anesthetic techniques that produce sensory anesthesia above T6 are not recommended because of the potential for decreasing expiratory reserve volume, impairing cough effort, and creating anxiety-provoking weakness.

Postoperative Implications

Postoperative care of patients with COPD is directed at minimizing the incidence and severity of pulmonary complications because such patients are at increased risk for the development of acute respiratory failure. Postoperative pulmonary complications most often are characterized by atelectasis followed by pneumonia and decreases in Pao_2.

Ambulation should be encouraged in order to increase functional residual capacity (FRC) and improve oxygenation via V/Q matching. Incentive spirometry with maintenance of peak inflation for 3 to 5 seconds reexpands collapsed alveoli. Expiratory maneuvers (e.g., floating of balls on an expiratory spirometer) generate pleural pressures that exceed airway pressures and thereby can cause alveolar collapse.

E. COR PULMONALE

Definition

The term *cor pulmonale* or *pulmonary heart disease* refers to patients exhibiting pulmonary arterial hypertension (PAH) resulting in progressive right ventricular hypertrophy, dilation, and eventual cardiac decompensation. This arises from disorders that affect ventilatory drive or musculoskeletal respiratory mechanics; pulmonary airway, infiltrative, fibrotic, or vascular diseases; and diseases that are primarily cardiac but affect the pulmonary circulation and the lungs.

Incidence and Prevalence

In individuals older than 50 years of age, cor pulmonale is the third most common cardiac disorder (after ischemic heart disease and hypertensive cardiac disease). The male-to-female ratio of incidence of the disease is 5:1; 10% to 30% of patients admitted to the hospital with coronary heart failure exhibit cor pulmonale.

The prognosis is determined by the pulmonary disease responsible for the increased pulmonary vascular resistance (PVR). In patients with COPD in whom Pao_2 can be maintained at near-normal levels, the prognosis is favorable. However, cor pulmonale associated with hypoxic lung disease is associated with a 70% rate of mortality within 5 years after onset of associated peripheral edema. The prognosis is poor for patients in whom cor pulmonale is the result of gradual obstruction of pulmonary vessels by intrinsic pulmonary vascular disease or pulmonary fibrosis. These anatomic changes cause irreversible alterations in the pulmonary vasculature, resulting in fixed elevations of PVR.

Pathophysiology

COPD is associated with the functional loss of pulmonary capillaries and the subsequent arterial hypoxemia; these events initiate pulmonary vasoconstriction, which is the leading cause of chronic cor pulmonale. Sustained pulmonary vasoconstriction produces hypertrophy of the smooth muscle in the tunica media and an irreversible increase in the PVR. In the presence of chronically elevated pulmonary capillary pressure, the lungs are increasingly resistant to pulmonary edema because lymph vessels expand and their ability to carry fluid away from the interstitial spaces increases. The lymphatic pumping action creates a suction effect, which results in a negative pleural pressure. The rate at which right ventricular dysfunction develops depends on the magnitude of pressure increase in the pulmonary circulation and on the rapidity with which this increase occurs. For example, PE may result in right ventricular failure in the presence of a mean PAP as low as 30 mmHg. By contrast, when PAH occurs gradually, as it does in COPD, right ventricular compensation occurs; congestive heart failure rarely occurs before mean PAP exceeds 50 mmHg.

Clinical Manifestations and Diagnosis

Clinical manifestations of cor pulmonale often are nonspecific and obscured by coexisting COPD. Right-sided heart catheterization usually is required for diagnosis. Cardiac catheterization combined with pulmonary angiography provides the most definitive information on the degree of PAH, cardiac reserve, and the effects of pulmonary vasodilator treatment. Symptoms of cor pulmonale are retrosternal pain, cough, dyspnea on exertion, weakness, fatigue, early exhaustion, and hemoptysis. Occasionally, hoarseness secondary to left recurrent laryngeal nerve compression by the enlarged pulmonary artery is present. Syncope on effort may occur, reflecting the inability of the right ventricular stroke volume to increase in the presence of a fixed elevation of PVR.

Physical signs of cor pulmonale include the following:

- Elevation of jugular venous pressure
- Cardiac heave or thrust along the left sternal border and S_3 gallop
- Presence of an S_4 secondary to significant right ventricular hypertrophy
- A widely split S_2
- Possible murmur of pulmonic and tricuspid insufficiency
- Hepatomegaly, ascites, and lower extremity edema (late signs)

Treatment

The three major drug classes for treatment of PAH are prostanoids, endothelin receptor antagonists, and phosphodiesterase inhibitors. The goals of treatment are decreasing the workload of the right ventricle, reducing PVR, preventing increases in PAP, and avoiding major hemodynamic changes. Improvement of gas exchange is the primary focus of treatment in COPD patients with cor pulmonale. Treatment includes supplemental administration of O_2 in order to maintain a Pao_2 of greater than 60 mmHg or an arterial O_2 saturation of greater than 90%. O_2 is the only vasodilator with a selective effect on pulmonary vessels that is not associated with a risk of worsening hypoxemia.

Heart–Lung Transplantation

A heart–lung transplantation may ultimately be needed when cor pulmonale progresses despite the provision of maximal medical therapy. In general, preoperative preparation of the patient with cor pulmonale includes the following:

- Elimination and control of acute or chronic pulmonary infections
- Reversal of bronchospasm
- Improvement in clearance of secretions

- Expansion of collapsed or poorly ventilated alveoli
- Hydration
- Correction of any electrolyte imbalance

Anesthetic Considerations

Regional anesthesia technique may be appropriate as long as a high sensory level of anesthesia is not required because any decrease in systemic vascular resistance in the presence of a fixed PVR may produce undesirable degrees of systemic hypotension.

General Anesthesia

Volatile agents decrease PVR. Studies have demonstrated that PAP is decreased by isoflurane. N_2O has been shown to increase PVR in patients with primary pulmonary hypertension (PPH). Intravenous agents, with the exception of ketamine, appear to have little effect on PVR. During all stages of anesthesia, manipulations that increase PAP must be avoided. Five key principles should be followed:

1. Keep the patient well oxygenated.
2. Avoid acidosis.
3. Avoid the use of exogenous and endogenous vasoconstrictors.
4. Avoid presenting stimuli that increase sympathetic tone.
5. Avoid hypothermia.

F. CYSTIC FIBROSIS

Definition

Cystic fibrosis is the most common life-shortening autosomal recessive disorder.

Incidence and Prevalence

Cystic fibrosis affects an estimated 30,000 persons in the United States, with 1000 new cases per year. Most are diagnosed between the ages of 3 months and 6 years, but 8% are not diagnosed until after 18 years. One in 31 Americans is an asymptomatic carrier of the defective gene. More than 80% of those born with cystic fibrosis are born to parents with no history of the disease.

Pathophysiology

Cystic fibrosis is caused by a mutation of a gene on chromosome 7. The result is defective chloride ion transport in epithelial cells in the lungs, pancreas, liver, gastrointestinal tract, and reproductive organs. This decrease in chloride transport results in a decrease of sodium and water transport. This results in dehydrated, viscous secretions that can cause obstruction, destruction, and scarring of exocrine glands.

Laboratory Results

Because cystic fibrosis is an expiratory airflow obstructive disease, most pulmonary function test results will be abnormal. The white blood cell count may be elevated because of frequent pulmonary infections.

Clinical Manifestations

Pancreatic insufficiency, meconium ileus at birth, diabetes mellitus, azoospermia, and obstructive hepatobiliary tract disease (cirrhosis and portal hypertension) are often present. The primary causes of morbidity and mortality are bronchiectasis and COPD. Typically, a cough, chronic purulent sputum production, and exertional dyspnea will be seen.

Treatment

Treatment is similar to that for bronchiectasis and focuses on alleviation of symptoms (mobilization and clearance of lower airway secretions and treatment of pulmonary infections) and correcting organ dysfunction (pancreatic enzyme replacement). Treatment of secretions is usually done by chest physical therapy with postural drainage. Bronchodilator therapy may also be instituted. Antibiotics are often given to relieve the increased secretions from pulmonary infections. If no pathogens are seen, bronchoscopy to remove lower airway secretions may be indicated if there is no response to common antibiotics.

Anesthetic Considerations

Management is based on the same principles as in patients with COPD and bronchiectasis. Elective procedures are delayed until optimal pulmonary function is ensured by controlling infections and removing secretions from the airways. Vitamin K may be given if liver function is poor or if absorption of fat-soluble vitamins is poor in the gastrointestinal tract. Preoperative sedation is probably unnecessary because of possible respiratory depression. Maintenance of anesthesia with a volatile agent and oxygen can decrease airway resistance by decreasing the bronchial smooth muscle tone. Volatile agents are also helpful in decreasing the responsiveness of hyperreactive airways. Humidified gases are also important to decrease the viscosity of secretions. Frequent suctioning is also necessary.

G. PNEUMOTHORAX AND HEMOTHORAX

Definition

Pneumothorax is the presence of air or gas in the pleural space. Hemothorax is the presence of blood in the pleural space.

Incidence and Prevalence

Spontaneous pneumothorax occurs unexpectedly in healthy persons, most often in men 20 to 40 years of age. Secondary pneumothorax and hemopneumothorax are generally the result of trauma.

Pathophysiology and Treatment

Pneumothorax

Pneumothorax can be subdivided into three categories, depending on whether air has direct access to the pleural cavity. In simple pneumothorax, no communication exists with the atmosphere. Additionally, no shift of the mediastinum or hemidiaphragm results from the accumulation of air in the intrapleural space. The severity of pneumothoraces is graded on the basis of the degree of collapse: collapse of 15% or less is small, collapse of 15% to 60% is moderate, and collapse of greater than 60% is large. Treatment of simple pneumothorax is determined by the size and cause of injury and may include catheter aspiration or tube thoracostomy; close observation of the patient with simple pneumothorax is essential.

In communicating pneumothorax, air in the pleural cavity exchanges with atmospheric air through a defect in the chest wall. Because the exchange of air through the site of injury may often be heard, this entity is commonly known as a "sucking chest wound." Treatment measures include administration of supplemental oxygen, tube thoracostomy, and intubation; mechanical ventilation may be indicated.

Tension pneumothorax develops when air progressively accumulates under pressure within the pleural cavity. If the pressure becomes too great, the mediastinum shifts to the opposite hemithorax, and this causes compression of the contralateral lung and great vessels. Tension pneumothorax is potentially lethal; therefore, immediate treatment is essential. Decompression of the chest can be performed with the insertion of a 16- or 18-gauge angiocatheter into the second or third interspace anteriorly or the fourth or fifth interspace laterally. A rush of air is heard when decompression occurs. The angiocatheter must be covered if the sucking of more air into the pleura is to be prevented.

Hemothorax

Hemothorax is the accumulation of blood in the pleural cavity. It usually is a result of trauma, but other causes include the rupture of small blood vessels in the presence of inflammation, pneumonia, tuberculosis, or erosion by tumors. The treatment of hemothorax consists of airway management as necessary, restoration of circulating blood volume, and evacuation of the accumulated blood. Thoracostomy may be indicated if the initial bleeding rate is greater than 20 mL/kg/hr. If bleeding subsides but its rate remains greater than 7 mL/kg/hr, chest radiographic findings worsen, or hypotension persists after initial blood replacement and decompression, thoracostomy is indicated.

Pathogenesis

Different presentations may be distinguished, according to the mechanism of injury, as described in the following sections.

Spontaneous

Pneumothorax usually is caused by rupture of alveoli near the pleural surface of the lung after a forceful sneeze or cough. This mechanism is most common in persons with a long, narrow chest and in those with emphysema.

Traumatic

Hemothorax, pneumothorax, and flail chest may occur after blunt chest trauma; however, they most frequently occur after rib fracture. Hemopneumothorax also may occur with penetrating injury.

Iatrogenic

Hemothorax and pneumothorax may occur after any of the following:

- Subclavian central line insertion (incidence is 2% to 16%)
- Supraclavicular block to the brachial plexus (incidence is 1%; hemothorax and pneumothorax can be complications of interscalene block but are rare with intercostal block)

- Barotrauma (from overdistention of the alveoli by PEEP; an abrupt deterioration of alveolar oxygen tension and cardiovascular function during PEEP administration should arouse suspicion of pulmonary barotrauma, especially pneumothorax)
- Exposure to high airway pressures (e.g., during mechanical ventilation)
- Other surgical procedures (e.g., mediastinoscopy, radical neck dissection, mastectomy, or nephrectomy)

Laboratory Results

The chest radiograph frequently shows subcutaneous emphysema, pneumomediastinum, and pneumopericardium. Free fluid, as with hemothorax, may be best seen on a cross-table lateral radiograph.

Anesthetic Considerations

Pneumothorax or hemothorax can significantly interfere with oxygenation and ventilation. Decreased cardiac output, as with tension pneumothorax, can exacerbate intrapulmonary shunting. Cyanosis indicates both cardiac and pulmonary involvement. Nitrous oxide can quickly expand the size of a pneumothorax if a chest tube is not in place. Nitrous oxide is acceptable for use if the chest tube is patent and functioning. A closed pneumothorax is a contraindication to the administration of nitrous oxide. Decreased pulmonary compliance (increased pulmonary inspiratory pressure) during administration of anesthesia to patients with a history of chest trauma may reflect the expansion of an unrecognized pneumothorax.

In the case of ventilator-related pneumothorax, the mortality rate is significantly reduced if a chest tube is placed in less than 30 minutes. Development of tension pneumothorax during general anesthesia is manifested by sudden hypotension, loss of pulmonary compliance, or decreased ventilating volume. Patients with significant trauma may require fluid resuscitation and cardiovascular support. Agents chosen should have minimal cardiac depressant effects.

H. PULMONARY ARTERIAL HYPERTENSION

Definition

Pulmonary arterial hypertension usually represents an advanced stage of a large number of cardiovascular diseases. The mortality rate associated with PAH is high. PAH exists if the mean level of PAP increases by 5 to 10 mmHg or if pulmonary artery systolic pressure exceeds 30 mmHg and mean PAP exceeds 20 mmHg.

Incidence

Pulmonary arterial hypertension may be (1) primary or idiopathic (unexplained) or (2) secondary to an associated condition. In young adults, the female-to-male incidence of primary pulmonary arterial hypertension (PPAH) is 4:1; this incidence is similar to that in older groups of men and women.

Pathophysiology

Pulmonary arterial hypertension may be caused by many associated conditions, including pulmonary venous hypertension caused by left atrial outflow obstruction or pulmonary venous occlusive disease and PAH caused by hyperdynamic circulation (e.g., secondary to burns or sepsis), vasoconstriction, viscosity, obstruction, and reactive vascular disease.

Pulmonary arterial hypertension is characterized by a rapidly progressive course with a 79% mortality rate within 5 years of clinical diagnosis. The degree of increase in pressure in the pulmonary circulation has an important influence on the patient's life expectancy. Resistant PAH has long been identified as a major cause of early death. The prognosis is largely determined by right ventricular integrity.

Pulmonary arterial hypertension is characterized by an increase in vascular tone and the growth and proliferation of pulmonary vascular smooth muscle. Initial reversible vasoconstriction may progress to muscle hypertrophy and irreversible degeneration.

Clinical Manifestations and Diagnosis

Pulmonary arterial hypertension may be either acute or chronic. In almost all patients with PAH, dyspnea and exercise intolerance usually are the first complaints. Patients also may have angina. Right atrial hypertrophy or right ventricular hypertrophy (or both) may be evident on ECG. Chest radiography may demonstrate an enlarged pulmonary artery. Cardiac catheterization combined with pulmonary angiography is most informative in assessment of PAH, cardiac reserve, and the effects of pulmonary vasodilator therapy. Vasodilator therapy is attempted when a vasoconstrictor component is identified. Vasodilator challenge may be performed with cardiac catheterization using a rapid and effective pulmonary vasodilator such as nitroglycerin, isoproterenol, nifedipine, prostaglandin E_1, prostacyclin, prostaglandin E_2, hydralazine, nitroprusside, or adenosine for evaluation of the reversibility of PAH. Frequently, open-lung biopsy is performed for assessment of the histopathologic composition of small pulmonary arteries. Noninvasive evaluation includes Doppler echocardiography for measurement of the velocity of tricuspid regurgitation (which correlates well with invasive PAP measurements) and pulmonic peak flow velocity.

Anesthetic Considerations

Attempts to alleviate PH disease states have had varied success. Vasodilator agents are used most commonly and may be helpful in patients with reversible vasoconstriction. A list of vasodilators used in PAH is provided in the table below. Possible beneficial effects of pulmonary arterial dilation are preservation of lung function; prevention of right ventricle deterioration; and, it is hoped, improved survival. The principal objectives during anesthesia in patients with PAH are prevention of increases in PAH and avoidance of major hemodynamic changes. Considerations that apply to the care of patients with cor pulmonale also apply to those with PAH. Information regarding PAH and intravenous induction agents is lacking; however, most agents either have little effect on PVR or decrease it. Ketamine, which causes an increase in PVR, may be the exception.

Key Points

- PH has been classified by the World Health Organization into five groups: (1) PAH, (2) PH with heart disease, (3) PH with lung disease, (4) PH with pulmonary thromboembolism, and (5) miscellaneous.

Updated Clinical Classification of Pulmonary Hypertension

Group 1
Pulmonary arterial hypertension (PAH)
Idiopathic PAH
Heritable
- BMPR2
- ALK1, endoglin (with or without hereditary hemorrhagic telangiectasia)
- Unknown

Drug and toxin induced
Associated with:
- Connective tissue diseases
- HIV infection
- Portal hypertension
- Congenital heart diseases
- Schistosomiasis
- Chronic hemolytic anemia

Persistent pulmonary hypertension of the newborn
Pulmonary veno-occlusive disease with left-to-right shunts or pulmonary capillary hemangiomatosis

Group 2
Pulmonary hypertension owing to left heart disease
Systolic dysfunction
Diastolic dysfunction
Valvular disease

Group 3
Pulmonary hypertension owing to lung diseases or hypoxia
Chronic obstructive pulmonary disease
Interstitial lung disease

Other pulmonary diseases with mixed restrictive and obstructive pattern
Sleep-disordered breathing
Alveolar hypoventilation disorders
Chronic exposure to high altitude
Developmental abnormalities

Group 4
Chronic thromboembolic pulmonary hypertension

Group 5
Pulmonary hypertension with unclear multifactorial mechanisms
Hematologic disorders: myeloproliferative disorders, splenectomy
Systemic disorders: sarcoidosis, pulmonary Langerhans cell histiocytosis: lymphangioleiomyomatosis, neurofibromatosis, vasculitis
Metabolic disorders: glycogen storage disease, Gaucher disease, thyroid disorders
Others: tumoral obstruction, fibrosing mediastinitis, chronic renal failure on dialysis

ALK1, Activin receptor-like kinase type 1; *BMPR2,* bone morphogenetic protein receptor type 2; *HIV,* human immunodeficiency virus.
From Simonneau G, Robbins IM, Beghetti M, et al. Updated clinical classification of pulmonary hypertension. *J Am Coll Cardiol* 2009;54:S43-S54.

- PAH has further been classified into (1) idiopathic IPAH, (2) heritable, (3) related to other conditions, (4) PPH of the newborn, and (5) pulmonary veno-occulusive disease (PVOD).
- Heritable PH has been associated with bone morphogenic protein receptor 2 (BMPR2), but mutations are not always associated with PH, indicating other defects or insults are required. Evidence also supports involvement of a voltage-gated potassium ion channel and serotonin transporter.
- The basis for treatment of IPAH stems from deficiencies in prostacyclin and nitric oxide release and excess endothelin-1 found in patients with PH.
- PH can be diagnosed to some extent by physical examination, chest radiography, ECG, and echocardiography, but establishing the diagnosis with certainty requires a right-sided cardiac catheterization, which can check for left heart failure and response to a pulmonary vasodilator.
- Therapy includes moderate exercise, warfarin, oxygen, and calcium channel blockers.
- Targeted therapy with the prostacyclins, phosphodiesterase inhibitors, and endothelin receptor antagonists has made major improvements in the lives of patients with PAH.

The natural history of patients with groups 2 and 3 PH are influenced by their left heart and lung disease. In most cases, the presence of PH in addition to the underlying disease portends a poor prognosis.

Pulmonary Arterial Hypertension: Determinants of Prognosis*

Determinants of Risk	Lower Risk (Good Prognosis)	Higher Risk (Poor Prognosis)
Clinical evidence of RV failure	No	Yes
Progression of symptoms	Gradual	Rapid
WHO class†	II, III	IV
6-minute walk test‡	Longer (>400 m)	Shorter (<300 m)
CPET	Peak Vo_2 >10.4 mL/kg/min	Peak Vo_2 <10.4 mL/kg/min
Echocardiography	Minimal RV dysfunction	Pericardial effusion, significant RV enlargement or dysfunction, RA enlargement
Hemodynamics	RAP <10 mmHg, CI >2.5 L/min/m^2	RAP >20 mmHg, CI <2.0 L/min/m^2
BNP§	Minimally elevated	Significantly elevated

BNP, Brain natriuretic peptide; *CI,* cardiac index; *CPET,* cardiopulmonary exercise testing; *peak Vo_2,* average peak oxygen uptake during exercise; *RA,* right atrium; *RAP,* right atrial pressure; *RV,* right ventricle; *WHO,* World Health Organization.

*Most data available pertain to idiopathic pulmonary arterial hypertension (PAH). Few data are available for other forms of PAH. One should not rely on any single factor to make risk predictions.

†WHO class is the functional classification for PAH and is a modification of the New York Heart Association functional class.

‡The 6-minute walk test is also influenced by age, gender, and height.

§Because there are currently limited data regarding the influence of BNP on prognosis and many factors including renal function, weight, age, and gender may influence BNP, absolute numbers are not given for this variable.

From McLaughlin VV, Archer SL, Badesch DB, et al. ACCF/AHA 2009 expert consensus document on pulmonary hypertension: a report of the American College of Cardiology Foundation Task Force on Expert Consensus Documents and the American Heart Association developed in collaboration with the American College of Chest Physicians; American Thoracic Society, Inc.; and the Pulmonary Hypertension Association. *J Am Coll Cardiol* 2009;53:1573-1619.

Nonspecific treatments of PH include loop diuretics, digoxin, and anticoagulant therapy with warfarin when indicated. Traditional therapies include dihydropyridine calcium channel blockers such as nifedipine or amlodipine, which can modestly decrease pulmonary arterial pressures in vasoresponsive patients but can also cause sudden death in nonvasoresponsive patients.

Drug Treatment Options for Patients with Pulmonary Hypertension

Drug or Drug Class	Rationale	Potentially Responsive Types of Pulmonary Hypertension	Limitations
Anticoagulants	Reduce risk of pulmonary thromboembolism	Primary PH and PH secondary to acute pulmonary thromboembolism, chronic pulmonary thromboembolism, and anorectic drugs	For primary hypertension, concomitant vasodilator treatment also required
	Vasodilators		
Calcium antagonists	Inhibit influx of calcium into smooth muscle cells with elevated vasomotor tone; preferentially act on pulmonary vasculature	Primary PH and PH secondary to connective tissue vascular disease and COPD	Initial treatment in specialized centers recommended to avoid severe adverse outcomes such as negative inotropic effects
Epoprostenol (Flolan)–prostacyclin	May replace deficiencies in endogenous prostacyclin; also inhibits smooth muscle proliferation and platelet aggregation	Primary, persistent pulmonary hypertension of the neonate and that secondary to ARDS, crises after heart surgery in infants, and connective tissue disease in adults	Peripheral adverse effects occur when administered by continuous IV infusion
Nitric oxide	Interferes with endogenous vasoconstrictor mechanisms	Primary, persistent PH of the neonate and that secondary to corrective cardiac surgery in children, lung or lung-heart transplant surgery in adults, and COPD	Potential adverse effects include increased bleeding times, negative inotropic effects, and formation of potentially toxic products (e.g., nitrogen dioxide, methemoglobin)

Continued

Drug Treatment Options for Patients with Pulmonary Hypertension—cont'd

Drug or Drug Class	Rationale	Potentially Responsive Types of Pulmonary Hypertension	Limitations
Alprostadil (prostaglandin E_1)	Interferes with endogenous vasoconstrictor mechanisms	Secondary to ARDS	Impaired pulmonary metabolism may result in systemic hypotension
Bosentan (Tracleer)	Oral endothelin receptor antagonist	Severe PH	Hepatotoxicity
Treprostinil (Remodulin)	Prostacyclin analog	Primary PH; classes II–IV	Given by continuous infusion via wearable infusion pump
Ambrisentan (Letairis)	Selective endothelin type A (ET_A) receptor antagonist	Treatment of symptomatic patients (WHO class II or III) with pulmonary arterial hypertension (PAH)	Peripheral edema, nasal congestion, and serious birth defects may occur
Sildenafil (Revatio)	Inhibits phosphodiesterase type 5	Treatment for PAH along with anticoagulant and a diuretic	Headaches, dyspepsia, and transient color vision
Iloprost (Ventavis)	Synthetic analog of prostacyclin PGI2	Treatment of PAH in patients with NYHA class III or IV symptoms	Requires inhalation administration six to nine times a day
Inhibitors of Vasoconstriction			
α-Adrenoceptor antagonists	Inhibit the formation of the vasoconstrictor angiotensin II	Persistent PH of the neonate (especially preterm infants) and that secondary to COPD	Can cause severe systemic adverse effects
ACE inhibitors	Inhibit the formation of the vasoconstrictor angiotensin II	Secondary to connective tissue disease, effects of high altitude, and congestive heart failure	Prolonged treatment required to obtain an effect

ACE, Angiotensin-converting enzyme; *ARDS,* acute respiratory distress syndrome; *COPD,* chronic obstructive pulmonary disease; *IV,* intravenous; *PH,* pulmonary hypertension.

Modified from Treprostinil (Remodulin) for pulmonary arterial hypertension. *Med Lett.* 2002;44:80-82; Sildenafil (Revatio) for pulmonary arterial hypertension. *Med Lett* 2005;47:165-167; Ambrisentan (Letairis) for pulmonary arterial hypertension. *Med Lett* 2007;49:87-90.

Other therapies include prostacyclins such as epoprostenol and treprostinil; both are pulmonary and systemic vasodilators but must be given by continuous intravenous infusion through an indwelling catheter or by subcutaneous injection (treprostinil). Iloprost is an inhaled form of prostacyclin apparently with fewer side effects that can improve exercise capacity and symptom scores, but it requires frequent dosing. Side effects and economic costs are significant obstacles to the use of all these agents. Bosentan is a nonselective endothelin receptor antagonist, and sitaxsentan is a selective endothelin receptor antagonist. Both improve functional status and physiologic measures in PH.

Sildenafil, which inhibits phosphodiesterase type 5 in the pulmonary vasculature, has also been approved for this indication based on results of a controlled trial that showed it improved 6-minute walk distance, New York Heart Association (NYHA) functional class, pulmonary artery pressure, cardiac index, and oxygenation. Sildenafil (2005) is also less expensive than the prostacyclins and endothelin receptor antagonists. Dipyridamole also has some phosphodiesterase type 5 activity.

Inhaled nitric oxide is a selective pulmonary vasodilator that is often used to treat persistent PH of the newborn. In adults with PH, a 2-year trial of inhaled nitric oxide therapy combined with dipyridamole demonstrated improvements in exercise capacity, symptoms, and hemodynamic measures. A European consensus panel has released guidelines for the use of nitric oxide in this condition.

Surgical therapies may be general (lung transplant) or specific, as in the repair of congenital shunting lesions, mitral stenosis, or atrial defects. Pulmonary thromboendarterectomy is effective in some patients with PH associated with saddle pulmonary embolus.

I. PULMONARY EDEMA

Definition

Pulmonary edema is the accumulation of excess fluid in the interstitial and air-filled spaces of the lung. The mechanisms responsible for its development include an increase in hydrostatic pressure within the pulmonary capillary system, an increase in the permeability of the alveolocapillary membrane, and a decrease in intravascular colloid oncotic pressure.

Pulmonary edema is classified as being either cardiogenic (high pressure, hydrostatic) or noncardiogenic (increased permeability).

TYPES

Cardiogenic Pulmonary Edema

Cardiogenic pulmonary edema is initiated by some type of left-sided heart incompetence or failure. Left ventricular failure implies that there is a decrease in left ventricular contractility, which ultimately leads to a reduction in both stroke volume and cardiac output. Incomplete left ventricular emptying elevates left ventricular end-diastolic volume, which, in turn, elevates left ventricular end-diastolic pressure. Increased left ventricular end-diastolic pressure is "reflected back," causing elevation of the left atrial, pulmonary venous, and pulmonary capillary pressures. When pulmonary capillary pressure reaches levels of 20 to 25 mmHg (normal range, 10–16 mmHg), the rate of fluid transudation often exceeds lymphatic drainage capacity, and alveolar flooding occurs.

Noncardiogenic Pulmonary Edema

Noncardiogenic pulmonary edema is associated with an increase in endothelial permeability caused by an insult that disrupts the barrier function of the blood–tissue interface. Noncardiogenic pulmonary edema is associated with the leakage of both fluid and protein from the vascular space. Because this respiratory membrane disruption cannot be easily or directly measured, noncardiogenic pulmonary edema is said to exist when suspicious chest radiographic evidence coexists with insufficient hemodynamic basis. The presence of pulmonary wedge pressure less than 12 mmHg and the absence of a significant history of cardiac disease generally suffice for exclusion of a hemodynamic mechanism.

Neurogenic Pulmonary Edema

Neurogenic pulmonary edema begins with a massive outpouring of sympathetic nervous system stimulation triggered by CNS insult. This centrally mediated CNS overactivity typically occurs in the hypothalamic area. Excessive sympathetic activation induces remarkable hemodynamic alterations, primarily systemic and pulmonary vasoconstriction. The left ventricle fails because of the inordinate pressure work imposed by the systemic hypertension, and pulmonary blood volume increases because of the functional imbalance between the failing left ventricle and the normal right ventricle. Although this sequence seems to parallel that of hemodynamic pulmonary edema, a permeability component exists, as evidenced by the high protein concentration found in the pulmonary secretions of these patients.

Uremic Pulmonary Edema

Uremic pulmonary edema is seen in those patients with renal insufficiency or failure. Overhydration and expansion of the circulating blood volume lead to increases in pulmonary capillary pressures. Again, a "leaky" component exists because of the metabolic abnormalities associated with uremia. Reducing the circulating blood volume of these patients by hemodialysis promotes the resolution of this type of pulmonary edema.

High Altitude–Related Pulmonary Edema

High altitude–related pulmonary edema may occur in the absence of left ventricular failure whenever someone overexerts himself or herself before acclimating to a high altitude. The pathogenesis of this form of pulmonary edema is unclear but may be the result of intense hypoxic pulmonary arterial vasoconstriction or massive sympathetic discharge triggered by cerebral hypoxia.

Pulmonary Edema Caused by Upper Airway Obstruction

Pulmonary edema resulting from upper airway obstruction is caused by the prolonged, forced inspiratory effort against an obstructed upper airway. The most common cause of this type of pulmonary edema in adults is laryngospasm after extubation and general anesthesia. In children, pulmonary edema after obstruction caused by croup, epiglottitis, and laryngospasm also is well documented. Vigorous inspiration against obstruction creates high negative intrathoracic, transpleural, and alveolar pressures that enlarge the pulmonary vascular volume and subsequently the interstitial fluid volume. The capacity of the lymphatics becomes overwhelmed, and interstitial fluid transudes into the pulmonary alveoli. Hypoxia causes a massive sympathetic discharge that results in systemic vasoconstriction and a translocation of fluid from the systemic circulation to the already expanding pulmonary vascular and interstitial spaces. Hypoxia also increases pulmonary capillary pressures. Because hypoxia alters myocardial activity, left atrial function and left ventricular function are reduced. During obstruction, vigorous inspiratory efforts are unsuccessful because of the airway obstruction. Unsuccessful expiration produces an increase in intrathoracic and alveolar pressures. Intrinsic PEEP also is produced during this stage. Relief of the obstruction results in cessation of intrinsic PEEP.

The consequence of these events is the sudden massive transudation of fluid from the pulmonary interstitium into the alveoli, which results in pulmonary edema. The severity of pulmonary edema is determined by the extent of prior alveolar and capillary damage and the immensity of hemodynamic and cardiovascular alterations.

Clinical Manifestations

Physical examination reveals an increased work of breathing. As water accumulates, the lungs become heavy and noncompliant, and a decrease in FRC occurs. This increase in the volume of extravascular lung fluid provides a potent stimulus for surrounding interstitial stretch receptors (j-receptors) whose activation results in tachypnea. Tachypnea is not relieved by the administration of oxygen and the return of arterial oxygen tension (Pao_2) to normal. Intercostal retractions and use of accessory muscles are apparent on physical examination. Signs of sympathetic stress stimulation such as hypertension, diaphoresis, and tachycardia often are noted. The expectoration of pink, frothy sputum signals that alveoli have been flooded.

The detection of basilar crackles on auscultation is the traditional hallmark of early pulmonary edema. In reality, by the time these crackles become audible, excess water has already flooded the alveoli and has overflowed into the terminal bronchioles. It is in the bronchioles, not in the alveoli, that the crackles of pulmonary edema are generated. The earliest and most often disregarded clinical sign is rapid, shallow breathing.

In cardiogenic pulmonary edema, heart size may be increased. High central venous pressures (CVPs), an S_3 or S_4 gallop, and jugular venous distention often are observed. Chest radiography is still the most reliable and expedient tool for early detection of pulmonary edema. In cardiogenic pulmonary edema, the cardiac silhouette may appear abnormal or enlarged; in noncardiogenic pulmonary edema, it can be enlarged or remain normal. Interstitial edema can be observed before the alveoli flood and the onset of clinical signs occurs. Pleural effusions are common, and a "whited-out" or "butterfly" appearance may be noted.

Arterial blood gas analysis reveals hypoxemia secondary to V/Q abnormalities. When right-to-left shunting is great, the Pao_2 can be affected by any change in the central venous oxygen content. Increases in oxygen consumption or decreases in cardiac output further reduce the Pao_2. The arterial carbon dioxide tension ($Paco_2$) may be low, normal, or elevated. The initial hypocarbia is related to tachypnea and high minute volumes; at later stages, hypercarbia is frequently secondary to muscle fatigue and exhaustion. Changes in pH usually reflect changes in $Paco_2$, but metabolic and V/Q or lactic acidosis may occur from tissue oxygen deficiency, low cardiac output, or sepsis.

Treatment and Anesthetic Considerations

Treatment includes prompt recognition of the condition, securing a patent airway, supportive therapy with oxygenation, and the administration of diuretics. Although the onset of pulmonary edema after laryngospasm usually is immediate, cases have been reported of the occurrence of pulmonary edema several hours after laryngospasm. Therefore, it is recommended that patients who develop laryngospasm be observed postoperatively longer than the typical 60 to 90 minutes. The diagnosis of pulmonary edema and its differentiation into cardiac and noncardiac categories require the taking of a detailed medical history, physical examination, chest radiography, and ABG analysis.

Pulmonary edema is considered a medical emergency, and immediate intervention is required for treating the underlying disease, supporting other failing organ systems, and optimizing oxygen delivery. Oxygen should be administered by nasal cannula, face mask, or ETT. If oxygenation does not improve with the administration of high fractions of inspired oxygen, positive-pressure ventilation with either PEEP or continuous PAP must be initiated. Institution of positive-pressure mechanical ventilation in patients with acute pulmonary edema usually results in a prompt increase in oxygenation and, in some cases, in cardiac output. Improvement occurs because of superior inflation and $\dot{V}/\dot{Q}$ matching.

Pharmacologic therapy includes the use of vasodilators, inotropes, steroids, and diuretics. Morphine sulfate has been used in the treatment of cardiogenic pulmonary edema because of its venodilatory properties. Nitroprusside is very effective at decreasing preload, afterload and left ventricular afterload. This may result in better cardiac function, with a subsequent lowering of left atrial pressures. Inotropic agents such as dopamine or dobutamine improve myocardial contractility and lower cardiac filling pressures. In patients with chronic congestive heart failure and pulmonary congestion, digitalis augments contractility and promotes decreases in left atrial and ventricular filling pressures.

Fluid balance is managed with both fluid restriction and diuresis. This therapy helps achieve a "negative" fluid balance in hydrostatic pulmonary edema. Potent diuretics such as furosemide not only lower left atrial filling pressure by decreasing systemic venous tone but also induce diuresis of the expanded extravascular volume. The type of fluid, whether crystalloid or colloid, that should be used in the presence of pulmonary edema remains controversial. Regardless of type used, it is generally agreed that fluid administration proceeds slowly.

J. PULMONARY EMBOLISM

Definition

Pulmonary embolism (PE) is considered by some to be a clinical manifestation of deep venous thrombosis (DVT) rather than a separate entity. Most emboli (90%) arise in the proximal deep veins of the lower extremities, with the remainder originating from pelvic veins. DVT at proximal sites is more likely to cause symptoms. Three major factors promote the formation of venous thrombi: stasis of blood flow, venous injury, and hypercoagulation states. Other less common causes of PE include air, tumor, bone, fat, catheter fragments, and amniotic fluid. Fillers used in illicit drug preparations by intravenous drug abusers also may cause PE. Of particular concern to anesthesia providers are air emboli caused by the opening of venous structures during surgery or by disconnected intravenous lines.

Risk Factors for Venous Thrombosis Based on Virchow Triad

Stasis	Congestive heart failure or cor pulmonale General anesthesia Immobility Obesity Prior venous thrombosis Varicose veins
Hypercoagulability	Disseminated intravascular coagulation Estrogen therapy or oral contraceptive use Infection Malignancy Nephrotic syndrome Pregnancy Thrombophilias: Anticardiolipin antibody, factor V Leiden mutation, protein C and S deficiencies, antithrombin III deficiency
Vascular injury	Trauma Surgery

Modified from Ozsu S, Oztuna F, Bulbul Y, et al. The role of risk factors in delayed diagnosis of pulmonary embolism. *Am J Emerg Med* 2011;29(1):26-32; Epley D: Pulmonary emboli risk reduction. *J Vasc Nurs* 2000;18(2):61-68, 69-70; Dijk FN, et al. Pulmonary embolism in children. *Paediatr Respir Rev* 2012;13(2):112-122.

Most pulmonary emboli resolve within 8 to 21 days of the initial presentation. Chronically unresolved emboli that lodge in major pulmonary arteries may become incorporated into the vascular walls and obstruct blood flow. Patients with such emboli are surgical candidates, representing approximately 1000 cases in the United States each year.

Pathophysiology

When a thrombus has formed, it rarely remains static. It can be dissolved through fibrinolysis, become "organized" into a vessel wall, or be released into the circulation. Because thrombi are most friable early in their development, it is then that the greatest risk for embolism exists. Emboli are most often seen in the lower lung lobes, which receive the greatest amount of blood flow. Fortunately, these lower lung lobes also tend to receive the least ventilation, so much of the $\dot{V}/\dot{Q}$ ratio is preserved in patients with small- to moderate-sized emboli. The three components of the Virchow triad—stasis, hypercoagulability, and vessel wall injury—lead to venous thrombosis.

Clinical Manifestations and Diagnosis

The patient's clinical presentation depends largely on the size of the embolus. Signs and symptoms of PE vary, and the differential diagnosis according to size of emboli may be difficult. Dyspnea of sudden onset appears to be the only common historical complaint. Hypoxia is a constant feature of PE, possibly owing to intrapulmonary shunting.

Massive emboli can produce sudden cardiac collapse. Preceding symptoms range from pallor, shock, and central chest pain to sudden loss of consciousness. In patients with cardiac collapse, the pulse becomes rapid and weak, blood pressure decreases, neck veins become engorged, and cardiogenic shock may be present or impending. Also, a decrease in P_{ETCO_2} and an increase in Pa_{CO_2} occur, with the difference between the values for these two indexes increasing as conditions worsen. If a pulmonary artery

Associated Factors in Patients with Pulmonary Embolism*

Finding	Incidence (%)
Dyspnea	96
Tachycardia	71
Acute onset of symptoms (<48 hr)	70
Syncope	35
Arterial hypotension (SBP <90 mmHg)	34
Congestive heart failure	32
History of venous thrombosis	29
Recent major operations (within 10 days)	27
Cancer	12
Major trauma or fracture within 10 days	11
Chronic pulmonary disease	11
Stroke	2

SBP, Systolic blood pressure.

*Data from 1001 patients with pulmonary embolism.

From Kasper W, Konstantinides S, Geibel A, et al. Management strategies and determinants of outcome in acute major pulmonary embolism: results of a multicenter registry. *J Am Coll Cardiol* 1997;30(5):1165-1171.

catheter is in place, PAPs are observed to increase rapidly; also, the ECG may begin to show right ventricular strain. The prognosis for these patients is very poor.

Diagnostic Testing

Few of the common preoperative tests indicate the presence of PE. A number of imaging and laboratory tests are now available for diagnosis as listed below. In patients with PE, ABG analysis generally reveals hypoxemia and increased differences between P_{ACO_2} and Pa_{CO_2}, which result from ventilation of unperfused alveoli.

Diagnostic Tests for Suspected Pulmonary Embolism

Test	Comments
Oxygen saturation	Nonspecific but suspect PE if there is a sudden otherwise unexplained decrement
Electrocardiogram	May be normal, especially in younger, previously healthy individuals; may provide alternative diagnosis, such as MI or pericarditis
Echocardiography	Best used as a prognostic test in patients with established PE rather than as a diagnostic test; many patients with larger PE will have normal echocardiography findings
Lung scanning	Usually provides ambiguous results; used in lieu of chest CT for patients with anaphylaxis to contrast agent, renal insufficiency, or pregnancy
Chest CT	Most accurate diagnostic imaging test for PE; beware if CT results and clinical likelihood are discordant
Pulmonary angiography	Invasive, costly, and uncomfortable; used primarily when local catheter intervention is planned
D-dimer	An excellent "rule out" test if normal, especially is accompanied by non-high clinical suspicion

Diagnostic Tests for Suspected Pulmonary Embolism—cont'd

Test	Comments
Venous ultrasonography	Excellent for diagnosing acute symptomatic proximal DVT but a negative test result does not rule out PE because a recent leg DVT may have embolized completely; calf vein imaging is operator dependent
MRI	Reliable only for imaging proximal segmental pulmonary arteries; requires gadolinium but does not require iodinated contrast agents.

CT, Computed tomography; *DVT,* deep venous thrombosis; *MI,* myocardial infarction; *MRI,* magnetic resonance imaging; *PE,* pulmonary embolism.
From Goldhaber SZ. Pulmonary embolism. In Bonow RO, Mann DL, Zipes DP, et al, eds. *Braunwald's Heart Disease.* 9th ed. Philadelphia: Saunders; 2012:1686.

Advantages and Disadvantages of Diagnostic Tests for Suspected Pulmonary Embolism

Diagnostic Test	Advantages	Disadvantages
Plasma D-dimer ELISA	A normal result makes PE exceedingly unlikely	Level is elevated in patients with many systemic illnesses that mimic PE, such as pneumonia and MI Level is elevated in patients with sepsis, cancer, postoperative state, and pregnancy
ECG	Universally available; may indicate ominous acute cor pulmonale or benign pericarditis	Acute cor pulmonale on ECG is not specific for PE; not a sensitive test
Chest radiography	Usually has minor abnormalities but occasionally pathognomonic; may suggest alternative diagnoses such as pneumothorax	Not specific
Venous ultrasonography	Excellent for detecting symptomatic proximal DVT; surrogate for PE	Cannot image iliac vein thrombosis; imaging of calf is operator dependent; DVT may have embolized completely, resulting in a normal result
Contrast venography	Used to be gold standard; excellent for calf veins; necessary for catheter-based interventions.	Can cause chemical phlebitis; uncomfortable; costly; may fail to result in diagnosis of massive DVT because veins are filled with thrombus and cannot be opacified
Lung scanning	High-probability scans are reliable for detecting PE; normal or near-normal scans are reliable for excluding PE	Most scans are neither high probability nor normal or near normal; ventilation scans are falling out of favor; most test results are equivocal

Continued

Advantages and Disadvantages of Diagnostic Tests for Suspected Pulmonary Embolism—cont'd

Diagnostic Test	Advantages	Disadvantages
Chest CT	New-generation scanners constitute the new gold standard for diagnosis	Older-generation scanners are insensitive for important but distal PE
MRI	Excellent for anatomy and cardiac function; contrast agent does not cause renal failure	In preliminary use; not widely available; experience very limited
Echocardiography	Excellent for identifying right ventricular dilatation and dysfunction that is not obvious clinically, thus providing an early warning of potentially adverse outcome	Not specific; many patients with PE have normal echocardiograms; the test cannot reliably differentiate causes of right ventricular dysfunction
Pulmonary angiography	Necessary for catheter-based interventions	Invasive, costly, uncomfortable

CT, Computed tomography; *DVT,* deep venous thrombosis; *ECG,* electrocardiogram; *ELISA,* enzyme-linked immunosorbent assay; *MI,* myocardial infarction; *MRI,* magnetic resonance imaging; *PE,* pulmonary embolism.

Massive PE is associated with severe hypoxemia and hypocapnia. An initial difference between $Paco_2$ and $Petco_2$ is common early during the embolic event. Some common conditions associated with an increased risk for DVT are listed as follows.

- Advancing age
- Obesity
- Previous venous thromboembolism
- Surgery
- Trauma
- Active cancer
- Acute medical illnesses (e.g., acute myocardial infarction, heart failure, respiratory failure, infection)
- Inflammatory bowel disease
- Antiphospholipid syndrome
- Dyslipoproteinemia
- Nephrotic syndrome
- Paroxysmal nocturnal hemoglobinuria
- Myeloproliferative diseases
- Behçet's syndrome
- Varicose veins
- Superficial vein thrombosis
- Congenital venous malformation
- Long-distance travel
- Prolonged bed rest
- Immobilization
- Limb paresis
- Chronic care facility stay
- Pregnancy or puerperium

- Oral contraceptives
- Hormone replacement therapy
- Heparin-induced thrombocytopenia
- Other drugs
- Chemotherapy
- Tamoxifen
- Thalidomide
- Antipsychotics
- Central venous catheter
- Vena cava filter
- Intravenous drug abuse

Treatment

Aggressive efforts at prevention have been successful in reducing the incidence of DVT in surgical patients. Treatment is mainly aimed at prevention of further embolism and at provision of ventilatory support as shown in the table below. Use of graded compression stockings, intermittent pneumatic compression, administration of various anticoagulants and thrombolytics, and ambulation are typical measures for preventing embolus formation. It must be remembered that PE is a mechanical disease caused by acute pulmonary obstruction in a previously healthy patient.

Prevention of Venous Thromboembolism

Condition	Strategy
Total hip or knee replacement; hip or pelvis fracture	Warfarin (Coumadin) (target INR, 2.5) for 4–6 wk
	LMWH/subcut (e.g., fondaparinux 2.5 mg subcut except for total knee replacement) or rivaroxaban 10 mg daily or dalteparin 2500–5000 units daily subcut where available
	IPC ± warfarin
Gynecologic cancer surgery	LMWH: consider 1 month of prophylaxis
Thoracic surgery	IPC *or* GCS *plus* UFH 5000 units bid or tid
High-risk general surgery (e.g., prior VTE, current cancer, or obesity)	IPC *or* GCS *plus* UFH 5000 units bid or tid LMWH
General, gynecologic, or urologic surgery (without prior VTE) for noncancerous conditions	GCS *plus* unfractionated heparin 5000 units bid or tid Dalteparin 2500 units subcut once daily Enoxaparin 40 mg subcut once daily
Neurosurgery, eye surgery, or other surgery when prophylactic anticoagulation is contraindicated	GCS ± IPC

bid, Twice a day; *GCS,* graduated compression stockings; *INR,* international normalized ratio; *IPC,* intermittent pneumatic compression; *subcut,* subcutaneous; *tid,* three times a day; *UFH,* unfractionated heparin; *VTE,* venous thromboembolism.

*Approved only for total hip replacement prophylaxis.

Modified from Goldhaber SZ. Deep vein thrombosis and pulmonary thromboembolism. In Fauci AS, Kasper DL, Braunwald E, et al, eds. *Harrison's Principles of Internal Medicine.* 17th ed. New York: McGraw-Hill; 2008:1651-1657; Goldhaber SZ. Pulmonary embolism. In Libby P, Bonow RO, Mann DL, et al, eds. *Braunwald's Heart Disease: A Textbook of Cardiovascular Medicine.* 8th ed. Philadelphia: Saunders; 2008:1879.

Treatment requires rapid intervention before vital signs are affected by hypoxia and mechanical failure of the heart. Guidelines for treatment of PE are summarized in the following box.

Guidelines for the Treatment of Pulmonary Embolism

1. Treat DVT or PE with therapeutic levels of unfractionated intravenous heparin, adjusted subcutaneous heparin, or low-molecular-weight heparin for at least 5 days and overlap with oral anticoagulation for at least 4 to 5 days. Consider a longer course of heparin (≈10 days) for massive PE or severe iliofemoral DVT.
2. For most patients, heparin and oral anticoagulation can be started together and heparin discontinued on day 5 or 6 if the INR has been therapeutic for 2 consecutive days.
3. Treat patients with reversible or time-limited risk factors for at least 3 months. Patients with a first episode of idiopathic DVT should be treated indefinitely. The approved regimen is warfarin (target INR, 2.0–3.0 for 6 months) followed by low-intensity warfarin (target INR, 1.5–2.0).
4. The use of thrombolytic agents continues to be highly individualized, and clinicians should have some latitude in using these agents. Patients with hemodynamically unstable PE or massive iliofemoral thrombosis are the best candidates.
5. Inferior vena caval filter placement is recommended when there is a contraindication to or failure of anticoagulation, for chronic recurrent embolism with pulmonary hypertension, and with concurrent performance of surgical pulmonary embolectomy or pulmonary endarterectomy.

DVT, Deep venous thrombosis; *INR,* international normalized ratio; *PTE,* pulmonary thromboembolism.
Modified from Goldhaber SZ. Deep vein thrombosis and pulmonary thromboembolism. In Fauci AS, Kasper DL, Braunwald E, et al, eds. *Harrison's Principles of Internal Medicine.* 17th ed. New York: McGraw-Hill; 2008:1651-1657.

Surgery

Surgical intervention often is indicated for patients who are unresponsive to other measures. Procedures that used to be the mainstay of this intervention, such as ligation of the inferior vena cava, are now rarely performed. Currently, the most common surgical procedure for patients with PE is placement of an umbrella filter, which traps thromboemboli. It is estimated that 30,000 to 40,000 patients receive such filters annually in the United States. The filter is placed in the inferior vena cava under fluoroscopic guidance, usually below the renal veins at the level of L2 to L3. Suprarenal placement is required when a thrombus directly involves the renal veins or has propagated above the level of the renal veins.

Anesthetic Considerations

Anesthesia for patients at risk for PE is aimed at supporting vital organ function and minimizing anesthetic-induced myocardial depression. The use of a high FIO_2 aids in prevention of pulmonary vasoconstriction, and the monitoring of PAP helps the anesthesia provider optimize right-sided heart function and assess the effects of anesthetic management on PVR. Many anesthesia providers choose not to place pulmonary artery catheters because of concerns about the possibility that these catheters will dislodge clots in the right side of the heart.

Intravenous fluid infusion must be adjusted so that right ventricular stroke volume is optimized in the presence of marked increase in afterload. A continuous catecholamine infusion may be needed to enhance cardiac contractility. Induction is often performed with etomidate or ketamine (for maintenance of hemodynamic stability), but ketamine must be titrated judiciously because it may increase PVR.

The use of N_2O is generally believed to be acceptable. However, this may not be possible with the use of a high F_{IO_2}. Use of N_2O should be discontinued if PVR increases. Obviously the use of N_2O is contraindicated in patients with venous air embolism. Patients with moderate to severe PE often are experiencing acute right-sided heart failure. Cardiac function can be optimized by the use of minimally depressing cardiac agents such as narcotics.

Persistent severe hypotension, such as that accompanying a massive PE, may necessitate the use of a cardiotonic agent. The goal is preservation of perfusion to the brain and heart until cardiopulmonary bypass is started and surgical removal of the clot attempted. As always, heparin should be readily available, and when needed, it should be administered into a central line while blood aspiration is verified before and after injection. Reports of operative mortality during pulmonary embolectomy range from 11% to 55%, with much higher rates among patients experiencing cardiac arrest.

Detection of Pulmonary Embolism During Anesthesia

In the intubated patient under general anesthesia, combinations of symptoms may occur. A decreasing P_{ETCO_2} and tachycardia usually are the first symptoms seen in PE. These can be followed by a decrease in Sa_{O_2} and the generation of ABG values that indicate unexplained arterial hypoxemia. Increased PAP and CVP can be seen in combination with a decrease in systolic and diastolic blood pressures. Bronchospasm may occur. Finally, ECG changes that indicate right axis deviation, incomplete or complete right bundle branch block, or peaked T waves may be observed in the presence or absence of an accompanying systolic ejection murmur.

Intraoperative Management

Several measures can be taken to support anesthetized patients with suspected PE. First and most important, an airway must be established by intubation if the patient is not already intubated. Second, delivery of the anesthetic agent must be discontinued, and administration of a 100% F_{IO_2} initiated. Next, the circulatory system should be supported with the infusion of intravenous fluids or blood (or both) as needed and the use of sympathomimetics (e.g., dobutamine or dopamine) initiated if necessary. Dysrhythmias should be treated with intravenous administration of lidocaine, and the patient should receive PEEP for optimization of O_2 transport across the alveolar membrane as blood pressure is adequate.

Patients with PE present particular management challenges in their postoperative courses, including reperfusion edema, persistent hypoxemia, pericardial effusion, psychiatric disorders, and pulmonary blood flow steal. The areas of the lung to which pulmonary artery flow has been restored are subject to development of reperfusion pulmonary edema, presumably as a manifestation of oxidant- and protease-mediated acute lung injury. Other possible causes are extracorporeal circulation, anticoagulation, and an increase in perfusion pressure in a previously obstructed pulmonary artery. Complications include immediate pulmonary hemorrhage and respiratory disturbance, and death may occur. This phenomenon has been labeled *pulmonary blood flow steal* and is believed to be caused by postoperative redistribution of regional PVR and not by rethrombosis or embolism. It may develop 3 to 5 days after surgery.

K. RESTRICTIVE PULMONARY DISEASES

Definition

Restrictive pulmonary disease is defined as any condition that interferes with normal lung expansion during inspiration. Typically, it includes disorders that increase the inward elastic recoil of the lungs or chest wall. Consequently, the alteration in pulmonary dynamics results in decreases in lung volumes and capacities and in lung or chest wall compliance. Some restrictive diseases produce ventilation abnormalities and V/Q mismatching, and others lead to impairment of diffusion. FEV_1 and FVC are both decreased owing to a reduction in TLC or a decrease in chest wall compliance or muscle strength. However, the FEV_1/FVC ratio is normal or elevated.

Incidence and Prevalence

Statistics vary according to the acute intrinsic, chronic intrinsic, or chronic extrinsic nature of the restrictive disease.

Pathophysiology

Impairment-producing restrictive pulmonary diseases can be classified as (1) acute intrinsic, (2) chronic intrinsic, or (3) chronic extrinsic. Acute intrinsic disorders are primarily caused by the abnormal movement of intravascular fluid into the interstitium of the lung and alveoli secondary to the increase in pulmonary vascular pressures occurring with left ventricular failure, fluid overload, or an increase in pulmonary capillary permeability. Examples of acute intrinsic disorders include pulmonary edema, aspiration pneumonia, and ARDS. Chronic intrinsic diseases are characterized by pulmonary fibrosis. Conditions that produce fibrosis of the lung include idiopathic pulmonary fibrosis, radiation injury, cytotoxic and noncytotoxic drug exposure, O_2 toxicity, autoimmune diseases, and sarcoidosis. Chronic extrinsic diseases can be defined as disorders that inhibit the normal lung excursion. They include flail chest, pneumothorax, atelectasis, and pleural effusions. They also include conditions that interfere with chest wall expansion, such as ascites, obesity, pregnancy, and skeletal and neuromuscular disorders.

Clinical Manifestations

Clinical manifestations depend on the disorder but may include tachypnea, dyspnea, cough, bronchospasm, pulmonary vascular vasoconstriction, PH, cor pulmonale, and arterial hypoxemia. The pulmonary function tests reveal decreased vital capacity with normal expiratory flow rates.

Treatment

Treatment also depends on the specific restrictive disorder and may include oxygen therapy, bronchodilators, corticosteroids, and mechanical ventilation with PEEP.

Anesthetic Considerations

- Restrictive pulmonary disease does not dictate drug choices for induction and maintenance of general anesthesia.
- Drugs should be selected and administered to avoid postoperative ventilatory depression.
- Regional anesthesia may be acceptable, but sensory levels of blockade above T10 may impair respiratory muscle function.
- Controlled ventilation may maximize oxygenation and ventilation.
- Poorly compliant lungs may require high inspiratory pressures.
- Postoperative mechanical ventilation may be necessary.
- Extubation should be done only when patients clearly meet the criteria.
- Decreased lung volumes may impair cough and interfere with postoperative secretion removal.

L. TUBERCULOSIS

Definition

Tuberculosis is a chronic granulomatous disease that is spread primarily by aerosol transmission.

Incidence and Prevalence

In the past and before specific antimicrobial therapy, tuberculosis was a significant cause of death and disability in North America. It currently affects approximately 28,000 persons in North America. Elderly, debilitated, and malnourished individuals, and people who are immunosuppressed and living in crowded conditions are most often affected.

Pathophysiology

Tuberculosis is caused by the acid-fast bacillus *Mycobacterium tuberculosis*. After being inspired, the bacilli multiply, causing nonspecific pneumonitis.

Some bacilli migrate to the lymph nodes, encounter lymphocytes, and precipitate the immune response. Phagocytes engulf colonies of bacilli in the lung, isolate them, and form granulomatous tubercles. Infected tissues inside the tubercles create caseation necrosis (a cheeselike material). Isolation of the bacilli is completed by formation of scar tissue around the tubercle. After approximately 10 days, the immune response is complete, and further bacilli multiplication is prevented. After isolation of bacilli and development of immunity, tuberculosis can remain dormant for life. Reactivation may occur if live bacilli escape into bronchi or in states of decreased immunity. Patients with laryngeal tuberculosis or lung cavitation have the highest infectivity rate.

Laboratory Results

Diagnosis is made by positive tuberculin skin (purified protein derivative) testing, chest radiography, and positive sputum culture. A positive skin test result alone for tuberculosis may indicate only exposure to the tuberculin bacteria and is not by itself evidence of active disease. Chest radiography findings consistent with tuberculosis in the presence of acquired immune deficiency (AIDS) may be atypical.

Clinical Manifestations

Many patients are asymptomatic. Common manifestations include a low-grade fever, fatigue, weight loss, anorexia, lethargy, and a worsening cough (i.e., purulent sputum). Some patients occasionally develop pleural effusions, meningitis, bone or joint disease, genitourinary abscesses, or peritonitis. Chest pain, dyspnea, and hemoptysis are not common.

Treatment

Drugs of choice for treatment include isoniazid, rifampin, streptomycin, and ethambutol.

Anesthetic Considerations

Patients are placed in respiratory isolation until such time or therapy that they are no longer transmitters of the disease. Whenever possible, disposable equipment (i.e., filters and anesthesia circuits) should be used. Nondisposable equipment must be thoroughly sterilized. Elective surgery should be postponed in actively infected patients until adequate chemotherapy has been administered (usually 3 weeks of treatment) and verified by a negative sputum sample result. The implications of organ dysfunction that may be secondary to the disease or its treatment must be considered. Although the disease most commonly affects the pulmonary system, chemotherapeutic agents used for treatment may lead to organ toxicity (i.e., liver, kidneys, or peripheral nervous system).

Other Conditions

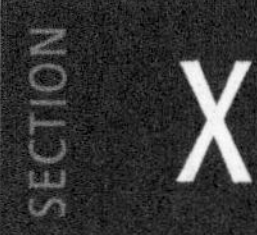

A. ALLERGIC REACTIONS AND HYPERSENSITIVITY

Definition

In some cases, the immune response to antigen is greatly exaggerated, a situation referred to as *hypersensitivity.* Anaphylaxis is a life-threatening response that a sensitized person develops within minutes after administration of a specific antigen. Hypersensitivity reactions are classified as types I, II, III, and IV.

TYPE I HYPERSENSITIVITY PATHOPHYSIOLOGY

Type I hypersensitivity is a rapidly developing reaction that results from antigen–antibody interaction in an individual who has been previously exposed and sensitized to the antigen. The responsible antigen, referred to as an *allergen,* reacts with specific IgE antibodies on tissue mast cells and circulating basophils to trigger mediator release and an allergic response. A key mediator of allergic symptoms is histamine, which is described in the following section. Chemically, allergens are usually proteins, and a multitude of environmental factors, including grass, pollen, dust, mites, molds, and animal dander, can generate type I hypersensitivity reactions.

Histamine

Histamine is a basic amine stored in granules within mast cells and basophils and secreted when allergen interacts with membrane-bound IgE or when complement components C3a and C5a interact with specific membrane receptors. Histamine produces symptoms of allergic reactions by acting on H_1- or H_2-receptors on target cells. The main actions of histamine in humans (via the receptors involved) are:

- Vasodilatation (H_1)
- Vascular permeability (H_1 and possibly H_2)
- Contraction of most smooth muscle other than that of blood vessels (H_1)
- Cardiac stimulation (H_2)
- Stimulation of gastric secretion (H_2)

Histamine causes the cutaneous "triple response," which includes erythema from local vasodilatation, wheal from increased vascular permeability and protein and fluid extravasation, and flare from an "axon" reflex in sensory nerves that releases a peptide mediator. The pathophysiologic effects of histamine can be blocked by H_1 receptor antagonists (diphenhydramine, hydroxyzine, cyclizine, loratadine) and H_2 receptor antagonists (cimetidine, ranitidine, famotidine).

Clinical Manifestations

Allergic reactions present with symptoms such as rhinitis, conjunctivitis, urticaria, pruritus, and possibly anaphylaxis. The term *anaphylaxis* refers to a severe, generalized, immediate hypersensitivity reaction that includes pruritus, urticaria, angioedema (especially laryngeal edema), hypotension, wheezing and bronchospasm, and direct cardiac effects (including arrhythmias). A shocklike state can develop from hypotension secondary to systemic vasodilatation and extravasation of protein and fluid. Clinical manifestations of an allergic reaction can occur in various combinations and usually occur within minutes of exposure to the precipitating antigen(s). In some cases, though, the onset of signs and symptoms may be delayed for 1 hour or longer. Signs and symptoms can be protracted and variably responsive to treatment. Biphasic anaphylaxis can also occur, in which early signs and symptoms clear, either spontaneously or after acute therapy, and symptoms reoccur several or many hours later. Generally, the severity of an anaphylactic event relates to the suddenness of its onset and to the magnitude of the challenge (i.e., the greater the provocative stimulus, the more severe is the reaction). However, anaphylaxis can occur after exposure to minute amounts of allergen in highly sensitive individuals.

Anaphylactoid reactions are caused by mediator release from basophils (but not from mast cells) in response to a non–immunoglobulin E (IgE)-mediated triggering event. Such reactions present with similar clinical manifestations as those with anaphylaxis; however, it has been reported that cutaneous symptoms are more frequent and cardiovascular collapse is less frequent in patients experiencing anaphylactoid reactions versus those experiencing anaphylactic reactions.

Tryptase is a marker for mechanistic delineation of an allergic response. It is an enzyme that is released from mast cells along with histamine and other inflammatory mediators during an allergic response. A significantly elevated tryptase level (>25 mcg/L) strongly suggests an allergic mechanism. The presence of a normal tryptase level, however, does not exclude an immunologic reaction because elevated tryptase levels are not found in almost one-third of anaphylactic cases. Although the diagnosis of anaphylaxis should not rely on a single test, the high positive predictive value of tryptase makes it useful medicolegally and for subsequent patient management.

TYPE II HYPERSENSITIVITY PATHOPHYSIOLOGY

Type II hypersensitivity reactions result when IgG and IgM antibodies bind to antigens on cell surfaces or extracellular tissue components such as basement membrane. The antigen–antibody reaction activates the complement cascade, causing production of C3a and C5a, which attract polymorphonuclear leukocytes and macrophages, and production of the C5b5789 membrane attack complex that inserts into target cell membranes. Examples of type II hypersensitivity reactions include transfusion reactions, autoimmune hemolytic anemia, myasthenia gravis, and Goodpasture's syndrome.

TYPE III HYPERSENSITIVITY PATHOPHYSIOLOGY

Type III hypersensitivity represents immune complex disease in which antigen–antibody complexes deposit in tissues and cause injury. Normally, immune complexes are cleared by the mononuclear phagocyte system shortly after their formation. In some situations, however, immune complexes persist and deposit in tissues. Protracted infections or autoimmune processes can lead to type III reactions. The mechanism of tissue injury is similar to that in type II reactions, involving activation of complement and recruitment of phagocytes. SLE, rheumatoid arthritis, and glomerulonephritis are examples of immune complex diseases.

TYPE IV HYPERSENSITIVITY PATHOPHYSIOLOGY

Type IV hypersensitivity is also referred to as *delayed-type hypersensitivity.* By strict definition, type IV reactions require at least 12 hours after contact with antigen. Migration of antigen-specific $CD4^+$ lymphocytes to the reaction site is followed by cytokine release and a local inflammatory response. Contact hypersensitivity is one form of type IV reaction and occurs where skin has come into contact with antigen. Contact dermatitis and the response to poison ivy are examples of contact hypersensitivity. Another form of type IV hypersensitivity is granulomatous hypersensitivity, in which chronic infection leads to the formation of granulomas in tissues. Granulomatous diseases include tuberculosis, sarcoidosis, and Crohn's disease.

DRUG REACTIONS

Incidence

Predicting who will react adversely to a drug or combination of drugs is difficult. Fortunately, life-threatening adverse reactions to drugs and products used during anesthesia and surgery are very uncommon, with the overall incidence estimated to be one in every 5000 to 10,000 anesthetics.

Pathophysiology

Adverse reactions to anesthetic agents have been found to be two-thirds immune mediated (anaphylactic reactions); the other third was classified as anaphylactoid reactions. Of anesthetic drugs that triggered anaphylactic reactions, neuromuscular blocking agents (NMBAs) do so most frequently. Anaphylactic and anaphylactoid reactions occurred more frequently in female patients, which is thought to be because of chemical epitopes that NMBAs and many cosmetics have in common. This observation may also explain why many patients generate an allergic response to NMBAs on their first exposure to the drug.

Persons who have an increased allergic tendency are termed *atopic* and exhibit a genetic predisposition to such events. Atopic patients frequently present with some history of hay fever, rhinitis, asthma, or food or drug allergy. A generalized history of allergy does not necessarily predispose a patient to anaphylactic or anaphylactoid reactions to anesthetic drugs. If a patient has a history of sensitivity to a particular anesthetic drug, such as a muscle relaxant, that individual may well be at increased risk for allergic responses to other agents in that class.

Anaphylactic reactions to local anesthetics are uncommon; ester local anesthetics are more likely than amide agents to elicit an allergic response. Ester local anesthetic metabolites, such as para-aminobenzoic acid, have been identified to be responsible for this higher incidence of allergic response. Local anesthetic solutions containing methylparaben and propylparaben as preservatives may induce allergic responses in susceptible individuals. Thus, administration of preservative-free local anesthetic solutions may reduce the likelihood of an allergic response. Recent theories suggest that allergies to various antioxidants and certain sulfite components may be responsible for some degree of allergic reactions to local anesthetic preparations.

Avoiding known causal agents (particularly those that induce histamine release), combined with careful selection and application of additional drugs, can reduce risk of adverse reactions. The most common causal agents are antibiotics (cephazolin), NMBAs, latex, opioids, protamine, propofol, and contrast dyes. A thorough history and discussion with the patient or the patient's guardian can usually reveal the potential for untoward drug effects and alert the anesthesia provider to avoid suspicious agents. Patients frequently mistake drug sensitivity or an unpleasant response for an allergy. This is especially true with local anesthetic solutions containing epinephrine or administered with opioids. Careful investigation and cautious interviewing techniques are usually beneficial in clarifying these questionable areas. Reviewing past procedural notes and anesthesia records and possible consultation with an allergist when appropriate can further help in determining situational specifics and facilitate appropriate planning. The administration of H_1- and H_2-receptor antagonists preemptively may prevent allergic reactions in many cases when a known or suspected sensitivity is present.

Treatment

Patients who do not appear to have life-threatening symptoms on initial presentation may nonetheless progress to life-threatening anaphylaxis. Early administration of medications may be beneficial in halting this progression. Standard therapy for non–life-threatening situations includes the following:

1. Epinephrine: The initial adult dose may range from 100 to 500 mcg subcutaneously or intramuscularly. This dose may be repeated every 10 to 15 minutes as needed up to a maximum of 1 mg per total dose. The dose in children is 10 mcg/kg up to a maximum of 500 mcg per total dose. The total dose can be repeated every 15 minutes for two doses and then every 4 hours as needed. Evidence indicates that more rapid systemic absorption and higher peak plasma levels occur after intramuscular administration than after subcutaneous administration.
2. Diphenhydramine: 1 to 2 mg/kg or 25 to 50 mg/dose (parenterally)
3. Steroids may also be administered. However, the efficacy of steroids in treating acute anaphylaxis or in reducing a late anaphylactic reaction has not been clearly established.

Life-threatening anaphylaxis requires immediate administration of epinephrine and may require other immediate measures for support of cardiorespiratory status. Cardiopulmonary resuscitation (CPR) should be instituted if there is loss of circulation or respiration. Oxygen (100%) should be administered and the airway secured. Hypotension should be addressed by administration of vasopressors and infusions of large volumes of intravenous fluids or colloids (or both) to compensate for peripheral vasodilation and intravascular fluid loss. Bronchospasm should be treated with inhaled bronchodilators, theophylline, or both.

Patients experiencing anaphylaxis may not always respond adequately to one injection of epinephrine. Epinephrine has a rapid onset but a short duration of action. At the same time, mediator release from mast cells and basophils may be prolonged, producing biphasic or protracted anaphylaxis. Moreover, patients who are taking β-adrenergic blocking agents may not respond to epinephrine and may require substantial fluid replacement. For patients with life-threatening anaphylaxis who are poorly responsive to initial doses of epinephrine, more frequent or higher doses may be required. If the patient does not respond to subcutaneous epinephrine, intravenous administration of epinephrine must be initiated. Bolus doses of 50 to 100 mcg should be titrated to effect. Epinephrine infusion should initially be administered at 1 mcg/min, which can be increased to 2 to 10 mcg/min. For refractory cardiorespiratory arrest in children, the initial intravenous epinephrine dose is 10 mcg/kg. Subsequent doses of 100 mcg/kg can be administered every 3 to 5 minutes, and if the patient is still refractory, the dose may be increased to 200 mcg/kg.

A good clinical response represents resolution of the allergic reaction. If there is partial resolution or concern about biphasic anaphylaxis, continuous monitoring is suggested. Additional history might reveal previous episodes of anaphylaxis or asthma. Antihistamines may be useful in the treatment of anaphylaxis, particularly for symptoms of urticaria and angioedema. An H_1 receptor antagonist, alone or in combination with an H_2 receptor antagonist, may be useful in reversing hypotension refractory to epinephrine and intravascular fluid replacement. Steroids, such as 200 mg of intravenous hydrocortisone, may reduce the risk of recurring or protracted anaphylaxis, although direct clinical evidence for this has not been clearly established.

TRANSFUSION REACTIONS

Incidence

Because of advances in technological capabilities and quality-control practices, blood transfusion reactions are, fortunately, not a common occurrence. Whereas the relative risk of an allergic transfusion reaction of mild severity (urticaria and pruritus) is approximately one in 500, a fatal hemolytic reaction occurs in approximately one in 250,000 to 600,000 transfusions administered nationally.

Pathophysiology

The mechanism responsible for most transfusion reactions involves ABO incompatibility. Transfusion of incompatible blood type causes recipient antibodies to react with donor red blood cells, causing their destruction and the potential for significant consequences. Disseminated intravascular coagulation, renal failure, and death are not uncommon after this type of reaction. Because the most common cause for a major hemolytic transfusion reaction is human error, it should never be assumed that another person is solely responsible for checking blood that one is preparing to administer to a patient.

Transfusion reactions are frequently masked, or at least delayed appreciably, during anesthesia. Hallmark symptoms of cardiovascular instability, such as hypotension, as well as fever, hemoglobinuria, and bleeding diathesis are indicative of a transfusion incompatibility and should be immediately treated.

Transfusion-related acute lung injury (TRALI) is the leading cause of transfusion-related morbidity and mortality. Recipient risk factors include higher interleukin-8 levels, liver surgery, chronic alcohol abuse, shock, higher peak airway pressure while being mechanically ventilated, current smoking, and positive fluid balance. Transfusion risk factors were recipient of plasma or whole blood from female donors, volume of human leukocyte antigens (HLA) class II antibody with normalized background ratio (NBG) greater than 27.5, and volume of anti-human neutropil antigens (HNA).

LATEX ALLERGY

Allergies to latex-containing products continue to be a source of significant problems for specific populations. Health care workers and certain patients, particularly those with congenital neural tube defects and those who have undergone multiple surgical procedures, have shown particular sensitivity to latex-containing products.

It has been estimated that approximately 0.8% of the general population has some form of sensitivity to latex. Atopic persons who react with skin dermatitis and who are allergic to certain fruits (particularly kiwi and bananas) should be further evaluated for latex allergy. Health care workers and patients who experience frequent exposure to devices and products that contain latex also exhibit such allergic reactions. The incidence of health care worker allergy to latex-containing products ranges between 8% and 25%. The most frequent clinical manifestations of latex reactions include some form of contact dermatitis, type I hypersensitivity reaction with the potential for anaphylaxis, or type IV hypersensitivity reaction.

Preventive procedures and recommended protocols have been established for the management of latex allergies that can have significant anaphylactic consequences. The incidence of latex allergies has increased proportionately with the 10-fold increase in medical glove usage to accommodate universal precautions and barrier protection during anesthesia, surgery, and obstetric care. Using gloves that do not contain latex (e.g., gloves processed from polyvinyl or neoprene) can prevent this source of latex exposure. Although skin prick, patch testing, and radioallergosorbent tests for latex allergy are available, all present various challenges in qualifying a conclusive diagnosis.

B. GERIATRICS

Definition

Geriatrics is the branch of medicine that deals with the physiologic effects of aging and the diagnosis and treatment of persons who are 65 years of age or older. By 2030, it has been estimated that approximately one in five people in the United States will be older than 65 years of age. Persons reaching age 65 years have an average life expectancy of an additional 18.4 years (19.8 years for women and 16.8 years for men).

Pathophysiology

Human organ function shows a linear decline with age. The rate constant for this decline is slightly less than 1% per year of the functional capacity present at age 30 years. As a consequence, a 70-year-old geriatric patient may have a 40% decrease in the function of any specific organ compared with that present at the age of 30 years.

Clinical Manifestations

Clinical manifestations include an increased prevalence of age-related concomitant disease (hypertension, renal disease, atherosclerosis, myocardial infarction, chronic obstructive pulmonary disease, cardiomegaly, diabetes, liver disease, congestive heart failure, angina, cerebrovascular accident). The commonly age-related anatomic and physiologic changes that occur are listed in the box on pg. 225.

Anesthetic Considerations

The choice of anesthetic technique should be based on the changes in organ system function in the patient, the pharmacokinetic and pharmacodynamic effects anticipated, the surgical requirements, and the needs and

Common Age-Related Anatomic and Physiologic Changes

General Changes
- Decreased organ function
- Increased body fat
- Decreased blood volume
- Loss of protective reflexes
- Decreased ability to retain body heat
- Decreased lean body mass
- Decreased skin elasticity
- Collagen loss
- Decreased intracellular water

Cardiovascular Changes
- Impaired pump function
- Prolonged circulation time
- Myocardial fiber atrophy
- Hypertension
- Depressed baroreceptor function
- Impaired cardiac adrenergic receptor quality
- Increased vagal tone
- Decreased sensitivity of adrenergic receptors
- Increased peripheral vascular resistance
- Decreased cardiac output
- Decreased organ perfusion
- Left ventricular hypertrophy
- Coronary artery disease

Pulmonary Changes
- Increased lung compliance
- Decreased forced expiratory volume
- Increased closing volume
- Increased incidence of dysrhythmias
- Decreased resting arterial oxygen tension
- Increased alveolar-arterial difference
- Ventilation/perfusion mismatch
- Decreased functional residual capacity
- Decreased total lung capacity

Central Nervous System Changes
- Decreased activity
- Decreased oxygen consumption
- Reduced number of functioning receptors
- Reduced production of neurotransmitters
- Neuronal loss
- Decreased cerebral blood flow

Renal Changes
- Decreased renal blood flow
- Decreased urine concentrating ability
- Decreased ability to conserve water
- Decreased elimination of drugs
- Decreased glomerular filtration rate

Hepatobiliary Changes
- Decreased hepatic blood flow
- Decreased plasma drug clearance

Endocrine Changes
- Decreased pancreatic function
- Increased incidence of diabetes
- Decreased tolerance to glucose load

predisposition of the patient. As a rule, geriatric patients are likely to be predisposed to hypotension as a result of reduced activity of the sympathetic nervous system and decreased intravascular volume. Decreased cardiac output and delayed drug clearance are likely to prolong the onset of drug effects and the duration of action (see the table below).

Age-Related Changes and Pharmacokinetics

Change	Effect
Contracted vascular volume	High initial plasma concentration
Decreased protein binding	Increased availability of free drug
Increased total body lipid storage sites	Prolonged action of lipid-soluble drugs
Decreased renal and hepatic blood flow	Prolonged action of drugs dependent on kidney and liver elimination

Regional, general, and monitored anesthesia care techniques are appropriate selections for geriatric patients. Each technique has its corresponding cadre of supporters. No conclusive study has demonstrated the superiority of any one specific anesthetic technique. With regional and local techniques, maintenance of consciousness during the surgical procedure may be associated with less confusion during the postoperative period. However, general anesthesia with endotracheal intubation may be advantageous for promoting bronchopulmonary toilet and facilitating surgical conditions. A progressive decrease in the reactivity of protective airway reflexes, such as coughing and swallowing, can be expected with age. Because elderly patients often are edentulous, a sealed fit with the anesthetic face mask may be difficult. These factors may increase the likelihood of regurgitation of gastric contents, with aspiration of vomitus into the lungs. The changes that accompany cervical arthritis and osteoarthritis, limiting extension and flexion of the neck, often make endotracheal intubation difficult.

It appears likely that the patient's preoperative health status and events during the course of the anesthetic that precipitate such physiologic changes as hypotension, hypoxia, hypercarbia, and hypertension do more to affect patient outcome than does anesthetic technique.

Great care must be taken to prevent trauma to the skin and bony prominences when geriatric patients are positioned for surgery on the operating table. Collagen loss and decreased elasticity of tissue make the skin more sensitive to damage from tape, monitoring devices, and contact with hard table surfaces. Additionally, any invasive procedure, including insertion of intravenous, spinal, and epidural catheters, should be accomplished with the goal of protecting the integrity of the skin.

Postoperative Implications

Postoperative complications in the elderly population are often related to cardiac and pulmonary dysfunction and decreased reserves. Monitoring with a pulse oximeter may permit detection of the need for supplemental oxygenation or ventilation during the postoperative period because ventilation–perfusion mismatch is common in geriatric patients. Elderly patients may be especially prone to regurgitation and aspiration from a reduction in airway reflexes. In addition, renal and hepatic dysfunction may prolong the duration of action of pharmacologic agents administered to the patient.

Elderly patients are also prone to postoperative heat loss. To encourage rewarming and prevent problems associated with shivering, the patient should be placed in a warmed environment. Geriatric patients may require special assistance in being oriented to time and place. Prolonged anesthetic effect may compound disorientation to an unfamiliar environment.

Postoperative delirium (PD) and cognitive dysfunction are higher in the elderly population. Postoperative delirium is a transient and fluctuating disturbance of consciousness that occurs shortly after surgery. Postoperative cognitive dysfunction is a more persistent change in cognitive performance diagnosed by neuropsychological tests.

Postoperative delirium in elderly adults leads to increased morbidity, delayed functional recovery, prolonged hospital stay, nursing home placement, and mortality. PD tends to occur between postoperative days 1 and 3 and usually resolves anywhere from hours to days. PD symptoms may persist for weeks to months. Patients at risk for PD are listed in the following box. Sedative–hypnotics, narcotics, benzodiazepines, and anticholinergics have been identified as the classes of drugs associated with PD. Protocols have been developed with effective interventions to decrease PD. Haloperidol has been successfully utilized in the treatment of immediate agitation. Benzodiazepines tend to worsen agitation unless the cause of delirium has been identified as alcohol withdrawal.

Surgical Patients at Risk for Postoperative Delirium

Age 70 years or older
History of delirium
History of alcohol abuse
Preoperative use of narcotic analgesics
Preoperative depression

C. GLAUCOMA OR OPEN GLOBE

Definition and Etiology

In glaucoma, intraocular pressure (IOP) is increased, resulting in impaired capillary flow to the optic nerve. If the condition is left untreated, loss of sight may result.

Pathophysiology

Types of Glaucoma

- Open-angle glaucoma: This is characterized by elevated IOP with an anatomically open anterior chamber. Sclerosed trabecular tissue impairs aqueous filtration and drainage. As treatment, miosis and trabecular stretching should be produced medically (eyedrops, epinephrine, timolol).
- Closed-angle glaucoma: The peripheral iris moves in direct contact with the posterior corneal surface, mechanically obstructing aqueous flow. This is caused by a narrow angle between the iris and posterior cornea and produces swelling of the crystalline lens.
- Congenital glaucoma is associated with some eye diseases (retinopathy of prematurity, aniridia, mesodermal dysgenesis syndrome). Surgical goniotomy or trabeculotomy should be performed to route aqueous flow into Schlemm canal. Cyclocryotherapy decreases aqueous formation by destroying the ciliary body by freezing tissue with a probe.

Open Globe

This condition usually follows traumatic injury.

Clinical Manifestations

The clinical manifestations of acute glaucoma are a dilated, irregular pupil and pain in and around the eye.

Diagnostic and Laboratory Findings

Normal IOP is 10 to 25 mmHg; abnormal elevated IOP is greater than 25 mmHg. Pressure becomes atmospheric when the globe is opened. Any sudden rise in IOP at this time may lead to prolapse of the iris and lens, extrusion of the vitreous humor, and loss of vision. Coagulation studies should be evaluated before retrobulbar block is instituted.

Treatment

Intraocular pressure is increased by the following: external pressure on the eye, including venous congestion associated with coughing, vomiting, or the prone position; scleral rigidity, which is increased in elderly persons; and changes in the intraocular structure or fluids. Pilocarpine hydrochloride decreases resistance to improve drainage of aqueous humor. Acetazolamide reduces the rate at which aqueous humor is formed.

Anesthetic Considerations

Drug therapy should be continued to maintain miosis. Anticholinergic drugs are acceptable in preoperative medication. Increases of IOP, hypercarbia, and central venous pressure should be avoided. Succinylcholine causes transient increases in IOP. Rapid-sequence induction generally is acceptable for patients with open globe and a full stomach. Awake intubations are not desirable because they may contribute to increases in IOP. Techniques and drugs associated with decreasing IOP include volatile anesthetics, intravenous anesthetics, hypocarbia, hypothermia, mannitol, glycerin, nondepolarizing muscle relaxants, and timolol. General anesthesia or retrobulbar blocks are acceptable for eye surgery. General anesthesia is typically used for open globe repair.

Drug interactions also must be considered. Echothiophate prolongs the effect of succinylcholine. Timolol may result in bradycardia. Etomidate may induce myoclonus.

Anesthetic Goals for Ophthalmic Surgery

The goals for ophthalmic surgery are akinesia, profound analgesia, minimal bleeding, avoidance of the oculocardiac reflex, control of IOP, awareness of drug interactions, and smooth induction and emergence without vomiting or coughing or bucking. If succinylcholine is necessary, a defasciculating dose of nondepolarizing agent will decrease muscle fasciculations and may not dramatically increase IOP.

D. MALNUTRITION

Definition

Malnutrition, or nutritional failure, is associated with protein depletion in the presence of adequate calories or with combined protein-calorie deficiency. Protein-calorie depletion is a frequent finding in surgical patients and in critically ill individuals.

Incidence and Prevalence

Critically ill patients experience negative caloric intake because of the hypermetabolic state produced by their illness. Trauma, fever, sepsis, and wound healing result in a drastically increased metabolism.

Pathophysiology

Basic energy requirements are an intake of 1500 to 2000 calories/day. An increase in body temperature of 1° C increases daily caloric requirements by 15%. Multiple fractures increase energy needs by 25%. Major burns cause the greatest increase in energy requirements: 100%. In addition, patients with large tumors may also have greatly increased energy requirements.

Clinical Manifestations

Protein depletion affects the protein content of all organs. The liver and the gastrointestinal tract are rapidly depleted; the brain is affected less than other organs. If protein depletion is severe, the gastrointestinal system will be unable to tolerate or digest food because protein is needed to produce digestive enzymes. Skeletal muscle is most affected and may lose as much as 70% of its protein. Patients with malnutrition are at increased risk of infections and complications in the postoperative period.

Diagnostic and Laboratory Findings

The lack of a specific test for protein-calorie malnutrition often makes diagnosis difficult. The best single index of malnutrition is evidence of weight loss from the patient's normal level of weight. Plasma albumin levels lower than 3 g/dL and transferrin levels less than 200 mg/dL have also been used to diagnose malnutrition. Nitrogen balance, which requires the careful collection of all drainage and excretions over 24 hours, may be used to evaluate nutritional status. Nitrogen balance provides an estimate of net protein degradation or synthesis.

Treatment

The steps in planning a nutritional regimen are first to identify the need for intervention, then to determine the route of delivery, and finally to adjust the amounts of macronutrients and micronutrients the patient requires.

Anesthetic Considerations

Enteral and parenteral are the two routes of choice. At times, these two routes are combined. Enteral supplements can be sipped or administered through a nasogastric feeding tube or gastrostomy tube. If the gastrointestinal tract is nonfunctional, intravenous (parenteral) nutrition is instituted. Isotonic solutions can be delivered through peripheral veins. However, if the solution is hypertonic because of a greater caloric need, a central line should be used.

Patients receiving exogenous nutritional support are prone to deficits or an overabundance of certain electrolytes. Careful evaluation of laboratory values preoperatively as well as of any function tests performed is imperative. Parenteral nutrition has the greatest potential for complications. Hypoglycemia and hyperglycemia are common. Increased carbon dioxide resulting from metabolism of large amounts of glucose may hinder early extubation postoperatively. Patients with compromised cardiac function are at risk of congestive heart failure related to fluid overload. Electrolyte abnormalities include hypokalemia, hypomagnesemia, hypocalcemia, and hypophosphatemia. If parenteral nutrition is continued intraoperatively, infusions of other fluids should be minimized. Malnutrition is a clinical finding that must be partially corrected preoperatively. Therapy must be maintained.

E. OBESITY

Definition

Obesity is a complex multifactorial chronic disease that develops from an interaction of genotype and the environment. Overweight is defined as a body mass index (BMI) of 25 to 29 kg/m^2 and obesity as a BMI of 30 kg/m^2, as shown in the table on pg. 230.

BMI can be calculated by:

$$\text{BMI} + \text{weight (kilograms)/height (meters)}^2$$

$$\text{BMI} + (\text{weight (pounds)/height (inches)}^2) \times 703$$

Classification of Overweight and Obesity by Body Mass Index

	Obesity Class	Body Mass Index (kg/m^2)	Risk of Disease
Underweight	–	<18.5	Increased
Normal	–	18.5–24.9	Normal
Overweight	–	25–29.9	Increased
Obese	I	30–34.9	High
	II	35–39.9	Very high
Extremely obese	III	>40	Extremely high
Super obese		>50	Extremely high
Super-super obese		>60	Extremely high

Data from National Institute of Health. *Clinical Guidelines on the Identification, Evaluation, and Treatment of Overweight and Obesity in Adults: the Evidence Report.* NIH publication no. 98-4083. Washington, DC: National Institutes of Health; September 1998; Klein S, Romijn J. Obesity. In Larsen PR, et al. *Williams Textbook of Endocrinology*. 10th ed. Philadelphia: Saunders; 2003: 1619-1641; Flier JS. Obesity. In Braunwald E, Fauci AS, Kasper DL, et al, eds. *Harrison's Principles of Internal Medicine.* 15th ed. New York: McGraw-Hill; 2001:479-486; Brodsky JB, Lemmens HJ. Is the super-obese patient different? *Obes Surg* 2004;14(10):1428.

Incidence and Prevalence

Obesity is a disease that affects more than one-third of the adult U.S. population. It is the second leading cause of preventable death in the United States. Current estimates are that 65% of adults in the United States are classified as overweight or obese and more than 30% of adults are classified as obese; this means the prevalence of obesity has doubled over the past 20 years. There are an estimated 23 million persons in the United States with a BMI of no less than 35 kg/m^2 and 8 million with a BMI of 40 kg/m^2 or higher. Obesity in children and adolescents has also increased significantly since the mid-1990s. In the United States, 30% of this population is overweight, and 15% is obese.

Pathophysiology

Genetic predisposition, believed to be a primary factor in the development of obesity, explains only 40% of the variance in body mass. The significant increase in the prevalence of obesity has resulted from environmental factors that increase food intake and reduce physical activity. Other factors such as socialization, age, sex, race, and economic status affect its progression. In the United States, food consumption has risen as a result of the supersizing of portions and the availability of fast food and snacks with high fat content. Physical activity has been reduced as a result of modernization (television and computers), a sedentary lifestyle, and work activities. Cultural and lifestyle variations play an important role in the development of obesity.

Clinical Manifestations

Manifestations include increased cardiac output, blood volume, oxygen consumption, minute ventilation, work of breathing, and carbon dioxide production, as listed in the following box. Obesity is associated with an increase in the incidence of more than 30 medical conditions. The risk of cardiovascular disease, certain cancers, diabetes, and disease overall is linearly related to weight gain. Type 2 diabetes, coronary heart disease, hypertension, and hypercholesterolemia are prominent conditions in overweight and obese patients. With increasing weight gain and increased adiposity, glucose tolerance deteriorates, blood pressure rises, and the lipid profile becomes more atherogenic. Hormonal and nonhormonal mechanisms contribute to the greater risk of breast, gastrointestinal, endometrial, and renal cell cancers. Psychological health risks often stem from social ostracism, discrimination, and an impaired ability to participate fully in activities of daily living. The physiologic changes associated with obesity are listed in the following box.

Physiologic Changes Occurring with Obesity

Cardiovascular Changes
- Increased cardiac output
- Increased blood volume
- Hypertension
- Pulmonary hypertension
- Ventricular hypertrophy
- Congestive heart failure

Metabolic Changes
- Increased metabolic rate
- Diabetes mellitus due to insulin resistance

Respiratory Changes
- Increased oxygen consumption
- Increased carbon dioxide production
- Increased work of breathing
- Increased minute ventilation
- Decreased chest wall compliance
- Decreased lung volumes (including functional residual capacity), restrictive pattern
- Arterial hypoxemia
- Obstructive sleep apnea
- Obesity hypoventilation syndrome

Gastrointestinal Changes
- Fatty liver infiltration
- Elevated intraabdominal pressure (gastroesophageal reflux disease, hiatal hernia)
- Increased gastric volume
- Increased gastric acidity

Other Changes
- Osteoarthritis

Diagnostic and Laboratory Findings

Findings include hypercholesterolemia, hypertriglyceridemia, and altered pulmonary function test results. Baseline arterial blood gases, chest radiography, electrocardiography, and echocardiography are used for diagnosis.

Treatment

A multimodal approach in the treatment of obesity includes dietary intervention, increased exercise, behavior modification, drug therapy, and surgery. Weight loss programs are individualized to each patient based on the degree of obesity and coexisting conditions. Drug therapy is initiated in patients with a BMI greater than 30 kg/m^2 or a BMI between 27 and 29.9 kg/m^2 with a coexisting medical condition. Medications that promote weight loss have limited efficacy. Despite the enormous potential market, efforts to develop effective drug therapies have been disappointing. The U.S. Food and Drug Administration's guidance for long-term weight loss drugs recommends that a 5% weight reduction be maintained for 12 months after treatment initiation. Two drugs are available for use: orlistat (Xenical and Alli) and phentermine (Adipex-P, others). When used in combination with a comprehensive weight loss program, they can occasionally be effective in producing weight loss in the range of 4 to 5.5 kg.

Orlistat is a lipase inhibitor that decreases the absorption of fat in the gastrointestinal tract. It has recently been released as an over-the-counter medication. Side effects are minor and most related to gastrointestinal discomfort. Phentermine, a sympathomimetic agent, is approved for short term use (up to 12 weeks) as a weight loss management drug. Tolerance, dependence, abuse, and a relatively high number of side effects limit its usefulness. Several antidepressants, antiepileptic, and antidiabetic drugs may promote weight loss and are used off label for this indication.

Surgical approaches designed to treat obesity can be classified as malabsorptive or restrictive. Malabsorptive procedures, which include jejunoileal bypass and biliopancreatic bypass, are rarely used at the present time. Restrictive procedures include the vertical banded gastroplasty (VBG) and gastric banding, including adjustable gastric banding (AGB). Roux-en-Y gastric bypass (RYGB) combines gastric restriction with a minimal degree of malabsorption. VBG, AGB, and RYGB can all be performed laparoscopically. RYGB, the most commonly performed bariatric procedure in the United States, involves anastomosing the proximal gastric pouch to a segment of the proximal jejunum and bypassing most of the stomach and the entire duodenum. It is the most effective bariatric procedure to produce short- and long-term weight loss in severely obese patients. Advances in laparoscopic surgery have significantly improved surgical procedure times, morbidity, and mortality related to bariatric surgery.

Pharmacologic Considerations

Obesity is associated with significant alterations in body composition and function that can alter the pharmacodynamics and pharmacokinetics of drugs. Alterations in the volume of distribution are related to the size of the fat organ, increased blood volume, increased cardiac output, increased total body weight, and alterations in protein binding and lipophilicity of the drug. Highly lipophilic drugs have an increased volume of distribution in obese persons compared with persons of normal weight. The increased volume of distribution requires higher doses of lipophilic drugs to produce the required pharmacologic effect and prolongs the elimination of certain drugs such as benzodiazepines. Factors such as protein binding and end-organ clearance affect volume of distribution.

There is no relationship for some highly lipophilic drugs (digoxin, remifentanil, and procainamide) between their solubility and distribution in obese patients. Dosing by ideal body weight is appropriate for these drugs. Drugs with weak or moderate lipophilicity are usually dosed based on ideal body weight or lean body mass. Recommendations for dosing commonly used anesthetics are listed in the table on pg. 233.

Elimination of drugs in obese individuals is normal or increased in phase I reactions (oxidation, reduction, and hydrolysis) and increased in phase II reactions (metabolism). Renal clearance is increased by the augmented renal blood flow and glomerular filtration rate.

Anesthetic Considerations

No demonstrable difference in emergence from inhalation versus narcotic technique has been discerned in obese patients. The use of short-acting water-soluble anesthetics facilitates smooth anesthetic induction, maintenance, and emergence from anesthesia. Objectives for maintenance of anesthesia in obese patients include strict maintenance of airway, adequate

Dosing Guidelines for Intravenous Anesthetics

Anesthetic Agent	Dosing	Guidelines
Midazolam (Versed)	TBW	Increased central Vd; increase initial dose to achieve therapeutic effect; prolonged sedation
Thiopental	TBW	Increased V_d; increase initial dose; prolonged time to awakening
Propofol	TBW: Initial and infusion	Increased V_d; increase initial dose; high affinity for fat; high hepatic extraction
Fentanyl	TBW	Increased V_d; increased elimination half-life
Sufentanil	TBW	Increased V_d; increased elimination half-life
Remifentanil	IBW	Consider age and lean body mass
Cisatracurium	TBW	No difference than those with normal weight
Vecuronium	IBW	Increased V_d; impaired hepatic clearance; prolonged duration of action
Rocuronium	IBW	Faster onset and similar duration of action
Succinylcholine	TBW	Increased plasma pseudocholinesterase activity; increase dose

IBW, Ideal body weight; *TBW*, total body weight; V_d, volume of distribution.

skeletal muscle relaxation, optimum oxygenation, avoidance of the residual effects of muscle relaxants, provision of appropriate intraoperative and postoperative tidal volume, and effective postoperative analgesia. Depending on the patient's condition, these can be achieved by either general or regional anesthesia regimens. An epidural anesthetic with concomitant "light" general anesthesia is frequently chosen. A light general anesthetic can facilitate management of the airway, ventilation, and the patient's level of consciousness, and the epidural anesthetic provides surgical analgesia and anesthesia. Combining these techniques accomplishes all of the objectives. The epidural catheter can be used for postoperative analgesic administration. This enhances earlier resumption of deep-breathing and coughing maneuvers.

Airway Evaluation

A thorough airway evaluation is warranted to determine the optimal airway management technique in overweight and obese patients. Most practitioners use evaluation of multiple patient physical characteristics to identify potential airway problems indicative of the unanticipated difficult airway. These include measurement of interincisor distance, thyromental distance, head and neck extension, Mallampati classification, body weight, and a history of difficult airway. Evaluation of the length of upper incisors, visibility of the uvula, shape of the palate, compliance of the mandibular space, and length and thickness of the neck provides further assessment. Increasing neck circumference and the Mallampati classification higher than grade III have been identified as the two most important factors in morbidly obese patients.

Anatomic aberrations of the upper airway induced by severe obesity include reduced temporomandibular and atlanto-occipital joint movement. Unsatisfactory mouth opening, presence of neck or arm pain, or inability to place the head and neck into "sniffing position" may indicate the need for awake fiberoptic intubation. Extreme airway narrowing, in conjunction with shortened mandibular–hyoid distance (less than three fingerbreadths), can complicate mask ventilation and intubation. Presence of a short, thick neck; pendulous breasts; hypertrophied tonsils and adenoids; and beards can contribute to a difficult ventilation or intubation. Marginal room air pulse oximeter saturations, abnormal arterial blood gas results, and previous history of complicated airway management also indicate a potentially difficult intubation, which occurs in at least 13% of severely obese patients.

Aspiration Prophylaxis

Of significance to the airway in anesthetized obese patients is the increased risk of regurgitation (passive and active) and subsequent pulmonary aspiration. Obese persons have greater volumes and more acidic gastric fluid than persons of normal weight. Gastroesophageal reflux and hiatus hernia, which are more prevalent in obese patients, also predispose them to esophagitis and pulmonary aspiration. Other conditions that cause delayed gastric emptying, such as diabetes mellitus or traumatic injury, further increase the risk of aspiration. For these reasons, obese patients are considered to have a "full stomach" even if the prescribed nothing-by-mouth intake restriction has been followed. Debate and controversy exist as to the relative risk of aspiration in obesity; most practitioners use techniques to attenuate this complication.

Timely preinduction administration of histamine-2 receptor and dopamine receptor antagonists coupled with oral administration of nonparticulate antacids decreases morbidity resulting from pulmonary aspiration and Mendelson syndrome. Head-up positioning of the patient, with application of the Sellick maneuver during rapid sequence induction, limits the volume of vomitus that enters the trachea if regurgitation occurs. Nasogastric or orogastric suctioning before emergence further reduces the amount of fluid available for aspiration.

Intubation

The obese patient should be positioned with the head elevated (reverse Trendelenburg position) on the operating room table. This position facilitates patient comfort, reduces gastric reflux, provides easier mask ventilation, improves respiratory mechanics, and helps to maintain functional residual capacity. The reduced functional residual capacity in obese patients contributes to the rapid desaturation that occurs with induction of general anesthesia. To attenuate the desaturation and to maximize oxygen content in the lungs, patients are preoxygenated with 100% mask oxygen for at least 3 to 5 minutes. The patient's head, neck, and shoulders should be carefully moved into "sniffing position" by using pillows, "doughnuts," or foam head supports.

Some practitioners advocate the use of an "awake look" to visualize the difficulty of the airway. Careful administration of sedative drugs, application of topical anesthesia to the oropharyngeal structures, and transtracheal and superior laryngeal nerve blocks are performed. Nasal oxygen is used as a supplement during awake laryngoscopy. If epiglottic and laryngeal architecture is easily visualized, successful asleep intubation can be done. If the airway structures cannot be visualized, airway management using a glidescope, intubating laryngeal mask airway, or awake fiberoptic intubation should be performed. The surgeon and another skilled anesthesia provider must also be in attendance during the induction. Muscle hypotonus in the floor of the mouth followed by rapid occurrence of soft tissue obstruction and hypoxia requires one person to support the mask and airway while another person bag ventilates the patient.

Volume Replacement

The normal adult percentage of total body water is 60% to 65%. In a severely obese patient, it is reduced to 40%. Therefore, calculation of estimated blood volume should be 45 to 55 mL/kg actual body weight rather than the 70 mL/kg apportioned to a nonobese adult. Use of reduced parameters for volume replacement and avoidance of rapid rehydration lessen cardiopulmonary compromise. Fluid management is guided by blood pressure, heart rate, and urine output measurements. Volume expanders, such as hetastarch (Hespan), should not be administered at greater than recommended volumes per kilogram of ideal body weight (20 mL/kg). Dilutional coagulopathy, factor VIII inhibition, and decreased platelet aggregability can result from excessive administration. Albumin 5% and 25% should be used as indicated to support circulatory volume and oncotic pressure. When replacing blood loss with crystalloid, the 3:1 ratio (3 mL of crystalloid to 1 mL of blood loss) is applicable to severely obese patients.

Intraoperative Positioning

Surgical positioning of morbidly obese patients necessitates extra precautions to prevent nerve, integumentary, and cardiorespiratory compromise. The type of surgery, combined with inordinate stretching or compression of nerve plexus, and prolonged immobility cause local tissue ischemia and damage that begins at the cellular level. Hypothermia, hypotension, table positioning, and the hydraulic pressure effect that the adipose patient places on orthopedic or cardiopulmonary structures potentiate impairment.

Regional Anesthesia

Regional anesthesia can be used as the primary anesthetic technique in selected cases or as an accompaniment to postoperative pain and mobility management. Difficulties are frequently encountered, however, in severely obese patients. Anatomic landmarks used to guide conduction blockade are not easily visualized or palpable.

Extubation

The risk of airway obstruction after extubation is increased in obese patients. A decision to extubate depends on evaluation of the ease of mask ventilation and tracheal intubation; length and type of surgery; and presence of preexisting medical conditions, including obstructive sleep apnea. Criteria for extubation include an awake patient; tidal volume and respiratory rate at preoperative levels; sustained head lift or leg lift for at least 5 seconds; strong, constant hand grip; effective cough; adequate vital capacity of at least 15 mL/kg; and inspiratory force of at least 25 to 30 cm H_2O negative. Patients must be placed with their heads up or in a sitting position. If doubt exists about the ability of the patient to breathe adequately, the endotracheal tube is left in place. Extubation over an airway exchange catheter or through a fiberoptic bronchoscope may be performed.

F. SCLERODERMA

Definition

Widespread, symmetric lesions that cause induration of the skin and are followed by atrophy and pigmentation changes characterize scleroderma. It is a systemic disease that affects muscles, bones, the heart, and the lungs. Intestinal and pulmonary changes also occur. Lung volumes, vital capacity, compliance, and dead space all decrease. The respiratory rate increases, and diffusion capacity is impaired. Pulmonary hypertension can occur.

Anesthetic Considerations

Tightening of the skin around the neck may limit mobility and mouth opening. Alternate methods to secure the airway (e.g., fiberoptic intubation) should be considered. Baseline pulmonary function tests and arterial blood gases may assist in optimizing these patients preoperatively, intraoperatively, and postoperatively. Postoperative ventilatory assistance may be needed. Be alert for vasospastic phenomena after induction of anesthesia; these should be treated with a plasma expander. Regional anesthesia is acceptable. Core temperature must be maintained. Gastrointestinal pretreatment (e.g., histamine blockers, metoclopramide) may be necessary because of poor gastric emptying.

G. SYSTEMIC LUPUS ERYTHEMATOSUS

Definition

Systemic lupus erythematosus (SLE) is a chronic inflammatory disorder of connective tissues that affects multiple organ systems with periods of remissions and exacerbations.

Incidence and Prevalence

Systemic lupus erythematosus occurs eight to 15 times more often in women than in men and affects approximately 75 in 1,000,000 persons every year. It occurs most often in Asians and in African Americans. Exacerbations are more common in spring and summer and during stresses such as infection, pregnancy, and surgery.

Pathophysiology

The origin of SLE is unknown. One theory is that it is an antibody–antigen autoimmune response. Another theory deals with predisposing factors that promote susceptibility to SLE. These factors include stressors such as infection, exposure to ultraviolet light, immunizations, and pregnancy. A third theory suggests that drugs such as procainamide, hydralazine, penicillin, anticonvulsants, oral contraceptives, and sulfa drugs may trigger SLE.

Clinical Manifestations

Clinical manifestations of SLE include arthritis of the upper and lower extremities as well as avascular necrosis of the femur. Systemically, SLE affects major organ systems (heart, lungs, kidneys, liver, neuromuscular system, skin). Pericarditis, myocarditis, tachycardia, arrhythmias, and congestive heart failure may develop. Left ventricular dysfunction and endocarditis have also been associated with SLE. About 50% of patients with SLE develop such cardiopulmonary abnormalities. Pneumonia, pleural effusions, cough, dyspnea, and hypoxemia are common. Glomerulonephritis and oliguric renal failure may result. Some patients develop lupoid hepatitis, which may be fatal. They may also incur intestinal ischemia. The neuromuscular system may be affected by myopathies. Psychological changes include schizophrenia and deterioration of the intellect. The skin may exhibit the typical lesion associated with SLE; this "butterfly rash" appears over the nose and is erythematous. Alopecia may also be seen clinically.

Diagnostic and Laboratory Findings

Complete blood count with differential may reveal anemia, a decreased white blood cell count, and a decreased platelet count. Specific tests for SLE include antinuclear antibodies, anti-DNA, and lupus erythematosus cell tests; urine analysis may reveal both red and white blood cells. Chest radiography may reveal pulmonary involvement, and electrocardiography may show conduction abnormalities.

Treatment

The usual treatment of SLE includes anti-inflammatory therapy with aspirin. Corticosteroids are often used to suppress adverse renal and cardiovascular system changes. For patients who do not respond well to steroids, immunosuppressive agents may be used. Antimalarial drugs, in small doses, have been found to be effective in treating arthritis and skin lesions.

Anesthetic Considerations

Anesthesia management is based on medications used to treat the disorder as well as the organ involvement. Care must be taken in positioning the patient to avoid hyperextension of the neck. These patients may be difficult to intubate because of their inflammatory changes, and they frequently have restrictive lung disease and therefore may be difficult to ventilate. Rapid rates with smaller tidal volumes may be helpful. Overall, a thorough preoperative evaluation should be performed to establish organ system involvement.

Cutaneous lesions on the nose and mouth may make mask fit difficult. Cricoarytenoid arthritis rarely occurs. Patients with advanced disease may be debilitated, and chest radiography findings, complete blood cell count, and electrolytes should be checked. Anemia and thrombocytopenic purpura have been identified. The partial thromboplastin time may be falsely elevated because antibodies of SLE react with phospholipids used to determine partial thromboplastin time. If renal dysfunction is advanced, drugs dependent on renal elimination should be avoided. If the patient is currently receiving steroids or has taken them within 6 months, a steroid bolus should be used.

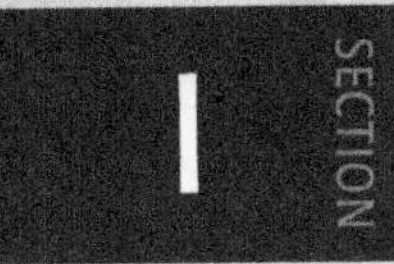

SECTION I Cardiovascular System

A. ABLATION PROCEDURES

MAZE and Mini-MAZE Procedures

The MAZE procedure is offered to patients at high risk for stroke who have unsuccessful attempts at pharmacologic treatment. It is an "open-heart" cardiac surgery procedure intended to eliminate atrial fibrillation (AF). The name refers to the series of incisions arranged in a mazelike pattern in the atria. The Cox MAZE III procedure is now considered to be the "gold standard" for effective surgical cure of AF. It may be performed concomitant with mitral valve repair or replacement for patients who also have mitral valve disease. MAZE is performed using pulmonary vein isolation and a number of incisions in the right and left atria. These incisions or cryoablations ultimately form scar tissue, thereby mechanically interrupting transmission of triggering impulses of AF. For open MAZE, it is necessary for the patient to have a sternotomy and cardiopulmonary bypass (CPB). All of the monitoring and medication necessary for CPB is required for the MAZE procedure. In addition to the lesions made in the atria, the left atrial appendage is often removed because it is thought to be a culprit in the stasis of blood flow, thereby increasing the possibility of thrombus formation and stroke. The term *mini-MAZE* is still sometimes used to describe an open-heart procedure requiring CPB, but it more commonly refers to minimally invasive epicardial procedures not requiring CPB.

The mini-MAZE procedure is performed using thoracoscopy on a beating heart. "Keyhole" incisions are used for the mini-MAZE, and the patient is placed in the lateral position. Routine monitoring with the addition of an arterial line and one-lung ventilation are adjuncts of this procedure.

Pulmonary Vein Isolation and Catheter Ablation for Persistent Atrial Fibrillation

Surgical management of rate-related cardiac rhythm anomalies has historically been provided by catheter ablation of the offending right atrial conduction pathways. For conditions such as Wolff-Parkinson-White syndrome, right atrial flutter, and supraventricular tachycardia, catheter ablation to permanently block impulses has been performed by groin catheterization similar to cardiac angiography. Until recently, AF has not been addressed in this manner.

Research on the contributing triggers for AF has illuminated the possibility that pulmonary vein isolation and ablation of offending fibers is an alternative when chemical means fail. Catheter ablation for AF has been performed with patients under general anesthesia. The procedure involves groin catheterization, continuing with a catheter puncture across the atrial septal wall and advancement of the catheter into the left atrium. A lesion is created with the catheter tip and using a specified energy. The lesion then prevents transmission of offending impulses that trigger the AF.

General anesthesia management includes an endotracheal tube, an arterial line, and resuscitative drugs. Hemodynamic instability, including multiple arrhythmias and blood pressure swings, may occur during this procedure. These are often short lived and resolve spontaneously without any intervention or with very little intervention on the part of the anesthesia provider.

B. AUTOMATIC INTERNAL CARDIOVERTER DEFIBRILLATOR

Definition

Automatic implantable cardioverter defibrillators are surgically implanted to prevent sudden cardiac death from malignant ventricular tachyarrhythmias. These are self-contained diagnostic devices that continuously monitor the patient's heart rate and electrocardiographic activity. They sense potentially lethal ventricular arrhythmias and treat them with electrical discharges. Whereas pacemakers use low-energy impulses measured in microjoules, these defibrillators release an electrical discharge of approximately 30 J after sensing periods of fibrillation lasting approximately 20 seconds. Most devices now can be programmed to reconfirm ventricular tachycardia or ventricular fibrillation after charging to prevent inappropriate shock therapy.

Indications

Patients considered for implantation are those who have had minimal success with standard antiarrhythmic drug therapy. The majority of patients have severe coronary artery disease with reduced left ventricular (LV) function, ischemic cardiomyopathy, or idiopathic cardiomyopathy.

Anesthetic Technique

1. Anesthetic management is best handled with monitored anesthesia care, but a brief period of general anesthesia might be used during defibrillator testing and programming of the device.
2. Prolonged periods of asystole are at times encountered and can cause cerebral and myocardial ischemia.
3. Vasoactive drugs are helpful for blood pressure stabilization.
4. If ventricular tachycardia occurs before clinical induction, lidocaine treatment should be avoided because it may result in the inability to induce ventricular tachycardia on demand during testing.
5. Standard monitoring should include electrocardiography (ECG) leads II and V_5 and an arterial line for continuous blood pressure assessment.
6. Intravenous (IV) sedation or general anesthesia may be used for these patients. Because of the stress associated with testing and the amount of sedation necessary for the procedure, some practitioners advocate that general anesthesia with a controlled airway is the best choice.

C. SURGERY FOR CORONARY ARTERY DISEASE

Coronary artery disease is the predominant cause of death in patients in the fourth and fifth decades of life and the most common cause of *premature* death in men ages 35 to 45 years. Annually, approximately 1.5 million individuals endure some level of myocardial insult. The most recent data show that more than 1,285,000 inpatient angioplasty procedures, 427,000 inpatient bypass procedures, 1,471,000 inpatient diagnostic cardiac catheterizations, 68,000 inpatient implantable defibrillators, and 170,000 inpatient pacemaker procedures are performed in the United States each year.

Coronary artery disease alters coronary blood flow, decreases coronary reserve, and increases the incidence of coronary artery vasospasm. Risk factors associated with the progression of coronary artery disease include age, gender, genetic predisposition, obesity, hyperlipidemia, hypertension, stress, diabetes mellitus, and smoking. Exacerbating the effects of coronary artery disease are combinations of peripheral vascular disease, carotid disease, and a compromised pulmonary system.

Patients with atherosclerotic coronary disease become symptomatic when 75% of the coronary vessel is occluded, resulting in a decrease in coronary blood flow. Ischemia depresses myocardial function and causes severe chest pain referred to as *angina pectoris*. In addition to pain, cells are subject to increased irritability and become increasingly vulnerable to fibrillation, alterations in the conduction pathways, and thrombus formation.

Anesthesic Technique

The goals of anesthetic management for coronary revascularization are directed toward producing analgesia, amnesia, and muscle relaxation; abolishing autonomic reflexes; maintaining physiologic homeostasis; and providing myocardial and cerebral protection. The avenues available to accomplish these goals include an effective preoperative evaluation, administration of modest doses of sedation and pain medication before any attempt at line placement is made; and use of O_2 in the preoperative setting. Administration of a balanced anesthetic with opioid, inhalation agents, sedative–hypnotics, and muscle relaxant provides a stable hemodynamic state for the difficult cardiovascular patient. The inhalation agents offer the additional advantage of anesthetic preconditioning, which is cardioprotective.

Preoperative Assessment

A thorough preoperative assessment of the patient should include a comprehensive review of systems, airway status, and laboratory data; physical examination; review of surgical history; and review of current medications. Actual reports of diagnostic procedures such as cardiac catheterization, echocardiography, and Doppler studies should be reviewed by the anesthesia provider.

Hemodynamic Status

Evaluation of cardiovascular status includes a discussion with the patient regarding his or her functional status.

Cardiac catheterization may be used for diagnostic assessment, electrophysiologic evaluation, or direct intervention for patients in cardiogenic shock. The catheterization evaluation provides information about pressures and oxygen saturations of the four chambers of the heart, pulmonary artery (PA) pressure, systemic pressure, body surface area, cardiac index (CI) ($L/min/m^2$), stroke index ($mL/beat/m^2$), LV fraction (EF), degree of stenosis in coronary vessels, and coronary dominance. The normal values are listed in the table on pg. 241.

Normal Intracardiac Pressures

	Notation	Range (mmHg)
Central venous pressure	CVP	0–8
Right atrial pressure	RAP	0–8
Right ventricular end-systolic pressure	RVESP	15–25
Right ventricular end-diastolic pressure	RVEDP	0–8
Pulmonary artery pressure (systolic)	PAP systolic	15–25
Pulmonary artery pressure (diastolic)	PAP diastolic	8–15
Pulmonary artery pressure (mean)	PAP	10–20
Pulmonary capillary wedge pressure; pulmonary artery occlusion pressure	PCWP; PAOP	6–12

An EF of 50% or greater in a patient with normal valve function is acceptable. If the patient has mitral regurgitation, an EF of 50% to 55% is considered to indicate LV dysfunction. An EF of less than 50% reflects a moderate reduction of ventricular function. Poor cardiac function relates to an EF below 30% and may stem from ventricular hypokinesis, akinesis, or dyskinesis.

Echocardiography is used to evaluate ventricular function by measuring wall motion during systole. It can permit a qualitative and quantitative assessment and reflects the four types of abnormal wall functions described previously.

Single-photon emission computed tomography (SPECT) is another diagnostic tool used in the preparation of patients for cardiac surgery. It is a noninvasive procedure that makes use of a radionuclide tracer to provide a three-dimensional picture of heart structures and function. It is capable of producing a measurement of rate and volume of blood flow, size and location of blockages or narrowing of vessels, and more accurate diagnosis of heart disease in women.

Laboratory Data

Laboratory examinations for patients with ischemic heart disease involving two or more associated risk factors (diabetes, obesity, family history, and smoking) should include a complete blood count; electrolytes; cardiac enzymes (including enzyme fraction for creatinine phosphokinase), serum creatinine, cholesterol; and coagulation screening profile.

Coagulation function studies are used to monitor patients receiving heparin therapy and warfarin products. Platelet inhibitors are often part of the drug regimens of patients who need cardiac surgery. These agents are associated with the risk of excess bleeding. However, no evidence suggests that surgery is contraindicated in this situation. It is recommended that 24 to 48 hours elapse before surgery is performed after these drugs are discontinued. The platelet inhibitors (glucoprotein IIb/IIIa receptor inhibitors) in use at this time include abciximab (ReoPro), eptifibatide (Integrilin), and tirofiban (Aggrastat). It should be emphasized that long-term heparin therapy results in prolonged bleeding times and may affect calculations of loading doses of heparin required for CPB. Other issues related to the cause and treatment of adverse bleeding are discussed later in this chapter.

Long-Term Use of Medications

Prevention of rebound hypertension and reduction of perioperative hemodynamic stress are primary considerations for continuation of antihypertensive therapy until the morning of surgery. Potential drug interactions with anesthetic agents should be anticipated and evaluated, and treatment should proceed accordingly.

Calcium channel blockers are used widely to control hypertension, angina, and arrhythmias in patients with cardiovascular disease. Their continued use up to the day of surgery is a common practice and provides the advantage of controlling dysrhythmias and preventing coronary spasm. Potential hazards associated with continued therapy include a reduction in patient responses to inotropes and vasopressors and atrioventricular (AV) conduction problems.

β-Adrenergic receptor–blocking agents play an important role in the therapy of cardiovascular patients and must be continued up to and during the preinduction period. β-Blockers allow for reduction in myocardial oxygen consumption by providing an overall decrease in sympathetic stimulation and catecholamine release. Because the heart rate is slowed, diastolic filling is improved. These drugs are helpful in controlling anginal symptoms, hypertension, tachycardia, and myocardial ischemia. Bronchospasm and decreased inotropic response to β stimulants in conjunction with greater vasoconstriction in response to sympathomimetics are potential disadvantages to continuation of β-blockade up to the time of surgery.

Digitalis therapy may be continued until the morning of surgery if it is used to treat rapid ventricular response to AF or flutter; otherwise, it may be discontinued because other inotropes with greater efficacy may be given preoperatively if needed. If potassium is used, its effects must be carefully monitored.

It is recommended that antidysrhythmics be continued until the day of surgery except for disopyramide, encainide, and flecainide, which should be discontinued except in the presence of the most life-threatening dysrhythmias. These agents have been associated with increased mortality, and postbypass myocardial infarction has been noted with their continuance. Disopyramide has been noted to cause difficulty in termination of CPB.

Antidepressants provide no advantage if continued up to the day of surgery and may interact negatively with sympathomimetics. However, as noted previously, it is important to give sedation and anxiolysis to these patients during the preoperative phase.

Anesthetic Technique

Electrocardiography and Noninvasive Blood Pressure

Leads II and V_5 can help in the diagnosis of dysrhythmias, ischemia, conduction defects, and electrolyte disturbances. None of the standard leads can detect posterior wall ischemia. The noninvasive blood pressure cuff must be placed on the same side as the arterial line to allow for correlation of blood pressure.

Radial Arterial Line

Sternal retraction may play a role in distorting the radial artery waveform. The right radial artery is usually selected in cases in which the left internal mammary artery is dissected for anastomosis and because radial arterial line monitoring may show a false low number because of compression of the left subclavian artery at the retractor. The brachial artery is contraindicated because it is an end artery of the arm.

Other Arterial Line Sites

Use of the brachial artery for monitoring is most commonly dismissed because it provides the bulk of circulation for the lower arm and is considered an end artery. The femoral artery is superficial and offers access to the central arterial tree. It also provides appropriate access if intraaortic balloon pump (IABP) placement is necessary. However, if the femoral artery is used, it should be noted that an alternative site may become necessary if use of IABP is instituted.

1. **Central venous pressure (CVP):** Use of the right internal jugular (IJ) vein is recommended because cannulation of the left IJ vein increases the risk of laceration of the left brachiocephalic vein. CVP lines may be used for monitoring, to provide a central line for fluid and drugs, and in situations in which a PA catheter is not used.
2. **PA catheter:** The PA catheter was historically used for all coronary artery bypass graft (CABG) procedures, but it is associated with complications and now has a more narrow range of uses. It is indicated for use in high-risk patients with an EF of less than 40%.
3. **Transesophageal echocardiography (TEE):** TEE allows continuous monitoring of the chambers of the heart, ascending and descending aorta, valvular function, chamber filling, and wall contractility and motion. Detection of gaseous or particulate emboli, identification of intracardiac shunting, diagnosis of aortic dissection, evaluation of saphenous vein graft flow, and confirmation of LV dimension (filling) during weaning are other potential applications for this monitoring method. TEE may predict or suggest myocardial ischemia as defined by regional wall motion abnormalities, valve replacement procedures, cardiac aneurysms, intracardiac tumors, aortic dissection, and repair of complex congenital lesions. Relative contraindications to the use of TEE include dysphagia, mediastinal radiation, upper gastrointestinal surgery or bleeding, esophageal stricture, tumor, varices, and recent chest trauma. In conjunction with the increased use of TEE, certain complications have been reported to occur during open-heart surgery. Cardiac arrhythmias, bronchospasm, and esophageal laceration are rare. The common cardiac formulas are listed in the table on pg. 244.
4. **Monitoring core temperature:** Accurate monitoring of core temperature is essential to control target hypothermia as well as to reestablish normothermia. The most accurate indicator of core temperature is at the thermistor of the PA catheter. Brain temperature is reflected in nasopharyngeal measurement, but a lag time occurs on rewarming. The probe should be inserted before heparinization to a depth of 7 to 10 cm through the nares. Tympanic temperature may also lag behind brain rewarmed temperature and is no better for monitoring of this parameter. Bladder or rectal temperature measurement is today considered inaccurate when renal and splanchnic blood flow is decreased. Brain temperature should not drop below 20° C because profound hypothermia (15° to 20° C) appears to cause a loss of cerebral autoregulation.
5. **Cerebral monitoring:** In addition to the monitoring of brain temperature, electrophysiologic monitoring is often used. Electroencephalography (EEG) is not an effective method for monitoring subtle changes, but any

Cardiac Formulas

Parameter	Notation	Formula	Normal Range
Stroke volume	SV	SV = CO ÷ HR	60–90 mL/beat
Stroke index	SI	SI = SV ÷ BSA	40–60 mL/beat/m^2
Cardiac output	CO	CO = SV × HR	5–6 L/min
Cardiac index	CI	CI = CO ÷ BSA	2.5–4 L/min/m^2
Mean arterial pressure	MAP	MAP = diastolic pressure + one third pulse pressure	80–120 mm Hg
Systemic vascular resistance	SVR	SVR = (MAP − CVP) ÷ (CO × 80)	700–1400 dyne/sec/cm^5
Pulmonary vascular resistance	PVR	PVR = (PAP − PCWP) ÷ (CO × 80)	50–300 dyne/sec/cm^5
Left ventricular stroke work index	LVSWI	LVSWI = 0.0136 × (MAP − PCWP) × SI	40–60 g × m/beat/m^2
Coronary perfusion pressure	CPP	CPP = DIA BP − LVEDP	mmHg
Ejection fraction	EF	EF = (EDV − ESV) ÷ EDV	55%–70%
Rate-pressure product	RPP	RPP = SYS BP × rate	>15,000
Triple index	TI	TI = SYS BP × rate × PCWP	>180,000

BSA, Body surface area; *CVP,* cardioventricular pacing; *DIA BP,* diastolic blood pressure; *EDV,* end-diastolic volume; *ESV,* end-systolic volume; *HR,* heart rate; *LVEDP,* left ventricular end-diastolic pressure; *PAP,* peak airway pressure; *PCWP,* pulmonary capillary wedge pressure; *SI,* stroke index; *SYS BP,* systolic blood pressure.

asymmetric EEG activity is considered a problem. Bispectral analysis monitoring *may* correlate with the depth of anesthesia; it is actually a derived parameter to assess the degree of wakefulness.

Perfusion Principles

The goal of CPB is to provide a motionless heart in a bloodless field while the vital organs continue to be adequately oxygenated. The CPB pump provides respiration (oxygenation and elimination of CO_2), circulation (maintenance of perfusion pressure), and regulation of temperature (hypothermia to preserve myocardium). Initiation of CPB subjects the circulating blood of the patient to significant physiologic and physical changes.

Anesthetic and perfusion management must address the impact of low flow indices, reduced metabolic requirements, changing viscosity of the patient's circulating volume, and postoperative inflammatory response. Multiple factors interact to create a substantially new environment for physiologic homeostasis.

Hemodynamic abnormalities that occur during CPB include endothelial dysfunction ("total body systemic inflammatory response"), which causes symptoms similar to those in patients with sepsis or trauma. Other abnormalities include persistent heparin effect, platelet dysfunction or loss, coagulopathy, fibrinolysis, and hypothermia.

Rapid recirculation of the total blood volume during CPB subjects blood and tissue components to a foreign environment that invites cellular trauma. The patient experiences tremendous alterations in core temperature, hematocrit (in the form of hemodilution), the coagulation cascade, and perfusion pressures (nonpulsatile perfusion).

As a result of excessive hemodilution, the platelet count decreases rapidly to 50% of the preoperative level but usually remains above 100,000 per microliter. Bleeding time is greatly prolonged, and platelet aggregation and function are impaired. Reductions occur in the plasma concentrations of coagulation factors II, V, VII, IX, X, and XII and are attributed to hemodilution.

Extracorporeal Circuit

The CPB (pump) circuit consists of separate disposable components bioengineered to interface with perfusion pumps, fluid-based thermoregulating systems, air-oxygen blenders, anesthetic vaporizers, pressure transducers, temperature monitors, and in-line oxygen and blood-gas analyzers. The pump components include venous cannulas from the right atrium or vena cava, which are usually fenestrated at the tip and reinforced. Venous tubing includes the venous return for the blood drained to the machine from the LV.

The venous drainage to the venous reservoir depends on gravity, patient intravascular volume, and the position of and resistance from the venous cannula. The table height can affect venous drainage to the pump. Drainage collects in the venous reservoir, where air bubbles are removed and drainage from other reservoirs is mixed together. If a low volume is allowed here, air can be entrained into the arterial circulation.

Blood suctioned from the heart, pericardium, and pleural spaces drains to the cardiotomy reservoir. The CPB circuit pushes blood forward and returns blood under pressure to the patient by means of either rollers (most common) or a centrifugal (vortex) pump.

Prime

A significant factor is the amount of crystalloid solution required to prime the tubing, reservoir, filters, and oxygenator. Establishment of an air-free circuit is essential for unimpaired fluid volume transport and prevention of air embolism.

Most circuits require at least 2000 mL of a solution such as Normosol, Plasmalyte A, or Isolyte S, with pH and electrolytes closely matching the composition of whole blood. Added to this base solution are heparin, sodium bicarbonate, mannitol, hetastarch, albumin, and possibly corticosteroids or antihyperfibrinolytic agents. This addition can result in priming volumes in excess of 2000 mL, which, when transfused to the patient at the onset of CPB, can cause a hemodilutional bolus of 30% to 50% of the patient's circulating blood volume.

Vascular Transport

The heart and lungs are isolated and bypassed from systemic blood flow. This function is accomplished by right atrial or vena caval cannulation with subsequent diversion of venous blood that is returning to the heart.

The venoatrial cannulas are connected to polyvinyl chloride tubing that extends from the surgical field to the venous reservoir situated at a level well below the patient's heart to facilitate gravity exsanguination.

Blood from the reservoir is propelled by roller or centrifugal pump to the oxygenator, where it becomes arterialized by interfacing with a membrane oxygenator.

A heat exchanger mounted on the oxygenator provides for control of blood temperature. Oxygenated blood passes through an arterial filter and an in-line arterial gas monitoring device.

Aortic cannula placement is distal to the sinus of Valsalva and proximal to the brachiocephalic (innominate) artery. The arterial line pressure of the extracorporeal circulation (ECC) depends on flow and resistance but usually is maintained below 300 mmHg.

Myocardial Protection Techniques

Injury to the myocardium is a complex occurrence and may result from numerous physiologic events. Tachycardia, hypertension or hypotension, and ventricular distention can all play a role in the events that produce an oxygen supply–demand imbalance.

Contractile function deteriorates rapidly after the initial insult of ischemia. Rapid cardioplegia-induced cardiac arrest, decompression of the ventricles, and hypothermia are the underlying techniques used to ensure myocardial protection during CPB.

The duration of aortic cross-clamping time, collateral coronary blood supply, frequency of cardioplegia delivery, and composition of cardioplegia are factors that influence the extent of reperfusion injury. Intermittent doses of cold crystalloid cardioplegia help to maintain cardiac arrest, hypothermia, and pH; counteract edema; wash out metabolite; and provide oxygen and substrate for aerobic metabolism.

Administration of inhalation anesthetics has been shown to produce protection against myocardial ischemia and reperfusion injury. This phenomenon is termed *anesthetic-induced preconditioning* (APC) and derives from positive effects on mitochondria, potassium adenosine triphosphate channels, reactive oxygen species, calcium overload, and inflammation. APC reduces myocardial necrosis and improves postoperative cardiac performance.

Cardioplegia

Cardioplegia is a potassium solution administered into the coronary circulation to provide diastolic arrest. It is composed of potassium (15–30 mEq/L), calcium to prevent ischemic contracture (stone heart), albumin or mannitol for osmolarity correction, and glucose or simple amino acids as a metabolic substrate.

The cardioplegia delivers oxygen and nutrients, removes waste products, and cools or rewarms the heart. It is administered in an antegrade manner into the aortic root, from which it distributes to the coronaries and into the myocardium. It may also be administered in a retrograde fashion into the coronary sinus, from which it distributes through veins, venules, and capillaries of the myocardium.

The cardioplegia composition is blood or crystalloid based. Blood-based cardioplegia is oxygenated blood that is diluted with fluid at a 4:1 ratio. It has a hematocrit of 16% to 18% and is given at 4° to 14° C.

Crystalloid-based solutions do not contain hemoglobin; therefore, they deliver dissolved O_2 only. Because of this, crystalloid solutions can be used only with myocardial hypothermic techniques. Intracellular cardioplegia has a low sodium content to produce loss of membrane potential by eliminating the sodium gradient across the membrane.

Extracellular solutions produce diastolic arrest by depolarization of the membrane with high potassium concentrations.

Anticoagulation

Initiation of CPB requires systemic heparinization to establish a safe level of anticoagulation. The currently accepted regimen is 300 units of heparin per kilogram of patient weight.

The heparin dose is usually calculated to maintain an activated clotting time (ACT) of 400 sec (the normal range is 130 sec or less).

Heparin is administered IV through the central venous port. Its peak effect occurs within 2 minutes, and verification is based on the ACT, which should be established 5 to 10 minutes after administration.

Special circumstances such as long-term heparinization, antithrombin III deficiency, heparin-induced thrombocytopenia (HIT), and excessive hemodilution may cause "heparin resistance," which alters the algorithm for calculating the loading dose.

Management of a patient with heparin-associated thrombocytopenia and thrombosis (HATT) presents a particular challenge. HIT is evident after exposure to heparin because the platelet count suddenly falls. The onset can be as soon as 2 days or as long as 5 days after institution of heparin therapy. Surgery should be postponed if at all possible, and heparin must be eliminated from the patient's medication regimen until the platelets are normal and do not aggregate in response to heparin. A polysulfated glycosaminoglycan (danaparoid) as well as a thrombin inhibitor (hirudin) have been used safely for CPB.

Prophylaxis and Treatment of Coagulopathy

Antifibrinolytics

Patients for CABG procedures on CPB receive an antifibrinolytic. First-time patients are treated with aminocaproic acid.

Aminocaproic Acid and Tranexamic Acid

Aminocaproic acid (Amicar) was initially proposed for the treatment of fibrinolysis associated with prostate and cardiac surgery. Tranexamic acid is considered to be more potent than aminocaproic acid. Antifibrinolytics are hemostatic agents given as an IV loading dose and then by continuous infusion before CPB.

The loading dose of aminocaproic acid is 100 to 150 mg/kg followed by an infusion dose of 10 to 15 mg/kg/hr. The dose of tranexamic acid is 10 to 15 mg/kg loading with an infusion of 1 to 1.5 mg/kg/hr. The drug has renal excretion and a plasma half-life of approximately 80 minutes. These drugs have proven effective in reducing bleeding after bypass.

Desmopressin

Desmopressin acetate (DDAVP) is a synthetic analog of vasopressin, which releases a variety of hemostatically active substances from the vascular endothelium. It is administered in doses of 0.3 mcg/kg intravenously, intranasally, or subcutaneously.

It has a half-life of 55 minutes (with clinical effects lasting from 5 to 6 hours) and results in an approximately fourfold increase in circulating levels of factor VIII, prostacyclin, tissue plasminogen activator, and von Willebrand factor.

The overall effect of desmopressin is hemostatic. DDAVP has also been used to treat uremia, cirrhosis, platelet disorders, and mild or moderate cases of hemophilia A (von Willebrand disease). Current evidence does not support the broad administration of DDAVP to cardiac surgical patients as prophylaxis for bleeding.

Pharmacologic Approaches to Blood Pressure Control

Blood pressure control during the perioperative phase may be accomplished with the use of pharmacologic agents independently or in combination. Vasodilators such as hydralazine, nitroglycerin, and nitroprusside are useful for control of blood pressure and improving peripheral blood flow.

α-Adrenergic agonists (e.g., clonidine) reduce stress-mediated neurohumoral responses to induction and CPB. They decrease heart rate and blood pressure and have sedative and antinociceptive characteristics, which may reduce opioid requirements without respiratory depression. They can be used independently or in conjunction with IV induction agents and opioids; they help to reduce the amount of agent required.

Careful use of β-blockers can decrease heart rate, contractility, and blood pressure, which works to reduce oxygen use. These drugs increase the duration of diastole to allow for a more complete oxygenation of the LV. They act synergistically with nitroglycerin and blunt tachycardia and decrease ischemia of the myocardium. They have the ability to reduce catecholamine-induced ventricular arrhythmias. The disadvantage associated with β-blockers is that they may precipitate bradyarrhythmias, heart block, or bronchospasm. β-Blockers available in IV form for use during cardiac surgery include esmolol, labetalol, metoprolol, and propranolol. Reversal of the effects of β-blockers can be achieved through use of β-agonists (isoproterenol) and cardiac pacing (unless emergent CPB initiation is possible).

Vasodilator therapy includes direct vasodilators (hydralazine, nitroglycerin, or nitroprusside), α-adrenergic blockers (labetalol, phentolamine), angiotensin-converting enzyme inhibitors (enalaprilat IV), central α-agonists (clonidine), or calcium channel blockers (nicardipine IV, verapamil, or diltiazem). Disadvantages include a slow onset of action or long duration of action, reflex tachycardias, and toxicity reactions. The drug therapy is to be selected individually for each patient and situation and administered judiciously for the desired effect.

Vasopressor therapy includes agents with selective direct effects (methoxamine, phenylephrine), α_1-agonist mixed agents (dopamine, ephedrine, epinephrine, noradrenaline), or vasopressin (direct peripheral vasoconstriction with no β-adrenergic effects).

Other drugs that work indirectly to increase blood pressure include the positive inotropic drugs (e.g., dobutamine, dopamine, and milrinone). Calcium reverses hypotension associated with the use of halogenated agents, calcium channel blockers, hypocalcemia, β-blockers, and CPB. When administered intravenously by central line, it can increase blood pressure as well as reverse the cardiac effects of toxicity resulting from hyperkalemia.

Preoperative Period

Considerations during the preoperative period include sedation and monitoring of the patient while placement of appropriate invasive monitoring lines ensues.

All equipment should be available and invasive lines inserted before the patient is brought to the operating room.

Invasive monitors are useful during induction and should be placed before induction except in emergency situations such as ruptured aneurysms, cardiac tamponade, or ventricle rupture.

Induction

Hemodynamic alterations occur at induction of anesthesia. The induction plan should take into consideration LV function. No single technique has been demonstrated as superior with regard to the prevention of postoperative myocardial infarction by intraoperative ischemia. It is important to control heart rate because this parameter is most likely to produce myocardial ischemia.

On induction, myocardial ischemia can be detected through the ECG, TEE, or PA wedge pressure readings.

Intraoperative events that are known to precipitate ischemia are listed in the following box.

Perioperative Events That May Elicit Ischemia

- Coronary spasm
- Endotracheal intubation
- Sympathetic stimulation
- Sternal split
- Light anesthesia
- Cannulation
- Initiation of bypass
- Incomplete revascularization
- Tachycardia
- Atherosclerotic plaque
- Hypertension
- Air or particulate thrombus formation
- Manipulation of heart
- Fibrillation

Methods for diminishing the incidence of ischemia include therapeutic interventions such as preoxygenation before induction, reduction of wall tension with nitroglycerin, control of heart rate with β-adrenergic blocking agents, reduction of the work of the myocardium through control of myocardial depression with increased anesthetic levels, and maintenance of coronary perfusion pressure through the use of a nonchronotropic agent such as phenylephrine.

Many cardiac patients have low circulating blood volume because of hypertensive vasoconstriction. A reduced plasma volume may necessitate fluid loading or prophylactic treatment with pressors such as phenylephrine before induction. Hypovolemia should be anticipated and can be monitored by observation of blood pressure alterations and CVP.

High or low cardiac output (CO) has a significant effect on the pharmacokinetics of anesthetic agents. The anesthetic ideally should not interfere with heart rate or metabolic demand for oxygen. Patients with disease of the left main coronary artery are more susceptible to insult during induction. Hemodynamic changes in these patients precipitate extension of already present ischemic effects.

A slow, methodic, balanced technique with combinations of midazolam, fentanyl or sufentanil, etomidate, thiopental, or propofol and a nondepolarizing muscle relaxant reduces hemodynamic changes and meets the goals of diminishing workload on the myocardium. The common opioid doses for maintenance during CPB are listed in the box on pg. 250.

Intraoperative Period

Incision to Bypass

After induction, the skin incision and sternal split constitute two very stimulating steps in the process of preparation for CPB.

A patient in whom anesthesia is adequate will show minimal response to these steps, thereby reducing the need for additional adjuncts. A continuous opioid infusion with "background" volatile agent or continuous infusion of propofol may help to maintain blood pressure and ensure amnesia as well as provide a smooth transition toward CPB.

Common Opioid Doses for Maintenance During Cardiopulmonary Bypass

	Loading Dose	Infusion Rate	Additional Bolus
Sufentanil	0.5–2 mcg/kg	0.5–1.5 mcg/kg/hr	2.5–10 mcg
Fentanyl	4–20 mcg/kg	2–10 mcg/kg/hr	25–100 mcg
Remifentanil	1–2 mcg/kg	0.1–1 mcg/kg/min	0.1–1 mcg/kg

During sternotomy, for approximately 15 to 20 seconds, the lungs must be deflated to prevent laceration or puncture. In most cases, the left internal mammary artery is dissected and mobilized for anastomosis to the left anterior descending artery. This requires placement of an internal mammary artery retractor on the left side of the operating table. When there is a left radial arterial line, careful attention to positioning of the wrist ensures that the arterial waveform is not damped. When only saphenous vein grafts are to be harvested, the pace of the operation may increase significantly, and cannulation of the aorta and right atrium may occur earlier.

Once the internal mammary and saphenous grafts are mobilized or harvested, the patient requires heparinization before cannulation of the aorta and right atrium. Bolus administration of heparin is administered in a central line and may decrease arterial pressure 10% to 20%. Anticoagulation is measured with ACT approximately 3 to 5 minutes after heparin administration. The ACT should be approximately 400 seconds before it is safe to institute CPB. The following box is a checklist for CPB.

Checklist for "Going on Pump"

- Heparin administered
- ACT checked and at least 350 to 400 seconds
- Muscle relaxant adequate (or infusion turned on to maintain)
- Inotropic infusions turned off
- Pupil symmetry assessed for later comparison (unilateral dilation may indicate unilateral carotid perfusion on cardiopulmonary bypass)
- PA catheter (if used) pulled back 5 cm
- Urinary output emptied before bypass (start anew with initiation of bypass)
- Proper functioning of all monitors ensured

Aortic cannulation is associated with a hypertensive response, probably because of direct stimulation of sympathetic nerves in the aortic arch. Reduction of mean arterial pressure (MAP) assists aortic cannulation and prevents laceration of the aorta. As a result of manipulation of the heart during cannula placement, venous cannulation (right atrium) may lead to fluctuations in arterial pressure. Right atrial cannulation drains the superior and inferior venae cavae; ventricular tachyarrhythmias may occur, and CO and blood pressure may decrease. If additional cannulation of the coronary sinus for retrograde cardioplegia delivery is required, severe hypotension may ensue and necessitate administration of volume by the perfusionist via the aortic cannula.

After the patient has been placed on extracorporeal support and adequate perfusion flow and pressure have been achieved, most surgeons prefer to stop ventilation to deflate the lungs and optimize surgical conditions. Some surgeons prefer to continue ventilation until the myocardium is motionless. CPB should not commence unless all of the parameters for institution of bypass have been addressed by the anesthesia provider.

Initiation of Bypass

Multiple events occur simultaneously and can cause a significant drop in blood pressure at the initiation of CPB. Hemodilution decreases blood viscosity and dilutes catecholamines in the plasma, contributing to the drop in pressure. Rapid cooling of the patient occurs to a target temperature of 28° C. When the target temperature is reached or spontaneous hypothermic fibrillation of the heart occurs, the aorta is cross-clamped. At times, the myocardial arrest may require retrograde administration of cardioplegia via the coronary sinus.

Cerebral and renal protection is important during CPB. Techniques for cerebral protection include metabolic suppression, which can be accomplished with hypothermia, burst suppression, use of calcium channel blockers to reduce the incidence of vasospasm, and decrease in intraoperative bleeding attained through use of antifibrinolytics. The perfusionist also plays a central role in providing cerebral protection. As core temperature is lowered, the pH rises, placing the patient in an alkalotic state. The alpha-stat system represents alkalotic management of cerebral perfusion, but pH-stat relies on hypercarbia to manage CBF. The essential difference is that alpha-stat management represents CBF that is not dependent on MAP and does not mandate the addition of exogenous CO_2 to maintain pH in the normal range.

Renal protection is best maintained by the preservation of renal blood flow and monitoring of urine production. Risk factors for renal dysfunction after CPB include prolonged bypass time (>3 hours) and low CO. Osmotic diuretics, low-dose dopamine, and fenoldopam are used during CPB in patients at risk for development of acute renal failure. Prevention of renal insufficiency postoperatively includes control of hypertension, control of hyperglycemia, reduction of "pump" time, maintenance of fluids, and the use of medications that promote urinary output. Urinary output is considered satisfactory if it measures 1 mL/kg/hr during CPB.

Bypass

During cardiac bypass, anesthesia is maintained with an opioid drip as well as the addition of volatile agent on the perfusion circuit.

Controversy exists regarding an acceptable mean blood pressure range during CPB. Keep in mind that CBF is autoregulated, as is flow to other organs. Because of hypothermia, the lower limit of autoregulation is further decreased. This fact, coupled with the presence of high perfusion pressures, can result in an increase in the possibility of emboli and bleeding on the surgical field; the use of 50 to 70 mmHg is promoted as a practical norm in most facilities.

ACT is checked every 20 to 30 minutes by the perfusionist and is maintained at greater than 400 seconds with the addition of heparin to the pump as necessary. Because of hemodilution, the hematocrit frequently falls to approximately 20 g/dL, which is an acceptable level in most patients. Hypokalemia can be problematic, and the perfusionist checks electrolytes frequently during the pump run. Fluids are kept to a minimum during the bypass phase, and the perfusionist often makes adjustments.

It is important to have open communications with the perfusionist, surgeon, and anesthesia provider during CPB so that coagulation, pressure maintenance, and adjustment of electrolyte imbalances are carefully regulated.

Weaning from Bypass

When a patient is being weaned from CPB, considerations should include the ventricular function of the heart before bypass and the length of time the aorta was cross-clamped. Below is a checklist for weaning from bypass.

Checklist for Weaning from the Pump

- Patient is warm (at least 35° C).
- Heart rhythm has returned.
- All monitors are functioning; ECG, PA tracing, arterial line tracing, and CVP reflect heart filling.
- Heart rate is 70 to 100 beats/min (<60 beats/min means reduced CO; >120 beats/min is detrimental to LV filling).
- Infusions are prepared as necessary.
- Inflate lungs (but keep them out of the surgeon's field).
- Pressures become pulsatile as ventricles fill.
- Draw blood for measurement of electrolytes, hematocrit, arterial blood gases, and activated clotting time.
- Surgeon clamps venous drain and removes cannula.
- Patient is off pump.

If the ventricle was in good condition before bypass and the cross-clamp time was less than 60 minutes, the initiation of inotropes is probably not necessary. Otherwise, an inotrope should be chosen in consultation with the surgeon. Additional parameters that should be verified include patient temperature, heart rhythm, monitor status, and adequacy of perfusion.

During weaning, the perfusionist partially occludes the venous line to increase right atrial pressure, blood flows into the right ventricle and out through the PA, and pressures become pulsatile.

The rate of rewarming must be limited to 1° C per 3 to 5 minutes to prevent formation of gaseous emboli in the circulatory system or the ECC.

Rewarming begins slightly before removal of the aortic cross-clamp, when the last distal anastomosis begins in multiple graft procedures, or when the valve sutures have been placed during valve replacement procedures. The temperature gradient between arterial and venous blood should be maintained below 10° C, and the time frame for rewarming is usually 30 minutes. Laboratory values, including arterial blood gases, electrolytes, and hematocrit, should be obtained. Patient ventilation is reinstituted.

An infusion of calcium chloride (1 g/100 mL 5% dextrose in water [D_5W]) is administered via a central line. After most of the calcium chloride has been given, a small test dose of protamine, usually 10 mg, is administered to test for an unexpected reaction before infusion. If the patient remains stable, protamine administration is initiated slowly over approximately 20 minutes to avoid hypotension. Protamine is given in a calculated dose that is approximately a 1:1 ratio of the initial heparin dose. When one-third of the dose of protamine has been given, the perfusionist should be told to stop collecting blood via suction from the operative field because this would clot the pump. Small increments of phenylephrine may be administered to maintain blood pressure within desired ranges. The surgeon can restart bypass throughout the weaning process as necessary. Communication is vital during the weaning process. The possibility always exists that the patient will have to be returned to bypass.

Notify the surgeon when the protamine has been completely administered and recheck the ACT. Recheck CO and pressures to establish postoperative baselines.

When bypass is completely discontinued, check ACT values and institute treatment if they are elevated. Bypass may have to be reinstituted if severe hypotension, excessive bleeding, or a persistently low CO is present. If the protamine is completely administered and a return to bypass is required, heparin (300 units/kg) may be readministered. At times, an IABP may be required.

In anticipation of the increased metabolic uptake associated with this phase of the operation, administration of amnestic agents and muscle relaxants to maintain appropriate anesthetic levels should be instituted. When the aortic cross-clamp is removed, reperfusion to the myocardium allows the heart to rewarm and flushes residual cardioplegic solution and accumulated metabolic byproducts out of the coronary vessels. Hypotension should be anticipated. Plasma levels of atrial natriuretic factor have been shown to decrease with the onset of aortic cross-clamping and either decrease or increase significantly when the cross-clamp is removed.

Sweating during the rewarming phase of CPB represents a normal thermoregulatory response that can be associated with cutaneous dilation that is caused by elevated skin temperatures. Postoperative shivering should be avoided to prevent increased oxygen demand and carbon dioxide production.

Protamine Administration

Protamine sulfate is the drug of choice for heparin reversal. It inactivates heparin by binding with it to form an inert salt. At the conclusion of CPB, the residual amount of heparin is assessed and appropriately neutralized.

Protamine is initiated after a test dose of 1 mg in 100 mL over 10 minutes before heparinization. It binds and inhibits the anticoagulation effects to circulating heparin.

Adverse reactions to protamine include histamine-releasing reactions, true anaphylaxis mediated by a specific antiprotamine antibody, or reactions in which release of thromboxane leads to pulmonary vasoconstriction or bronchoconstriction. In the presence of increased risk factors, heparinase I may be given.

Protamine Reversal of Heparin

- 10 mg protamine reverses 1000 units heparin.
- 10 mg protamine = 1 mL of protamine.
- 1 mL of protamine reverses 30 mL heparin (an average initial dose).
- Protamine reversal is 1:1 ratio with heparin dose.

Complications of Cardiac Bypass

Separation from Cardiopulmonary Bypass

Preexisting ventricular dysfunction or myocardial insult associated with CPB complicates the process of weaning the patient from extracorporeal support. Separation from bypass presents a tremendous challenge in providing appropriate pharmacologic and mechanical support sufficient for the recovery of ventricular function. The major pharmacologic interventions include the use of both inotropic and vasodilator treatment of systolic or diastolic dysfunction.

Tachycardia and arrhythmias must be prevented, arterial blood pressure maintained, and myocardial contractility promoted while constraints on oxygen demand are maintained. The ideal regimen for pharmacologic therapy includes drugs that have rapid onset and termination, have a neutralizing effect on ischemia, and are nontoxic to the myocardium.

Catecholamines have variable effects on heart rate, rhythm, and metabolism. Milrinone, epinephrine, norepinephrine, dobutamine, dopamine, and isoproterenol are selected based on targeted functions. Dopamine increases pulmonary vascular resistance, PA pressure, and LV filling pressures; however, chronic heart failure can lead to a depletion of neurotransmitters, making indirect-acting catecholamines such as dopamine less effective. The impact of high-dose dopamine on renal perfusion cannot be ignored, and low (renal dose) levels may be required if concern for α-adrenergic–mediated constriction of renal or tissue beds exists.

Calcium may be beneficial on termination of CPB and should be administered just before weaning when ionized calcium levels are deficient and inotropic assistance is required.

Phosphodiesterase inhibitors such as milrinone may be helpful in providing prophylactic inotropic support in anticipation of ventricular failure. In conjunction with decreased LV wall tension, milrinone promotes cardiac function without increasing myocardial oxygen demand. Milrinone is similar to dobutamine in its effects on myocardial contractility, myocardial oxygen consumption rate, systemic vascular resistance (SVR), and pulmonary vascular resistance; however, patients are less susceptible to biochemical changes in neurohumoral regulation, which may reduce the efficacy of β-agonists.

Blood from the pump is sequestered into the cell saver device and concentrated to be returned to the patient via IV infusion after separation from CPB. This assists in bolstering the blood pressure without the administration of large amounts of crystalloid or pressors. In addition, colloid may be included to decrease the incidence of hypotension. Monitoring devices should be recalibrated before separation from the CPB, and the lungs should be expanded and mechanical ventilation instituted before weaning. This is done to assess the possibility of atelectasis, pneumothorax, and hydrothorax.

Pacing

Usually during rewarming, fibrillation of the myocardium occurs with a gradual progression to normal sinus rhythm. If defibrillation does not occur spontaneously, antiarrhythmic therapy, electrical cardioversion, or both are used. Control of heart rate and rhythm may be effected through the use of atrial, ventricular, AV sequential, or overdrive pacing in addition to necessary antiarrhythmic drugs. Epicardial electrode placement on the wall of the atrium is routine for cardiac surgery. Pacemakers allow for rapid adjustment of decreased CO when the conduction pathway is damaged or highly irritable.

Atrial contraction determines CO by controlling the volume of blood ejected into the ventricle. Atrial volume, ventricular volume and compliance, and the pattern of atrial contraction influence ventricular filling. If ventricular pacing is used alone, CO may decrease because of loss of the atrial "kick," but AV pacing alters the AV interval in relation to the PR interval, thereby improving CO.

Left Ventricular Dysfunction

Left ventricular dysfunction may be indicated by a rise in PA pressure in conjunction with depressed systemic arterial blood pressure. The causes of LV failure can be varied and may include preoperative markers such as a diminished LV EF and LV hypokinesis or akinesis.

Transesophageal echocardiography is an invaluable tool for confirming and isolating hypodynamic ventricular wall motion. If depressed contractility results from lack of appropriate inotropic and pharmacologic support, this should be remedied immediately. In some cases, the myocardium may be "stunned" and may require additional support through the reengagement of CPB, resting of the heart, and examination of the anastomosis for leaks and the grafts for air emboli or kinking.

In the event that cardiac depression remains unresolved or worsens, a mechanical assist device such as an IABP may be percutaneously introduced to provide diastolic augmentation and decreased afterload.

Right Ventricular Dysfunction

An inflammatory mediated response from the ECC or acute anaphylactic reaction caused by protamine sulfate or blood product transfusion may lead to increased pulmonary vascular resistance, resulting in depressed right ventricular function.

Pharmacologic intervention to reduce pulmonary vasoconstriction includes nitric oxide–based vasodilators and β_2-adrenergic agonists. For cases in which conventional treatment fails, intervention may include the use of prostaglandin E_1.

Left atrial injection of norepinephrine has been demonstrated to increase systemic pressures while avoiding the first-pass effects on the pulmonary vascular system. When right ventricular failure is unrelated to pulmonary vascular resistance, phosphodiesterase inhibitors may be beneficial for resolving the condition while avoiding the vasodilatory effects of prostaglandins.

Failure to Wean

The quality of the surgical correction and the quality of myocardial preservation are important determinants of the success in weaning from CPB. Failure to wean can be attributed to multiple factors, including heart block or ventricular dysfunction resulting from hyperkalemia, interruption of coronary flow (because of air, fat, or particulate emboli), extended CPB and aortic cross-clamp times, and arrhythmias associated with reperfusion injury.

Failure to wean on the primary attempt may lead to significant damage or distention of the heart. Systemic hypotension may promote metabolic acidosis and organ damage or failure. Additional inotropic support may be required for returning to bypass under these conditions and may result in the additional administration of blood products as a result of excessive hemodilution. If return to CPB becomes necessary, an additional heparin bolus may be required.

These situations are always emergent and require extreme caution in ensuring that the patient is being ventilated and adequately anticoagulated and that anatomic reconnection to ECC is achieved before bypass is reengaged. Preparations should include an avenue for mechanical support (e.g., IABP, ventricular assist device) if the need arises.

Intraaortic Balloon Pump

In the event of LV failure or myocardial hypokinesia resulting from CPB or ischemic insult, insertion of an intraaortic balloon may be necessary to provide diastolic counterpulsation for the patient.

The intraaortic balloon is a distensible polyurethane catheter that is percutaneously inserted through the femoral artery using the Seldinger technique for large-diameter catheter placement. The tip of the catheter allows aortic pressure monitoring and is threaded to the descending thoracic aorta with the tip at the distal aortic arch. The balloon (size 34, 40, or 50 mL) is inflated with helium or carbon dioxide gas. Balloon deflation can be triggered by the R wave of the ECG or by the arterial pressure waveform, atrial pacing mode, AV sequential pacing mode, or internal asynchronous timing (not recommended).

Inflation of the intraaortic balloon is timed to occur during diastole, forcing blood into the coronary arteries and periphery. It deflates during systole to promote ventricular ejection. Diastolic augmentation is achieved during inflation and results in increased coronary perfusion pressure as well as increased flow to the great vessels arising from the aorta. In most instances, this diastolic augmentation results in pressures greater than the patient's systolic pressure. Afterload reduction results when the balloon is rapidly deflated before ventricular ejection, reducing ventricular wall tension and therefore myocardial oxygen demand.

Ventricular Assist Devices

The placement of a ventricular assist device is an option when termination of bypass cannot be tolerated by the patient and no other options to ensure survival exist. This effort in most cases represents a bridge to cardiac transplantation or allows for additional resting time to promote recovery of severely compromised cardiac contractile function. Most institutions have established protocols and criteria for considering a patient as a candidate for this device. Age, pulmonary function, and organ system viability are factors in this selection process.

Cardiopulmonary bypass is reinstituted to prepare the circuit and cannulation sites for transfer from the ECC to a centrifugal assist device. Cannulation depends on which ventricle requires support and represents a mechanically assisted atrial-aortic shunt of blood flow to circumvent the impaired ventricle. This is a simple circuit with no oxygenator or heating element component; therefore, during the transfer from the ECC to the mechanical assist device, the patient must be ventilated. Appropriate pharmacologic support is essential.

Extubation

The current trend is toward early extubation of the postoperative cardiac surgical patient. Controversy surrounds the efficacy of extubation within 2 to 4 hours of closure. However, "fast tracking," a term used to describe early extubation and discharge from the intensive care unit, has become popular as a cost-effective technique associated with this major surgical procedure. The patient population for fast-track cardiac anesthesia must be a "less sick" group to prevent precipitation of hypertensive episodes and increased postoperative myocardial ischemia. Ideally, fast-track candidates are younger than 70 years of age; have normal ventricular and valvular function and an uncomplicated surgery; and are free of renal, neurologic, and coagulation disorders in the immediate postoperative period.

The selection of agents for fast tracking starts in the preinduction phase with agents that have a short duration of action. Lower doses of opioids are supplemented with low-dose inhalation agents and propofol infusions. α-Agonists are used as adjuncts because of their ability to blunt neurohumoral stress responses. Postoperative analgesia can be accomplished with the use of low-dose morphine, nonsteroidal anti-inflammatory drugs, patient-controlled analgesia, and thoracic epidurals with short-acting opioids.

Extubation criteria include a warm patient, low-dose or no inotropic drugs or vasoactive drips, no balloon pump, and bleeding less than 100 mL/hr. The patient must be awake, pain free, and hemodynamically stable and must meet all conventional metabolic criteria for extubation. Regardless of the anesthetic technique used, the key to optimizing patient recovery is postoperative pain management, which facilitates early mobility and nutritional intake.

D. MINIMALLY INVASIVE CORONARY ARTERY BYPASS TECHNIQUES

Port-Access Coronary Artery Bypass Grafting

To minimize postoperative pain and to speed recovery, some cardiovascular surgeons have used a port access method of coronary artery bypass (PACAB). In these procedures, multiple ports are placed in the chest wall for video-assisted surgery in addition to performance of a mini-thoracotomy in some patients. The Heartport system used during PACAB necessitates the femoral artery approach and uses an endoaortic balloon occlusion for instillation of cardioplegia. One-lung ventilation and extensive monitoring are required during the internal mammary artery (IMA) dissection. The indirect visualization of the heart through echocardiography, video (endoscopy), and fluoroscopy makes the procedure somewhat cumbersome and tedious for the surgeon.

Anesthetic techniques include all monitors and considerations for CPB as well as the need for one-lung ventilation. Patient benefits from this port-access technique include less postoperative pain, a reduced intensive care unit stay, an accelerated recovery time, improved postoperative pulmonary function, and a reduced need for inpatient cardiac rehabilitation. Aortic atherosclerotic disease is a contraindication for PACAB procedure. Heartport has a long bypass run for single vessel CABG, which maximizes the risk of stroke even though the sternotomy is eliminated.

Procedures that benefit from port access include multivessel CABG, mitral valve procedures, aortic valve replacements, and some congenital heart defect procedures. Concerns remain regarding aortic dissection as well as stroke and embolism because the surgeon does not have direct access to the surgical field and cannot directly suction air from the heart. Patient selection is an important factor in safety of the procedure.

Minimally Invasive Direct Coronary Artery Bypass

Minimally invasive direct coronary artery bypass (MIDCAB) follows the basics of conventional CABG procedures but does not require CPB, cardioplegia, or a large incision. Through a small incision (10–12 cm) and under direct vision, the graft is anastomosed while the heart is still beating. This procedure is beneficial to the patient because of the smaller incision, the absence of CPB and its inherent complications, and the reduced need for blood transfusions. The disadvantages include the fact that it is limited to use for only one or two arteries and that one-lung ventilation often is requested by the surgeon. Because the heart continues to beat, the anastomoses are difficult to suture, and significant ischemia may occur, precipitating hemodynamic compromise of the patient. The perfusionist and CPB equipment must be immediately available for urgent conversion to coronary bypass is necessary. Anesthetic management is closely related to that for off-pump coronary artery bypass procedures with normal sternotomies.

Off-Pump Coronary Artery Bypass

Surgical techniques in this area, along with advances in equipment, allow multivessel procedures with median sternotomy to be performed. Because CPB is not used, hearts of patients undergoing off-pump coronary artery bypass (OPCAB) are normothermic, and maintenance of coronary perfusion and hemodynamic stability are absolutely necessary. Communication between the surgeon and the anesthesia provider is of paramount importance. The anesthesia provider is a crucial member of the team who should be as observant of the surgical field as the surgeon. Unlike CPB cases, during OPCAB procedures, the grafting phase requires involvement and vigilance on the part of the anesthesia provider.

The patients undergoing OPCAB are anesthetized with the intent of "early" extubation. A modified fast-track approach that avoids ischemia while facilitating early extubation is desirable. The choice of an anesthetic must take into consideration that a slow heart rate facilitates the surgical procedures and reduces myocardial oxygen demand. A narcotic–oxygen–muscle relaxant technique facilitates minute-to-minute control of hemodynamics. Maintenance of the systolic pressure promotes hemodynamic stability when the heart position is changed during exposure of the different vessels. It is recommended that the systolic pressure be maintained above 100 mmHg. Prudent volume loading and positioning of the patient in the Trendelenburg position with a right rotation promote recovery of blood pressure when retraction is used in exposure of the posterior pericardium.

Extensive invasive monitoring is indicated, along with a large-bore peripheral IV and a right IJ triple-lumen catheter capable of handling continuous thermodilution CO and transvenous pacing. Multiple central ports must be available for continuous infusion of various vasoactive medications. Temperature monitoring is vital. It is necessary to maintain fluids and any other drips or instillations at warm temperatures, to use a forced air-warming device on the head and neck, and to maintain a warm room temperature. If the grafts are completely arterial, as is often the case in OPCAB procedures, the anesthesia provider should investigate the possibility of placing a forced air warmer on the patient's lower extremities.

The muscle relaxant chosen should be one without histamine-releasing effects. Some anesthesia providers insist that a neuromuscular blocker such as pancuronium, which independently causes tachycardia, should be avoided. However, when potent narcotics such as sufentanil are used, the synergistic effects of these two drugs should be considered and used. A target heart rate of not greater than 70 beats/min can be achieved with the addition of an esmolol drip. Because surgical manipulation itself precipitates arrhythmias, antiarrhythmic medications (lidocaine, magnesium, or amiodarone) for treatment of these problems must be readily available. In addition to drugs, it is appropriate to let the surgeon know what impact surgical manipulations have on the myocardium and to ask the surgeon to stop temporarily, if possible, when the situation warrants it. If bradycardia becomes a problem, treatment with medications as well as epicardial or transvenous pacing may be necessary.

The use of antifibrinolytics is controversial because some surgeons are concerned about graft thrombosis associated with the use of these agents. Anticoagulant therapy is facility specific but usually directed at a target ACT of 300 seconds and incomplete coagulation reversal. When protamine is given, it is usually at a reduced dose to achieve an anticoagulation level 25% to 50% above the control ACT. When instilling protamine, the ACT should be checked one-third and two-thirds of the way through the dose to avoid overshooting the target ACT. In off-pump procedures, the coagulation system is normal because it has not been exposed to the ECC and its effects; therefore, the possibility of pulmonary embolus, graft clotting, and so on exists just as in other major vascular procedures.

For OPCAB patients to be extubated, they must be warm, awake, pain free, and receiving no or low-dose inotropes and vasoactive drugs; no balloon pump must be in use; bleeding must be less than 100 mL/hr; and patients must be hemodynamically stable and meet conventional metabolic and mechanical criteria for extubation. The table on pg. 260 shows some monitoring approaches for OPCAB and MIDCAB.

Monitoring Approaches for OPCAB and MIDCAB

Monitor	Advantages	Disadvantages	Comments
ECG	Universal Simple Inexpensive Recognized criteria	Insensitive Position dependent (lead and heart) Incision dependent Loss of V4-V5 (MIDCAB)	Best if multi-lead Should be calibrated ST-segment treading helpful
Central venous pressure	Simple Inexpensive	Insensitive for LV dysfunction No cardiac output	Important for drug infusions Affected by position of heart and patient Use of "introducer" allows rapid insertion of PAC
Pulmonary artery catheter	LV filling pressure Cardiac output Options may be helpful (SVo_2, CCO, pacing)	Expensive Insensitive for acute regional dysfunction Postoperative nuisance	Controversial monitor May prolong ICU stay because of "abnormal numbers"
Trans-esophageal echocardi-ography	Gold standard for acute ischemia Verify restoration of function Guide surgical cannula placement	Expensive User dependent Distracting May not have good view of heart	Requires expertise May give false sense of security
Cardiac output (bioimped-ance, aortic flow, CO_2 rebreathing)	Less invasive than PAC Can give beat-to-beat flow	Expensive No measure of LV filling May be user dependent	Bioimpedance questionable with open chest Cannot get readings on all patients

CCO, Continuous cardiac output; *ICU*, intensive care unit; *LV*, left ventricular, *MIDCAB*, minimally invasive direct coronary artery bypass grafting; *OPCAB*, off-pump coronary artery bypass grafting; *PAC*, pulmonary artery catheter, SVo_2, mixed venous oxygen saturation.
From Hensley FA, Martin DE, Gravlee GP, eds. *A Practical Approach to Cardiac Anesthesia. 2008*. 4th ed. Philadelphia: Lippincott Williams & Wilkins; 2008.

E. PACEMAKERS

Indications

1. Sick sinus syndrome or symptomatic bradycardia.
2. Heart blocks
   a. AV block including third-degree heart block and type 2 second-degree heart block
   b. Fascicular block including symptomatic bifascicular block and trifascicular block
3. Temporary pacemakers are indicated for same reasons as permanent pacemakers. They may serve as a bridge until permanent pacing is available or until the cardiac condition stabilizes, such as after coronary artery bypass grafting.

Preoperative Assessment

1. Assess the patient's current cardiac status and symptoms.
2. Determine the original reason for the pacemaker.
3. Determine the type of pacemaker and the settings. If unknown, the specific model number and manufacturer may be obtained by radiography of the pace generator.
4. Determine the location of the generator. Usually it is located in the upper chest, but occasionally it may be located in the abdomen.
5. Pacemaker wires may become easily dislodged in the first 6 weeks after placement. Central line placement may need to be done under fluoroscopy to avoid lead disruption.
6. Magnetic resonance imaging (MRI) is contraindicated in patients with pacemakers because of the potential for pacemakers to dysfunction unless the pacemaker is MRI compatible.

Perioperative Management

Although most pacemakers now are resistant to electromagnetic interference (EMI) from the use of electrocautery, it can occasionally occur. The pacemaker output may be inhibited, or the pacemaker may be reset to a preset pacing mode (DOO or VOO).

If EMI occurs, a doughnut magnet can be applied directly over the pacemaker, which will cause it to convert to an asynchronous mode or a committed mode. Most pacemakers will automatically convert to an asynchronous mode when prolonged EMI is detected, so the magnet intervention is rarely needed.

Heart rate should be monitored with a precordial or esophageal stethoscope, pulse oximeter, or arterial line or by palpating the pulse during electrocautery.

Postoperatively, pacemaker function is not routinely checked unless interference was detected or the surgical procedure involved primary insertion or generator change.

Pacemaker Insertion

Insertion sites can be the subclavian vein or through the cephalic vein in the deltopectoral groove. Leads are placed through the subclavian vein through the tricuspid valve into the right atrium or dual chamber leads may be placed with one in the right atrium and one in the right ventricle. Anesthetic requirements are usually local anesthesia administered by the surgeon and IV sedation.

Common complications during placement include dysrhythmias. Less common potential complications include pneumothorax, dislodging of electrodes, and cardiac tamponade.

Pacemaker Types (Definitions and Nomenclature)

Unipolar pacing involves a negative electrode in the atrium or ventricle and a positive ground far from the heart. These are rarely used and are more prone to interference from electrocautery and other devices such as microwaves.

Bipolar pacing involves placement of both electrodes in the chamber being paced or sensed. Asynchronous generators simply provide electrical impulses without sensing. Synchronous generators have both pulse-sensing and generating circuits. A five-letter code describes the functions and settings of the pacemaker (see the table on pg. 262).

Pacemaker Codes and Function

I Chamber Paced	II Chamber Sensed	III Response Mode	IV Program Function	V Special Function
A = Atrial V = Ventricular D = Dual chamber	Atrium Ventricle Both	I = Inhibited T = Triggered D = Dual 0 = None R = Reverse	P = Program M = Multiprogram C = Communicating	B = Bursts N = Norm rate S = Scanning E = External

	Assigned Function
DDD	Atrial and ventricular sensing and pacing
VDD	Programmable AV interval: senses both chambers, paces ventricle
DVI	Programmable AV interval: senses ventricles paces atrium at fixed rate. Ventricular pacing occurs if no QRS is sensed within time interval needed to match the set rate of pacemaker.
VVT	Programmable escape interval: senses ventricle and paces ventricle. If a QRS is sensed, the pacer will generate an impulse with the sensed beat.
VVI	Inhibited output from sensed ventricle: demand ventricular pacing. Senses ventricular and paces ventricles. If QRS is sensed, the pacer will be inhibited from firing.
V00	Asynchronous ventricular pacing
AAT	Programmable escape interval: senses atrium and paces atrium. If a P wave is sensed, the pacer will generate an impulse with the sensed beat.
AAI	Inhibited output from sensed atrium: demand atrial pacing. Senses atrium and paces atrium. If a P wave is sensed, the pacer will be inhibited from firing.
A00	Asynchronous atrial pacing

The two most common types of pacemakers are VVI and DDD.

Automatic Internal Cardiac Defibrillator

Internal cardiac defibrillators (ICDs) are used in populations that are at high risk of sudden death from cardiac tachydysrhythmias.

Internal cardiac defibrillators consist of two defibrillating electrodes or patches and separate electrodes that are used for pacing and sensing. The patches are placed near the pericardium. The generator is implanted in either the abdomen or chest wall.

All ICDs are extremely sensitive to EMI used in electrocautery. EMI is detected as ventricular fibrillation by the device and delivers a shock to the patient. Magnet application will cause the device to suspend detection, but it will not interfere with the pacing function. Intraoperatively, if ventricular fibrillation occurs, the magnet can simply be removed, and the device can deliver a shock, usually within 10 seconds. External defibrillators should always be readily available in case of failure.

The ICD can be turned off manually for the duration of the operation before the patient is taken into the operating room, and it can be turned back on in the postanesthesia care unit. Personnel trained in the use of an external cardiac defibrillator should be readily available while the device is turned off.

If only bipolar cautery is used, the device can usually remain on.

F. VALVULAR HEART DISEASE

Aortic Stenosis

Disease of the aortic valve may present as aortic valvular stenosis, insufficiency, or a combination of both. Valvular heart disease is usually caused by rheumatic disease, but it may also occur secondary to calcific degeneration in elderly patients. Endocarditis and congenital abnormalities of the bicuspid valve account for most of the remainder. It is rarely possible to repair the aortic valve; therefore, most conditions require valve replacement.

Pathophysiology

Chronic obstruction to LV ejection results in concentric LV hypertrophy and myocardium that is highly susceptible to ischemia (even in the absence of coronary artery disease). Aortic stenosis is severe when the valve area is less than 0.6 cm^2 and the pressure gradient is greater than 70 torr.

Hemodynamic Goals

Left ventricular filling is dependent on atrial contractions, heart rate, and normal intravascular volume. Decreases in SVR are dangerous because of the fixed ventricular ejection; decreased SVR results in decreased blood pressure, coronary perfusion pressures, and resultant ischemia. Extreme and rapid increase in SVR increases LW workload and further decrease stroke volume through the stenotic aortic valve.

Dysrhythmias

Dysrhythmias should be aggressively treated. Because the ventricle is stiff, atrial contraction is critical for ventricular filling and stroke volume.

Anesthetic Technique

Induction

1. Usually a high-dose narcotic technique is used: fentanyl, etomidate, and a muscle relaxant.
2. Avoid anesthetic agents that reduce vascular tone. Vasopressors should be available for induction.
3. Maintain intravascular volume and sinus rhythm.
4. Maintain heart rate; avoid decreased SVR and blood pressure.
5. External cardiac massage is not effective in these patients. Ventricular tachycardia and fibrillation are usually fatal.

Maintenance

Use a high-dose narcotic, a low-dose volatile agent, oxygen, and air.

After Bypass

1. The patient may have higher filling pressures because of the noncompliant ventricle. Inotropic support is commonly required.
2. The patient may be hyperdynamic or require vasodilators for hypertension.
3. The drug of choice for hypotension is ephedrine

Aortic Regurgitation

Pathophysiology

The incompetent aortic valve results in a decrease in forward LV stroke volume because part of the ejected LV volume regurgitates back into the LV from the aorta, resulting in chronic volume overload of the LV and eccentric hypertrophy.

Aortic regurgitation causes a decrease in aortic diastolic blood pressure and decreased coronary artery perfusion pressures, resulting in subendocardial ischemia and angina (even in the absence of coronary artery disease). The magnitude of regurgitation is dependent on the duration of flow and the pressure gradient across the valve. Regurgitation can be reduced by increasing heart rate and decreasing SVR.

In chronic aortic regurgitation, as end-diastolic volume increases, stroke volume increases so that the EF is well maintained until LV failure occurs. When failure occurs, CO decreases, end-diastolic volume increases, and pulmonary edema results.

In acute aortic regurgitation, the sudden increase in LV volume without ventricular hypertrophy results in sudden cardiac failure.

Anesthetic Technique

Maintenance of adequate ventricular volume in the presence of mild vasodilation and increases in heart rate is most likely to optimize forward LV stroke volume.

Avoid increases in SVR and BP; avoid decreases in heart rate.

Mitral Stenosis

Pathophysiology

Increased left atrial pressure and volume overload occur as a result of the narrowed mitral orifice. Persistent increases in the left atrial pressure are reflected back through the pulmonary circulation, leading to right ventricular hypertrophy and failure, tricuspid regurgitation, and perivascular edema in the lungs. The left atrial enlargement predisposes the patient to formation of thrombi and systemic emboli, especially with the development of AF.

Anesthetic Technique

Tachycardia results in inadequate LV filling and concomitant hypotension. Continued preoperative administration of digitalis and β-antagonists, the selection of anesthetics with a minimal propensity to increase heart rate, and achievement of an anesthetic depth sufficient to suppress sympathetic nervous system responses are recommended.

Induction agents should be administered slowly to avoid drug-induced reductions in SVR and resultant hypotension in the presence of a fixed LV stroke volume. Avoid ketamine because of the increase in heart rate associated with this drug.

Preoxygenation and brief laryngoscopy reduce the potential for hypoxia, hypercarbia, and acidosis. (These potentiate pulmonary vasoconstriction, which will potentiate right-sided heart failure.) Avoid increases in heart rate; avoid decreases in myocardial contractility, SVR, and blood pressure.

Mitral Regurgitation

Pathophysiology

Chronic volume overload of the left atrium occurs, resulting in a decreased LV stroke volume because of part of the stroke volume's regurgitation through the incompetent valve. The increase in left atrial pressure results in elevated pulmonary pressures and right-sided heart failure. LV hypertrophy results to compensate for the decreased CO. PA capillary wedge pressure overestimates LV end-diastolic pressure. The amount of regurgitation depends on the size of the valve orifice, the heart rate, and the pressure gradient across the valve.

Mild increases in heart rate improve LV stroke volume. Bradycardia results in acute volume overload of the left atrium.

The drug of choice for hypotension is ephedrine.

The pressure gradient across the valve is determined by the compliance of the LV and the impedance to LV ejection into the aorta. Reducing SVR can improve forward flow.

Anesthetic Technique

1. Select agents that promote vasodilation and increase heart rate.
2. Avoid myocardial depression, which will decrease CO.
3. Barbiturates, benzodiazepines, etomidate, and succinylcholine are good choices.
4. Maintain normocarbia and oxygen saturation to prevent increases in pulmonary hypertension associated with pulmonary vasoconstriction.

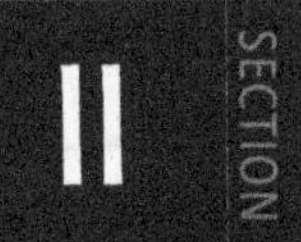

SECTION II Gastrointestinal System

A. ANAL FISTULOTOMY AND FISTULECTOMY

1. Introduction

Most perianal fistulas arise as a result of infection within the anal glands located at the dentate line (cryptoglandular fistula). Fistulas may also arise as the result of trauma, Crohn's disease, inflammatory processes within the peritoneal cavity, neoplasms, or radiation therapy. The ultimate treatment is determined by the cause and the anatomic course of the fistula and can include fistulotomy and fistulectomy. The primary goal is palliation, specifically to drain abscesses and prevent their recurrence. This is often accomplished by placing a Silastic seton (a ligature placed around the sphincter muscles) around the fistula tract and leaving it in place indefinitely. In the absence of active Crohn's disease in the rectum, attempts at fistula cure may be undertaken.

2. Preoperative assessment

a) History and physical examination
   (1) Respiratory: A careful evaluation of respiratory status is important. If the patient has significant respiratory disease, the lithotomy position is better tolerated than the prone or jackknife positions.
   (2) Musculoskeletal: Pain is likely at the surgical site and should be considered when positioning the patient for anesthetic induction. (If the patient has pain while sitting, regional anesthesia should be performed with the patient in the lateral decubitus position.)
   (3) Hematologic: If regional anesthesia is planned and the patient is taking acetylsalicylic acids, nonsteroidal anti-inflammatory drugs (NSAIDs), or dipyridamole, check the platelet count and bleeding time.

b) Patient preparation
   (1) Laboratory tests: As indicated per history and physical examination
   (2) Diagnostic tests: As indicated per history and physical examination
   (3) Medication: Standard premedication

3. Room preparation

a) Monitoring equipment: Standard
b) Drugs
   (1) Standard emergency drugs
   (2) Standard tabletop
   (3) Intravenous (IV) fluids: 18-gauge IV line, normal saline or lactated Ringer solution at 4 to 6 mL/kg/IM

4. Anesthetic technique

General anesthesia, local anesthesia with sedation, and spinal or epidural techniques may be used.

5. Perioperative management

a) Induction: Standard. Procedures done with the patient in the jackknife or prone position may require endotracheal intubation for airway control if a regional technique is not performed.

b) Maintenance
   (1) Standard
   (2) Position: Use chest support or bolster to optimize ventilation in the jackknife position; take care in positioning the patient's extremities and genitals after turning the patient into the jackknife position. Avoid pressure on the eyes and ears after turning the patient. Avoid stretching the brachial plexus. Limit abduction to 90 degrees.

c) Emergence: No special considerations are needed. The patient is extubated awake and after return of airway reflexes.

6. Postoperative implications

a) Lithotomy position, possibly leading to damage to the peroneal nerve, which can lead to foot drop
b) Urinary retention
c) Poor wound healing
d) Atelectasis
e) Cauda equina syndrome with spinal anesthesia in lithotomy position

B. CHOLECYSTECTOMY

1. Introduction

Surgery of the upper abdomen is used in the treatment of gallstones and other diseases of the gallbladder. Open cholecystectomy is performed in patients with adhesions, previous surgical procedures, infection, or major medical problems. An intraoperative cholangiogram may be done to determine if there are gallstones present within the biliary tree. The mortality rate for elective cholecystectomy is less than 0.5%. In patients older than 70 years of age, the mortality rate rises to 2% to 3%, mostly because of preexisting cardiopulmonary disease. Presently, the surgical approach used during cholecystectomy is laparoscopic.

2. Preoperative assessment

a) History and physical examination
   (1) Standard
   (2) Gastrointestinal assessment: Pain is localized in the right subcostal region. The patient may experience referred pain in the back at the shoulder level. Anorexia, nausea, and vomiting are common. Infection and fever are rare.

b) Diagnostic tests: These are as indicated by the patient's history and medical condition.

c) Preoperative medication and IV therapy
   (1) Use an antimicrobial to prevent bacteremia.
   (2) Narcotics must be used with caution to minimize potential spasm in the biliary tract and sphincter of Oddi. Medications used to inhibit sphincter of Oddi spasm include nitrates, glucagon, Narcan, and anticholinergics.
   (3) Use a single, large-bore (18-gauge) IV catheter with fluid replacement. Patients may be dehydrated and require generous IV hydration before induction.
   (4) Use prophylactic antiemetics and aspiration prophylaxis.

3. **Room preparation**
   a) Monitoring equipment: Standard
   b) Pharmacologic agents
      (1) Standard
      (2) Caution advised with use of narcotic agents because of potential changes in biliary pressure
   c) Position: Supine
4. **Anesthetic technique**

General endotracheal anesthesia with muscle relaxation is used.

5. **Perioperative management**
   a) Induction: Rapid-sequence induction with oral endotracheal intubation if the patient is considered to have a full stomach
   b) Maintenance
      (1) No specific requirements
      (2) Muscle relaxation per abdominal surgery
      (3) Antiemetic administration
      (4) Potential intraoperative complications include hemorrhage, gas embolism, symptomatic bradycardia, pneumothorax, and subcutaneous emphysema.
   c) Emergence: Awake extubation after airway reflexes are adequate
6. **Postoperative implications**
   a) Retraction in the right upper quadrant during surgery can lead to atelectasis in the right lower lobe; postoperative pain and splinting may lead to impaired ventilation.
   b) Right intercostal nerve blocks improve postoperative pain management.
   c) Use patient-controlled analgesia for pain management.

C. COLECTOMY

1. **Introduction**

Colectomy is performed most commonly for adenocarcinomas and diverticulosis. Other indications include penetrating trauma, ulcerative and ischemic colitis, volvulus, and inflammatory bowel disease.

2. **Preoperative assessment and patient preparation**
   a) History and physical examination: Assess hydration status, nutritional level, and electrolyte state.
   b) Diagnostic tests: These are as indicated by the patient's condition.
   c) Preoperative medication and IV therapy
      (1) Patients may be receiving steroid therapy or immunosuppressant drugs.
      (2) Bowel preparation is usually indicated with electrolyte preparations except in emergencies.
      (3) Expect fluid shifts requiring moderate to large fluid resuscitation. Two large-bore IV access tubes are indicated.
      (4) IV antibiotic therapy should be initiated before incision
3. **Room preparation**
   a) Monitoring equipment: Standard with warming modalities
   b) Pharmacologic agents: Standard
   c) Position: Supine with the arms extended
4. **Anesthetic technique**
   a) Epidural (T4 level) with "light" general anesthetic
   b) General anesthesia with oral endotracheal tube (most common)

5. **Perioperative management**
   a) Induction: Consider the possibility of a full stomach; rapid-sequence induction may be indicated. If the colectomy is performed for perforation of the bowel from any cause, septicemia must be suspected. Extreme hemodynamic variability with severe hypotension is possible.
   b) Maintenance
      (1) Muscle relaxation is required.
      (2) Closely monitor fluid and hydration status and blood loss.
      (3) Avoid nitrous oxide, which may cause bowel distention.
   c) Emergence: This involves awake extubation after rapid-sequence induction or placement of a nasogastric tube.
6. **Postoperative implications**
   a) Pain and splinting may lead to hypoventilation and decreased postoperative ventilation.
   b) Control pain with epidural or patient-controlled analgesia.
   c) If massive transfusion and significant cardiovascular and or respiratory pathophysiology exists, postoperative ventilation is warranted.

D. COLONOSCOPY

1. **Introduction**

Colonoscopy is used to examine the colon and rectum to diagnose inflammatory bowel disease, including ulcerative colitis and granulomatous colitis. Polyps can be removed through the colonoscope. The colonoscope is also helpful in diagnosing or locating the source of gastrointestinal bleeding; a biopsy of lesions suspected to be malignant may be performed.

2. **Preoperative assessment and patient preparation**
   a) History and physical examination: Assess the patient's hydration status, nutritional level, and electrolyte state.
   b) Diagnostic tests: These are as indicated by the patient's condition.
   c) Preoperative medication and IV therapy
      (1) Patients may be receiving steroid therapy or immunosuppressants.
      (2) Bowel preparation is required for visualization of the mucosa. Colon electrolyte lavage preparations (Colyte, GoLYTELY) are given the night before the procedure.
      (3) One 18-gauge IV tube is used; adequate fluid replacement is ensured.
      (4) The patient is lightly sedated with midazolam because the procedure lasts less than 30 minutes and is an outpatient procedure.
3. **Room preparation**
   a) Monitoring equipment: Standard
   b) Pharmacologic agents
      (1) Standard
      (2) Glucagon
   c) Position: Left lateral decubitus; position changes sometimes required to aid advancement of the scope at the descending sigmoid colon junction and splenic fixture.
4. **Anesthetic technique**
   a) Monitored anesthesia care
   b) IV sedation: Midazolam (Versed), fentanyl, or propofol in sedative doses

5. **Perioperative management**
   a) Induction: Oxygenation of the patient with the use of nasal cannula or a face mask
   b) Maintenance: No specific indications
   c) Emergence: No specific indications
6. **Postoperative implications**

Complications of the procedure include perforation of the bowel, abdominal pain and distention, rectal bleeding, fever, and mucopurulent drainage.

E. ESOPHAGEAL RESECTION

1. **Introduction**

Esophagectomy is commonly performed for malignant disease of the middle and lower third of the esophagus. It may also be indicated for Barrett's esophagus (peptic ulcer of the lower esophagus) and for peptic strictures that do not respond to dilation and end-stage achalasia. Whereas lesions in the lower third are usually approached through a left thoracoabdominal incision, middle-third lesions are best approached by the abdomen and thoracotomy. Resections of the esophagogastric junction for malignant disease are best performed through a left thoracoabdominal approach in which a portion of the proximal stomach is removed along with a celiac node dissection. In a transhiatal approach, the esophagus is exposed through abdominal and neck incisions.

Total esophagectomy may be done through an abdominal and right thoracotomy approach with colonic interposition and anastomosis in the neck. Either the right or the left side of the colon can be mobilized for interposition. Both depend on the middle colic artery and the marginal artery of the colon for their vascular supply.

2. **Preoperative assessment**
   a) History and physical examination
      (1) Cardiovascular: The patient may be hypovolemic and malnourished from dysphagia or anorexia. Chemotherapeutic drugs (daunorubicin, doxorubicin [Adriamycin]) may cause cardiomyopathy. Chronic alcohol abuse may also produce toxic cardiomyopathy.
      (2) Respiratory: A history of gastric reflux suggests the possibility of recurrent aspiration pneumonia, decreased pulmonary reserve, and increased risk of regurgitation and aspiration during anesthetic induction. If a thoracic approach is planned, the patient should be evaluated to ensure that one-lung ventilation can be tolerated. Patients with upper esophageal tumors or mediastinal lymphadenopathy may need tracheal or bronchial compression. Difficult airway and respiratory compromise are possible. Many patients with esophageal cancer have a long history of smoking, with consequent respiratory impairment.
         (a) Chemotherapeutic drugs (bleomycin) may cause pulmonary toxicity that can worsen with high concentrations of oxygen.
         (b) Pulmonary function tests and arterial blood gases can be helpful in predicting the likelihood of perioperative pulmonary complications and whether the patient may require postoperative mechanical ventilation. Patients with baseline hypoxemia or hypercarbia on room air arterial

blood gases have a higher likelihood of postoperative complications and a greater need for postoperative ventilatory support. Severe restrictive or obstructive lung disease will also increase the chance of pulmonary morbidity in the perioperative period.

b) Patient preparation
   (1) Laboratory tests: Type and cross-match packed red blood cells, electrolytes, glucose, blood urea nitrogen, creatinine, liver function test, complete blood count, and platelet count. Prothrombin time, partial thromboplastin time, urinalysis, arterial blood gases, and other tests as indicated by the patient's history and physical examination.
   (2) Diagnostic tests: Chest radiography, electrocardiography, pulmonary function tests, and other tests are as indicated by the patient's history and physical examination. If congestive heart failure or cardiomyopathy is suspected, consider cardiac or medical consultations.
   (3) Medications: For premedication, consider aspiration prophylaxis.

3. Room preparation

a) Monitoring equipment
   (1) Standard monitoring equipment
   (2) Arterial line and central venous pressure or pulmonary arterial catheter as indicated

b) Additional equipment: Patient warming device, fiberoptic scope to confirm the double-lumen tube (DLT) if used.

c) Drugs
   (1) Standard emergency drugs
   (2) Standard tabletop
   (3) IV fluids: Two 14- to 16-gauge IV lines normal saline or lactated Ringer solution at 8 to 12 mL/kg/hr; warmed fluids
   (4) Blood loss can possibly be significant; blood should be immediately available.

4. Anesthetic technique

General endotracheal anesthesia with or without epidural anesthetic for postoperative analgesia is administered. If the thoracic or abdominothoracic approach is used, placement of a double-lumen tube is indicated because one-lung anesthesia provides excellent surgical exposure. If the patient is clinically hypovolemic, intravascular volume should be restored before induction and carefully titrate the induction dose of sedative–hypnotic agents.

5. Perioperative management

a) Induction
   (1) Patients with esophageal disease are often at risk for pulmonary aspiration; therefore, rapid-sequence induction is indicated.
   (2) If a difficult airway is anticipated, awake intubation can be done using a fiberoptic bronchoscope.

b) Maintenance
   (1) Standard maintenance uses a narcotic, inhalation agent, or both. Avoid nitrous oxide.
   (2) A combined technique with general and epidural anesthesia may be used. If epidural opiates are used for postoperative analgesia, a loading dose should be administered at least 1 hour before the conclusion of surgery.

(3) Position: The patient is supine, with checked and padded pressure points. Avoid stretching the brachial plexus. Limit abduction to 90 degrees. If the lateral decubitus position is used, an axillary roll and arm holder are needed. Check pressure points, including ears, eyes, and genitals. Check radial pulses to ensure correct placement of the axillary roll (a misplaced axillary roll will compromise distal pulses). Problems that can arise include brachial plexus injuries and damage to soft tissues, ears, eyes, and genitals from malpositioning.

(4) Maintain normal volume status euvolemia as significant third spacing can occur

(5) Transient compression of the myocardium can occur (i.e., thoracic approach) and cause dysrhythmias or hypotension. An arterial line is recommended to maintain blood pressure.

c) Emergence: The decision to extubate at the end of surgery depends on the patient's underlying cardiopulmonary status and the extent of the surgical procedure. The patient should be hemodynamically stable, warm, alert, cooperative, and fully reversed from any muscle relaxants before extubation. With patients who require postoperative ventilation, the double-lumen tube should be changed to a single-lumen endotracheal tube before transport to the postanesthesia intensive care unit. Weaning from mechanical ventilation should begin when the patient is awake and cooperative, is able to protect the airway, and has adequate pulmonary function.

6. Postoperative implications

a) For atelectasis or aspiration, recover the patient in Fowler position.

b) Hemorrhage: Check coagulation times; replace factors as necessary.

c) Pneumothorax or hemothorax: Decreased partial oxygen pressure, increased partial carbon dioxide pressure, wheezing, and coughing are noted; confirm with chest radiography and institute chest tube drainage as necessary. In an emergency (tension pneumothorax), use needle aspiration, supportive treatment, oxygen, vasopressors, endotracheal intubation, and positive-pressure ventilation.

d) Hypoxemia or hypoventilation: Ensure adequate analgesia and supplemental oxygen. Determine the cause.

e) Esophageal anastomotic leak: Begin surgical repair for an esophageal anastomotic leak.

f) Pain management: Patient-controlled analgesia or epidural analgesia is used; the patient should recover in the intensive care unit or in a hospital unit accustomed to treating the side effects of epidural opiates (respiratory depression, breakthrough pain, nausea, and pruritus).

g) Recurrent laryngeal nerve injury: hoarse voice, respiratory distress

F. ESOPHAGOSCOPY AND GASTROSCOPY

1. Introduction

Flexible, diagnostic esophagogastroduodenoscopy, a common procedure in pediatrics, is usually performed with the patient under deep sedation in an endoscopy suite or special procedure area. Rigid esophagoscopy is usually performed for therapeutic indications, such as removal of a foreign body, dilation of an esophageal stricture, or injection of varices. The procedure is similar for each diagnosis and is generally performed with endotracheal intubation. Foreign body removal is normally a short procedure, but dilation and variceal injection can be prolonged and may require multiple insertions or removals of the endoscope. Compression of the trachea distal to the endotracheal tube by the rigid esophagoscope is common.

2. Preoperative assessment

Esophagoscopy for foreign body removal is usually performed in healthy infants and children, although esophageal lodging of a foreign body can occur in any age group. All of these patients should be treated with full-stomach precautions. Esophageal dilation usually is performed in two distinct patient populations: those with prior tracheoesophageal fistula repair and those with prior ingestion of a caustic substance.

- a) History and physical examination
  - (1) Cardiovascular: Patients with tracheoesophageal fistulas may have congenital cardiac anomalies.
  - (2) Respiratory: Patients with prior caustic ingestion may have a history of pulmonary aspiration, with resultant chemical pneumonitis, fibrosis, or both. Prolonged intubation after tracheoesophageal fistula repair may lead to subglottic stenosis. Check any recent anesthesia records for endotracheal intubation.
- b) Patient preparation
  - (1) Laboratory tests: As indicated per the patient's history and physical examination
  - (2) Diagnostic tests: As indicated per history and physical examination
  - (3) Medications: For foreign body removal, IV access may be necessary before induction. No premedication is used if the patient is younger than 1 year old.

3. Room preparation

- a) Monitoring equipment: Standard
- b) Drugs
  - (1) Standard emergency drugs
  - (2) Standard tabletop
  - (3) IV fluids: One 20- to 22-gauge IV line with normal saline or lactated Ringer solution at 4 to 6 mL/kg/hr

4. Anesthetic technique

General anesthesia with an endotracheal tube. Room temperature can be maintained at 65° to 70° F as long as the patient is covered.

5. Perioperative management

- a) Induction: Rapid-sequence induction is usually appropriate for this patient population unless the patient is presenting for dilation alone and has no evidence to suggest reflux.
- b) Maintenance
  - (1) Maintain anesthesia with a volatile agent, nitrous oxide, and oxygen. Opiates are unnecessary because postprocedural pain is negligible. Maintain neuromuscular blockade. Movement must be avoided, particularly with rigid esophagoscopy. Consider the use of dexamethasone to treat airway edema.
  - (2) Position: Supine. Pressure points are checked. Arms are positioned at less than 90°. Avoid stretching the brachial plexus.
  - (3) Warming modalities for pediatric patients: Increased room temperature, warming blankets, and a Humidivent.
- c) Emergence: Extubate when the patient is fully awake. Do not attempt reversal of neuromuscular blockade until first twitch of train-of-four has returned.

6. **Postoperative implications**
   a) Pneumothorax: Esophageal perforation is more common with rigid esophagoscopy and will lead to pneumothorax.
   b) Aspiration
   c) Accidental extubation
   d) Stridor secondary to subglottic edema
   e) Postoperative pain is negligible; if the patient reports marked substernal discomfort, suspect esophageal perforation.

G. GASTRECTOMY

1. **Introduction**

Total gastrectomy is annually performed for gastric cancer.

2. **Preoperative assessment and patient preparation**
   a) History and physical: Assess fluid and hydration status. The patient may be vomiting or bleeding or may have anorexia.
   b) Diagnostic tests
      (1) Abdominal radiography
      (2) Laboratory tests include a complete blood count, electrolytes, blood urea nitrogen, glucose, magnesium, calcium, phosphate, prothrombin time, and partial thromboplastin time. Perform other tests based on history and physical examination.
   c) Preoperative medication and IV therapy
      (1) Expect a moderate fluid shift with moderate to large fluid losses. Two large-bore IV catheters (14- to 16-gauge) are indicated.
      (2) Antibiotic therapy is indicated.
      (3) Blood transfusions are given.
3. **Room preparation**
   a) Monitoring equipment
      (1) Standard
      (2) Active warming measures
      (3) Foley catheter
   b) Pharmacologic agents: Standard
   c) Position: Supine with the arms extended
4. **Anesthetic technique**
   a) General anesthesia
   b) Epidural for intraoperative or postoperative pain management (or both)
5. **Perioperative management**
   a) Induction: Most patients are considered to have full stomachs; therefore, rapid-sequence induction with cricoid pressure.
   b) Maintenance
      (1) Muscle relaxation is required.
      (2) A narcotic or inhalation agent (or both) is administered.
      (3) Closely monitor hydration status and blood loss.
      (4) Avoid nitrous oxide to minimize gastric or colonic distention.
      (5) A nasogastric tube may be inserted.
      (6) Prophylactic antiemetics because of the risk of postoperative nausea and vomiting
   c) Emergence: Awake extubation is performed after rapid-sequence induction or placement of a nasogastric tube.

6. Postoperative implications

Pain may lead to hypoventilation, reduced cough, splinting, and atelectasis.

H. GASTROSTOMY

1. Introduction

A gastrostomy involves the placement of a semipermanent tube through the abdominal wall directly into the stomach. These tubes are used for gastric decompression or for feeding. It may be temporary or permanent. A percutaneous endoscopic gastrostomy is often performed. Feeding gastrostomy tubes are indicated in patients unable to feed by mouth but able to absorb enteral nutrition, such as patients with advanced malignancy and intestinal obstruction, inadequate oral intake, and neurologic impairment.

2. Preoperative assessment

Patients undergoing gastrostomy may have neurologic impairment caused by a stroke and head injury. This compromises their ability to handle oral secretions and increases their risk for aspiration.

a) History and physical examination
   (1) Cardiac: Patients are likely to be hypovolemic secondary to chronically poor oral intake and malnutrition.
   (2) Respiratory: Patients may have difficulty swallowing and inadequate laryngeal reflexes, placing them at high risk for aspiration of gastric contents and associated pneumonitis. Hypoxemia and decreased pulmonary reserve can be caused by prior pulmonary infections.
   (3) Neurologic: The patient is often neurologically impaired and debilitated.
   (4) Renal: Long-term indwelling urinary catheters increase the risk of infection.

b) Patient preparation
   (1) Laboratory tests: As indicated by the patient's history and physical examination
   (2) Diagnostic tests: As indicated by the patient's history and physical examination

3. Room preparation

a) Monitoring equipment: Standard monitoring equipment
b) Drugs: Standard emergency drugs
c) Standard tabletop
d) IV fluids: One 18-gauge IV line with normal saline or lactated Ringer solution at 5 to 8 mL/kg/hr

4. Anesthetic technique

IV sedation or monitored anesthesia care with local anesthesia is used.

5. Perioperative management

a) Induction
   (1) If general anesthesia is planned, use rapid-sequence induction with cricoid pressure.
   (2) Titrate narcotics (fentanyl) or benzodiazepines (midazolam) as indicated.

b) Maintenance
   (1) General anesthesia: Muscle relaxation may be necessary.
   (2) Position: Supine with pressure points padded

c) Emergence: Tracheal extubation is performed after the return of protective laryngeal reflexes.

6. Postoperative implications

Mild to moderate postoperative pain intensity may be controlled with parenteral narcotics or intercostal blocks. Postoperative complications include aspiration pneumonia, wound infection, and atelectasis.

I. HEMORRHOIDECTOMY

1. Introduction

Hemorrhoids are masses of vascular tissue found in the anal canal. Internal hemorrhoids are found above the pectinate line, arise from the superior hemorrhoidal venous plexus, and are covered with mucosa. External hemorrhoids are found below the pectinate line, arise from the inferior hemorrhoidal venous plexus, and are covered by anoderm and perianal skin. Treatment includes hemorrhoidectomy.

2. Preoperative assessment and patient preparation

a) History and physical examination: Signs include bright red blood on toilet paper or the surface of the stool, iron-deficiency anemia, a prolapsed mass of tissue that protrudes from the anus, and thrombosis (blood clot within the hemorrhoidal vein) causing pain.

b) Diagnostic tests: A complete blood count is indicated.

c) Preoperative medication and IV therapy

(1) A narcotic with premedication is considered if the patient experiences pain.

(2) An 18-gauge IV line with minimal fluid replacement

3. Room preparation

a) Monitoring equipment: Standard

b) Position: Prone, prone jackknife, or lithotomy

4. Anesthetic technique

a) Regional anesthesia, local anesthesia with sedation, or general anesthesia

b) Regional blockade: S_2-S_5 sensory level block

(1) Hypobaric spinal: Lithotomy position

(2) Hyperbaric spinal: Flexed prone or knee chest position

c) General anesthesia: Mask or laryngeal mask airway in lithotomy position (endotracheal intubation necessary for prone position)

5. Perioperative management

a) Induction

(1) Prone: General anesthesia induction is performed while the patient is on the stretcher.

(2) Position the patient on the operating table with adequate support and padding of the extremities, head, and neck.

b) Maintenance: General anesthesia: An adequate depth of anesthesia is required to relax the anal sphincter. Angiospasm during anal dilation can occur.

c) Emergence: If the prone position is used and general anesthesia is administered, patients are repositioned onto the stretcher before emergence.

6. Postoperative implications

Bearing down to void will be painful; keep fluids to a minimum.

J. HERNIORRHAPHY

1. Introduction

Inguinal hernias are defects in the transverse abdominal layer; a direct hernia comes through the posterior wall of the inguinal canal, and an indirect hernia comes through the internal inguinal ring. Femoral hernia occurs when the hernia sac is exposed as it exits the preperitoneal space through the femoral canal. Incisional hernias can occur after any abdominal incision, but they are most common after midline incisions. Factors leading to herniation are ischemia, wound infection, trauma, and inadequate suturing. Treatment is with herniorrhaphy.

2. Preoperative assessment

Predisposing factors for hernia often include increased abdominal pressure secondary to chronic cough, bladder outlet obstruction, constipation, pregnancy, vomiting, and acute or chronic muscular effort. The patient population may range from premature infants to elderly adults, with the possibility of various medical problems.

- a) History and physical examination: These are as indicated by the patient's condition.
  - (1) Musculoskeletal: Pain is likely in the area of the hernia; evaluate bony landmarks if regional anesthesia is planned.
  - (2) Hematologic: If regional anesthesia is planned, check the patient's coagulation status.
  - (3) Gastrointestinal: Hernias may become incarcerated, obstructed, or strangulated and can result in septicemia requiring emergency surgery. Fluid and electrolyte imbalance should be assessed.
- b) Patient preparation
  - (1) Laboratory tests: Complete blood count, electrolytes, and other tests as indicated by the history and physical examination
  - (2) Diagnostic tests: These are indicated by the history and physical examination.
  - (3) If necessary, use standard premedication.

3. Room preparation

- a) Monitoring equipment: Standard
  - (1) Standard anesthetic and emergency drugs
  - (2) Standard tabletop
  - (3) IV fluids: One 18-gauge IV line with normal saline or lactated Ringer's solution at 5 to 8 mL/kg/hr

4. Anesthetic technique

General, regional, and local anesthesia with sedation are all appropriate. The choice depends on such factors as site of incision, the patient's physical status, and the preference of both the patient and surgeon. General anesthesia may be preferred for incisions made above T8. Profound muscle relaxation may be needed for exploration and repair. If a laparoscopic approach is desired, general anesthesia and intubation are required.

5. Perioperative management

- a) Standard induction: General anesthesia by mask or laryngeal mask airway may be suitable for the patient with a simple chronic hernia. If there is obstruction, incarceration, or strangulation, rapid-sequence induction with endotracheal intubation is indicated. General endotracheal anesthesia is indicated in the patient with wound dehiscence.

b) Maintenance
   (1) Standard: Muscle relaxants may be necessary to facilitate surgical repair.
   (2) Position: While the patient is supine, pressure points should be checked and padded. Avoid stretching the brachial plexus. Limit abduction to 90 degrees.

c) Emergence: Consider extubating the trachea while the patient is still anesthetized to prevent coughing and straining. Patients who are at risk for pulmonary aspiration and who require awake extubation after rapid-sequence induction are not candidates for deep extubation.

6. Postoperative implications
   a) Wound dehiscence may occur with coughing or straining.
   b) Urinary retention: Patients with urinary retention may require intermittent catheterization until urinary function resumes.
   c) Pain management: Surgical field block or regional anesthesia should provide sufficient analgesia postoperatively.

K. LAPAROSCOPIC APPENDECTOMY

1. Introduction

Appendectomy is performed for acute appendicitis, and a laparoscopic approach is most commonly used.

2. Preoperative assessment and patient preparation
   a) History and physical examination
      (1) Gastrointestinal: Patients point to localized pain at McBurney point, which is midway between the iliac crest and umbilicus; rebound tenderness, muscle rigidity, and abdominal guarding are noted.
      (2) Pregnancy: Alder sign is used to differentiate between uterine and appendiceal pain. The pain is localized with the patient supine. The patient then lies on his or her left side. If the area of pain shifts to the left, it is presumed to be uterine.
   b) Diagnostic tests
      (1) The white blood cell count is elevated, with a shift to the left: 10,000 to 16,000 mm^3; 75% neutrophils. Increased body temperature may indicate ruptured appendix and septicemia.
      (2) Urinalysis shows a small number of erythrocytes and leukocytes.
      (3) Computed tomography and abdominal radiography are used.
      (4) Other laboratory tests include electrolytes, glucose, hemoglobin, and hematocrit. Perform tests as indicated from the history and physical examination. Vomiting will contribute to volume depletion and electrolyte abnormalities.
   c) Preoperative medication and IV therapy
      (1) An antibiotic is given for enteric anaerobic gram-negative bacilli.
      (2) A single 18-gauge IV catheter is used because the patient is dehydrated from fever, anorexia, and vomiting.

3. Room preparation
   a) Monitoring equipment
      (1) Standard
      (2) Fetal heart tone monitoring with pregnancy

b) Pharmacologic agents
    (1) Standard
    (2) For fetal safety, avoid teratogenic anesthetic during the first trimester.
c) Position
    (1) Supine
    (2) Left uterine displacement with pregnancy

4. Anesthetic technique

General anesthesia: Endotracheal intubation required

5. Perioperative management

a) IV rehydration is necessary
b) Induction
    (1) Use general anesthesia with rapid-sequence induction because patients may have a nasogastric tube or are considered to have a full stomach (emergency).
    (2) In the pregnant patient, special care should be taken to prevent aspiration pneumonitis.
c) Maintenance
    (1) No specific indications exist.
    (2) Muscle relaxation is necessary.
d) Emergence: Awake extubation secondary to rapid-sequence induction

6. Postoperative implications

None is reported

L. LAPAROSCOPIC CHOLECYSTECTOMY

1. Introduction

Laparoscopic cholecystectomy is a minimally invasive surgical procedure used in the treatment of gallstones and diseases of the gallbladder. The laparoscopic approach is contraindicated in uncorrectable coagulopathy, severe chronic obstructive pulmonary disease, and severe cardiac disease secondary to increased abdominal pressures.

2. Preoperative assessment and patient preparation

a) History and physical examination: These are as indicated by the patient's history and medical condition
b) Diagnostic tests: These are as indicated by the patient's history and medical condition.
c) Preoperative medication and IV therapy
    (1) Preoperative antibiotics are used.
    (2) Narcotics must be used with caution to minimize potential spasm in the biliary tract and sphincter of Oddi.
    (3) Use a single, large-bore (18-gauge) IV catheter for fluid replacement. Use a fluid warmer.
    (4) Administer prophylactic antiemetics and aspiration prophylaxis.

3. Room preparation

a) Monitoring equipment: Standard monitors
b) Pharmacologic agents: Standard
c) Position
    (1) Supine
    (2) Exposure of the operative site optimized with the reverse Trendelenburg position and by tilting the table to the left. Possible decrease in venous return, maintain adequate mean arterial pressure for cerebral perfusion.

4. Anesthetic technique

General endotracheal anesthesia with muscle relaxation

5. Perioperative management

a) Induction: Standard or rapid-sequence induction and endotracheal intubation with cricoid pressure is required.

b) Maintenance

(1) Muscle relaxation with appropriate reversal is used.

(2) The peritoneal cavity is insufflated for surgical exposure. Insufflation with carbon dioxide causes a rise in the carbon dioxide partial pressure.

(3) Controlled ventilation is required. Abdominal insufflation may lead to hypercarbia with inadequate ventilation. Special attention should be paid to possible adjustments in ventilator settings with insufflation and exsufflation.

(4) Basal measurements should be sufficient to control carbon dioxide partial pressure.

(5) Routine insufflation pressure is 15 mmHg (can decrease to 10–12 mmHg). Insufflation leads to increased intraabdominal pressure, increased afterload, and decreased preload. An intraabdominal pressure greater than 20 cm H_2O can decrease cardiac output, dramatically increase peak airway pressures, and cause hypotension. Insufflation to a pressure of approximately 15 mmHg is routine.

(6) All maintenance anesthetic drugs may be used. Avoid nitrous oxide secondary to bowel distention, which leads to decreased surgical exposure.

c) Complications include pneumoperitoneum hypercarbia, pneumothorax, pneumomediastinum, endobronchial intubation, decreased blood pressure, hemorrhage, dysrhythmias, visceral injury, hypothermia, and subcutaneous emphysema.

d) Emergence: Awake extubation is performed after the patient's airway reflexes are adequate.

6. Postoperative implications

a) Pain management: This approach offers the benefit of reduced postoperative pain secondary to smaller abdominal incisions. Patients may experience shoulder pain from the pneumoperitoneum, which is usually self-limiting. Use of IV narcotics, ketorolac or other NSAIDs are warranted.

b) Postoperative nausea and vomiting: Antiemetic prophylaxis is used.

M. LIVER RESECTION

1. Introduction

Patients presenting for hepatic surgery may have primary or metastatic tumors from gastrointestinal and other sources. Liver function may be entirely normal in these patients. Hepatocellular carcinoma is common in men older than 50 years and is associated with chronic, active hepatitis B and cirrhosis. Although most major liver resections can be performed by a transabdominal approach, some surgeons prefer a thoracoabdominal approach. The liver is transected by blunt dissection using the Cavitron ultrasonic suction aspirator and argon beam laser coagulator. Newer ablation devices include hydro jet and ultrasonic pulses.

As the principles and techniques of hepatic surgery have evolved, the overall mortality and morbidity rates have improved considerably. Because the normal liver can regenerate, it is possible to resect the right or left lobe along with segments of the contralateral lobe. In patients with cirrhosis, the regeneration process is limited; thus, uninvolved liver should be preserved.

2. Preoperative assessment

The following preoperative considerations are for patients without hepatic cirrhosis:

a) History and physical examination: These are as indicated by the patient's history and medical condition.

b) Patient preparation
   (1) Laboratory tests: Complete blood count, coagulation profile, liver function test, albumin, creatinine, blood urea nitrogen, blood sugar, bilirubin, and electrolytes are obtained. Perform other tests as indicated by the history and physical examination.
   (2) Diagnostic tests: Chest radiography, ultrasonography, computed tomography, and magnetic resonance imaging are used as indicated by the history and physical examination.
   (3) Medications: Standard premedication that accounts for the reduced ability of the liver to metabolize drugs is given. Other preoperative medications include antiemetics.

3. Room preparation

a) Monitoring equipment
   (1) Standard monitoring equipment
   (2) Arterial line and central venous pressure as clinically indicated

b) Additional equipment
   (1) Cell saver can be used for patients when malignancy is not a concern.
   (2) Possibly a rapid transfusion device

c) Drugs
   (1) Standard emergency drugs
   (2) Standard tabletop
   (3) IV fluids: 14- or 16-gauge IV lines (two) with normal saline at 10 to 20 mL/kg/hr; warmed fluids
   (4) Two units of packed red blood cells should be available. Blood loss can be significant, and massive transfusions may be required. Appropriate blood products also include 2 units of fresh-frozen plasma and 10 units of platelets.

4. Perioperative management and anesthetic technique

a) Induction
   (1) General endotracheal anesthesia with rapid sequence intubation is used.
   (2) Restore intravascular volume before anesthetic induction. If the patient is hemodynamically unstable, consider etomidate (0.2–0.4 mg/kg) or ketamine (1–3 mg/kg).

b) Maintenance
   (1) Standard
   (2) Combined epidural and general anesthesia: Be prepared to treat hypotension with fluid and vasopressors. General anesthesia is administered to supplement regional anesthesia and for amnesia. Coexisting coagulation abnormalities can increase the risk of epidural hematoma in these patients with preexisting coagulopathies.

(3) Position: The patient is supine, with checked and padded pressure points. Avoid stretching the brachial plexus. Limit abduction to 90 degrees.

c) Emergence

(1) For major hepatic resections, the patient is best cared for in an intensive care unit.

(2) Consider keeping the patient mechanically ventilated until the patient's condition is hemodynamically stable and ventilatory status is optimized.

(3) If surgical resection was minimal, the patient can be extubated awake and after reflexes have returned.

5. Postoperative implications

a) Decreased liver function: Patients with normal preoperative liver function may have significant postoperative impairment of liver function secondary to loss of liver mass or surgical trauma.

b) Pulmonary insufficiency (atelectasis, effusion, and pneumonia): More than 90% of patients will develop some form of respiratory complication.

c) Hemorrhage

d) Disseminated intravascular coagulation

e) Electrolyte imbalance

f) Hypoglycemia

g) Hypothermia

N. LIVER TRANSPLANTATION

1. Introduction

Liver transplantation is the treatment of choice for patients with acute and chronic end-stage liver disease. The liver transplant operation can be divided into three stages: (1) hepatectomy; (2) anhepatic phase, which involves the implantation of the liver; and (3) postrevascularization, which involves hemostasis and reconstruction of the hepatic artery and common bile duct. Hepatectomy can be associated with marked blood loss. Contributing factors include severe coagulopathy, severe portal hypertension, previous surgery in the right upper quadrant, renal failure, uncontrolled sepsis, retransplantation, transfusion reaction, venous bypass–induced fibrinolysis, primary graft nonfunction, and intraoperative vascular complications.

The anhepatic phase may be associated with significant hemodynamic changes. This stage consists of implantation of the liver allograft with or without venovenous bypass. Benefits of using the venovenous bypass system include improved hemodynamics during the anhepatic phase, decreased blood loss, and possible improvement of perioperative renal function. Complications of using the system include pulmonary embolism, air embolism, brachial plexus injury, and wound seroma or infection.

Before revascularization, the liver must be flushed with a cold solution (i.e., albumin 5%) through the portal vein and out the infrahepatic vena cava. The reperfusion of the liver may be the most critical part of the operation. Patients may experience pulmonary hypertension followed by right ventricular failure and profound hypotension. The hepatic artery reconstruction is performed after stabilization of the patient after revascularization. The last part involves hemostasis, removal of the gallbladder, and reconstruction of the bile duct.

2. Preoperative assessment

Patients requiring liver transplantation often have multiorgan system failure. Because of the emergency nature of the surgery, there may be insufficient time available for customary evaluation and correction of abnormalities.

a) History and physical examination
   (1) Cardiovascular: These patients can present with a hyperdynamic state, with increased cardiac output and decreased systemic vascular resistance. Many of these patients present with dysrhythmias, hypertension, pulmonary hypertension, valvular disease, cardiomyopathy (alcoholic disease, hemochromatosis, Wilson disease), and coronary artery disease.
   (2) Respiratory: Patients are often hypoxic because of ascites, pleural effusions, atelectasis, ventilation–perfusion mismatch, and pulmonary arteriovenous shunting. This normally results in tachypnea and respiratory alkalosis. Pulmonary infection usually is a contraindication to surgery. Adult respiratory distress syndrome usually is not.
   (3) Hepatic: Hepatitis serology and the cause of hepatic failure should be determined. Albumin is usually low, with consequent low plasma oncotic pressure leading to edema and ascites. The magnitude of action and duration of drugs may be unpredictable, although these patients generally have an increased sensitivity to all drugs, and the drug actions are prolonged.
   (4) Neurologic: Patients are often encephalopathic and may be in hepatic coma. In fulminant hepatic failure, increased intracranial pressure is common, accounting for 40% mortality (herniation), and may require prompt treatment (e.g., mannitol, hyperventilation).
   (5) Gastrointestinal: Portal hypertension, esophageal varices, and coagulopathies increase the risk of gastrointestinal hemorrhage. Gastric emptying is often delayed.
   (6) Renal: Patients are often hypervolemic, hyponatremic, and possibly hypokalemic. Calcium is usually normal. Metabolic alkalosis is often present. Preoperative dialysis should be considered.
   (7) Endocrine: Patients are often glucose intolerant or diabetic. Hyperaldosteronism may be present.
   (8) Hematologic: Patients are often anemic secondary to blood loss or malabsorption. Coagulation is impaired because of decreased hepatic synthesis function, abnormal fibrinogen production, impaired platelets, fibrinolysis, and low-grade disseminated intravascular coagulation.

b) Patient preparation
   (1) Laboratory tests: Complete blood count, coagulation profile, liver function tests, albumin, creatinine, blood urea nitrogen, blood sugar, bilirubin, and electrolytes are obtained. Perform other tests as indicated by the history and physical examination.
   (2) Diagnostic tests: Chest radiography, pulmonary function tests, electrocardiography, echocardiogram, and cardiac catheterization are obtained.
   (3) Medication: Standard premedication and aspiration prophylaxis are used, but the dose may be modified based on the patients preexisting mental and hemodynamic status.

3. Room preparation

a) Monitoring equipment
   (1) Standard
   (2) Arterial line, transesophageal echocardiography, central venous pressure, or pulmonary artery catheter as indicated

b) Additional equipment
   (1) Patient warming devices
   (2) Rapid infusion system
   (3) Blood warmers

c) Drugs
   (1) Standard tabletop
   (2) Standard emergency drugs
   (3) IV fluids: 14- to 16-gauge catheters (two), often placed in the right antecubital fossa or the left or right internal/external jugular. The left arm is avoided because the axillary vein is used for venovenous bypass.
   (4) Blood loss can be significant; blood should be immediately available.

4. Anesthetic technique

General anesthesia is used. These patients are challenging to manage during the various stages of the surgery. Hemodynamic instability, massive blood loss, electrolyte imbalance (hypocalcemia, hyperglycemia, hypernatremia, hyperkalemia), and coagulopathy may occur.

5. Perioperative management

a) Induction
   (1) Rapid-sequence induction with oral endotracheal tube is used.
   (2) May use a narcotic (fentanyl, 2–5 mcg/kg) just before induction.

b) Maintenance
   (1) Standard maintenance is with fentanyl, 10 to 50 mcg/kg, or an inhalation agent (or both) titrated according to individual patient response.
   (2) Antibiotics and immunosuppressants are given at the surgeon's request.
   (3) Position the patient supine and pad pressure points. Avoid stretching the brachial plexus greater than 90 degrees.
   (4) Reperfusion syndrome (which occurs during the revascularization phase) is characterized by decreased heart rate, hypotension, conduction defects, and decreased systemic vascular resistance while right ventricular pressures increase. The cause is unknown. Cardiac output can be maintained. An increase in serum potassium can lead to cardiac arrest.

6. Postoperative implications

a) Monitoring of hepatic function using laboratory data: Serial liver function tests, prothrombin time, partial thromboplastin time, ammonia levels, lactate, and bile output

b) Possible complications: Bleeding, portal vein thrombosis, hepatic artery thrombosis, biliary tract leaks, primary nonfunction, rejection, infection, pulmonary complications, electrolyte imbalances, hypertension, alkalosis, renal failure, peptic ulceration, and neurologic complications

O. PANCREATECTOMY

1. Introduction

Whereas distal pancreatectomy is performed for tumors in the distal half of the pancreas, subtotal pancreatectomy involves resection of the pancreas from the mesenteric vessels distally, leaving the head and uncinate process intact. In about 95% of patients with pancreatic cancer, the cancer is ductal adenocarcinoma, and most of these tumors occur in the head of the pancreas. Insulinoma is the most commonly occurring endocrine tumor of the pancreas.

Pancreatic cancer may appear as a localized mass or as a diffuse enlargement of the gland on computed tomography of the abdomen. Biopsy of the lesion is necessary to confirm the diagnosis. Complete surgical resection is the only effective treatment of ductal pancreatic cancer.

2. Preoperative assessment

Patients requiring pancreatic surgery can be divided into four groups: (1) those with acute pancreatitis in whom medical treatment has failed in the past, (2) patients with adenocarcinoma of the pancreas, (3) patients with neuroendocrine-active or -inactive islet cell tumors, and (4) patients with the sequelae of chronic pancreatitis (abscess or pseudocyst).

a) History and physical examination
   (1) Cardiovascular: Patients with acute pancreatitis may be hypotensive and may require aggressive volume resuscitation with crystalloid and even blood before surgery. Severe electrolyte disturbances may be associated with acute pancreatitis and some hormone-secreting tumors of the pancreas. Hypocalcemia is often present and can cause dysrhythmias and hypotension.
   (2) Respiratory: Respiratory compromise such as pleural effusions, atelectasis, and adult respiratory distress syndrome progressing to respiratory failure may occur in up to 50% of patients with acute pancreatitis.
   (3) Gastrointestinal: Jaundice and abdominal pain are common symptoms in this group of patients. The presence of ileus or intestinal obstruction should mandate full-stomach precautions and rapid-sequence induction. Electrolyte disturbances are common in acute pancreatitis and may include hypochloremic metabolic alkalosis, decreased calcium and magnesium, and increased glucose. These abnormalities should be corrected preoperatively.
   (4) Endocrine: Many patients with acute pancreatitis may have diabetes secondary to loss of pancreatic tissue. Hormone-secreting tumors of the pancreas are occasionally associated with multiple endocrine neoplasia syndromes. Insulinoma is the most common hormone-secreting tumor of the pancreas and can result in hypoglycemia.
   (5) Renal: Patients should be evaluated for renal insufficiency.
   (6) Hematologic: Hematocrit may be falsely elevated because of hemoconcentration or hemorrhage. Coagulopathy, including disseminated intravascular coagulation, may occur.

b) Patient preparation
   (1) Laboratory tests: Complete blood count, prothrombin time, partial thromboplastin time, platelet count, electrolytes, blood

urea nitrogen, creatinine, blood sugar, calcium, magnesium, amylase, and urinalysis, as well as other tests as indicated by the history and physical examination

(2) Diagnostic tests: Chest radiography, pulmonary function tests, electrocardiography, and computed tomography of the abdomen, as well as other tests as indicated by the history and physical examination

(3) Medication: Standard premedication with consideration for aspiration prophylaxis

3. **Room preparation**
   a) Standard monitoring equipment
   b) Arterial line, central venous pressure, or pulmonary artery catheter: As clinically indicated
   c) Additional equipment: Patient warming devices
   d) Drugs
      (1) Standard emergency drugs
      (2) Standard tabletop
      (3) IV fluids: 14- to 16-gauge IV lines (two) with normal saline or lactated Ringer solution at 10 to 20 mL/kg/hr; warmed fluids
      (4) Blood loss possibly significant; blood should be immediately available

4. **Perioperative management and anesthetic technique**

General endotracheal anesthesia is used; consider an epidural technique for postoperative analgesia.

   a) Induction
      (1) This is standard, with consideration of rapid-sequence intubation as indicated.
      (2) Restore intravascular volume before anesthetic induction.
      (3) If the patient is hemodynamically unstable, consider etomidate (0.2–0.4 mg/kg) or ketamine (1–3 mg/kg).
   b) Maintenance
      (1) Standard maintenance: This involves a narcotic, inhalation agent, or both.
      (2) Avoid nitrous oxide to minimize bowel distention.
      (3) Combined epidural and general anesthesia: Be prepared to treat hypotension with fluid and vasopressors.
      (4) Titrate epidural anesthesia as indicated by patient's response.
      (5) General anesthesia is administered to supplement regional anesthesia and for amnesia. If a patient is not a candidate for epidural, low-dose ketamine infusion is an option. Also, gabapentin 600 to 1200 mg orally once before surgery can decrease post pain.
      (6) Position: The patient is supine, with checked and padded pressure points. Avoid stretching the brachial plexus. Limit abduction to 90 degrees.
      (7) If patient has insulinoma, the most common endocrine tumor of the pancreas, anticipate potential uncontrolled insulin release.
   c) Emergence: The decision to extubate at the end of the operation depends on the patient's underlying cardiopulmonary status and the extent of the surgical procedure. Patients should be hemodynamically stable, warm, alert, cooperative, and fully reversed from any muscle relaxants before extubation.

5. Postoperative implications

Significant third-space and evaporative losses contribute to hypovolemia. Major hemorrhage can occur during dissection of the pancreas from the mesenteric and portal vessels. Total pancreatectomy is associated with diabetes that can be difficult to control. Subtotal resections lead to varying degrees of hyperglycemia. The patient should recover in an intensive care unit or hospital ward accustomed to treating the side effects of epidural opiates.

Tests for postoperative management include electrolytes, calcium, glucose, complete blood count, platelets, and other tests as indicated. Electrolyte disturbances are common in acute pancreatitis and may include hypochloremic metabolic alkalosis, decreased calcium and magnesium, and increased glucose. These abnormalities should be corrected preoperatively.

P. SMALL BOWEL RESECTION

1. Introduction

Small bowel resection is performed for various diseases, including intestinal obstruction, small bowel tumors, abdominal trauma, stricture, adhesions, Meckel's diverticulum, Crohn's disease, and infection.

2. Preoperative assessment and patient preparation

a) History and physical examination: Assess fluid and hydration status. The patient may be vomiting or bleeding or may have third spacing, diarrhea, dehydration, or sepsis.

b) Diagnostic laboratory tests should include a complete blood count, electrolyte panel, coagulation panel

c) Preoperative medication and IV therapy

(1) Patients may be receiving steroid therapy or immunosuppressant drugs.

(2) Expect fluid shifts requiring moderate to large fluid resuscitation. Two large-bore IV access lines are indicated.

(3) Preoperative hydration is essential.

3. Room preparation

a) Monitoring equipment: Standard with full warming modalities

b) Pharmacologic agents: Standard

c) Position: Supine with arms extended

4. Anesthetic technique

a) Epidural (T2–T4 level) with a "light" general anesthetic

b) General anesthesia with an endotracheal tube is necessary for small bowel resections that use a laparoscopic-assisted approach.

5. Perioperative management

a) Induction: Most patients are considered to have full stomachs; therefore, rapid-sequence induction is indicated. Medications used for aspiration prophylaxis should be administered.

b) Maintenance

(1) Muscle relaxation is required.

(2) Closely monitor hydration status and blood loss; anticipate large fluid shifts.

(3) Avoid nitrous oxide, which may cause bowel distention.

c) Emergence: Awake extubation is performed after rapid-sequence induction or placement of a nasogastric tube.

6. **Postoperative implications**
   a) Pain may lead to hypoventilation, reduced cough, splinting, and atelectasis.
   b) Pain control is with epidural or patient-controlled analgesia.

Q. SPLENECTOMY

1. **Introduction**

Patients presenting for splenectomy can be divided into two groups: trauma patients and patients with myeloproliferative disorders and other varieties of hypersplenism. Anesthetic management is individualized based on the individual patient's medical condition. Patients who have received chemotherapy must be assessed for potential organ system complications. Laparoscopic-assisted splenectomy best suited for normal and slightly enlarged spleens. The laparoscopic approach is unusually contraindicated in patients with cancer, large hilar lymph nodes, and portal hypertension. The only absolute contraindication to laparoscopic splenectomy is massive splenomegaly (spleen >30 in longitudinal axis).

2. **Preoperative assessment**
   a) History and physical examination
      (1) Cardiovascular: Patients with systemic disease may be chronically ill and have decreased cardiovascular reserve. Patients who have received doxorubicin (Adriamycin) may have a dose-dependent cardiotoxicity that can be worsened by radiation therapy. Manifestations include decreased QRS amplitude, congestive heart failure, pleural effusions, and dysrhythmia.
      (2) Respiratory: Patients may have a degree of left lower lobe atelectasis and altered ventilation. If they are treated with bleomycin, pulmonary fibrosis may occur. Methotrexate, busulfan, mitomycin, cytarabine, and other chemotherapeutic agents may cause pulmonary toxicity. A laparoscopic approach may be contraindicated in patients with severe cardiac or respiratory disease.
      (3) Neurologic: Patients may have neurologic deficits after taking chemotherapeutic agents. Vinblastine and cisplatin can cause peripheral neuropathies. Any evidence of neurologic dysfunction should be documented.
      (4) Hematologic: Patients are likely to have splenomegaly secondary to hematologic disease (Hodgkin's disease, leukemia). Cytopenias are common.
      (5) Hepatic: Some chemotherapeutic agents (methotrexate, 6-mercaptopurine) may be hepatotoxic. Evaluation of liver function tests should be considered in patients considered at risk.
      (6) Renal: Some chemotherapeutic drugs (methotrexate, cisplatin) are nephrotoxic. Patients exposed to such agents may have renal insufficiency.
   b) Patient preparation
      (1) Laboratory tests: Complete blood count, prothrombin time, partial thromboplastin time, bleeding time, platelet count, electrolytes, blood urea nitrogen, creatinine, urinalysis, and other tests are obtained as indicated by the history and physical examination. A type and screen should be obtained due to the potential for major blood loss.

(2) Medication: Standard premedication. Consider aspiration prophylaxis. Administer steroids (25–100 mg hydrocortisone) if the patient has received them as part of a chemotherapeutic or medical treatment.

3. **Room preparation**
   a) Monitoring equipment: Standard and others as indicated by the patient's status
   b) Additional equipment: Patient warming device
   c) Drugs
      (1) Standard emergency drugs
      (2) Standard tabletop
      (3) IV fluids: 16- to 18-gauge IV lines (two) with normal saline or lactated Ringer solution at 10 to 15 mL/kg/hr; warmed fluids

4. **Anesthetic technique**

General endotracheal anesthesia with or without an epidural for postoperative analgesia is used.

5. **Perioperative management**
   a) Induction
      (1) This is standard, with consideration of rapid-sequence intubation as indicated.
      (2) Restore intravascular volume before anesthetic induction. If the patient is hemodynamically unstable, consider etomidate or ketamine.
   b) Maintenance
      (1) Standard regimens are used; if bleomycin has been administered as part of the chemotherapeutic treatment, an oxygen concentration above 30% is indicated to decrease the potential for acute lung injury.
      (2) Combined epidural and general anesthesia: See the earlier discussion of pancreatectomy.
      (3) Position: The patient is supine, with checked and padded pressure points. Avoid stretching the brachial plexus. Limit abduction to 90 degrees. For the laparoscopic approach, the patient should be on a beanbag in 45-degree lateral decubitus position and full lateral decubitus position.
   c) Emergence: The decision to extubate at the end of the operation depends on the patient's underlying cardiopulmonary status and the extent of the surgical procedure. Patients should be hemodynamically stable, warm, alert, cooperative, and fully reversed from any muscle relaxants before extubation.

6. **Postoperative implications**
   a) Bleeding
   b) Atelectasis, usually in the left lower lobe
   c) Pain management: Multimodal approach with epidural local anesthetics, patient-controlled analgesia, or opiates (or a combination of these)

R. WHIPPLE RESECTION

1. **Introduction**

Whipple resection consists of a pancreatoduodenectomy, pancreatojejunostomy, hepaticojejunostomy, and gastrojejunostomy. On entering the peritoneal cavity, the surgeon determines the resectability of the pancreatic lesion. Contraindications to resection include involvement of mesenteric vessels, infiltration by tumor into the root of the mesentery, extension into the porta hepatis with involvement of the hepatic artery, and liver metastasis. If the tumor is deemed resectable, the head of the pancreas is further mobilized. The common duct is transected above the cystic duct entry, and the gallbladder is removed. When the superior mesenteric vein is freed from the pancreas, the latter is transected with care taken not to injure the splenic vein. The jejunum is transected beyond the ligament of Treitz, and the specimen is removed by severing the vascular connections with the mesenteric vessels. Reconstitution is achieved by anastomosing the distal pancreatic stump, bile duct, and stomach into the jejunum. Drains are placed adjacent to the pancreatic anastomosis. Some surgeons stent the anastomosis until it has healed.

2. **Preoperative assessment**
   a) History and physical examination: See the earlier discussion of pancreatectomy.
   b) Patient preparation
      (1) Laboratory tests: See the earlier discussion of pancreatectomy.
      (2) Diagnostic tests: See the earlier discussion of pancreatectomy.
      (3) Medication: See the earlier discussion of pancreatectomy.

3. **Room preparation**

See the earlier discussion of pancreatectomy.

4. **Anesthetic technique**

General endotracheal anesthesia with an epidural for postoperative analgesia is used. See the earlier discussion of pancreatectomy.

5. **Perioperative management**

See the earlier discussion of pancreatectomy.

6. **Postoperative implications**

See the earlier discussion of pancreatectomy.

Genitourinary System

A. CYSTECTOMY

1. Introduction

The bladder is usually removed for cancer but may also be removed for severe hemorrhagic or radiation cystitis. In a radical cystectomy for invasive cancer in women, the uterus, fallopian tubes, ovaries, and a portion of the vaginal wall are removed. In men, the ampulla of the vas deferens, prostate, and seminal vesicles are removed. There is also pelvic lymph node dissection, and a urinary diversion is created (through the intestine).

2. Preoperative assessment

a) Cardiac, respiratory, neurologic, and endocrine systems: Assessment is routine.
b) Renal: Gross hematuria may be a symptom. Check renal function tests as well as evidence of a urinary tract infection.
c) Gastrointestinal: Patients are at risk for fluid and electrolyte imbalance because of bowel preparation.

3. Patient preparation

a) Laboratory tests: Complete blood count, electrolytes, blood urea nitrogen, creatinine, glucose, prothrombin time, partial thromboplastin time, type and screen for 2 to 4 units of blood, and urinalysis
b) Diagnostic tests: Electrocardiography and chest radiography for most of this patient population
c) Medication: Sedation as needed

4. Room preparation

a) Monitors: Standard, arterial line, and central venous pressure; urine output not measurable during this procedure; two large-bore, reliable intravenous (IV) lines available
b) Additional equipment: Epidural insertion and infusion supplies (if using), and warming devices for the patient and fluids
c) Position: Supine
d) Drugs and fluids: 6 to 10 mL/kg/hr of crystalloid for maintenance; 2 to 4 units of blood readily available

5. Perioperative management

Combined general and epidural or general anesthesia with standard induction is used. The patient may be anemic because of hematuria and hypovolemic because of bowel preparation. Attempt to correct these conditions before induction. Maintenance is routine, with special attention paid to fluid calculations and keeping the patient warm. Plan to extubate immediately postoperatively unless the patient is unstable during the procedure or when prior respiratory complications prevent early extubation.

6. Postoperative implications

Epidural or patient-controlled analgesia should be planned for preoperative use. Watch the patient for signs of hypovolemia, anemia, or pulmonary edema resulting from fluid shifts intraoperatively.

B. CYSTOSCOPY

1. Introduction

Cystoscopy is the use of instrumentation to examine the urinary tract. A cystoscope may be used for diagnostic or therapeutic procedures such as for workup of hematuria, stricture, and tumor; removal and manipulation of stones; placement of stents; and follow-up of therapy. Retrograde pyelography and other dye studies may be used. This procedure is usually performed on an outpatient basis.

2. Preoperative assessment and patient preparation

a) History and physical examination: Standard
b) Diagnostic tests: Standard
c) Preoperative medication and IV therapy
 (1) Prophylactic antibiotics
 (2) 18-gauge IV catheter with minimal fluid replacement

3. Room preparation

a) Monitoring equipment: Standard
b) Pharmacologic agents: Indigo carmine, methylene blue
c) Position: Lithotomy

4. Anesthetic technique

The technique of choice is regional blockade or general anesthesia.

a) IV sedation: Midazolam (Versed), fentanyl, or propofol in sedation doses
b) Regional blockade: Analgesia to J10 required
c) General anesthesia: Laryngeal mask airway or oral endotracheal tube

5. Preoperative management

a) Induction: No specific indications
b) Maintenance
 (1) Diagnostic dyes may be administered. Use indigo carmine dye (α-sympathomimetic effects) cautiously in patients with hypertension or cardiac ischemia. Methylene blue dye may cause hypertension. Oxygen saturation readings may be altered by dye administration.
 (2) Persistent erection may occur in younger male patients, thus preventing manipulation of the cystoscope. Use deeper anesthesia.
 (3) Water or irrigation solution may be used to distend the bladder. See the discussion of transurethral resection of the prostate later in this section.
 (4) Quadriplegic or paraplegic patients may undergo repeated cystoscopies. Autonomic hyperreflexia is possible if the injury is above level T5.
c) Emergence: No specific indications

6. Postoperative implications

Postoperative care is standard.

C. EXTRACORPOREAL SHOCK WAVE LITHOTRIPSY

1. Introduction

Extracorporeal shock-wave lithotripsy (ESWL) is a technique that uses high-energy shock waves to fragment renal calculi into small particles. A biplanar fluoroscopy unit is used to focus the shock wave on the target stone. The shock wave is repeated several thousand times and causes the stone to disintegrate. The focused, reflected shock wave passes through the water and enters the body through the flank.

Modern lithotriptors do not require the patient to be submerged in water. Although they do use water for the production of shock waves, a membrane over the shock-wave generator encapsulates the fluid. Transmission of shock waves to the patient is ensured by the use of coupling gel between the patient and the generator membrane.

2. **Preoperative assessment and patient preparation**
   a) Routine preoperative assessment with laboratory tests based on any abnormalities found in the history and physical examination. Consider cardiac status; many hemodynamic changes are associated with this procedure.
   b) Absolute contraindications are pregnancy bleeding disorders and abnormal coagulation parameters. Relative contraindications include these active urinary tract infection and a urinary tract obstruction distal to the stone that prevents passage of stone fragments.
   c) Relative contraindications include aortic aneurysm, spinal tumors, orthopedic implants in the lumbar region, morbid obesity, AILD (automatic implantable cardioverter-defibrillator), uncontrolled arrhythmias, and coagulation disorders.
   d) Ureteral stent placement before ESWL may be used to move the stone upward in the ureter, where it is amenable to therapy.
   e) Adequate IV hydration aids in the passage of stone fragments.
   f) Prophylactic antibiotics may be given.
   g) Electrocardiography, automated cuff measurement of blood pressure, and pulse oximetry are indispensable during lithotripsy.
   h) The electrocardiograph must be of good quality because the R wave is used to trigger the shocks. Synchronization of the shock wave to the electrocardiograph has reduced the incidence of cardiac dysrhythmias but has not totally eliminated them. These dysrhythmias are attributed to mechanical stimulation of the heart. Supraventricular premature complexes and premature ventricular complexes are the most common dysrhythmias noted. Atropine or glycopyrrolate may be given to increase the heart rate and thus the shock-wave rate.
3. **Anesthetic technique**
   a) Patient movement: For lithotripsy to be most effective, the stone must remain at the focal point. Because patient movement and patterns of respiration can change kidney and stone position, movement must be minimized and ventilation carefully controlled. The number and intensity of shock waves can be reduced when stone movement is minimized.
   b) Anesthetic techniques: Various anesthetic techniques have been used for ESWL. General anesthesia is advantageous because of its rapid onset and control of patient movement. Other techniques include spinal or epidural anesthesia, patient-controlled analgesia, monitored anesthesia care, and topical anesthesia with eutectic local anesthetics. Continuous infusions of propofol, methohexital, ketamine, and alfentanil have been used alone or with midazolam for ESWL anesthesia.

Spinal anesthesia has the advantage of a rapid onset, and a pure opiate spinal using sufentanil is a common technique. Disadvantages include hypotension, spinal headache, and the inability to reinforce the block.

Although epidural anesthesia is associated with a slower onset, hypotension is less, and the block can be reinforced as needed. A dermatomal level of T4 or T6 must be achieved as renal innervation is derived from T10 to L2.

c) Side effects associated with ESWL
   (1) Hypothermia, hyperthermia
   (2) Cardiac dysrhythmias
   (3) Hemorrhagic blisters of skin
   (4) Renal edema
   (5) Renal hematoma
   (6) Lung injury
   (7) Flank pain
   (8) Hypertension, hypotension
   (9) Autonomic hyperreflexia
   (10) Nausea, vomiting
   (11) Hematuria
   (12) External petechia

D. LAPAROSCOPIC NEPHRECTOMY

1. Introduction

Indications for nephrectomy include calculus, hemorrhage, hydronephrosis, hypertension, neoplasms, transplantation, trauma, chronic infection, and vascular disease. Partial nephrectomy is performed to preserve as much renal function as possible. Surgery of the kidney is usually accomplished through a flank incision.

2. Preoperative assessment and patient preparation

a) History and physical examination: Individualized for the patient's condition
b) Diagnostic tests
   (1) IV pyelography with nephrotomography: Identify a renal mass.
   (2) Ultrasonography: This differentiates simple cysts from solid tumors.
   (3) Arteriography: This determines whether the kidney is suitable for renal transplantation.
   (4) Computed tomography
   (5) Laboratory tests
      (a) Prothrombin time, partial thromboplastin time, complete blood count, electrolytes, and glucose
      (b) Glomerular filtration rate: Blood urea nitrogen, plasma creatinine, and creatinine clearance
      (c) Renal tubular function: Urine concentration ability, sodium secretion, proteinuria, hematuria urine sediment, and urine volume
c) Preoperative medications and IV therapy
   (1) Identify the date of last hemodialysis.
   (2) Epidural catheter: Perform a test dose in the preoperative area.
   (3) Administer antibiotics.

(4) Use small incremental doses of benzodiazepines to facilitate anxiolysis.
(5) Have a minimum of two peripheral IV tubes (16 to 18 gauge) with moderate fluid replacement.
(6) In patients with renal failure, administer hypotonic solutions: 5% dextrose in water or 5% dextrose and 0.45% saline.
(a) Avoid normal saline: It may increase sodium levels.
(b) Avoid plasmalyte or lactated Ringer's solution: It may increase potassium levels.
(c) Restrict fluids and consider using microdrip tubing.

3. **Room preparation**
a) Monitoring equipment
(1) Standard
(2) An arterial line and central venous pressure monitoring may be necessary to trend volume status, especially if the patient is elderly with coexisting medical disease.
(3) A noninvasive blood pressure cuff should not be placed in an arm with an arteriovenous fistula.
b) Pharmacologic agents
(1) Dopamine: Low dose (2–5 mcg/kg/min) to increase urinary output
(2) Furosemide (Lasix), mannitol, or both for stimulation of urinary output
(3) Indigo carmine (hypertension resulting from an α-agonist) or methylene blue (hypotension and interference with the pulse oximeter) administration (IV to assess urinary flow)
(4) Hetastarch (Hespan) or albumin
(5) Heparin and protamine with donor kidneys
c) Position
(1) A lateral decubitus position is used, with the kidney bar raised.
(2) With low calcium levels, skin and nerve damage occur easily.
(3) Inadequate support of the head may lead to Horner syndrome (ptosis, enophthalmos, miosis, and anhidrosis) postoperatively.
(4) Evaluate the radial pulse after placement of an axillary roll.
(5) Respiration is impaired secondary to ventilation–perfusion mismatching, decreased functional reserve capacity, decreased vital capacity, and decreased thoracic compliance.
(6) Reassess breath sounds after movement; an endotracheal tube may migrate into the mainstem bronchus during positioning.

4. **Anesthetic technique**
a) See the discussion of radical prostatectomy later in this section.
b) Consider rapid-sequence induction because renal patients may be considered to have a full stomach.

5. **Perioperative management**
a) Induction
(1) Opioids can be used because only a small amount of the drug is excreted unchanged by the kidneys.
(2) Succinylcholine is contraindicated if the potassium is elevated.
(3) Cisatracurium does not require a functional kidney because it is degraded by Hofmann elimination and is a good choice for muscle relaxation. Laudanosine is a metabolite and is associated with seizures. This is not a concern with short-term perioperative use.

(4) Vecuronium and rocuronium may be used for muscle relaxation.
(5) Regardless of blood volume status, renal patients may respond to induction of anesthesia as if they are hypovolemic.
(6) Induction of anesthesia and intubation of the trachea can be safely accomplished with IV drugs plus a nondepolarizing muscle relaxant.
(7) Propofol is highly protein bound, and this may necessitate a reduced dosage. Propofol is exclusively metabolized by the liver, and metabolites are inactive.
(8) Ketamine is less protein bound with less than 3% renal excretion.
(9) Etomidate is 75% protein bound and does not require adjustment.

b) Maintenance
(1) Maintain normal end-tidal carbon dioxide levels.
(2) If working on a donor nephrectomy, the eleventh rib may be removed; pneumothorax is a complication; therefore, nitrous oxide is best avoided.
(3) Maintain urinary output; use medications if necessary.
(4) Inhalation anesthetic is used to control intraoperative hypertension.

c) Emergence
(1) If hypertension occurs on emergence, administer a vasodilator.
(2) Renal patients are considered to have a full stomach; some practitioners require an "awake" patient before extubation.
(3) Initiate regional blockade through the epidural catheter for postoperative analgesia before the end of the case.

6. **Postoperative implications**
a) Continue to assess volume status.
b) Obtain a chest film. Rule out pulmonary edema and pneumothorax, which may occur after administration of large volumes of fluid in the flank position or from removal of the eleventh rib, respectively.
c) For patients with renal failure, normeperidine, the major metabolite of meperidine, may accumulate and result in prolonged depression of ventilation and seizures.

E. LAPAROSCOPIC UROLOGIC SURGERY

1. **Introduction**

Laparoscopy is the process of inspecting the abdominal cavity through an endoscope. Some examples of surgical procedures that can be done laparoscopically include varicocelectomy, percutaneous stone retrieval, nephrectomy, transplants, and radical prostatectomy.

2. **Anesthetic technique**

Carbon dioxide is used to insufflate the abdominal cavity to facilitate view during this procedure. Several pathophysiologic changes can occur after carbon dioxide pneumoperitoneum and extremes of patient positioning required for the procedure.

Unique problems specific to urologic surgery are listed below.

a) The urogenital system is a retroperitoneal system. As such, carbon dioxide insufflated in this space communicates freely with the thorax and subcutaneous tissue. Subcutaneous emphysema can occur and may extend to the head and neck. In severe cases, it may lead to submucous swelling and airway compromise in the unprotected airway.
b) In long cases, carbon dioxide may not be reabsorbed and acidosis may develop. Because carbon dioxide insufflation coupled with steep Trendelenburg position and long procedures may increase intraabdominal and intrathoracic pressure, controlled ventilation is mandatory.
c) Increased pressure exerted by the insufflation may also affect renal and hepatic function. The pneumoperitoneum can cause renal cortical vasoconstriction because of activation of the sympathetic nervous system. Decreased renal perfusion activates the renin–angiotensin–aldosterone system, which causes vasoconstriction. These effects are additive to those seen with surgical stress. Renal and hepatic perfusion may be altered.
d) Some suggestions to minimize the impact of positive pressure pneumoperitoneum are (1) lowering insufflation pressures, (2) operating in a gasless environment, (3) substituting inert gas for carbon dioxide, (4) using drugs to antagonize the neuroendocrine response, (5) volume expansion, and (6) using mechanical devices. It has been reported that the use of intermittent sequential pneumatic compression activated over the lower limbs 15 minutes after the pneumoperitoneum improves splanchnic and renal perfusion. This technique augments cardiac output and lowers systemic vascular resistance.

F. PENILE PROCEDURES

1. Introduction

Penile procedures are commonly performed for the following three indications: (1) to repair congenital defects such as hypospadias (typically a pediatric procedure), which is usually a pediatric procedure; (2) for penectomy or penile resection as a result of penile cancer; and (3) for implants to compensate for impotence. Organic impotence is often secondary to diabetes, hypertension or side effects from the systemic treatments or spinal cord trauma.

2. Preoperative assessment

Assessment is individualized based on the patient's condition.

3. Patient preparation

a) Standard preoperative laboratory testing is as indicated.
b) Preoperative medications are individualized.

4. Room preparation

a) Monitoring: Standard
b) Position: Supine
c) Drugs and tabletop: Adult or pediatric setup

5. Anesthetic technique and perioperative management

a) For pediatric patients, an inhalation induction is typical for general anesthesia. Intubation is often desired because hypospadias repair generally takes longer than 2 hours.

b) For penectomy or prosthetic insertion, a regional or general anesthetic may be used, depending on the preferences of the patient, and presence of comorbidities medical condition. Muscle relaxation is not required, and blood loss is minimal.
c) Some practitioners perform a caudal block for pediatric patients just before awakening for postoperative pain control.

6. Postoperative implications

Urinary retention is common and may be intensified with the use of a regional anesthetic.

G. PERCUTANEOUS NEPHROLITHOTOMY

1. Introduction

Removal of kidney stones 25 mm or smaller can also be accomplished through percutaneous nephrolithotomy. This procedure requires general anesthesia and postoperative hospitalization. Stones are removed via a rigid operating scope inserted in the lower calyx of the kidney under fluoroscopy. After being located, calculi are pulverized using laser, electrohydraulic, or ultrasound probes placed directly on the stones. The procedure is performed with the patient in the prone position; therefore, associated anesthetic considerations apply.

H. RADICAL PROSTATECTOMY

1. Introduction

Open prostatectomy refers to removal of the prostate with or without the prostatic capsule. Several surgical approaches may be used, including suprapubic, transvesical, retropubic, perineal, and transcoccygeal. In suprapubic or transvesical procedures, the prostate is removed through the cavity of the bladder. Retropubic prostatectomy is performed through a low abdominal incision without opening the bladder. The transcoccygeal approach allows maximal surgical access to the posterior lobes of the prostate. Perineal prostatectomy is most often performed for cancer of the prostate when it is confined to the capsule. This procedure may also be done with the assistance of a robot.

2. Preoperative assessment and patient preparation

a) History and physical examination: These are individualized based on the patient's condition; assess for symptoms of metastatic disease.
b) Diagnostic tests
   (1) Plasma concentration of prostate-specific antigen is increased in prostate cancer.
   (2) Blood urea nitrogen, creatinine, electrolytes, complete blood count, coagulation profile, and type and cross-match are obtained.
   (3) Ultrasonography is used.
c) Preoperative medication and IV therapy
   (1) Bowel preparation will render the patient in a dehydrated state.
   (2) Have a minimum of two peripheral IV lines (18 and 16 gauge) with moderate fluid replacement.
   (3) Epidural catheter: Perform a test dose in the preoperative area.

(4) Administer antibiotics.
(5) Small incremental doses of benzodiazepines may be given to ease patient preparation.

3. Room preparation

a) Monitoring equipment
(1) Standard
(2) Arterial line and central venous pressure monitoring may be necessary to trend volume status, especially if the patient is elderly with coexisting medical diseases. Central venous pressure monitoring may also be indicated for potential of venous air embolism related to positioning of the patient.
(3) Warming modalities are used.

b) Pharmacologic agents
(1) Although controversial, low-dose dopamine (2 to 5 mcg/kg/min) may be initiated to increase urinary output.
(2) Hetastarch (Hespan) and albumin

c) Position: Supine; the surgeon may request use of kidney rest and for the patient's body to be partially flexed. Expect the need to rotate the patient from side to side for optimal surgical viewing.

4. Anesthetic technique

a) Regional blockade, general anesthesia, or a combination of both
b) Technique of choice: General anesthesia with endotracheal intubation
c) Regional blockade: Epidural catheter placement in preoperative area; analgesia to T6 to T8
d) General anesthesia: Endotracheal intubation
e) Regional blockade with general anesthesia: Smaller doses of each with the combination technique

5. Perioperative management

a) Induction: The patient may be dehydrated and show an exaggerated response to medications.

b) Maintenance
(1) Initiate warming modality and use fluid warmers.
(2) Position
(a) Radical retropubic: Supine with the operating room table broken in the midline or kidney rest to provide slight hyperextension; a slight Trendelenburg position until the patient's legs are parallel to the floor
(b) Radical perianal: Exaggerated lithotomy position combined with flexion of the trunk and a Trendelenburg tilt
(3) The Foley catheter is discontinued during the case, and volume status (blood loss) is difficult to quantify.
(4) Muscle relaxation is necessary.
(5) Methylene blue or indigo carmine is administered after reanastomosis of the urethras. A momentary and artificial decrease in the pulse oximetry reading will occur.

c) Emergence
(1) Initiate regional blockade through the epidural catheter for postoperative analgesia before the end of the case.
(2) Base extubation on the patient's general health, amount of blood loss, and overall status after the procedure.
(3) An awake or deep extubation may be appropriate.

6. **Postoperative implications**
   a) Obtain hemoglobin and hematocrit.
   b) Continue to trend volume status.
   c) For postoperative pain management, consider patient-controlled analgesia, epidural techniques, or a combination of ketorolac and opiates.
   d) Early postoperative complications include deep venous thrombosis, pulmonary embolus, and wound infection.
   e) Late complications include incontinence, impotence, and bladder neck contracture.
   f) Rhabdomyolysis is seen with the extreme lithotomy position and may progress to acute renal failure. Monitor urine output and maintain at more than 0.5 mL/kg/hr.

I. RENAL TRANSPLANT

1. **Introduction**

Renal transplantation has been performed for nearly a century and is an accepted means of replacing kidney function in patients with end-stage renal disease who are on maintenance dialysis. In this procedure, the donor kidney is placed extraperitoneally in the recipient's iliac fossa. The renal artery is anastomosed to the internal iliac artery, the renal vein to either the external or the common iliac vein and the ureter to the bladder. The anesthesia provider plays a vital role in management of the viability of the transplanted kidney. Three interrelated variables affect surgical outcomes: management of the donor, preservation of the harvested organ, and perioperative care of the transplant recipient. Additionally, improved surgical and immunosuppressive techniques have contributed to better outcomes in terms of graft survival.

2. **Preoperative assessment and patient preparation**
   a) Harvested organ preservation
      (1) Ischemic time, beginning with the clamping of the donor's renal vessels and ending with the vascular anastomosis in the recipient, is a crucial factor in graft preservation. When renal ischemic time is less than 30 minutes, diuresis begins quickly, but if it is 2 hours or longer, a variable period of oliguria or anuria may occur. The definition of renal ischemic times for warm and cold preservation techniques is noted in the following table.

Definition of Ischemic Time

	Warm	Cold
Begins	Clamping of donor vessels; initial placement in recipient	Perfusion of harvested organ with cold preservation solution; storage at 4° C
Ends	Vascular anastomosis in recipient; interrupted with perfusion of cold preservation solution	Perfusion by recipient

b) Donor preparation
   (1) Choice of anesthesia for the living, related donor is not critical.
   (2) Adequate amounts of balanced salt solution should be administered to ensure a brisk diuresis from the donor kidney and to offset reduced venous return resulting from use of the flank position.
   (3) The greatest risk to the donor is hemorrhage.
   (4) Adequate IV access and blood must be available in the event that transfusion becomes necessary.
   (5) If the donor kidney is obtained from a brain-dead patient, preservation of graft function is the highest priority. The loss of sympathetic tone after brain death may produce mild hypotension despite adequate volume replacement. Many patients with irreversible cerebral dysfunction are hypovolemic and require vigorous fluid resuscitation.
   (6) If pharmacologic support of the cardiovascular system is necessary, a dopamine infusion at a rate of 1 to 3 mcg/kg/min is recommended. Renal vasoconstrictive properties of high-dose vasopressors reduce immediate allograft function and increase the risk of kidney damage. Maintenance of urinary output is paramount and may warrant the use of diuretics and a low-dose dopamine infusion.

c) Recipient preparation
   (1) Because cadaveric kidneys can be preserved for 36 to 48 hours with cold perfusion, time is sufficient for optimal preparation of the transplant recipient.
   (2) The recipient should be free of acute illness and infections because of the likelihood of their spread during immunosuppressive therapy.
   (3) Acute alterations in fluid and electrolyte balance should be corrected with dialysis carried out 24 hours before transplantation. Postdialysis laboratory values should be checked, and the serum potassium (K^+) level should be below 5.5 mEq/L. Coagulation studies and acid–base status should be normal. Serum creatinine concentration should be below 10 mg/dL and blood urea nitrogen level below 60 mg/dL after dialysis.
   (4) Anesthetic considerations are summarized in the following box.

Anesthesia for Renal Transplant

I. Preoperative assessment and preparation
   A. Clinical evaluation
      1. Evaluate status of coexisting diseases
         a. Diabetes mellitus
         b. Hypertension
         c. Cardiac disease
         d. Hyperparathyroidism
         e. Pericardial tamponade
      2. Perform dialysis within 24 hours of transplantation; check weight
      3. Evaluate tolerance to chronic anemia
   B. Laboratory evaluation
      1. Complete blood count with platelet count
      2. Prothrombin time, partial thromboplastin time, bleeding time

Continued

Anesthesia for Renal Transplant—cont'd

3. Blood urea nitrogen, creatinine, calcium, fluid balance
4. Electrocardiography; chest radiography

C. Type and cross-match 2 units of washed packed red blood cells
D. Determine current drug regimen
E. Premedication
1. Benzodiazepines, narcotics
2. Antacids, histamine-2 antagonists, metoclopramide

II. Monitors
A. Electrocardiography
B. Indirect or direct blood pressure measurement
C. Precordial, esophageal stethoscopy
D. Neuromuscular blockade evaluation
E. Foley catheter
F. Central venous, pulmonary capillary wedge pressure measurement if required

III. Anesthetic management
A. Regional techniques
1. Continuous spinal or epidural
2. Advantages
a. No need for muscle relaxants
b. Potential respiratory tract infection from intubation is avoided
c. Amount of local anesthetic required is small
d. Patients are awake and comfortable postoperatively
3. Disadvantages
a. Patient anxiety
b. Uncomfortable surgical positions, especially for donor
c. Coagulation abnormalities present
d. Fluid management with sympathetic blockade is a challenge
e. Unprotected airway in patients with delayed gastric emptying

B. General anesthesia
1. Induction with thiopental propofol or etomidate
2. Maintenance with volatile anesthetic (isoflurane or desflurane) or narcotic-based technique
3. Neuromuscular blockers
a. Succinylcholine
b. Atracurium and *cis*-atracurium
c. Vecuronium

IV. Miscellaneous drugs
A. Mannitol or furosemide
B. Prednisone or methylprednisolone
C. Azathioprine
D. OKT3
E. Cyclosporine

(5) Chronic anemia is common, and transfusion is not required if oxygen delivery is adequate. Because of the danger of volume overload, anemia should be corrected during dialysis with transfusion of packed red blood cells.

(6) Abnormal platelet function, as well as ineffective production of factor VIII and von Willebrand factor, accounts for the syndrome of uremic coagulopathy seen in patients with renal failure. Correction of coagulation abnormalities has been accomplished through dialysis and administration of conjugated estrogen and desmopressin.

(7) Patients should fast for 6 to 8 hours before surgery if possible.
(8) Premedication may include narcotics or benzodiazepines in usual to reduced doses, depending on the status of the patient.
(9) The use of antacids, H_2 antagonists, and metoclopramide should be considered if gastric emptying is delayed; however, reduced doses should be considered because these drugs depend on the kidney for excretion, and metoclopramide is partially excreted unchanged in the urine.

3. Anesthetic technique

a) Regional anesthesia
(1) Both regional and general anesthesia have been used successfully for renal transplantation.
(2) Spinal and epidural anesthesia are both satisfactory, and because the procedure is extraperitoneal and in the lower half of the abdomen, the block can be kept low.
(3) Advantages of regional anesthesia include a more aseptic technique, avoidance of the use of muscle relaxants and other drugs excreted by the kidney, and the fact that endotracheal intubation is not required. Intubation may increase the risk of nosocomial pneumonia. Pulmonary infection occurs in 10% to 15% of transplant recipients and is associated with a high mortality rate. An additional advantage of regional anesthesia is postoperative analgesia.
(4) Disadvantages of regional anesthesia techniques in these patients include hypotension associated with sympathetic blockade, the length of the procedure, and heparinization of the kidney. Sympathetic blockade can make control of blood pressure difficult in patients who may be hypovolemic.
(5) Because transplantation procedures may last several hours, large amounts of sedation may be needed to supplement regional techniques. Because local heparinization of the kidney is often used, the use of continuous regional techniques may be contraindicated. For these reasons, general anesthesia is now the preferred approach in patients who undergo transplantation.

b) General anesthesia
(1) When general anesthesia is used, nitrous oxide combined with volatile agents, particularly isoflurane, or short-acting opiates is well tolerated.
(2) The skeletal muscle relaxant properties and minimal metabolism make isoflurane an attractive choice.
(3) Reductions in cardiac output secondary to the negative inotropic effects of volatile drugs must be minimized to avoid suboptimal tissue oxygenation in these anemic patients.
(4) The choice of muscle relaxant must take into consideration the unpredictable nature of renal function after transplantation. Relaxants that are independent of renal function for plasma clearance, such as atracurium and *cis*-atracurium, are excellent for this patient population.
(5) The pharmacokinetics of anticholinesterase drugs used for antagonizing nondepolarizing muscle relaxants is unchanged within 1 hour after renal transplantation.
(6) Succinylcholine can be used to facilitate intubation if serum K^+ level is normal.

c) Other drugs and considerations
   (1) Mannitol is included in many transplant protocols. It does not depend on renal tubular concentrating mechanisms to promote urinary formation, and it facilitates urinary output and a reduction in tissue and intravascular volume.
   (2) The effect of low-dose dopamine administration on cadaver graft function has also been evaluated. An infusion rate of 1 to 3 mcg/kg/min preoperatively does not affect early or late graft function. In normovolemic and hemodynamically stable patients without severe vascular disease and in patients who do not receive kidneys subjected to prolonged hypertension, preservation, or anastomotic times, infusion of dopamine at a rate of 1 to 3 mcg/kg/min perioperatively does not affect early or late graft function. In these circumstances, early graft function is dependent on ischemic changes, and late graft function is dependent on the management of rejection.
   (3) Cardiac arrest has been reported after completion of the renal artery anastomosis to the transplanted kidney. Arrest occurred at the time the occlusion clamp was released and was attributed to hyperkalemia from washout of the K^+-containing solutions used to preserve the kidney. If clamping of the external iliac artery is necessary during the procedure, K^+ can be released from the ischemic limb. Unclamping may also result in hypotension from the release of vasodilating substances from ischemic limbs and the subsequent increase in vascular capacity.

d) Immunosuppressants
   (1) Tacrolimus (Prograf) is indicated for the prophylaxis of organ rejection in patients receiving allogeneic liver or kidney transplants. It is recommended that tacrolimus be used concomitantly with adrenal corticosteroids. Because of the risk of anaphylaxis, tacrolimus injection should be reserved for patients unable to take tacrolimus capsules orally. To avoid excess nephrotoxicity, tacrolimus should not be used simultaneously with cyclosporine. The recommended starting oral dosage of tacrolimus is 0.2 mg/kg/day administered every 12 hours in two divided doses. The initial dose of tacrolimus may be administered within 24 hours of transplantation but should be delayed until renal function has recovered (as indicated, for example, by a serum creatinine <4 mg/dL). In patients unable to take oral tacrolimus capsules, therapy may be initiated with tacrolimus injection. The initial dose of tacrolimus should be administered no sooner than 6 hours after transplantation. The recommended starting dose of tacrolimus injection is 0.03 to 0.05 mg/kg/day as a continuous IV infusion.
   (2) Sirolimus (Rapamune) is indicated for the prophylaxis of organ rejection in patients receiving renal transplants. It is recommended that sirolimus be used initially in a regimen with cyclosporine and corticosteroids. In patients at low to moderate immunologic risk, cyclosporine should be withdrawn 2 to 4 months after transplantation and the sirolimus dose should be increased to reach recommended blood concentrations. Sirolimus inhibits T lymphocyte activation and proliferation that occurs in response to antigenic and

cytokine (interleukin [IL]-2, IL-4, and IL-15) stimulation by a mechanism that is distinct from that of other immunosuppressants. Sirolimus also inhibits antibody production. Sirolimus should be administered orally once daily at 2 mg after initial loading.

(3) Mycophenolate mofetil (Cellcept) inhibits immunologically mediated inflammatory responses and tumor development. Selective, noncompetitive, and reversible inhibitor of inosine monophosphate dehydrogenase, mycophenolic acid, the active metabolite, inhibits the de novo synthesis pathway of guanosine nucleotides without being incorporated into DNA. Mycophenolate mofetil is indicated for the prophylaxis of organ rejection in patients receiving allogeneic renal, cardiac, or hepatic transplants. It should be used concomitantly with cyclosporine and corticosteroids. Mycophenolate mofetil IV is an alternative dosage form to mycophenolate mofetil capsules, tablets, and oral suspension; it IV should be administered within 24 hours after transplantation. Mycophenolate mofetil IV can be administered for up to 14 days; patients should be switched to oral mycophenolate mofetil as soon as he or she can tolerate oral medication.

(4) Azathioprine (Imuran) is a bone marrow–toxic derivative of 6-mercaptopurine. Although its mechanism of action is unknown, a single dose of 5 mg/kg is administered intravenously at the time of transplantation. The drug is added to an IV drip chamber and administered over 10 to 30 minutes. Maintenance doses of 2 mg/kg/day are used thereafter if leukocyte count is greater than 4000 white blood cells per microliter. Imuran is associated with dose-dependent neutropenia and occasionally with thrombocytopenia.

(5) Orthoclone (OKT3) is a mouse monoclonal antibody to the T3 antigen or human lymphocyte. It is administered daily by slow IV injection. A standard dose in patients who weigh more than 25 kg is 5 mg given by slow IV push. This drug is given only intravenously and is administered for 14 days. Patients receiving OKT3 are given antibiotics to minimize the risk of opportunistic infection. Risks associated with the use of this drug include anaphylaxis, pulmonary capillary leak, and fluid overload.

(6) Cyclosporine is a fungal metabolite that suppresses IL-II production and amplification of cell-mediated immunity. Side effects include nephrotoxicity, hypertension, hirsutism, tremor, and anaphylaxis. Use of the drug early after transplantation delays recovery of allograft function. It is not administered until renal allograft function has reduced serum creatinine level to half of the admission value. The induction dose is 12 mg/kg in two divided doses, and plasma levels are maintained by periodic IV or oral doses. The anesthetic action of drugs may be altered in individuals who receive even a single dose of cyclosporine. Several animal studies have shown that a single dose of this immunosuppressant increases the hypnotic effects of phenobarbital and the analgesic effect of fentanyl. The drug also enhances the neuromuscular blockade produced by vecuronium and atracurium.

(7) Steroid administration is common in patients who undergo renal transplantation. Both prednisone and methylprednisolone sodium succinate (Solu-Medrol) have potent anti-inflammatory and immunosuppressive effects. They are also associated with impaired fibroblast proliferation and function and with impaired wound healing. Prednisone administration is initiated with a dose of 2 mg/kg/day and slowly tapered to maintenance doses. Adjustments in the dosage of prednisone must be made according to the clinical situation. Methylprednisolone is used prophylactically in a dose of 2 mg/kg intravenously. It is also used for treatment of acute allograft rejection at a dose of 0.5 to 1 g/day for 3 days. The maximum dose is 6 g.

4. Perioperative management

a) Monitoring considerations

(1) In addition to routine monitors, a Foley catheter is inserted for the assessment of graft function.

(2) Central venous pressure lines are not routinely inserted; their use may indirectly improve graft function by improving the assessment of hydration status.

(3) A pulmonary artery catheter is useful if cardiac compromise is suspected or if the kidney is expected to have delayed graft function.

(4) Protection of vascular access and fistula patency is of prime importance with the use of blood pressure cuffs or if arterial cannulation is necessary.

(5) Sterile precautions during insertion of invasive lines are extremely important because transplant patients are immunocompromised.

(6) Strict adherence to aseptic technique is mandatory in the management of these lines, catheters, and endotracheal tubes. Commitment to aseptic technique on the part of the entire team may make the difference between safe transplantation and death for the patient.

b) Fluid therapy

(1) Fluid management may be generous or conservative.

(2) Fluid replacement should be with normal saline or with dextrose in saline, generally at a maintenance infusion rate.

(3) Immediate function of the transplanted kidney cannot be guaranteed, and excessive intraoperative fluid replacement can lead to pulmonary edema and swelling of the grafted kidney.

J. ROBOTIC UROLOGIC SURGERY

1. Introduction

Robotic-assisted surgery is an emerging technique for management of various urologic procedures such as prostatectomy. One of the commercially available systems is the da Vinci surgical system (Intuitive Surgical, Mountain View, CA). It consists of a surgeon's console for surgical work, a surgical cart that houses the video and lighting equipment, and a robotic tower that supports three or four robotic arms.

The surgeon's console provides the surgeon with a three-dimensional, 10×–magnified view through a binocular viewpoint. Interaction is through "masters" into which the surgeon's hands are inserted. Free movement is possible from the masters to robotic instruments. Endoscopic instruments include graspers, hooks, scissors, knives, and surgical energy devices.

2. **Anesthetic technique**

Robotic surgery requires a coordinated approach by anesthetist and surgeon because the surgery is performed using a modified laparoscopic technique and can be very long in duration.

a) The Trendelenburg position is used. Major complications of surgery in the Trendelenburg position include: (1) neuropathies; (2) central venous pressure elevation; (3) intraocular or intracranial pressure elevation; (4) increased pulmonary venous pressure; (5) decreased pulmonary compliance; (6) reduced functional residual capacity; and (7) swelling of the face, eyelids, conjunctiva, and tongue.
b) Major anesthetic considerations for robotic procedures are summarized in the following box.

Anesthesia for Robotic Surgery

There is risk of thromboembolism during lengthy procedures in the Trendelenburg position. Use thromboembolic stockings to reduce risk.
Maximize protection over pressure areas to avoid nerve injury.
General anesthesia or combined general and regional anesthesia may be used.
Difficulties inherent in patients having prolonged surgery in the Trendelenburg position with the lower limbs in lithotomy are present.
Difficulties with peritoneal insufflation are present.
Blood pressure augmentation with vasoconstrictors may be necessary. This is probably because of prolonged pneumoperitoneum.
A high volume requirement is required.
Oliguria is common and generally responds to a fluid challenge.

K. SCROTAL PROCEDURES

1. **Introduction**

Scrotal procedures are considered minor operative procedures and can be performed on an outpatient basis. In adults, most elective scrotal procedures can be performed under local anesthesia with sedation. The most common procedures include surgery for infertility, hydrocele, and undescended testicle and orchiectomy for cancer.

The most common emergency scrotal operation is for testicular torsion. These patients will be in acute pain and should be considered to have a full stomach.

2. **Preoperative assessment**

a) Most patients who present for infertility concerns, hydrocele, and minor procedures are essentially healthy.
b) Those who present for orchiectomy require careful preoperative evaluation for possible metastasis.
c) No specific laboratory tests or medications are required except those that are suggested from the preoperative evaluation.

3. **Room preparation**

a) Monitoring: Standard
b) Position: Supine. The patient's arms usually are out at the sides. The lithotomy position may be requested.

c) Drugs and tabletop: Sedatives and narcotics. The tabletop should be set up for emergency general anesthesia.

4. **Anesthetic technique and perioperative management**
   a) Local anesthesia with sedation, regional anesthesia, or general anesthesia, may be selected depending on the patient's condition and the anesthesia provider's preference.
   b) There are no specific considerations because muscle relaxation is not required, and blood loss is minimal.
5. **Postoperative implications**

Pain management may be commenced intraoperatively by the use of narcotics, ketorolac, or both. Some patients, especially if being treated for malignancy, may experience nausea and vomiting.

L. TRANSURETHRAL RESECTION OF THE PROSTATE

1. **Introduction**

Transurethral resection of the prostate (TURP) is one of the most commonly performed surgical procedures in men older than 60 years of age. These patients are often at greater anesthetic risk because they are more likely to have cardiovascular or pulmonary problems. The procedure consists of opening the outlet channel from the bladder with the use of a resectoscope in the urethra for electrically cutting away the obstructing median and lateral lobes of prostate tissue. Bleeding is controlled with a coagulation current. For visualization of the surgical field continuous irrigation is used to wash away blood and dissected prostatic tissue and to distend the bladder.

Various types of irrigating fluid have been used. Although distilled water is associated with the least optical impairment, hemolysis of red blood cells is an unacceptable side effect. Normal saline or lactated Ringer solution is highly ionized and promotes dispersion of high current from the resectoscope. For these reasons, irrigating solutions typically consist of sorbitol (2.70 g) and mannitol (0.54 g) in 100 mL of water (Cytal) or glycine 1.5%. Glycine is slightly hypoosmolar to the blood but is used widely because of its low cost. Average features of a TURP are listed in the following table.

Average Parameters with a TURP

Parameter	Average
Resection time	<77 min
Resectate mass	20-48 g
Absorbed volume	1 L
Blood loss	175-534 mL
Speed of TURP syndrome onset	15 min
Serum sodium nadir	132-135 mmol/L

Adapted from Gravenstein D, Hahn RG. TURP syndrome. In Lobato EB, Gravenstein N, Kirby, RR, et al, eds. *Complications of Anesthesiology.* Philadelphia: Lippincott Williams & Wilkins; 2008: 474-491.

2. **Anesthetic technique**
   a) Spinal anesthesia and general anesthesia have both been used for TURP procedures. Some clinicians believe that spinal anesthesia is ideal because the signs and symptoms of hypervolemia and bladder perforation are more easily detected. A T10 sensory level is necessary for adequate anesthesia. There is no consensus as to the superiority of either technique.
   b) Although general anesthesia may mask early complications, it may be desirable in select patients who need pulmonary support or cannot tolerate a fluid load for compensation of a loss of sympathetic tone or when other contraindications to spinal anesthesia exist.
   c) Some key points for anesthesia management of TURP are listed in the following box.

Key Points for Anesthesia Management of Transurethral Resection of the Prostate

- TURP syndrome is caused by disturbance of intravascular volume or serum osmolality.
- Four questions to ask before a TURP:
  1. What is the irrigation fluid?
  2. What is the bag height over the prostate?
  3. What type of resectoscope is being used?
  4. In what mode is the resectoscope being used?
- Techniques for detection of pending TURP syndrome include measurement of serum sodium, measurement of breath alcohol levels by inserting 1% ethanol in the irrigating solution, and volumetric fluid balance.
- Treat symptomatic patients (those with mental status changes, seizures, or hypotension) aggressively; treat asymptomatic aberrant values (hyponatremia, hyperglycemia) very slowly, if at all.
- Sodium loss is an important source of hyponatremia a few hours after a TURP during which absorption of an electrolyte-free irrigating fluid has occurred.

Adapted from Gravenstein D, Hahn RG. TURP syndrome. In Lobato EB, Gravenstein N, Kirby RR, et al, eds. *Complications of Anesthesiology.* Philadelphia: Lippincott Williams & Wilkins; 2008: 474-491.

3. **Perioperative management**
   a) Complications: A number of complications are associated with resection of the prostate as listed in the following box.

Complications of Transurethral Resection of the Prostate

Hypervolemia
Hyponatremia
Bladder perforation
Hemorrhage
Glycine toxicity
Ammonia toxicity
Electrical hazards
Hypothermia
Bacteremia

b) Fluid absorption: Large amounts of irrigating solution can be absorbed through venous sinuses. The amount absorbed and the rate of absorption depend on the size of the gland to be resected, the congestion of the gland, the duration of resection, the pressure of the irrigating solution, the number of sinuses open at any one time, and the experience of the resectionist.
   (1) An average of 10 to 30 mL of fluid can be absorbed per minute of resection time, and 6 to 8 L can be absorbed in cases that last up to 2 hours. In general, limiting resection time to 1 hour is desirable.
   (2) *TURP syndrome* is a general term used to describe complications specifically related to absorption of irrigating fluid include volume overload with pulmonary edema and dilutional hyponatremia.
   (3) Central nervous system (CNS) symptoms associated with hyponatremia include restlessness, headache, irritability, confusion, visual disturbances, nausea, coma, and seizures.
   (4) Serum sodium (Na^+) concentrations of 120 mEq/L appear to be borderline for the development of severe symptoms. Electrocardiographic changes characterized by widening of the QRS complex and ST-segment elevation are seen when the serum level decreases to 115 mEq/L.
   (5) At levels less than 100 mEq/L, ventricular tachycardia and fibrillation can occur.
   (6) CNS symptoms can be detected more easily in patients receiving regional anesthesia.
   (7) Progressive increases in blood pressure, central venous pressure, or pulmonary artery wedge pressure (when monitored) suggest hypervolemia.
   (8) Hyponatremia in such cases results from water excess rather than from Na^+ loss. Fluid restriction, serial electrolyte screening, and airway and cardiac support are initial treatments for TURP syndrome. Hypertonic saline (3%–5% sodium chloride) and diuretics (furosemide, 0.15–0.5 mg/kg).

c) Bladder perforation
   (1) Perforation of the bladder is another complication of prostatic surgery.
   (2) Symptoms vary, depending on whether the rupture is intraperitoneal or extraperitoneal, as shown in the following box.

Symptoms of Bladder Perforation

Extraperitoneal
Periumbilical, inguinal, or suprapubic pain
Lower abdominal distention
Pain

Intraperitoneal
Abdominal rigidity, distention, pain
Referred shoulder pain
Hiccup, shortness of breath
Tachycardia
Hypotension or hypertension
Diaphoresis
Vomiting

(3) These symptoms are better recognized when the patient has regional anesthesia if the regional technique does not produce a high block. With general anesthesia, only the surgeon can appreciate the inability to recover bladder fluid as a sign of perforation. Intraperitoneal fluid will be excreted by the kidney.

(4) If hemodynamic instability occurs, suprapubic drainage is effective for removal of excess intraperitoneal fluid.

d) Glycine, which can also be used as bladder irrigation, can produce toxicity when absorbed.

(1) Glycine, an amino acid normally found in the body, is a major inhibitory transmitter.

(2) Signs and symptoms include nausea, vomiting, fixation and dilation of the pupils, weakness, and muscle incoordination.

(3) Transient blindness after TURP has been attributed to edema of the cortex, atropine, and hyponatremia.

(4) Glycine may also result in CNS toxicity as a consequence of its biotransformation to ammonia. Ammonia toxicity results in encephalopathy and delayed awakening in the postoperative period. NH_3 yields glutamine, which is metabolized to the inhibitory neurotransmitter serotonin. Hyperammonemia also decreases the production of dopamine and norepinephrine, which are central excitatory neurotransmitters.

e) Skin burns

(1) The use of high voltage for cutting and coagulation during TURP may result in skin burns.

(2) Electrocardiography pads may be placed at other sites so that potential burns are avoided.

f) Blood loss

(1) Blood loss during TURP generally is related to the weight of the resected tissue, operating time, and skill of the surgeon.

(2) Assessment of blood loss is difficult because of the dilution of blood in irrigating fluid.

(3) Hematocrit may be increased, decreased, or unchanged, depending on the amount of fluid in the intravascular space at the time.

(4) Blood transfusion should be based on preoperative hematocrit, the duration and difficulty of resection, and a general assessment of the patient.

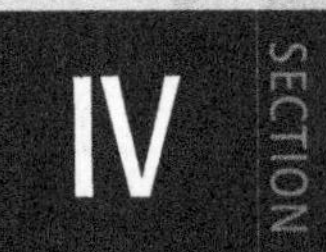

Head and Neck

A. CLEFT PALATE AND LIP

Cleft Palate

1. Introduction

Cleft palate repair is usually performed in stages, depending on the extent of the defect. For the more severe deformities, the initial operation repairs the lip and anterior portion of the hard palate. The soft palate and other deformities are usually corrected later after 6 months of age. Infants with cleft lip deformities can have difficulty feeding and may be prone to malnutrition and congenital (heart) anomalies and disease.

2. Anesthetic technique

a) Intubation may be difficult because the laryngoscope blade can slip into the cleft. However, packing the cleft with gauze may prevent this from occurring.

b) An oral RAE tube or flexible connector is used and secured at the midline of the lower lip.

c) A specialized mouth gag is used to hold the mouth open and the endotracheal tube (ETT) in place during cleft palate surgery.

d) All air bubbles should be carefully removed from intravenous (IV) lines to prevent an air embolus because of the incidence of associated cardiac anomalies, such as an atrial ventricular defect (AVD), which may lead to air crossing from the venous to the arterial circulation.

e) Congenital heart diseases may influence drugs that are selected for maintenance of anesthesia and for infiltration of the operative site, particularly if epinephrine is selected.

f) Care must be implemented to protect the child's eyes because accidental damage may occur during the surgical procedure.

g) Before emergence, a suture is often placed through the tip of the tongue, and the suture is taped to the cheek. This suture eliminates the need for an oral airway and prevents damage to the palatal repair.

h) If soft tissue obstruction occurs during emergence or recovery, traction on the suture can alleviate the problem. If edema occurs, a more aggressive and immediate airway management technique should be used.

i) Copious secretions, suctioning the stomach, and blood may cause laryngospasm after extubation; therefore, a clear airway is imperative.

Cleft Lip

1. Anesthetic technique

a) Management of unilateral cleft lip repair consists of routine induction followed by oral intubation using an oral RAE tube or a flexible connector.

b) Secure the tube to the lower lip and midline via tape. To decrease tension on the surgical sutures at the end of the procedure, the surgeon may place a Logan bow across the upper lip of the patient.

c) When the Logan bow is placed, mask ventilation during emergence will become impaired or impossible.
d) Extubation must be performed only with the patient fully awake and reflexes intact.
e) The child's surgical site must also be protected from finger and hand manipulation. Some hospitals recommend the use of hand mittens or taping the extremities onto armboards during the postoperative period.
f) Close monitoring of respiration should proceed into the postoperative period.

B. DACRYOCYSTORHINOSTOMY

1. Introduction

Dacryocystorhinostomy is performed for patients who have chronic tearing or obstruction at the level of the nasolacrimal duct. This procedure restores drainage into the nose from the lacrimal sac. The surgeon injects lidocaine 1% with 1:100,000 epinephrine, bupivacaine (Marcaine) 0.75%, and hyaluronidase (Wydase) in the operative site along the lacrimal crest. An additional injection may be given along the medial orbital wall, anesthetizing the ethmoidal nerve. This block may cause a temporary dilated pupil or medial rectus muscle paralysis.

A small incision is made near the medial canthus to allow a subperiosteal dissection to the lacrimal sac. The bone between the lacrimal fossa and middle fossa is broken and cut, making a small canaliculi. The mucosa of the lacrimal sac is anastomosed to the mucosa of the nose. To prevent closure of the newly formed path by scarring, a silicone tube may be placed inside the duct. Muscles and tissues in the area are then closed. The patient is then asked to open the eyelids, and when the proper height is obtained, the incision is closed.

2. Preoperative assessment and patient preparation

a) History and physical examination: This procedure may be done in patients of varying age. The patient's cardiac history should be determined because epinephrine is to be used for vasoconstriction. Infections in the surgical area should be treated with antibiotics for several days before surgery. Because of the inaccessibility of the anesthesia provider to the head, patients with obstructive sleep apnea (OSA) should also be identified and anesthesia planned accordingly.
b) Patient preparation
   (1) Laboratory tests: As indicated by the history and physical examination
   (2) Diagnostic tests: Electrocardiography (ECG) as indicated by the history and physical examination
   (3) Premedication: Standard

3. Room preparation

a) Monitoring equipment: Standard
b) Additional equipment: An end-tidal carbon dioxide sensing nasal cannula may be used to give additional information about ventilation.
c) An extra-long circuit should be available because of turning of the table 90 to 180 degrees.
d) Drugs: Standard emergency and standard tabletop agents are used.

e) IV fluids: An age-appropriate IV line and fluid are used for pediatric patients. One 18-gauge IV line is used for adults with normal saline or lactated Ringer solution at 2 mL/kg/hr (blood loss should be minimal because of the use of epinephrine).

4. Perioperative management and anesthetic technique

Most of these procedures can be done with local anesthesia with sedation; general anesthesia is rarely used. The choice depends on the preferences of the surgeon and the patient preference.

a) Induction is routine for general surgery and the patient's preference.
b) For local anesthesia with sedation, short-acting agents are best because these procedures are usually done on an outpatient basis.
c) Maintenance is routine.
d) Emergence: For general anesthesia, the patient should be extubated while awake unless the condition dictates otherwise (i.e., reactive airway disease).

5. Postoperative implications

There may be some temporary dilation of the pupil or medial rectus paralysis.

C. DENTAL RESTORATION

1. Introduction

Dental restoration procedures are performed under general anesthesia for a multitude of reasons. These include rampant cavities, history of mental disability, and an uncooperative patient who is not an appropriate candidate for local anesthetic and an office procedure.

2. Anesthetic technique

a) Mentally disabled patients often develop a close personal relationship with either a family member or their long-term health care worker. It is often suggested that this individual accompany the patient to decrease anxiety and communicate a health history to the anesthesia provider.
b) A thorough airway assessment should be performed before considering induction.
c) Oral midazolam (0.5 mg/kg) or ketamine (3–4 mg/kg IM) is most effective in sedating mentally disabled children in the preoperative arena.
d) Because many patients requiring dental restoration have congenital anomalies, it is common to find a patient with a small oropharynx, enlarged tonsils, a large tongue, and increased secretions.
e) Atlantoaxial instability and congenital heart disease should also be considered in the preoperative preparation and anesthetic management.
f) Preparation and appropriate airway management must be planned and implemented for these patients.
g) Patients who receive phenytoin to control seizures may have gingival hyperplasia. Because the gingiva is highly vascular, any surgical manipulation during restoration may lead to significant blood loss.
h) In patients with normal airways, a standard induction is appropriate and a nasal intubation usually facilitates the dental procedure.
i) The application of a topical vasoconstrictive nasal spray during the preoperative period reduces or prevents bleeding during the insertion of the nasotracheal tube.

j) After loss of consciousness, lubricated intranasal trumpets may be inserted into the most patent nasal airway. Starting with a smaller nasal trumpet, several are placed in increasing sizes to dilate the airway. When full dilation of the nares has occurred, a well-lubricated ETT is passed through the nose into the trachea, either blindly or assisted by Magill forceps under direct laryngoscopy.
k) The nasal ETT is preferably placed on the side opposite where the surgeon will be working. The ETT is often sewn to the nasal septum by the surgeon.
l) Throat packs may be placed to prevent blood from entering the stomach and causing nausea and vomiting; monitoring their removal is essential to preventing respiratory obstruction after extubation.

D. ENDOSCOPY

1. **Introduction**
   a) Endoscopic surgery includes panendoscopy, laryngoscopy, microlaryngoscopy (laryngoscopy aided by an operating microscope), esophagoscopy, and bronchoscopy. All of these procedures can be performed by using a rigid or flexible endoscope. If the rigid laryngoscope is used, the laryngoscope may be suspended from an arching support anchored to the patient's abdomen or chest or from a Mayo stand over the patient.
   b) One of the most common endoscopic procedures performed is endoscopic sinus surgery. Endoscopic sinus surgery is often associated with multiple and seasonal allergies leading to polyps. Patients undergoing surgery are often also being evaluated for such pathology responsible for hoarseness, stridor, or hemoptysis. Other possible reasons for endoscopic examination include foreign body aspiration, papillomas, trauma, tracheal stenosis, obstructing tumors, and vocal cord dysfunction. Several complications can arise with endoscopic surgery; eye trauma, epistaxis, laryngospasm, bronchospasm, and excessive plasma levels of local anesthesia and epinephrine have been reported.
2. **Anesthetic technique**
   a) Preoperatively, the patient should be examined for any signs of airway obstruction and proper measures taken to ensure safe and controlled airway management. Knowledge of the location and size of a mass is important, and discussion with the surgeon about chest radiography, magnetic resonance imaging (MRI), and computed tomography (CT) scan results can be invaluable.
   b) Light sedation is suggested for premedication because older children and adults may experience respiratory depression and worsening of airway obstruction. The airway must be protected from aspiration of gastric contents, especially during prolonged airway manipulation and deeper sedation.
   c) Premedication with an antisialagogue to dry secretions and a full regimen of acid aspiration prophylaxis in aspiration-prone patients may be indicated.
   d) An awake oral or nasal intubation with minimal sedation and topical anesthesia of the oral cavity, pharynx, larynx, and nasopharynx may be indicated.

e) For shorter ear, nose, and throat (ENT) procedures, anesthesia should be maintained with short-acting inhalation and IV agents to avoid patient movement and vocal cord movement and to control sympathetic nervous system response to brief periods of extreme stimulation as in laryngoscopy.
f) Good muscle relaxation of the vocal cords is an essential part of anesthesia management for microsurgery of the larynx. A short-acting relaxant or infusion may be considered for brief cases.
g) If the procedure is expected to last 30 minutes or more, use of an intermediate-duration neuromuscular blocking drug such as vecuronium, atracurium, cis-atracurium, or rocuronium for the initial tracheal intubation allows the return of muscle strength and spontaneous respiration to meet extubation criteria at the end of the surgical procedure.
h) Emergence should include adequate oropharyngeal suctioning, humidified oxygenation, and observation in the postanesthesia care unit for laryngeal spasm or postextubation croup.

3. **Perioperative management**
   a) Airway considerations
      (1) One of the greatest management challenges during endoscopic procedures is to share the airway continuously with the surgeon.
      (2) Several methods have been used to provide oxygenation and ventilation during the procedures. One method is to control the airway by using a small cuffed ETT (5.0–6.0 mm for an adult). Because the 5.0- and 6.0-mm ETTs are designed for smaller patients, a better ETT selection might include the microlaryngeal ETT (MLT).
      (3) The MLT in similar sizes (5.0–6.0 mm) has a cuff that is larger than the small standard ETTs (5.0–6.0 mm), allowing for a larger cuff distribution across the surface of the trachea and is the same length as an adult sized tube.
      (4) There are some distinct advantages of an ETT; these include a secure airway with easily controlled ventilation, a cuff to protect the lower airway from debris, monitoring of end-tidal CO_2, and the ability to administer inhalational anesthetics.
      (5) Several drawbacks include the potential for extubation and loss of airway, complications during laser surgery, and interference with the operative field by the ETT.
      (6) Intermittent apnea is also used as a technique to ventilate patients in this shared space. The anesthesia provider or the surgeon repeatedly removes the ETT, operates during a brief period of apnea, and then allows the anesthesia provider to reintubate and ventilate the patient. One advantage of the technique is that no special equipment is needed to ventilate the patient.
      (7) Many of the patients having these procedures have a long history of heavy smoking and alcohol use, which predisposes them to cardiovascular disease and labile vital signs. Some of the disadvantages of this approach include difficulty in reintubation of the patient and the time allotment between ventilations while preventing desaturations. The procedure must be interrupted frequently to ventilate the patient, and the airway is unprotected while the ETT is removed. During this technique, the blood pressure and heart rate tend to fluctuate widely. The procedure

resembles a series of stress-filled laryngoscopies and intubations separated by varying periods of minimal surgical stimulation. IV administration or topical application of agents such as lidocaine; small doses of alfentanil, remifentanil, sufentanil, or fentanyl; or β-adrenergic receptor blocking drugs such as esmolol may help moderate the sympathetic response.

(8) After the procedure, suctioning blood out of the stomach will help to decrease nausea and vomiting.

E. FOREIGN BODY ASPIRATION

1. Introduction

Aspiration of foreign bodies is a common problem. There is a high morbidity and mortality, particularly in children, who aspirate foreign objects. Some common aspirants include peanuts, popcorn, jelly beans, coins, and bites of meat and hot dogs. The majority of aspirated items are food particles; however, beads, pins, and small toys are not unusual. A common site of foreign body aspiration is the right bronchus. If the patient is supine when the aspiration occurs, the object will most likely be found in the right upper lobe. If the patient is standing, the right lower lobe is most likely to be affected. Signs of aspiration include wheezing, choking, coughing, tachycardia, aphonia, and cyanosis. These signs indicate an obstructive severe irritation and swelling in the airway. As a result of the swelling, air may be trapped in the lungs, not allowing adequate expiration.

2. Anesthetic technique

a) The anesthetic management depends on the location of the airway obstruction, the size and location of the object, and the severity of the obstruction. If it is located at the level of the larynx, a simple laryngoscopy with Magill forceps should allow for easy removal of the object.

b) Care must be taken not to dislodge the object and allow the object to fall deeper into the airway. If the foreign body is located in the distal larynx or the trachea, the patient should have an inhalation induction performed in the operating room, maintaining spontaneous respiration. With the patient spontaneously breathing, the surgeon will most likely use a rigid bronchoscope for extraction of the foreign body.

c) A mask induction without cricoid pressure or positive-pressure ventilation is the preferred induction technique. The anesthesia provider should not assist with respirations because this may cause the object to move further into the airway and compromise ventilation with occlusion. Patients should be placed in the sitting position because it is known to produce the least adverse effect on airway symptoms.

d) An antisialagogue, H_2 antagonist, and metoclopramide are often administered intravenously to decrease secretions and promote gastric emptying; the secretions may obscure the view through the bronchoscope.

e) Patients with full stomachs who are induced with a rapid sequence must be prepared for complete occlusion of the airway.

f) Direct and sometimes rigid laryngoscopy is typically performed. A rigid bronchoscope is also used and passed through the vocal cords into the trachea. Ventilation is accomplished through a side port of the laryngoscope or bronchoscope that can be attached to the anesthesia circuit.

g) If a foreign body is present, the telescope eyepiece within the bronchoscope is removed and optical forceps are inserted through the bronchoscope for retrieval of the item. While the telescopic eyepiece is being changed, a leak is present in the ventilation system and protracted periods can lead to hypoxia.
h) When an anesthesia gas machine circuit is used, high fresh gas flow rates, large tidal volumes, and high concentrations of inspired volatile anesthetic agents are often necessary to compensate for leaks around the ventilating bronchoscope.
i) Coughing, bucking, or straining during instrumentation with the rigid bronchoscope may cause difficulty for the surgeon and result in damage to the patient's airway; these must be avoided.
j) The best anesthesia technique for rigid laryngoscopy and bronchoscopy is total IV anesthesia (TIVA), which allows greater control of cardiovascular stability and relaxation for short periods, as well as ventilation with 100% oxygen, which allows longer periods of hypoventilation without hypoxia.
k) A rigid bronchoscopy can lead to several complications, including damage to dentition, gums, and upper lips as well as chipped or damaged teeth, all of which can be prevented to some degree with the use of a mouth guard and vigilance.
l) Vagal stimulation may be noted from the extreme head extension, and tracheal tears can occur with the introduction of the bronchoscope. Inadequate ventilation manifests as hypoxemia, hypercarbia, barotrauma, and dysrhythmias.
m) The surgeon must be prepared to perform an emergency tracheostomy or cricothyrotomy if a partial obstruction suddenly becomes complete.
n) At the conclusion of the procedure, patients can be intubated to provide ventilation until returning to consciousness. Allow the patient to return to consciousness as quickly as possible with airway reflexes intact before extubation.
o) Laryngeal and subglottic edema may occur for 24 hours after removal of a foreign body. To check for airway edema, the cuff of the ETT can be deflated if not contraindicated, and the lumen of the ETT should be occluded for one or two breaths during inspiration and expiration while listening for air movement around the tube. If there is no air escaping around the ETT, postoperative sedation and ventilation might be considered. Dexamethasone can be administered prophylactically to decrease airway edema.
p) Close observation and use of humidified oxygen are suggested during the recovery period. Some additional supportive measures that can alleviate some of the postoperative complications that occur include racemic epinephrine, bronchodilators, and steroids.

F. INTRAOCULAR PROCEDURES

1. Introduction

Intraocular procedures may refer to vitrectomy, glaucoma drainage, corneal transplant, and open eye injury. These procedures involve entry into the vitreous humor. It is crucial to avoid increases in intraocular pressure (IOP) with all intraocular procedures.

The most common of these procedures, vitrectomy, is performed by making three openings into the vitreous cavity. One of these openings is used to instill balanced salt solution; another is made for insertion of a fiberoptic light. The third opening is made for the insertion of various instruments used to remove abnormal tissue from the vitreous cavity. Frequently, a gas bubble is introduced during vitrectomy to tamponade retinal tears.

2. **Preoperative assessment**
   a) History and physical examination: Individualized based on patient's history and medical condition
   b) Patient preparation
      (1) Laboratory and diagnostic tests: These are as indicated from the history and physical examination.
      (2) Medications: Midazolam, 1 to 2 mg, may be given intravenously in divided doses as a premedication. The anesthesia provider must be aware that ocular drugs applied topically can have systemic effects. These include hypertension, arrhythmias, nausea and vomiting, agitation, excitement, disorientation, seizures, hypotension, and metabolic acidosis.
3. **Room preparation**
   a) Monitoring equipment is standard.
   b) Additional equipment includes standard emergency drugs, a long breathing circuit (table will be turned), and right-angled ETTs.
   c) IV fluids: One 18-gauge IV line with normal saline or lactated Ringer solution at 2 to 4 mL/kg/hr is used.
   d) A Hudson hood may be used to provide oxygen to the patient if a regional block with sedation is to be used. Care must be taken if there is any electrocautery because the hood will create an oxygen-rich environment under the drape and increase the risk of fire.
4. **Perioperative management and anesthetic technique**
   a) These procedures can be done with the patient under general anesthesia or under a regional block (retrobulbar or peribulbar block) with sedation.
   b) General anesthesia with endotracheal intubation is indicated for infants; young children; patients with severe claustrophobia; patients who are unable to cooperate, communicate, or lie flat for long periods; and patients with a history of acute anxiety attacks.
   c) Most adult patients do well with a regional block with sedation, which is the preferred anesthetic technique. If this method of anesthesia is used, it is important to determine the patient's response to sedatives and narcotics before administration of the block. After the table is turned and the patient is draped, it may be difficult to maintain a patent airway or a secure one if necessary. Care must be taken to avoid oversedation. If oversedated, patients tend to be startled when they arouse and may be confused and move about. A short-acting hypnotic (propofol) may be useful immediately before administration of the block. The surgeon needs to have the patient's cooperation during the block because the surgeon may ask the patient to look from side to side.
   d) General ETT anesthesia is also appropriate.
      (1) Induction: Standard IV induction. Ketamine is not a drug of choice because increased IOP is to be avoided. Care must be

taken to avoid pressure on the eyes with the mask. Nondepolarizing muscle relaxants are used for intubation and continued throughout the procedure titrated to patient response. It is imperative that the patient not move during the procedure. All connections in the breathing circuit should be secured.

(2) Maintenance: Continuous IV anesthesia is an option. Another option is the use of inhalational agents. Nitrous oxide (N_2O) may or may not be used. If used, however, and the surgeon performs a gas-fluid exchange, the N_2O should be discontinued 5 to 10 minutes before this exchange. Consider an antiemetic because of the high incidence of postoperative nausea and vomiting.

e) Bradycardia and hypotension can be caused by the oculocardiac reflex.

f) Emergence: Smooth emergence and extubation are important. Coughing, bucking, and straining should be avoided to prevent increasing the IOP. Consider deep extubation, although care must be taken not to place pressure on the operative eye with the face mask.

5. Postoperative implications

Again, coughing, bucking, and straining should be avoided. The patient may be positioned prone or to one side (as ordered by the surgeon) for correct positioning of the gas bubble. The patient's respiratory status should be ensured before the patient is turned postoperatively.

G. JET VENTILATION

1. Introduction

Jet ventilation has been used extensively for laryngeal surgery. When the trachea is not intubated, a metal needle mounted in the operating laryngoscope or passed through the cords can be used for jet ventilation. Jet ventilation may be performed manually using a simple hand valve attached to an appropriate oxygen source or with the use of various mechanical devices that allow for adjustment of rate and oxygen concentration. Because oxygen can support combustion, the anesthesia provider should consider as low a concentration of oxygen as is possible. Many patients will tolerate an Fio_2 of 30% or less; however, oxygen requirements for each patient should be considered for their individual needs. Also, using lower levels of oxygen will minimize the risk of fire.

a) High-frequency jet ventilation: High-frequency jet ventilation (HFJV) was originally used as a technique to provide adequate oxygenation and alveolar ventilation for rigid bronchoscopy and laryngeal surgery. HFJV is typically ventilation at low tidal volumes with high respiratory rates. A needle connected to a high-pressure hose with a regulator to adjust rate and volume is used to deliver the ventilation. With the tip of the needle either above or below the glottis, the anesthesia provider directs a high-velocity jet stream of oxygen into the airway lumen. The lungs are ventilated as the mixture of oxygen forces air into the lumen. Introduction of high-pressure (up to 60 psi) jet-injected oxygen entrains room air into the lung, allowing the jet stream of gases into the airway for ventilation. Although inspiration is accomplished by HFJV pressurizing gas into the airway, the expiration is passive. Therefore, some pauses in ventilation may be necessary to provide adequate time for expiration, particularly in patients with severe respiratory disease.

If an airway mass lies above the level of delivery of the gas jet, it may be easy to force the gas down the trachea during inspiration. But the gases will be trapped during expiration. This air trapping can lead to increased airway pressure, subcutaneous emphysema, and pneumothorax, particularly in patients with bullae. The anesthesia provider or surgeon may also find it difficult to aim the jet into the airway lumen, leading to hypoxia. If the jet is not accurately aimed, gastric distention, subcutaneous emphysema, or barotrauma may result. Patients with decreased pulmonary compliance or increased airway resistance from bronchospasm, obesity, or chronic obstructive pulmonary disease (COPD) are at high risk for developing hypercarbia with jet techniques. Jet ventilation is contraindicated in any situation in which an unprotected airway is a concern (e.g., full stomach, hiatal hernia, or trauma).

Adequacy of ventilation is assessed by observing chest movement, auscultation with the precordial stethoscope, and a pulse oximeter. TIVA is the primary anesthesia technique used with HFJV because volatile agents cannot be delivered and environmental contamination is a concern. TIVA with short-acting agents such as propofol, alfentanil, fentanyl, and remifentanil provide an excellent anesthetic for these procedures.

H. LARYNGECTOMY

1. Introduction

Most cancers of the upper respiratory tract are squamous cell carcinomas. When the laryngeal musculature or cartilage is invaded, total laryngectomy is performed. Intractable aspiration, with resultant pneumonia that has been unresponsive to other treatments, is another indication for laryngectomy.

a) Surgical procedures
   (1) *Total laryngectomy* involves removal of the vallecula and includes the posterior third of the tongue if necessary. Surgical exposure is from the hyoid bone to the clavicle. A tracheostomy is performed, and an anode tube is placed. The larynx is usually transected just above the hyoid bone. The trachea is brought out to the skin as a tracheostomy without the need for an ETT or tracheostomy tube as the pharynx is closed.
   (2) *Supraglottic laryngectomy* leaves the true vocal cords by resection of the larynx from the ventricle to the base of the tongue. Surgical exposure is similar to that for total laryngectomy. The specimen includes the epiglottis, the false vocal cords, the supraglottic lesions, and a portion of the base of the tongue. The thyroid perichondrium is approximated to the base of the tongue along with the strap muscles for closure. A temporary tracheostomy is required.
   (3) *Hemilaryngectomy* or vertical partial laryngectomy retains the epiglottis but involves removal of a unilateral true and false vocal cord. Surgical exposure is similar to that of supraglottic laryngectomy, and a tracheostomy is required.
   (4) *Near-total laryngectomy* involves removal of the entire larynx. One arytenoid is used to construct a phonatory shunt for speaking. A permanent or temporary tracheostomy is created, and the procedure may be combined with neck dissection and pharyngectomy with flap reconstruction.

The table below describes the structures removed, structures remaining, and postoperative conditions for the types of surgical procedures.

Laryngectomy

Structures Removed	Structures Remaining	Postoperative Conditions
	Total Laryngectomy	
Hyoid bone Entire larynx (epiglottis, false vocal cords, true vocal cords) Cricoid cartilage Two or three rings of trachea	Tongue Pharyngeal wall Lower trachea	Loses voice; breathes through tracheostomy; no problem swallowing
	Supraglottic or Horizontal Laryngectomy	
Hyoid bone Epiglottis False vocal cords	True vocal cords Cricoid cartilage Trachea	Normal voice; may aspirate occasionally, especially liquids; normal airway
	Vertical (or Hemi-) Laryngectomy	
One true vocal cord False vocal cord Arytenoid Half of the thyroid cartilage	Epiglottis One false vocal cord One true vocal cord Cricoid	Hoarse but serviceable voice; normal airway; no problem swallowing
	Laryngofissure and Partial Laryngectomy	
One vocal cord	All other structures	Hoarse but serviceable voice; occasionally almost normal voice; no airway problem; no problem swallowing
	Endoscopic Removal of Early Carcinoma	
Part of one vocal cord	All other structures	May have a normal voice; no other problems

2. Preoperative assessment

Most patients are older and have a long history of tobacco and alcohol abuse. Associated medical problems may include COPD, hypertension, coronary artery disease, and alcohol withdrawal.

a) History and physical examination: Individualized

(1) Respiratory: Smoking (more than 40 packs/year) is associated with bronchitis, pulmonary emphysema, and COPD, which impair respiratory function. Arterial blood gases may reveal carbon dioxide retention and hypoxemia. Pulmonary function tests demonstrate decreased forced expiratory volume, forced vital capacity, and the ratio of forced expiratory volume to forced vital capacity. Preoperative airway assessment is imperative because edema may distort airway anatomy, and tumor and edema may cause airway compromise. Tracheal deviation must be considered. Fibrosis, edema, and scarring from prior radiation therapy may distort the airway as well.

(2) Assess for signs of alcohol withdrawal (altered mental status, tremulousness, and increased sympathetic activity).
(3) Gastrointestinal: Weight loss, malnutrition, dehydration, and electrolyte imbalance can be significant.
(4) Hematologic: Anemias or coagulopathies may be present.

3. Patient preparation

a) Laboratory tests: Baseline arterial blood gases; electrolytes; hemoglobin; hematocrit; prothrombin time; partial thromboplastin time; and, if indicated from the history and physical examination, hepatic function tests are obtained.
b) Diagnostic tests: Chest radiography, ECG, pulmonary function testing, echocardiography, and stress tests are as indicated from the history and physical examination. Indirect and direct laryngoscopies preoperatively and review of CT may help in planning intubation.
c) Medications: Treatment with a long-acting hypnotic, such as chlordiazepoxide or diazepam, as a precaution for delirium tremens can be considered unless sedation would be contraindicated because of concerns of airway compromise. An IV antisialagogue (glycopyrrolate, 0.2 mg) facilitates endoscopy by the surgeon.

4. Room preparation

a) Monitoring equipment
(1) Standard
(2) Foley catheter
(3) Arterial line: Useful for serial laboratory and arterial blood gas studies
(4) Central venous pressure (CVP) catheter: If indicated by coexisting disease (prefer basilic or cephalic vein)
b) Additional equipment
(1) Regular operating table: May be turned 180 degrees
(2) Extension tubes
(3) Fluid warmer and humidifier
(4) Fiberoptic laryngoscope with anticipated difficult airway or potential for airway obstruction
(5) Tracheostomy under local anesthesia occasionally necessary for severe airway management.
c) Drugs
(1) Standard emergency drugs
(2) Standard tabletop
(3) IV fluids
(4) Two 16- to 18-gauge or larger IV lines with normal saline or lactated Ringer solution at 3 to 5 mL/kg/hr
(5) No sudden large blood losses; transfusion usually not necessary

5. Perioperative management and anesthetic technique

General endotracheal anesthesia is used.

a) Induction: Standard IV induction is appropriate with a normal airway. The choice of an induction drug should be based on the patient's medical condition. If airway difficulty is possible, direct laryngoscopy can be performed while the patient is breathing spontaneously, and a muscle relaxant may be administered when the glottis is visualized. In more difficult cases, awake intubation or fiberoptic laryngoscopy may be required.
b) Maintenance: The patient is in the supine position, with the head elevated 30 degrees; standard maintenance is used, considering the

patient's preexisting medical problems. An inhalation agent and supplemental narcotics benefit patients with reactive airway disease. Use of nondepolarizing muscle relaxants should be discussed with the surgeon because nerve stimulation for facial nerve localization may be performed.

c) Emergence: Many patients undergo tracheostomy. If a tracheostomy is not performed, the amount of airway edema and distortion needs to be discussed with the surgeon before determining extubation. Gradual emergence with stable hemodynamic parameters is an important consideration in the patient with coronary artery disease.

6. **Postoperative implications**
   a) Injury to the facial nerve can cause facial droop. Recurrent laryngeal nerve injury can result in vocal cord dysfunction; diaphragmatic paralysis may result from phrenic nerve injury.
   b) Pneumothorax may occur with low neck dissection.
   c) Airway impingement results from restrictive neck dressings or hematoma development.
   d) Communication difficulties occur after laryngectomy.

I. LASER SURGERY

1. **Introduction**

Specific issues during ENT surgery are described. The term *laser* is an acronym for light amplification by stimulated emission of radiation.

a) Laser technology

The two most common lasers used in ENT surgery are the CO_2, Nd:YAG (neodymium-doped yttrium aluminum garnet), and recently the argon laser. Laser light is different from standard light. Whereas standard light has a variety of wavelengths, lasers have only one wavelength (monochromatic); laser light oscillates in the same phase or all of the photons are moving in the same direction (coherent), and its beam is parallel (collimated). The wavelength of the Nd:YAG laser beam is shorter as it passes through the garnet than that of the CO_2 laser. The shorter wavelength allows less absorption by water and therefore less tissue penetration. For example, whereas the shorter wavelength of the Nd:YAG allows the laser light to pass through the cornea, the longer wavelength of the CO_2 laser would burn the cornea.

Laser light emits a small amount of radiation and can be infrared, visible, and ultraviolet in the spectrum. Lasers enable very precise excision, produce minimal edema and bleeding, and are favored by surgeons for resection of tumors and other obstructions of the airway. For operations in and around the larynx, the CO_2 laser is most often used because of its shallow depth of burn and extreme precision. The CO_2 laser produces a beam with a relatively long wavelength that is absorbed almost entirely by the surface of these tissues, vaporizing cellular water. Intermittent bursts of the CO_2 laser produce intense, precisely directed energy that results in a clean cut through the target tissue with minimal amount of penetration of surrounding tissue. A low-energy helium–neon laser is commonly used to aim or direct CO_2 laser beams.

Compared with the CO_2 laser, the Nd:YAG laser is poorly absorbed by water but easily absorbed by hemoglobin and pigmented tissues. The Nd:YAG laser light is capable of producing deep tissue penetration that may not be apparent for hours or days after exposure to the laser. The Nd:YAG laser allows debulking of larger tumors within body cavities. For this reason, the Nd:YAG laser is best suited for resection of bronchial, esophageal, bladder, hepatic, and splenic tumors. Laser light beams are primarily used for their thermal effect and can be used to cut, coagulate, or vaporize tissues. The exact tissue interaction of a laser is dependent on several variables, including the types of tissues being irradiated, the wavelength of the emitted beam, and the power of the beam.

2. Perioperative management

a) Safety guidelines: The use of laser technology mandates taking measures to ensure the safety of the patient and operating room personnel. These measures are listed in the box below. Specific concerns include eye protection with appropriate colored glasses, avoidance of the dispersion of noxious fumes, and fire prevention. Stray or reflected beams of the Nd:YAG laser are capable of traversing the eye to the retina; therefore, green-lensed eye protection for all personnel is mandatory during its use. All persons in the operating room must wear goggles specifically designed to absorb Nd:YAG laser beams. The required protective eyewear for CO_2 can be any clear glass or plastic that surrounds the face. Orange-red eye protection is required for the potassium-titanyl phosphate (KTP) laser and orange glasses for the argon laser.

General Safety Protocol for Surgical Lasers

1. Post warning signs outside any operating area: "WARNING: LASER IN USE."
2. Protect the patient's eyes with appropriate colored glasses, wet gauze, or both.
3. Use matte-finish (black) surgical instruments to reduce beam reflection and dispersion.
4. Use the lowest concentration of oxygen possible.
5. Avoid using N_2O because it supports combustion.
6. Place lasers in standby mode when not in use.
7. Use an endotracheal tube specifically prepared for use with lasers.
8. Inflate cuff of laser tube with normal saline.
9. Shield all adjacent tissues with wet gauze to prevent damage by reflected beams.
10. Suction the plume, and evacuate it from the surgical field.

When tissues are cut by a laser, the smoke and vapors that are formed are called laser "plume." This plume is an environmental concern and potentially toxic to operating room personnel. When the tissues vaporized by the laser are malignancies or viral papilloma, the concern arises as to whether these vapors are even more dangerous to operating room personnel if not removed from the environment. Because this issue remains under investigation, it is judicious to suction the laser plume and not allow it to circulate into the room.

3. Anesthetic technique

a) The prevention of combustion within the airway is of primary concern to the anesthesia provider. Fire in the airway is relatively uncommon (0.4%), and it is usually caused by penetration of the laser through the ETT, which exposes the beam to a rich oxygen supply.

b) N_2O, although not flammable, also supports combustion and can propagate the flame. Positive-pressure ventilation in the presence of intraluminal combustion produces a blowtorch effect with serious damage to the respiratory tract of the unfortunate patient. An Fio_2 of 30% or less is recommended for laser surgery that takes place in the airway.

c) Steps to reduce the possibility of fire include using the lowest concentration of oxygen appropriate for a particular patient, avoiding paper surgical drapes, spraying the flame with a 60-mL syringe filled with normal saline, and using water-based rather than oil-based lubricants.

d) When a flame has been ignited, extinguish the flame, discontinue oxygen administration, and immediately remove the ETT and replace it with a new ETT large enough to allow the surgeon to assess the lungs with a bronchoscope. The advantages and disadvantages of ETTs for use with lasers are listed in the following table.

Advantages and Disadvantages of Commonly Available Laser-Resistant Tracheal Tubes

Tube Type	Advantages	Disadvantages
Metal	Atraumatic external surface Double cuff maintains seal even if punctured by laser Kink resistant	Thick-walled nonflammable cuff reflects laser and transfers heat Cuff difficult to deflate if punctured Metal may reflect beam onto nontargeted tissue
Polyvinyl chloride (PVC)	Inexpensive Nonreflective Maintains shape well Double cuff maintains seal after proximal cuff puncture	Burns vigorously and yields pulmonary toxin (hydrogen chloride) Cuffed version contains flammable material
Red rubber	Wrapping protects flammable material but dries tube Maintains structure Nonreflective	Red rubber itself is highly flammable Tubes are thick walled
Silicone rubber	Wrapping protects flammable material Methylene blue aids in detection of cuff perforation Nonreflective	Contains flammable material Turns to toxic ash Single cuff is vulnerable to laser damage

J. LE FORT PROCEDURES

1. Introduction

a) The usual preoperative diagnosis for patients with maxillary fractures is facial trauma. Le Fort fractures are frequently associated with other skull fractures, zygoma fractures, and possible intracranial fractures and thus with cerebrospinal fluid rhinorrhea.

b) The fractures are divided into Le Fort I, II, and III. The Le Fort I fracture is a horizontal fracture of the maxilla extending from the floor of the nose and hard palate through the nasal septum and through the pterygoid plates posteriorly. The palate, maxillary alveolar bone, lower pterygoid plate, and part of the palatine bone are all mobilized. The Le Fort II fracture is a triangular fracture running from the bridge of the nose through the medial and inferior wall of the orbit beneath the zygoma and through the lateral wall of the maxilla and the pterygoid plates. The Le Fort III fracture totally separates the midfacial skeleton from the cranial base, traversing the root of the nose, the ethmoid bone, the eye orbits, and the sphenopalatine fossa.

2. Preoperative assessment and patient preparation

The airway is a priority. If the airway cannot be managed, emergency intubation becomes necessary. Avoid blind nasal intubation in patients with cerebrospinal fluid rhinorrhea, periorbital edema, "raccoon's eyes" bruising, or other evidence of nasopharyngeal trauma.

a) Neurologic: Document any neurologic deficit; intracranial trauma may require invasive monitoring.
b) Laboratory tests: Hematocrit and any other tests are as indicated by the history and physical examination.

3. Room preparation

a) Monitoring equipment: Standard
b) Additional equipment: Fiberoptic cart, a long breathing circuit (the table will be turned 180 degrees)
c) Drugs
   (1) Standard emergency
   (2) Standard tabletop
d) IV fluids: One 18-gauge line with normal saline or lactated Ringer solution at 6 to 8 mL/kg/hr

4. Perioperative management and anesthetic technique

General endotracheal anesthesia is used.

a) Induction: Fiberoptic laryngoscopy should be performed if there is any doubt about the ease of intubation. Patients with mandibular and maxillary (Le Fort I and II) fractures should undergo intubation. Patients with nasal, orbital, or zygomatic fractures usually are intubated orally. Consider using anode or right-angled ETTs. A Le Fort type II or III fracture is a relative contraindication for nasal intubation or nasogastric tube placement.
b) Maintenance
   (1) Muscle relaxation is usually required. Consider the prophylactic use of antiemetics for patients with wired jaws.
   (2) Position: The patient is supine; check and pad pressure points. Avoid stretching the brachial plexus, and limit abduction to 90 degrees. Protect the patient's eyes with ophthalmic ointment.
   (3) Blood loss can become significant. Intraoperative measurement of hemoglobin and hematocrit is necessary.
   (4) Administration of dexamethasone is frequently requested by the surgery.
c) Emergence: Extubation should be performed when the patient is fully awake in the case of difficult airway or wired jaws. A wire cutter should be available at all times. Verify that throat packing has been removed before extubating. Patients with facial or airway swelling and those involved in multiple trauma may need continued postoperative intubation and ventilation. An orogastric tube should be inserted to the stomach to suction blood before jaw wiring.

5. Postoperative implications

a) For airway obstruction, wire cutters must be available.

b) Aggressive treatment of nausea and vomiting is important.
c) Pain management includes narcotics, as well as antiemetics as needed.
d) Cerebrospinal fluid leak may occur.

K. MAXILLOFACIAL TRAUMA

1. Introduction

Traumatic disruption of the bony, cartilaginous, and soft tissues of the face and upper airway challenge the anesthesia provider to recognize the nature and extent of the injury and consequent anatomic alteration. It is imperative to create an anesthetic plan for securing the airway without promoting further damage or compromising ventilation. Possible mechanisms by which the upper or lower airway may become obstructed include edema; bleeding from the oral mucosa and palate; intraoral fracture sites; the presence of foreign bodies such as avulsed teeth, blood clots, or bony fragments; distortion of the nasal passages; injury of the pharynx and sinuses; and open lacerations.

Two common causes of maxillofacial fractures are blunt and penetrating trauma and gunshot wounds. Because of the intense forces required to cause facial fractures, other traumas (e.g., subdural hematoma, pneumothorax, cervical spine injury, and intraabdominal bleeding) often occur simultaneously with these fractures.

2. Anesthetic technique

a) Initial management of the airway depends on the situation at hand. In the case of severe facial or neck trauma, alternative methods of tracheal intubation such as fiberoptic laryngoscopy, retrograde wire placement, jet ventilation via a cricothyrotomy, or emergent tracheostomy may be necessary to secure the airway.
b) Injuries of the head and neck should alert the anesthesia provider to possible cervical spine injury. Although a complete evaluation of all cervical vertebrae is ideal, inspection of a lateral radiograph of the cervical spine is judicious to determine the presence or absence of dislocations and fractures. All seven cervical vertebrae must be visible. The seventh cervical vertebra is the most common site for traumatic fracture of the spine. Physical assessment is also required to rule out the presence of neck injury. Pain, deformation, and range of motion after radiographic studies are confirmed to be normal are also ceased.
c) Vertebral artery injury must be suspected with a cervical injury because these fractures can lead to vertebral artery tear or occlusion. If deteriorating respiratory function requires immediate airway management and intubation, the head should be maintained in a fixed position before any manipulation of the airway is performed. The use of manual in-line axial stabilization (MAIS) (by a qualified assistant) or a rigid cervical collar in place is recommended. The removal of the anterior segment of the collar can facilitate intubation and manipulation of the soft tissues of the neck.
d) Blunt trauma to the face or anterior neck may produce rapid airway occlusion secondary to soft tissue edema or hematoma formation secondary to trauma of the vascular structures of the neck. If a hematoma is discovered in the vascular structures of the neck, an ENT surgeon must be notified immediately. A patient exhibiting

smoke or blistering in the area of the mouth and nares or with a history of inhalation of toxic byproducts of combustion should be intubated immediately. Edema of the face and glottis, which may lack symptoms in the early stages, has the potential to produce serious airway compromise several hours after injury. Securing the airway by either oral or nasal intubation is preferable to tracheostomy, which is associated with a higher incidence of complications. It is imperative to avoid intubation in patients who may have sustained a basilar skull fracture.

L. MYRINGOTOMY AND TUBE PLACEMENT

1. Introduction

A myringotomy allows the pressure to equalize between the middle ear and the atmosphere, reducing the pressure in the middle ear compartment. Simple tubes with a lumen are placed through the patient's tympanic membrane to alleviate the pressure created in the middle ear usually seen with chronic serous otitis media or recurrent otitis media. These tubes function as an escape for the ostium and enable nonstop drainage of this pressure. Chronic otitis media is manifested as fluid in the middle ear. Recurrent otitis media, a common pediatric disorder, is defined as six or more episodes of otitis media over the prior year. Untreated otitis media may lead to permanent middle ear damage and hearing loss; therefore, prompt treatment is necessary. Children with chronic otitis media frequently have accompanying recurrent upper respiratory infections (URIs). Intervals between URIs may be brief. The patient is usually on a regimen of antibiotics. Thus, scheduling surgery during these interludes is often impractical. Often the eradication of middle ear fluid and inflammation resolves the URI; therefore, surgery should not be delayed.

2. Anesthetic technique

a) Bilateral myringotomies with tube insertions are typically very short operations.
b) Sedative premedications may outlast the procedure and are usually not necessary.
c) Mask or IV induction and maintenance using oxygen, N_2O, and agent such as sevoflurane is routinely used.
d) If IV access is established, it is usually after mask induction in children and may include fluid therapy or an injection cap for temporary access and administration of drugs. Because most patients scheduled for myringotomics are young and healthy, IVs are not usual necessary unless another procedure is performed in addition to positron emission tomography.
e) N_2O is often avoided in surgeries that involve the middle ear because it is 34 times more soluble in blood than nitrogen and can create pressure in the closed space. Because the myringotomy surgical procedure is relatively short and a tube will be placed through the tympanic membrane into the middle ear to relieve the pressure, the effects of N_2O are often not relevant.
f) For bilateral procedures, the inhalation anesthetic is discontinued during the second myringotomy to facilitate prompt emergence. N_2O is continued until the completion of the surgery.
g) Intubation is performed only if airway difficulties are anticipated or encountered. However, the airway equipment is always prepared

and available. The procedure is typically short and without much risk of bleeding.

h) The patient is supine with the head turned to expose the ear to the microscope. An ear speculum is inserted into the ear canal, cerumen is removed, and an incision is made in the tympanic membrane. Fluid is sometimes suctioned from the middle ear. Then a tympanostomy tube is inserted through the incision into the middle ear, straddling the tympanic membrane.

i) Upon completion of the tube insertion, antibiotic and steroid eardrops frequently are inserted into the external auditory canal. The surgeon moves to the other side of the table, the microscope is repositioned, the head is turned, and the procedure is repeated in the other ear.

M. NASAL SURGERY

1. Introduction

Nasal surgery is often performed to restore the caliber of the nasal airway or for cosmetic purposes. Whether for rhinoplasty, septoplasty, or septorhinoplasty, the nasal cavity can be anesthetized by placing 4% cocaine–soaked pledgets up each nostril for 5 to 10 minutes. To ensure vasoconstriction and minimize bleeding, the site is infiltrated with 1% lidocaine and 1:100,000 epinephrine. A hypertensive technique may also be initiated to control bleeding.

An incision is made in the septum down to the cartilage with elevation of a submucoperichondrial flap. This may be repeated on the contralateral side. Bone and cartilaginous deformities may be resected or weakened on the face. They may also be removed first, shaped, and then replaced. When the surgeon is satisfied with the resection, the incision is closed with an absorbable suture. In rhinoplasty, depending on the area needing work, the nasal contours can be remodeled by tip remodeling, humps can be reduced, bone osteotomies can be performed to shape the contour of the nose, or combinations thereof can be done. After surgery, both nasal cavities are packed, and external splints may be used.

2. Preoperative assessment and patient preparation

Generally, these procedures are elective and can be performed on an outpatient basis. It is important to identify patients with obstructive apnea. These patients often have chronic airway obstruction, redundant pharyngeal tissues, or both. Such patients, as well as patients with asthma, should undergo arterial blood gas and pulmonary function testing. Ketorolac and acetylsalicylic acid should be avoided in patients who also have nasal polyps because they often are hypersensitive to acetylsalicylic acid, a condition that can precipitate bronchospasm.

a) History and physical examination: Carefully evaluate cardiovascular status because the use of local vasoconstrictors may cause dysrhythmia, coronary artery spasm, hypertension, and seizures.

b) Patient preparation
   (1) Laboratory tests: As indicated by the history and physical examination
   (2) Diagnostic tests: As indicated by the history and physical examination
   (3) Standard premedication

3. Room preparation
- a) Monitoring equipment: Standard
- b) Additional equipment: Regular operating table, turned 90 to 180 degrees; anesthesia circuit extension available
- c) Drugs
  - (1) Standard emergency
  - (2) Standard tabletop
- d) IV fluids: Two 18-gauge lines with normal saline or lactated Ringer solution at 4 to 6 mL/kg/hr

4. Perioperative management and anesthetic technique
Use general endotracheal or local anesthesia with sedation; the choice depends on the preferences of the surgeon and the patient as well as on the acetylsalicylic acid status of the patient.
- a) Induction: Routine. Use of an oral right-angled ETT is convenient for the surgeon but is not necessary. If a sedation technique is chosen, short-acting agents are best because these procedures are usually minor, and patients are usually sent home.
- b) Maintenance is routine.
- c) Emergence: Counsel patients that the nose will be packed with bandaging and possibly splinted, so mouth breathing will be necessary on awakening. To decrease the incidence of coughing during extubation, lidocaine may be given.

5. Postoperative implications
- a) Elevate the head of the bed.
- b) Nasal packing and swallowed blood may contribute to postoperative nausea and vomiting.
- c) Mild analgesics after discharge are usually sufficient.

N. OPEN-EYE PROCEDURES

1. Introduction
Intraocular pressure is determined by the balance between production and drainage of aqueous humor and by changes in choroidal blood volume. Resistance to outflow of aqueous humor in the trabecular tissue maintains IOP within physiologic range. Normal IOP is 12 to 16 mmHg in the upright posture and increases by 2 to 3 mmHg in the supine position.

When the globe is open, the IOP is equal to ambient pressure. If the volume of choroid and vitreous should increase while the eye is opened, the vitreous may be lost. Any deformation of the eye by external pressure on the globe will cause an apparent increase in intraocular volume. This discussion is of open-eye procedures.

2. Preoperative assessment and patient preparation
- a) History and physical examination: Standard; the patient may come in as an emergency with a full stomach; ensure that the patient has no other injuries.
- b) Diagnostic and laboratory tests: These are as indicated by the history and physical examination.
- c) Preoperative medication and IV therapy
  - (1) Aspiration prophylaxis is used.
  - (2) Atropine or glycopyrrolate reduces oral secretions and may inhibit the oculocardiac reflex.
  - (3) Avoid narcotics, which may cause nausea and vomiting.

(4) Sedatives are given in the preoperative hold area and are titrated to effect.
(5) One 18-gauge IV tube with minimal fluid replacement is used.

3. Room preparation

a) Monitoring equipment: Standard
b) Pharmacologic agents: Standard; lidocaine and atropine
c) Position: Supine; the table may be turned for the surgeon's access

4. Anesthetic technique and perioperative management

General anesthesia with endotracheal intubation because a retrobulbar block causes a transient rise in IOP, which may cause intraocular contents to be expelled.

a) Induction (general)
(1) The goal is to avoid increasing IOP.
(2) When preoxygenating, avoid pressing the face mask onto the eyeball.
(3) Awake intubation is contraindicated because it may cause coughing and bucking.
(4) IV lidocaine, 1 mg/kg, may eliminate coughing and bucking.
(5) The use of succinylcholine in open eye globe injuries is controversial. If the use of succinylcholine is necessary, administration of a defasciculatiing dose of a nondepolarizing agent is warranted; it is a safe combination for rapid-sequence induction in the open eye in a patient with a full stomach.
(6) Induction may be with propofol and a large dose of a nondepolarizing muscle relaxant.
(7) Use of ketamine is contraindicated; it causes a moderate increase in IOP and nystagmus or blepharospasm.

b) Maintenance
(1) Inhalation agents cause dose-related decreases in IOP; the degree of IOP reduction is proportional to the depth of anesthesia.
(2) Oculocardiac reflex
(a) This is caused by traction on the extraocular muscles (medial rectus), ocular manipulation, or manual pressure on the globe.
(b) Signs and symptoms are bradycardia and cardiac dysrhythmias.
(c) Treatment is to stop surgical stimulus, ensure that dysrhythmia is not the result of hypoxia (by oxygen saturation confirmation) or ventilation, and administer atropine if needed.

c) Emergence
(1) The goal is to avoid excessive coughing and bucking.
(2) Empty the patient's stomach with a nasogastric tube and suction the pharynx while the patient is still paralyzed or deeply anesthetized.
(3) Administer an antiemetic before the end of surgery.
(4) Administer lidocaine, 1 mg/kg, to prevent coughing during emergence.
(5) Extubate the trachea before the patient has a tendency to cough.

5. Postoperative implications

a) Transport the patient to the recovery room with the head up 10 to 20 degrees to facilitate venous drainage from the eye.

b) The patient can be placed on the side with the operative side upward.
c) Shivering and pain can increase IOP and should be prevented.

O. ORBITAL FRACTURES

1. Introduction

Surgical access to the orbit may be needed to repair orbital fractures. The orbit may be divided into several compartments, including the peripheral surgical space, subperiosteal space, central surgical space, and subtenon space. The approach for orbital wall fractures depends on the location and the pathologic process involved. The common approach to these fractures is the transperiosteal or extraperiosteal approach. A skin incision is made in the desired quadrant just outside the orbital rim. The periosteum is identified and incised and is then resected from the wall and orbital margin.

2. Preoperative assessment and patient preparation

a) History and physical examination: Patients are usually healthy aside from the underlying trauma. Evaluation should focus on any coexisting disease and systemic manifestations of the trauma.
b) Laboratory tests: As indicated by the history and physical examination
c) Diagnostic tests: As indicated by the history and physical examination
d) Premedication: Standard

3. Room preparation

a) Monitoring equipment: Standard
b) Additional equipment: Regular operating table that is turned 90 to 180 degrees; availability of an anesthesia circuit extension is required
c) Drugs: Standard emergency and standard tabletop
d) IV fluids: One 18-gauge IV line with normal saline or lactated Ringer solution at 4 to 6 mL/kg/hr

4. Perioperative management and anesthetic technique

a) Use general endotracheal anesthesia for patients with orbital fractures identified as Le Fort II or III; nasal intubation is contraindicated.
b) Induction: Standard; an oral right-angled ETT may be preferred.
c) Maintenance: Standard; muscle relaxation is not required.
d) Position: Supine; check and pad pressure points. The table is turned 90 degrees; have extension tubes or long tubes for an anesthesia circuit. Check the patient's eyes and tape or use ointment (or do both).
e) Potential complication
   (1) Oculocardiac reflex is triggered by pain, direct pressure on the eye, and pulling on the extrinsic muscle of the eye. It has both trigeminal afferent and vagal efferent pathways. Bradycardia caused by the oculocardiac reflex is the most common manifestation, although junctional rhythm, atrioventricular block, ventricular premature contractions, ventricular tachycardia, and asystole also can occur.
   (2) To treat, tell the surgeon to stop the stimulus, ensure adequate oxygenation and ventilation, evaluate the depth of anesthesia, and administer atropine as needed. Lidocaine infiltration near the eye muscles may help to attenuate the reflex, which is self-limiting (i.e., it will tire itself with repeated manipulations).

5. Postoperative implications

a) For nausea and vomiting, begin prophylactic treatment before the end of the surgical procedure.

b) For pain management, use acetaminophen and parenteral opiates as needed.

P. ORTHOGNATHIC SURGERY

1. Introduction

Orthopedic orthognathic procedures often require a sagittal splitting of the mandible to move the lower jaw either forward or back. A Le Fort I or Le Fort II osteotomy may be performed to move the maxilla in any direction to correct anomalies. Many of these patients have anomalies of the mandible and maxilla, small mouth openings, and appliances that make intubation difficult and airway management challenging.

2. Anesthetic technique

a) Because most of the malocclusions are treated orally, a nasal ETT is usually preferred over an oral intubation. Securing the nasotracheal tube away from the surgical field without causing necrotic injury of the nares is vital.

b) Blood loss during these procedures can be extensive; the patient is typed and crossmatched and deliberate hypotensive anesthetic techniques are often used.

c) Rigid external or internal fixation devices are used to maintain stability in both the mandible and maxilla postoperatively; therefore, the proper cutting tools should be at the patient's bedside for emergency airway issues.

d) The anesthesia provider must also consider that edema will many times be extensive and progress over the first 24 hours after orthognathic surgery. To prevent postoperative respiratory problems, the patient may remain intubated for several days. If extubation is necessary, it should only be done when the patient is awake and in full command of his or her reflexes. Suctioning the stomach to remove blood and providing antiemetics can help the incidence of postoperative nausea and vomiting.

Q. PTOSIS SURGERY

1. Introduction

If ptosis is severe, the function of the levator palpebrae is poor. Most frequently, ptosis surgery involves shortening or reattaching the muscle at its site of insertion on the superior tarsus. The upper eyelid is marked at the desired height so it matches the opposite eyelid. Local anesthetic is injected by the surgeon. The skin is incised along the upper eyelid crease, and dissection proceeds until the orbicularis oculi is reached. At the medial and lateral ends of the tarsus, scissors incisions are made, and a clamp is placed between the two incisions. The levator muscle is resected as desired, and the eyelid height is evaluated. The skin incision is then closed, with any excess being excised.

2. Preoperative assessment and patient preparation

a) This type of procedure in adults is preferably performed using local anesthesia so the patient can keep the eyes open and the eyelid position can be adjusted.

b) History and physical examination are routine.

c) Patient preparation
   (1) Laboratory tests: As indicated by history and physical examination
   (2) Diagnostic tests: As indicated by history and physical examination
   (3) Premedication: Light sedation as needed
   (4) IV fluids: One 18- or 20-gauge needle with normal saline or lactated Ringer solution; keep vein open; blood loss is normally minimal

3. Perioperative management and anesthetic technique
   a) Patients are kept awake such that they are able to open their eyes to facilitate adjustment of the eyelids.
   b) Deep sedation is required for only localization; then the patient is kept awake.
   c) Patients are positioned upright or supine with the ability to sit upright during surgery. The table is rotated 90 to 180 degrees.

4. Postoperative implications
   a) Antibiotic steroid ophthalmic ointment is applied to the suture line.
   b) Sometimes an eye pad is applied or the patient receives iced saline pads in the postanesthesia care unit.

R. RADICAL NECK DISSECTION

1. Introduction

Radical neck dissection is required when cancerous tumors have invaded the musculature and other structures of the head and neck. These tumors are often friable and bleed readily. These patients are frequently heavy drinkers and smokers who have bronchitis, pulmonary emphysema, or cardiovascular disease. If the tumor interferes with eating, then weight loss, malnutrition, anemia, dehydration, and electrolyte imbalance can be significant. Patients who have had radiation treatments of the neck and jaw before surgical intervention will have soft tissues that are less mobile, making intubation more difficult. Many of these patients are older. The number of complications in patients age 65 years and older is nearly double that of younger patients. Consultation with a surgeon as to the nature, extent, and location of the tumor; therapy administered (radiation or chemotherapy); CT results; history and physical examination; and so on remains important in determining the appropriate techniques for airway management.

Head and neck reconstruction is an integral part of surgical removal of head and neck tumors. Traditional methods of reconstruction include regional pedicle flaps with microvascular reconstruction. These flaps include pectoralis major myocutaneous flap; trapezius flap; and local rotational flaps, such as forehead flap. Additionally, small bowel may be harvested to reconstruct the oropharynx and esophagus. The anesthesia team plays an important role in maximizing the overall success rate of a free flap and microvascular flow of the flap. The anesthesia provider must communicate with the surgeon regarding the planned donor site, which limits the available sites to place lines necessary for monitoring and venous access. Although the choice of monitoring is largely dependent on the general condition of the patient, the placement of a CVP line, a Foley catheter, and an arterial line (beat-to-beat and arterial blood gas trends) is suggested, particularly if deliberate hypotension during anesthesia is used. A pulmonary artery catheter may be useful if a history of cardiac problems is present. The internal jugular approach should be avoided because of proximity to the surgical site. Sites commonly used for CVP and pulmonary catheter placement when the internal jugular is not accessible are the subclavian and femoral veins, respectively.

2. **Anesthetic technique**
   a) Maintenance of anesthesia is often performed with an inhalation agent and supplemental narcotics. The use of a nondepolarizing muscle relaxant should be discussed with the surgical team preoperatively because the surgeon frequently uses a nerve stimulator to locate nerves distorted by the tumor during the procedure.
   b) Significant blood loss can be a problem, so hypertension should be avoided and treated aggressively. Sometimes a controlled hypotension technique may be requested. At least one (and preferably two) large-bore peripheral IV lines (14 to 16 gauge) should be in place. The patient's blood should be typed and crossmatched, with blood readily available. Monitoring estimated blood loss and measuring the hematocrit may provide some guidelines for replacement of blood.
   c) A positive fluid balance in the postoperative phase can result in edema and congestion of the flap, predisposing it to vascular compromise. Colloids may be used to help limit the amount of crystalloid required during the procedure. Patients undergoing a radical neck dissection are frequently hypovolemic and have electrolyte imbalances. This requires some fluid replacement and electrolyte balance intraoperatively to maintain cardiovascular stability.
   d) In preparation for a tracheostomy or total laryngectomy to be performed during the surgical procedure, the patient should receive 100% oxygen. The trachea will be transected by the surgeon, which requires that the anesthesia provider suction the airway and remove the ETT only to a level above the tracheal incision. After the tracheostomy tube has been placed by the surgeon and ventilation validated, the ETT can then be completely removed. A reinforced tube is usually placed in the distal airway by the surgeon and connected to the anesthesia machine. A reassessment of the ventilation should be performed, including the entire procedure of listening to bilateral breath sounds and observing chest excursion, end-tidal CO_2, and positive inspiratory pressure or negative inspiratory pressure. After the anesthesia provider has validated tube placement, the ETT is sutured to the chest wall for the entire surgical duration. At the end of surgery, the reinforced tube may be switched for a tracheostomy cannula.
   e) During radical lymph node dissection of the neck for carcinoma, manipulation of the carotid sinus may elicit a vagal reflex, causing bradycardia, hypotension, or cardiac arrest. Small doses of local anesthetic injected near the carotid sinus or administration of an anticholinergic agent may block vagal reflexes.
   f) Due to the long duration of the surgery and interruption of venous flow, venous thrombus is commonly seen in patients who are undergoing radical neck dissection. Venous air embolism may also occur during radical neck dissection from the head-up position and open neck veins during surgery. Careful monitoring with precordial Doppler sonography or transesophageal echocardiography provides the best detection of air embolism. Immediate removal of the air through the CVP is essential.

g) Laryngeal edema, vascular occlusion, and obstruction can also occur as a result of the venous stasis that follows major disruptions in venous flow during surgery or with trauma. Continuous review of complications and follow-up treatments are necessary.
h) Postoperative considerations consist of tracheostomy care; controlled ventilation; chest radiography to rule out pneumothorax, hemothorax, and pulmonary edema; and monitoring for laryngeal edema induced by thrombosis. It is suggested that these patients be admitted overnight in the intensive care unit because they have undergone major fluid and electrolyte shifts and altered ventilation–perfusion status and have spent an extensive time under the influence of anesthesia.

S. RHYTIDECTOMY OR FACELIFT

1. Introduction

Rhytidectomy is a reconstructive plastic procedure in which the skin of the face and neck is tightened, wrinkles (rhytid) are removed, and the skin is made to appear firm and smooth. In the preoperative area, the surgeon marks where the planned incisions will be made; before incision, the surgeon localizes the area. Typically, lidocaine 1% with 1:100,000 epinephrine is infiltrated along the incision lines, and lidocaine 0.5% with 1:400,000 epinephrine is infiltrated into the anticipated dissection line.

The facelift incision begins in the temporal scalp area about 5 cm above the ear and 5 cm behind the hairline, curves down parallel to the hairline toward the superior root, and continues caudally in the natural preauricular skin crease. The dissection begins in the temporal hair-bearing area; dissection continues through temporoparietal fascia and down to the loose areolar layer. The facial nerve branches and enters the facial muscles on their deep surface; dissection during this procedure must be done carefully. The only large sensory nerve that is important is the great auricular nerve. This nerve crosses the surface of the sternocleidomastoid muscle below the caudal edge of the auditory canal and is found posterior to the external jugular.

2. Preoperative assessment and patient preparation

a) History and physical examination
   (1) Most patients are older and have some effects of aging, but the age range may be anywhere from 40 to 70 years. Therefore, cardiovascular status should be evaluated because of the use of epinephrine in the local anesthetic.
   (2) Because of the inaccessibility of the face to the anesthesia provider and the need for sedation, careful airway evaluation and a history of sleep apnea should be identified.

b) Patient preparation
   (1) Laboratory tests: As indicated by the history and physical examination
   (2) Diagnostic tests: ECG if indicated by the history and physical examination
   (3) Premedication: Standard

3. Room preparation

a) Monitoring equipment is standard, including an end-tidal carbon dioxide nasal cannula or a second nasal cannula attached to the capnograph.

b) Additional equipment: An extra long anesthesia circuit should be available because of the turning of the table 90 to 180 degrees, and an oral right-angled ETT is indicated if general anesthesia is to be used.
c) Drugs: Standard emergency and standard tabletop agents are used.
d) IV fluids: Because of the use of vasoconstrictors in local anesthesia, blood loss should be minimal.
e) One 18-gauge IV line with normal saline or lactated Ringer solution at 2 mL/kg/hr is used or the vein is kept open with replacement of the NPO (nothing by mouth) deficit.

4. **Perioperative management and anesthetic technique**
   a) Most facelifts are done with deep sedation. The surgeon needs the patient to remain asleep throughout the procedure.
   b) The choice depends on the patient and surgeon's preference.
   c) If a general anesthetic technique is chosen, an oral right-angled ETT may be used to facilitate exposure of the surgical field.
   d) If a local anesthetic with IV sedation is the technique chosen, a nasal airway may be placed if the patient easily obstructs.
   e) Induction: Routine. If a local anesthetic with sedation is chosen, a short-acting agent (i.e., propofol) should be used because most of these surgical procedures are done on an outpatient basis with the patient going home the same day.
   f) Before administration of local anesthetic, the patient must be motionless and deeply sedated.
   g) Maintenance: Routine. Deep sedation can be maintained with an infusion. Hypertension should be controlled because this may result in hematoma. Vital signs should be maintained within normal limits. Depending on the patient's anatomy and the skill and experience of the surgeon, this procedure could last up to 6 hours. The surgeon may perform facial nerve monitoring. If so, paralysis should be avoided with a general anesthetic technique.
   h) Emergence: If a general anesthetic is used, emergence should be smooth, preventing coughing and bucking to limit the risk of hematoma formation.
5. **Postoperative implications**
   a) Hematoma is the most common complication of this procedure, usually occurring at the end of the procedure, but it may also present within the first 10 to 12 hours.
      (1) The cause of this is usually intraoperative hypertension.
      (2) This complication most commonly presents itself with the patient's appearing restless and having unilateral pain to the face or neck.
      (3) However, if these symptoms are noticed, the surgeon should be notified because treatment must be surgical.
      (4) If left untreated, this could compromise the patient's respiratory status.
      (5) A general anesthetic technique or IV sedation technique may be done for evacuation of the hematoma. If the hematoma is large, a general technique may be performed if the patient is restless and anxious.
   b) This procedure disrupts branches of the sensory nerves to the face. Numbness may last several months postoperatively, usually 2 to 6 months. The numbness is usually limited to the area of the lower two-thirds of the ear, the preauricular area, and the cheeks.

c) Nausea and vomiting can contribute to hematoma formation, so prophylaxis should be administered. Dexamethasone 4 to 8 mg is often used and has the additional benefit of reduced swelling. A serotonin receptor is also commonly administered.
d) Postoperative pain is usually mild.

T. SINUS AND NASAL PROCEDURES

1. Introduction

Sinus and nasal procedures for drainage of chronic sinusitis, polyp removal, repair of deviated septum, or closed reduction of fractures generally involve a young and healthy patient population. Many of the patients having sinus and nasal surgery have chronic environmental and drug allergies; therefore, there is an increased incidence of reactive airway disease in these patients. The use of fiberoptics or functional endoscopic sinus surgery for nasal and sinus surgery is indicated for treatment of chronic sinusitis.

2. Anesthetic technique

a) Nasal surgery may be successfully accomplished with local, monitored anesthesia care, or general anesthesia. All three methods of

Topical Anesthetic Drugs

Drug	Concentration	Dose	Notable Features
Cocaine	4%	3 mg/kg	Only local anesthetic with vasoconstrictive ability Blocks reuptake of norepinephrine and epinephrine at adrenergic nerve endings
Lidocaine	2% and 4% solution 2% viscous solution 10% aerosol 2.5%, 5%, 10%, 15%, 20% ointment	4 mg/kg plain 7 mg/kg epinephrine 250-300 mg	Rapid onset Suitable for all areas of the tracheobronchial tree
Benzocaine	Cetacaine contains 14% benzocaine, 2% butamben, and 2% tetracaine		Short duration of action (10 min) Can produce methemoglobinemia
Bupivacaine	0.25%, 0.5%, 0.75%	2.5 mg/kg plain	Slow hepatic clearance Long duration of action
Mepivacaine	1%, 2%	4 mg/kg	Intermediate potency with rapid onset
Dyclonine	0.5%, 1%	300 mg maximum	Topical spray or gargle Frequent use for laryngoscopy Absorbed through both skin and mucous membranes

anesthesia require profound nasal vasoconstriction. The mucous membranes of the sinuses and nose are highly vascular, and blood loss may be significant if vasoconstriction is not used. The surgeon may select to control vasoconstriction with epinephrine or cocaine, as shown in the table on pg. 339.

b) The anesthesia provider may be asked to use a hypotensive technique or slight head elevation (10–20 degrees) during the procedure. Using general anesthesia has been associated with an increased blood loss even with the use of an epinephrine injection. This exaggerated blood loss may be related to the vasodilatory properties of the inhalation agents.

c) Delivering general anesthesia for sinus surgery with propofol as well as other IV anesthetic techniques for the maintenance of anesthesia has been associated with less blood loss than occurs with the use of volatile agents for maintenance.

d) The placement of an oropharyngeal pack and light suctioning of the stomach at emergence may attenuate postoperative retching and vomiting. After all of the packing is removed, extubation should be performed on the awake patient who has regained control of protective reflexes. The use of IV or topical lidocaine may reduce some of the coughing before extubation, reducing bleeding in the postoperative period.

U. STRABISMUS REPAIR

1. Introduction

Strabismus repairs are performed to correct ocular malalignment. This malalignment may be esotropia (eyes deviate inward) or exotropia (eyes deviate outward). This procedure straightens the eyes cosmetically and allows the patient binocular vision by the lengthening or shortening of individual muscles or pairs of muscles. The specific muscles involved are the horizontal rectus and the oblique muscles.

A forced duction test is performed by the surgeon after induction and intubation by manipulating the sclera of the operative eye to aid the surgical plan. An incision is made through the conjunctiva in the area of the muscle to be manipulated. The muscle is then isolated and sewn back farther on the globe if the muscle tension is to be increased. If the muscle tension needs to be decreased, a segment of the muscle is removed.

2. Preoperative assessment

Strabismus repair is the most common ophthalmic surgical procedure performed on children. These children are usually otherwise healthy. There is, however, a higher incidence of strabismus in children with cerebral palsy and myelomeningocele with hydrocephalus. Malignant hyperthermia also is more common with children undergoing strabismus repair.

a) History and physical examination
   (1) A careful family history should be obtained preoperatively, including any history of family problems with anesthesia.
   (2) Respiratory: For patients with signs and symptoms of an acute respiratory infection, surgery should be postponed because these children are at greater risk for laryngospasm and bronchospasm.

b) Patient preparation
   (1) Laboratory tests: These are as indicated by the history and physical examination. Caffeine and halothane contracture tests

may be indicated if the patient is believed to be susceptible to malignant hyperthermia.
(2) Diagnostic tests: As indicated by the history and physical examination
(3) Medications: Midazolam, 0.5 to 0.7 mg/kg orally, is given as a premedication.

3. **Room preparation**
   a) Monitoring equipment: Standard
   b) Additional equipment
      (1) Standard emergency drugs (including lidocaine and atropine)
      (2) Pediatric standard tabletop
      (3) IV fluids: One 20- or 22-gauge IV line with normal saline or lactated Ringer solution at 5 to 10 mL/kg/hr
4. **Perioperative management and anesthetic technique**
   a) Induction: General endotracheal anesthesia is the technique of choice. Nondepolarizing muscle relaxants may be used after the forced duction test is performed by the surgeon. Bradycardia is common owing to the oculocardiac reflex, so atropine is commonly indicated. If the oculocardiac reflex occurs, ask the surgeon to stop ocular manipulation and reassess anesthesia depth and hemodynamic stability before proceeding with the procedure.
   b) Maintenance: Routine. Watch for signs and symptoms of malignant hyperthermia.
   c) Emergence: Nausea and vomiting are very common. Prophylactic antiemetics are recommended.
5. **Postoperative implications**

Aggressive prophylaxis and treatment of postoperative nausea and vomiting are required. Minimal analgesia is necessary.

V. TONSILLECTOMY AND ADENOIDECTOMY

1. **Introduction**

Tonsillectomy and adenoidectomy are among the most common surgical procedures performed in the United States, especially for children. Such surgical procedures are indicated for the treatment of hypertrophic tonsils and adenoids and for recurrent or chronic upper respiratory tract and ear infection and OSA.

The lateral tonsils, tonsillar tissue at the base of the tongue, and adenoids form a tonsillar "ring" around the oropharynx that can lead to significant airway challenges after surgical intervention. An adenotonsillectomy, although often considered a simple procedure, requires a great degree of finesse by the anesthesia provider.

2. **Anesthetic technique**
   a) Considerations of airway obstruction, shared airway, mechanical suspension of the airway, management of intubation and extubation, pain management, and the desire for a rapid awakening are all subtleties of anesthesia that challenge the anesthesia provider.
   b) In adult patients, a tonsillectomy may also accompany a uvulopalatopharyngoplasty (UPPP) for Pickwickian syndrome or OSA. OSA is typically seen with obesity and redundant pharyngeal tissue. Patients with OSA can also present with a history of right heart failure, cor pulmonale, and congestive heart failure, which is not uncommon.

c) The patient undergoing a tonsillectomy or adenoidectomy will probably have a higher incidence of airway obstruction because of the hypertrophied tissues. Chronic obstruction and infections of the tonsils can lead to potential systemic involvement, producing additional cardiac and respiratory anomalies.

d) In the case of suspected airway obstruction, the clinician must choose wisely among routine IV induction, inhalation induction, awake intubation, or fiberoptic-assisted intubation before induction. Adult patients with severe OSA may require a tracheostomy under local anesthesia in advance to secure the airway before the induction of general anesthesia. Such determination is based on the degree of obstruction, physical examination of the airway, and clinical judgment of the anesthesia provider. Regardless of the induction technique chosen, the use of an antisialagogue is strongly encouraged to reduce oral secretion to improve visualization during intubation and surgery.

e) In children, anesthesia is usually induced with an inhalation agent, oxygen, with or without N_2O by mask. Some institutions allow parental presence in the operating room during induction to prevent separation anxiety in the child. Tracheal intubation in children is best accomplished under deep inhalation anesthesia or aided by a short-acting nondepolarizing muscle relaxant. The airway generally is secured with an oral RAE or reinforced tube. A cuffed tube is recommended in patients older than 8 to 10 years of age, with continued attention to inflation pressures of the cuff. A properly sized pediatric ETT should allow a leak at 20 cm H_2O airway pressure, which reduces the likelihood of postoperative croup and tracheal edema. The tube must be secured midline. A simple yet effective method of securing the oral RAE tube is to apply a strip of tape directly to the chin, incorporating the ETT and another strip of tape over the tube. The first strip provides a secure base for the second strip, which actually holds the tube.

f) After the airway is secured, the mouth gag is inserted by the surgeon. An adequate depth of anesthesia is needed to facilitate gag insertion. The gag, designed to maintain an open mouth and tongue retraction, is equipped with a groove for the ETT to rest in. The airway should be reevaluated at the time the gag is placed to ensure that the tube has not been moved from its original position and that occlusion of the ETT has not occurred as a result of compression from the gag. The table is frequently turned 45 to 90 degrees away from the anesthesia provider just before incision.

g) The choice of techniques varies for the maintenance of anesthesia. There are four major goals to consider when choosing an anesthetic: (1) provide a depth of anesthesia adequate to blunt strong reflex activity elicited by the procedure, (2) a rapid and smooth emergence to facilitate the return of protective reflexes, (3) good postoperative analgesia, and (4) reduced postoperative bleeding.

h) The use of intermediate-acting muscle relaxants is acceptable, but their action must be completely reversed at the end of the case. Judicious narcotic supplementation will reduce the total amount of inhalation agent required and provide analgesia with minimal postoperative respiratory depression. Although postoperative bleeding has been a concern in the past regarding the use of ketorolac, it has been successfully used as an alternative to opioids, has not been found to increase bleeding, and has lead to shortened hospital stays after tonsillectomy.

i) Blood loss during tonsillectomy is difficult to assess but has been estimated to average 4 mL/kg or 5% of blood volume. Average blood loss during UPPP is slightly higher because the procedure frequently is performed in conjunction with adenotonsillectomy. Replacement for blood loss of less than 10% of the calculated volume may be accomplished with the administration of 3 mL of crystalloid per milliliter of blood loss. Although younger, healthier patients can tolerate greater volumes of blood loss, transfusion should be considered if blood loss exceeds 10% of calculated preoperative blood volume.

j) At the end of the surgical procedure, the surgeon may release tension on the mouth gag to ensure that all bleeding has been controlled. The insertion of an orogastric tube and some irrigation may be used to remove blood and secretions from the stomach and oropharynx. This is thought to reduce the incidence of postoperative nausea and vomiting. Suctioning of the oropharynx and nares should be done very gently and briefly by avoiding the surgical beds and to prevent disruption of and prevent mucosal bleeding. Vigorous suctioning may also induce laryngospasm and bronchospasm.

k) During emergence from anesthesia after tonsillectomy or UPPP, the anesthesia provider should ensure that all protective reflexes have returned, the airway is free of blood and debris, and an adequate breathing pattern is present before the removal of the ETT. A topical spray of 2% lidocaine (maximum, 3 mg/kg) on the glottic and supraglottic areas before intubation prevents postextubation stridor and laryngospasm after adenotonsillectomy. This approach has proved as effective as administering lidocaine, 1 mg/kg IV before extubation, but without higher sedation scores.

3. **Postoperative implications**

a) The postoperative tonsillectomy patient should be transported to the recovery room in the "tonsil position" (i.e., on one side with the head slightly down). This allows blood or secretions to drain out of the mouth rather than flow back onto the vocal cords.

b) Adults frequently prefer a middle or high Fowler position after UPPP. This position aids in ventilation and feeling of asphyxiation in the immediate postoperative period. The anesthesia provider must ensure that the patient is awake enough to manage his or her own airway.

c) One hundred percent oxygen with a high-humidity mist is given by face mask or face tent to hydrate the airway. The pharynx should be rechecked directly for bleeding and edema before discharge from the recovery room.

Bleeding Tonsil

The incidence of posttonsillectomy bleeding that requires surgery is 0.3% to 0.6%. Approximately 75% of the postoperative tonsillar hemorrhages that occur are within 6 hours of the surgical procedure. The remaining 25% of the postoperative bleeds occur within the first 24 hours of surgery, although bleeding may be noted up until the sixth postoperative day. Because the cautery is used for control of bleeding instead of ligatures, a slow oozing of the tonsillar bed is far more common than profuse bleeding.

One concern is that these patients may swallow large volumes of blood before bleeding is actually discovered. The patient may present with signs of hypovolemia, which are evidenced by tachycardia, hypotension, and agitation. If the blood is swallowed, the patient may have nausea and vomiting.

Appropriate laboratory tests (e.g., hemoglobin and hematocrit) should be performed to determine replacement. If reoperation is deemed necessary, restoration of intravascular volume or blood (or both) based on the volume lost should precede induction. It is important to evaluate the adequacy of IV access before induction (two IV lines may be appropriate), assess the coagulation variables, and be prepared to transfuse blood. All such patients should be assumed to have a significant amount of blood in the stomach, and an awake intubation of the trachea should be an initial consideration to maintain reflexes.

At induction of anesthesia, an additional person should be available to provide suctioning of blood from the oropharynx. If an awake technique is not practical, a rapid-sequence induction with cricoid pressure should be implemented. The patient should be placed in a slight head-down position to protect the trachea and glottis from aspiration of blood. A nasogastric tube may be placed to remove stomach contents before induction and then removed after induction. The induction agent selected is based on the hemodynamics and condition of the patient.

W. TRACHEOTOMY

1. Introduction

Tracheotomy is an incision into the trachea to form a temporary or permanent opening, the latter of which is called a tracheostomy. The incision is made through the second, third, or fourth tracheal ring, and a tube is inserted through the opening to allow passage of air and the removal of tracheobronchial secretions. Except in cases of head, neck, and face trauma, tracheotomy is rarely performed as an emergency procedure.

- a) Indications for tracheostomy
  - (1) To relieve upper airway obstruction
    - (a) Foreign body
    - (b) Trauma
    - (c) Acute infection: acute epiglottitis, diphtheria
    - (d) Glottic edema
    - (e) Bilateral abductor paralysis of the vocal cords
    - (f) Tumors of the larynx
    - (g) Congenital web or atresia
  - (2) To improve respiratory function
    - (a) Fulminating bronchopneumonia
    - (b) Chronic bronchitis and emphysema
    - (c) Chest injury with or without flail chest
  - (3) Respiratory paralysis
    - (a) Unconscious head injury
    - (b) Bulbar poliomyelitis
    - (c) Tetanus
    - (d) Prolonged intubation
- b) Tracheostomy technique
  - (1) Patient positioned supine with sandbag between scapulae
  - (2) Transverse cervical skin incision 1 cm above the sternal notch
  - (3) Incision extending to the sternocleidomastoid muscles
  - (4) Dissection through fascial planes and retraction of anterior jugular veins
  - (5) Retraction of the strap muscles
  - (6) Division of the thyroid isthmus and oversewing to prevent bleeding

(7) Placement of a cricoid hook on the second tracheal ring
(8) Stoma fashioned between the third and fourth tracheal rings
(9) Removal of the anterior portion of the tracheal ring
(10) No advantage in creating a tracheal flap
(11) ETT withdrawn to the subglottis
(12) Tracheostomy tube inserted using an obturator
(13) When correct position confirmed, removal of the ETT
(14) Securing of the tube with tapes

2. Preoperative assessment and patient preparation

a) History and physical examination: These patients may or may not be already intubated. If the patient is not intubated, his or her airway should be carefully assessed. Information regarding any abnormal pathologic features that may make intubation difficult should be sought from the surgeon or reports from specific tests such as triple endoscopy. If intubated, the patient's respiratory status and the following should be assessed: vent settings, peak airway pressures, respiratory rate, amount and color of tracheal secretions, need for and frequency of suctioning, lung sounds, arterial blood gases, chest radiography, and the presence of pulmonary infections.

b) Diagnostic tests
(1) ECG and chest radiography: As indicated by the patient's medical condition.
(2) Laboratory tests: As indicated by the patient's medical condition

c) Preoperative medication and IV therapy
(1) Preoperative medication as tolerated by patient.
(2) One 16- or 18-gauge IV line with minimal fluid replacement

3. Room preparation

a) Monitoring
(1) Monitoring is routine, with a CVP or pulmonary arterial catheter, as well as an arterial line as indicated by the patient's history.
(2) If peak airway pressures are greater than 60 mmHg, the patient may need a ventilator from the intensive care unit.
(3) A sterile 6-inch connector is used to attach the ETT to the vent or sterile circuit.
(4) Consider a bronchial adapter. Patients frequently have a bronchoscopy after tracheotomy placement.
(5) Warming modalities are used.

b) Pharmacologic agents: No special considerations

4. Anesthetic technique and perioperative management

Use general anesthesia and skeletal muscle paralysis or local anesthesia.

a) Induction: If a difficult airway is anticipated, awake fiberoptic intubation should be performed. The surgeon should be on standby for an emergency tracheotomy in the event that intubation attempts are unsuccessful. If the patient is already intubated, titrate anesthetic agents to the patient's need or convert sedation to general anesthesia.

b) Maintenance
(1) Adjust the oxygen and air mixture to maintain saturation at greater than 95%.
(2) If the patient is stable, an inhalation agent, and a narcotic may be introduced.
(3) Attempt to maintain the oxygen concentration at 30% to decrease the chance of airway fires.

(4) If an airway fire occurs
   (a) Pour saline into the pharynx to absorb the heat.
   (b) Temporarily discontinue the oxygen source.
   (c) Extubate and reintubate with a new ETT.
   (d) Follow up with chest radiography, bronchoscopy, steroids, and blood gas measurements.

(5) Maintain constant communication with the surgeon. Use a team approach. Use hand ventilation with 100% oxygen during insertion of the tracheotomy tube. The surgeon will ask the anesthesia provider to gently pull back the oral ETT before insertion of the tracheostomy tube.

c) Emergence
   (1) The patient may be transferred to the intensive care unit after the procedure. The nondepolarizing muscle relaxant may not have to be reversed if prolonged ventilation is planned.
   (2) The patient has 100% oxygen through an Ambu bag with monitoring devices functioning and is returned to the unit.

5. Postoperative implications

a) Assess patients for any symptoms associated with pneumothorax, pneumomediastinum, aspiration of blood, cardiac tamponade, hemorrhage, and subcutaneous emphysema.
b) Suction the airway as often as necessary to maintain airway and remove secretions.

X. UVULOPALATOPHARYNGOPLASTY

1. Introduction

Uvulopalatopharyngoplasty is performed primarily for the treatment of OSA. Tonsillectomy is often performed concurrently. Nasopharyngeal airway obstruction is relieved by removing redundant and obstructing tissues of the posterior pharynx.

Inspiratory muscle tone is lost during rapid eye movement sleep, resulting in relaxation of the pharyngeal muscles and thus creating airway obstruction. Adults with OSA are often obese.

2. Preoperative assessment

a) History and physical examination
   (1) Cardiac: Hypoxia and hypercapnia may lead to pulmonary hypertension, right ventricular hypertrophy, cor pulmonale, cardiac arrhythmias, and failure of the right side of the heart.
   (2) Respiratory: Frequent nocturnal arousals (up to 50 times per hour) are common. Periods of apnea may last up to 2 to 3 minutes. These patients often have a long history of snoring.
   (3) Neurologic: Loss of rapid eye movement sleep results in excess daytime somnolence, fatigue, and impaired judgment.
   (4) Gastrointestinal: These patients may have increased incidence of gastroesophageal reflux disease and hiatal hernia and should be considered to have full stomachs.

b) Patient preparation: Medical management includes weight reduction in obese patients, decreasing alcohol consumption, and nasal continuous positive airway pressure.
   (1) Laboratory tests: As indicated by the history and physical examination. These patients often develop polycythemia from chronic hypoxemia.

(2) Diagnostic tests: As indicated by the history and physical examination
(3) Medications: Use minimal preoperative narcotics or sedatives because these patients have heightened sensitivity to them. Anticholinergics are helpful to decrease secretions.

3. **Room preparation**
   a) Monitoring equipment: Standard
   b) Additional equipment: Airway adjuncts, difficult airway cart
   c) Operating room table: Ensure an appropriate weight limit.
   d) Drugs
      (1) IV fluids: 0.9% normal saline or lactated Ringer solution, 4 mL/kg/hr through an 18-gauge IV line
      (2) Blood: Type and screen
      (3) Tabletop: Rapid-sequence induction setup
4. **Perioperative management and anesthetic technique**
   a) Induction
      (1) Awake fiberoptic laryngoscopy and intubation may be indicated.
      (2) Inhalation agents are used with maintenance of spontaneous respiration and succinylcholine only after visualization of the larynx.
      (3) IV rapid-sequence induction is performed after 3 to 4 minutes of preoxygenation, cricoid pressure, and elevation of the head of the bed.
   b) Maintenance
      (1) Inhalation agent: Isoflurane or desflurane
      (2) 50% oxygen (may require high fractional inspired oxygen)
      (3) Position: Supine, shoulder roll, head extension
      (4) Operating table turned 90 to 180 degrees
   c) Emergence
      (1) Lidocaine, 1 to 1.5 mg/kg before extubation
      (2) As with tonsillectomy, the surgeon may release the mouth gag to see whether there is any uncontrolled bleeding. At this time, the patient should have an orogastric tube placed, and the stomach should be suctioned. The nasal cavity and oropharynx should also be gently suctioned and care taken not to dislodge any clots that may precipitate bleeding and cause laryngospasm.
      (3) Extubation criteria
         (a) The patient is awake, alert, and following verbal commands.
         (b) Muscle relaxant reversal is adequate.
         (c) Respiratory mechanics are acceptable. Premature extubation can lead to loss of the airway from laryngospasm or airway obstruction.
5. **Postoperative implications**
   a) Head of the bed elevated
   b) Humidified oxygen
   c) Hemoglobin and hematocrit if blood loss was excessive
   d) Careful titration of narcotics
   e) Postoperative complications: Airway obstruction resulting from swelling is the most common postoperative complication of uvulopalatopharyngoplasty. Typically, the patient will receive a dose of steroids intraoperatively to aid in reducing this swelling. Patients who undergo this procedure are usually admitted to the hospital, where their respiratory and airway status may be monitored carefully. If the tonsils have been removed, the possibility of recurrent bleeding must also be considered.

V SECTION Intrathoracic and Extrathoracic

A. BREAST BIOPSY

1. Introduction
Breast cancer is diagnosed by excisional breast biopsy (by needle aspiration or open excision) followed later by a more definitive surgical procedure designed to decrease tumor bulk and thus enhance the effectiveness of systemic therapy (chemotherapy, hormonal therapy, or radiation). Carcinoma of the breast is an uncontrolled growth of anaplastic cells. Types include ductal, lobular, and nipple adenocarcinomas.

2. Preoperative assessment and patient preparation
- a) History and physical examination
  - (1) The most common initial sign of carcinoma of the breast is a painless mass.
  - (2) Bloody discharge is more indicative of cancer than is spontaneous unilateral serous nipple discharge.
  - (3) Signs of advanced breast cancer include dimpling of skin, nipple retraction, change in breast contour, edema, and erythema of the breast skin.
- b) Diagnostic tests
  - (1) Mammography, thermography, and ultrasonography are used.
  - (2) Metastases to bone are frequent; therefore, a bone scan and measurement of alkaline phosphatase may be indicated.
  - (3) Laboratory tests are as indicated by the patient's medical condition.
- c) Preoperative medications and IV therapy
  - (1) The patient may be receiving hormone therapy.
  - (2) Use light sedation and short-acting narcotics preoperatively because the procedure lasts less than 1 hour.
  - (3) One 18-gauge IV line with minimal fluid replacement is used.

3. Room preparation
- a) Monitoring equipment
  - (1) Standard
  - (2) Noninvasive blood pressure cuff on the side opposite of surgery
- b) Pharmacologic agents: Standard
- c) Position: Supine; may need to tuck the surgical arm to the side

4. Anesthetic technique
- a) Local infiltration and general anesthesia are used.

5. Perioperative management
- a) Induction: Consider rapid-sequence induction and endotracheal intubation with a patient who is obese or has a full stomach.
- b) Maintenance: No indications are needed.
- c) Emergence: If rapid-sequence induction is used, perform an awake extubation.

B. BRONCHOSCOPY

1. Introduction

Bronchoscopy permits direct inspection of the larynx, trachea, and bronchi. Indications include collection of secretions for cytologic or bacteriologic examination, tissue biopsy, location of bleeding and tumors, removal of a foreign body, and implantation of radioactive gold seeds for tumor treatment. A common indication for bronchoscopy is suspicion of bronchial neoplasm.

2. Preoperative assessment

- a) History and physical examination
  - (1) Respiratory: Evaluate for chronic lung disease, wheezing, atelectasis, hemoptysis, cough, unresolved pneumonia, diffuse lung disease, and smoking history.
  - (2) Cardiac: Question underlying dysrhythmias because they may arise with stimulation from the scope or could be a sign of hypoxemia during the procedure.
  - (3) Gastrointestinal: Assess the patient's drinking history and nutritional intake.
- b) Diagnostic tests
  - (1) Chest radiography
  - (2) CT
  - (3) Pulmonary function test with lung disease
  - (4) Laboratory tests, including a complete blood count, electrolytes, glucose, and others as indicated by the patient's medical condition
- c) Preoperative medications and intravenous (IV) therapy
  - (1) The patient may already be taking sympathomimetic bronchodilators and aminophylline. The patient may benefit from administration of an inhaled bronchodilator preoperatively.
  - (2) Sedatives and narcotics are to be used with caution in patients with poor respiratory reserve.
  - (3) Cholinergic blocking agents reduce secretions.
  - (4) IV lidocaine, 0.5 to 1.5 mg/kg, decreases airway reflexes.
  - (5) Topical anesthesia involves 4% lidocaine using a nebulizer to anesthetize the airway by spraying the palate, pharynx, larynx, vocal cords, and trachea.
  - (6) One 18-gauge peripheral IV line with minimal fluid replacement is used.

3. Room preparation

- a) Monitoring equipment is standard: An arterial line is used if thoracotomy is planned or the patient is unstable.
- b) Pharmacologic agents: Lidocaine and cardiac drugs are used.
- c) Position: Supine; the table may be turned. One must manage an upper airway that is shared with the surgeon.

4. Anesthetic technique

- a) Local infiltration or general anesthesia is used.
- b) The technique of choice is general anesthesia. One must discuss with the surgeon whether a rigid or flexible fiberoptic bronchoscopy will be performed (see the box on pg. 350).

Consideration for Rigid Versus Fiberoptic Bronchoscopy

Rigid

1. Has been used extensively for removal of foreign bodies
2. In moderate or massive hemoptysis, provides better opportunity to suction
3. When airway patency is compromised by granulation tissue or tumor, instrument is able to pass the point of obstruction
4. Preferred for visualization of the carina and for the assessment of its mobility and sharpness
5. Allows the endoscopist to obtain a larger bronchoscopy specimen
6. Preferred in infants and small children

Fiberoptic

1. May require fragmentation of the aspirated object
2. Provides a better yield than rigid bronchoscopy in diagnosing bronchogenic carcinoma
3. Allows detailed visualization of the tracheobronchial tree
4. Facilitates intubation in patients who have difficult anatomic features
5. Improves patient comfort
6. Provides video imaging

c) Nerve blocks
   (1) Transtracheal: 2 mL of 2% plain lidocaine through the cricothyroid membrane using a 22-gauge needle attached to a small syringe
   (2) Superior laryngeal: 25-gauge needle anterior to the superior cornu of the thyroid cartilage
d) If topical anesthesia is used, consider total dosage of local anesthetic and be prepared to treat local anesthetic toxicity.

5. **Perioperative management**
   a) Induction
      (1) Flexible bronchoscopy
         (a) The endotracheal tube (ETT) must be large enough (8–8.5 mm) to permit the endoscope to pass easily.
         (b) Do not administer oxygen through the suction channel of the flexible bronchoscope (to avoid gas trapping and inducing barotrauma).
      (2) Rigid bronchoscopy
         (a) Conventional ventilation
            (i) Ventilation through the side port requires high gas flow rates and an intact glass eyepiece.
            (ii) Suction, biopsy, and foreign body manipulation require removal of the glass and loss of ventilation.
         (b) Jet ventilation
            (i) Give patients high fraction of inspired oxygen and hyperventilate them before apneic oxygenation.
            (ii) Perform jet ventilation through the side port of a catheter alongside the bronchoscope.
            (iii) Place the tracheal tube to the left side of the mouth because the surgeon will insert the scope down the right side.
            (iv) The ETT must be smaller in diameter to allow surgical access.
            (v) Consider total IV anesthesia when using jet ventilation.

(3) After preoxygenation, general anesthesia is induced with the insertion of an oral ETT.
(4) Succinylcholine may be contraindicated if the patient has severe muscle spasm, wasting, or complains of myalgia.

b) Maintenance
(1) General anesthesia must provide good muscle relaxation without patient movement such as coughing, laryngospasm, or bronchospasm. Because of the extensive sensory innervation in the trachea and bronchi, a deep plane of anesthesia must be maintained to avoid coughing, bucking, and exaggerated hemodynamic response.
(2) Cardiac dysrhythmia (i.e., supraventricular tachyarrhythmias, premature ventricular contraction, and atrial dysrhythmias) may be a problem. Plan appropriate treatment modalities.
(3) Inhalation anesthetics are useful to provide adequate suppression of upper airway reflexes and permit high inhaled concentrations of oxygen.
(4) Air leaks around the bronchoscope may be minimized by having an assistant externally compress the patient's hypopharynx.
(5) Spontaneous ventilation is preferred in cases of foreign body removal; positive airway pressure could push the foreign body deeper into the bronchial tree.

c) Emergence
(1) The patient should be awakened rapidly with complete return of airway reflexes before extubation.
(2) The patient needs to have a cough to clear secretions and blood from the airway.

6. Postoperative implications

a) If nerve blocks are administered, keep the patient from eating or drinking for several hours postoperatively; the blocks cause depression of airway reflexes.
b) Subglottic edema may be treated with aerosolized racemic epinephrine 2.25% (0.05 mL/kg) and IV dexamethasone (0.1 mg/kg).
c) Chest radiographs are obtained to detect atelectasis or pneumothorax.
d) Complications: A toxic reaction to local anesthetic is possible.

C. BULLAE

1. Introduction

Bullae are air-filled spaces of lung tissue resulting from the destruction of alveolar tissues and consolidation of alveoli into large pockets. They offer low resistance to inspiration and tend to increase in size with positive pressure ventilation. A valvelike mechanism may be present that causes air trapping on expiration. Enlarging bullae compress normal lung tissue and vasculature to the point of causing hypoxemia, polycythemia, and cor pulmonale. Overdistended bullae can rupture and cause pneumothorax or tension pneumothorax with cardiopulmonary collapse, requiring insertion of a chest tube. A chest tube may show a large, continuous air leak, and ventilation may be difficult.

2. **Anesthetic technique**
   a) A double-lumen tube (DLT) is indicated when a thoracotomy is planned to resect bullous tissue. This allows for separate ventilation of each lung and the ability to use adequate tidal volumes (VTS) on the healthy lung without risking further rupture of bullae.
   b) In the event of a pneumothorax, the unaffected lung can be ventilated while a chest tube is placed or the incision is made. When the surgery is nearing completion, each lung can be separately checked for air leaks.
   c) During general anesthesia for bullous disease, spontaneous ventilation is desirable until the chest is opened to reduce the risk of rupture of bullae. Patients with severe cardiopulmonary disease may not be able to ventilate adequately under general anesthesia, and positive-pressure ventilation may be required.
   d) Small VTS, high respiratory rates, and high FIO_2 can be delivered by gentle manual ventilation to keep airway pressures below 10 to 20 cm H_2O.
   e) An alternative to positive-pressure ventilation is high-frequency jet ventilation, which is used to decrease the chance of barotrauma.
   f) Nitrous oxide should be avoided in bullous disease because it rapidly enlarges the air-filled spaces.
   g) The choice of other anesthetic agents depends on the patient's cardiopulmonary status and the anesthesia provider's desire to maintain spontaneous ventilation.
   h) After excision of the bullae, normal lung tissue rapidly expands, and compliance and gas exchange rapidly improve. Care must still be taken with positive-pressure ventilation if some unresectable bullae remain.

D. MASTECTOMY

1. **Introduction**

Total mastectomy (simple or complete mastectomy) removes only the breast; no axillary node dissection is involved. It is used for the treatment of ductal carcinoma in situ. Radical mastectomy involves removal of the breast, underlying pectoral muscles, and axillary lymph nodes. There are two major alternatives to radical mastectomy: modified radical mastectomy and wide local excision of the tumor (partial mastectomy or lumpectomy) with axillary dissection. This treatment is followed by postoperative radiation therapy to the remaining breast.

2. **Preoperative assessment**

Patients often have no other underlying medical problems. The anesthetic implications of metastatic spread to bone, brain, liver, lung, and other areas should be considered. Preoperative assessment should be routine, with special consideration to the following:
   a) Cardiac: Cardiomyopathies may result from chemotherapeutic agents such as doxorubicin ($>$550 mg/m^2). Patients exposed to this type of drug may experience cardiac dysfunction, and a cardiac consultation may be needed to determine ventricular function.
   b) Respiratory: If the patient has undergone radiation therapy, there may be some respiratory compromise. Drugs such as bleomycin ($>$200 mg/m^2) can cause pulmonary toxicity and necessitate

administration of a low fractional of inspired oxygen (<0.30). However, a higher fraction of inspired oxygen is warranted if necessary to keep SpO_2 at 88% to 92% or greater.

c) Neurologic: Breast cancer often metastasizes to the central nervous system, and there could be signs of focal neurologic deficits, altered mental status, or increased intracranial pressure. If mental status is altered, a full medical workup should be undertaken without delay. Surgery should be postponed until the cause is found.

d) Hematologic: The patient may be anemic secondary to chronic disease or chemotherapeutic agents.

3. Room preparation

Monitors and equipment are standard. If the procedure is for a superficial biopsy, monitored anesthesia care with sedation can be used. Be sure to place the blood pressure cuff on the arm opposite the operative site. The patient is placed in the supine position during the procedure.

4. Perioperative management and anesthetic technique

a) Routine induction and maintenance are used.

b) Pressure dressings are often applied with the patient anesthetized and "sitting up" at the conclusion of the procedure. Communicate with the surgeon if this type of dressing will be used to time emergence more appropriately. If there are no further considerations, the patient may be extubated in the operating room.

5. Postoperative implications

a) If the patient is unstable hemodynamically (which may suggest a tension pneumothorax), place a 14-gauge angiocatheter in the second intercostal space while the surgeons prepare for chest tube placement.

b) Postoperative chest radiography may be needed if a pneumothorax is suspected.

c) Complications

(1) Deep surgical exploration may inadvertently cause a pneumothorax. The patient should be monitored for signs and symptoms of pneumothorax, which include increased peak inspiratory pressures, decreased arterial carbon dioxide pressure, asymmetric breath sounds, hemodynamic instability, and hyperresonance to percussion over the affected side.

(2) Diagnosis is concluded by chest radiography.

(3) Treatment includes placing the patient on a fractional inspired oxygen of 100% and insertion of a chest tube.

E. MEDIASTINAL MASSES

1. Introduction

Masses in the mediastinum can compress vital structures and cause changes in cardiac output, obstruction to air flow, atelectasis, or central nervous system changes. Masses can include benign or cancerous tumors, thymomas, substernal thyroid masses, vascular aneurysms, lymphomas, and neuromas. Surgical procedures for diagnosis or treatment of these masses may include thoracotomy, thoracoscopy, and mediastinoscopy.

Tumors within the anterior mediastinum can cause compression of the trachea or bronchi, increasing resistance to air flow. Changes in airway dynamics with supine positioning, induction of anesthesia, and positive-pressure ventilation can cause collapse of the airway with total obstruction to flow. Manipulation of tissue intraoperatively, edema, and bleeding into masses can increase their size and effects on airways or vasculature. As a result, total airway obstruction can occur at any phase of anesthesia, including during positioning, induction, intubation, emergence, or recovery. Positive pressure ventilation may be impossible even with a properly placed ETT if the mass encroaches on the airway distal to the ETT. Localization of the mass by computed tomography (CT) or bronchoscopy may facilitate placement of the ETT distal to the mass. Maintenance of spontaneous ventilation retains normal airway-distending pressure gradients and can maintain airway patency when positive pressure will not. Maintenance of spontaneous ventilation is the goal when managing these patients.

2. Clinical manifestations

Signs and symptoms of respiratory tract compression should be sought preoperatively. Many patients with mediastinal masses are asymptomatic or characterized by vague signs such as dyspnea, cough, hoarseness, or chest pain. The common symptoms are listed in the following box.

Symptoms of Mediastinal Mass

Sweats	Inability to lie flat
Syncope	Chest pain or fullness
Orthopnea	Superior vena cava obstruction
Hoarseness	Cough (especially when supine)

Data from Slinger P, Karsli C: Management of the patient with a large anterior mediastinal mass: recurring myths. *Curr Opin Anaesthesiol* 2007;20(1):1-3.

a) Wheezing may represent air flow past a mechanical obstruction rather than bronchospasm.
b) Shortness of breath at rest or with exertion and coughing are other symptoms. Symptoms may be positional, worsening in the supine or other position.
c) A chest radiograph may show airway compression or deviation.
d) CT, transesophageal echocardiography, and magnetic resonance imaging may further delineate the size and effects of masses.
e) Subclinical airway obstruction may be revealed by flow-volume loops, which demonstrate changes in flow rates at different lung volumes.
f) Decreased maximal inspiratory or expiratory flow rate alerts the anesthesia provider to increased risk of obstruction perioperatively.
g) Comparison of flow rates obtained with the patient in the upright and supine positions can reveal whether the supine position will exacerbate obstruction intraoperatively.
h) If any sign of respiratory obstruction is present, surgery for the biopsy of masses should be performed with the patient under local anesthesia whenever possible.
i) Radiation to decrease mass bulk in radiosensitive tumors is recommended before surgery to reduce the risk of airway obstruction.

3. Anesthetic technique

a) In the case of mediastinal masses, awake fiberoptic bronchoscopy and intubation enable the anesthesia provider to evaluate the large airways for obstruction and to place the ETT beyond the obstruction while maintaining spontaneous ventilation.

b) The effect of positional changes can be checked with the bronchoscope. Spontaneous ventilation should be maintained as long as possible or throughout the procedure if feasible.
c) The ability to effectively provide positive-pressure ventilation should be proven before administration of muscle relaxants.
d) The use of a helium–O_2 mixture can improve air flow during partial obstruction. The use of this low-density gas decreases turbulence past a stenotic area, improving flow and decreasing the work of breathing.
e) Emergency strategies that may become necessary in the case of airway compromise include repositioning or awakening the patient, rigid bronchoscopy to establish a patent airway beyond the obstruction, or (in the case of life-threatening compromise), sternotomy with manual decompression of the mass off of the airway.
f) Mediastinal masses can cause compression of great vessels or cardiac chambers. Compression of the pulmonary artery is rare because it is a higher pressure vessel than the pulmonary vein and is somewhat protected by the arch of the aorta. Compression of this vessel, however, can lead to sudden hypoxemia, hypotension, or cardiac arrest. Patients with any cardiac or great vessel involvement should receive only local anesthesia whenever possible, remain in the sitting position, and maintain spontaneous respirations. If general anesthesia is required, prior establishment of the means for extracorporeal ventilation should be established.
g) Superior vena cava syndrome is venous engorgement of the upper body caused by compression of the superior vena cava by a mass. It leads to the following signs and symptoms: dilation of collateral veins of the upper part of the thorax and neck; edema and rubor of the face, neck, and upper torso and airway; edema of the conjunctiva with or without proptosis; shortness of breath; headache; visual distortion; or altered mentation. Placement of IV lines in the lower extremities is preferred because insertion in sites above the superior vena cava could delay the drug effect as a result of slow distribution. Fluids should be administered with caution because large volumes can worsen symptoms.

F. MEDIASTINOSCOPY

1. Introduction

Mediastinoscopy involves passing a scope into the mediastinum via an incision above the suprasternal notch. The scope is passed anterior to the trachea in close proximity to the left common carotid artery, left subclavian artery, innominate artery, innominate veins, vagus nerve, left recurrent laryngeal nerve, thoracic duct, superior vena cava, and aortic arch.

2. Anesthetic technique

a) Large-bore IV access should be in place, and banked blood should be immediately available in the event of a tear in a major blood vessel, which is the most common severe complication.
b) Air embolism is also a risk if a venous tear occurs.
c) Arrhythmias such as bradycardia are possible with manipulation of the aorta or trachea during blunt dissection.

d) The mediastinoscope can place pressure on the innominate brachiocephalic artery as it passes through the upper thorax, causing a decrease in blood flow to the right common carotid artery and the right vertebral artery and a decrease in subclavian flow to the right arm. The decrease in cerebral flow could be detrimental, especially if the patient has a history of cerebrovascular disease.
e) Monitoring perfusion to the right arm with a pulse oximeter or radial artery catheter can detect decreased flow to the right arm and signal concurrent loss of flow to the brain via the innominate artery.
f) Repositioning of the mediastinoscope is required to reestablish flow to the brain.
g) A noninvasive blood pressure cuff placed on the left arm enables continued monitoring of systemic blood pressure during periods of innominate artery compression.
h) Complications of mediastinoscopy include pneumothorax, hemorrhage resulting from tearing of major vessels, arrhythmias, bronchospasm resulting from manipulation of the airway, laceration of the esophagus, and chylothorax secondary to laceration of the thoracic duct.

G. ONE-LUNG VENTILATION

1. **Introduction**
   a) Indications for lung separation: The ability to provide distinct ventilation to the separate lungs facilitates pulmonary surgery by providing a quiet surgical field. This is particularly helpful in the case of thoracoscopic surgery, in which visualization and the ability to manipulate the operative lung are limited. Thoracic surgeons commonly consider lung separation an absolute requirement for pulmonary surgery. However surgery can be performed on a lung that is being ventilated, and thoracic surgery alone is not an absolute indication for one-lung ventilation (OLV). Certain situations, such as infectious contamination of one lung, are absolute indications for OLV. Most common thoracic surgeries create relative indications for lung separation because they can safely be accomplished without it. Indications for lung separation are noted in the following section.
   b) Indications for separation of the two lungs (DLT intubation) or OLV
      (1) Absolute
         (a) Isolation of one lung from the other to avoid spillage or contamination
            (i) Infection
            (ii) Massive hemorrhage
         (b) Control of the distribution of ventilation
            (i) Bronchopleural fistula
            (ii) Bronchopleural cutaneous fistula
            (iii) Surgical opening of a major conducting airway
            (iv) Giant unilateral lung cyst or bulla
            (v) Tracheobronchial tree disruption
            (vi) Life-threatening hypoxemia related to unilateral lung disease
         (c) Unilateral bronchopulmonary lavage
            (i) Pulmonary alveolar proteinosis

(2) Relative
  (a) Surgical exposure: High priority
    (i) Thoracic aortic aneurysm
    (ii) Pneumonectomy
    (iii) Thoracoscopy
    (iv) Upper lobectomy
    (v) Mediastinal exposure
  (b) Surgical exposure: Medium (lower) priority
    (i) Middle and lower lobectomies and subsegmental resections
    (ii) Esophageal resection
    (iii) Procedures on the thoracic spine
  (c) Postcardiopulmonary bypass pulmonary edema or hemorrhage after removal of totally occluding unilateral chronic pulmonary emboli
  (d) Severe hypoxemia related to unilateral lung disease

2. **Perioperative management**
   a) Methods of lung separation: Several devices have been developed to enable isolation of one lung and ventilation of the other. The single-lumen endobronchial tube provides a simple approach by advancing a 7.5-mm, 32-cm ETT over a fiberoptic scope into one bronchus (see the table below).

Summary of Lung Separation Devices and Recommendations for Placement

Device	Indication	Tube Size	Placement and Confirmation
Left-sided DLT	Majority of elective left or right thoracic surgical procedures	Determined by measurements of the tracheal width from chest radiograph	Fiberoptic bronchoscopy
Right-sided DLT	Left bronchus—distorted anatomy; left pneumonectomy		Fiberoptic bronchoscopy with guided technique
Fogarty occlusion catheter	Critically ill patient; small bronchus; difficult airway; nasotracheal intubation	Standard ETT ≥6 mm in diameter	Fiberoptic bronchoscopy
Univent blockers	Selective lobar blockade; difficult airway requiring lung separation		Fiberoptic bronchoscopy
WEB	Critically ill patients; selective lobar blockade; difficult airway; nasotracheal intubation requiring lung separation	Standard endotracheal tube ≥8 mm in diameter	Fiberoptic bronchoscopy with guided technique

DLT, Double-lumen endotracheal tube; *ETT,* endotracheal tube; *WEB,* wire-guided endobronchial blocker.
From Campos JH. Lung separation techniques. In Kaplan JA, Slinger PD, eds. *Thoracic Anesthesia.* 3rd ed. Philadelphia: Churchill Livingstone; 2003.

(1) Bronchial blockers consist of catheters with an inflatable balloon that blocks the bronchus. A separate ETT is then placed into the trachea. Bronchial blockers are very useful in patients in whom the securing of the airway is anticipated to be difficult. Current options for stand-alone bronchial blockers include the 8 Fr-Fogarty embolectomy catheter and the wire-guided endobronchial blocker (WEB). The Fogarty catheter is useful in pediatric patients because it comes in smaller sizes. These blockers are inserted through a conventional ETT and guided into the appropriate bronchus using a bronchoscope.

(2) The Univent tube consists of an integrated ETT with a second lumen for a deployable bronchial blocker. After intubation of the trachea has been performed, the blocker is advanced into the bronchus with the aid of the fiberoptic bronchoscope. This tube is as easy to pass into the trachea as a single-lumen tube. The Univent tube is available in sizes from 6 to 9 mm internal diameter (although accounting for the blocker channel, the outer diameter is greater than that of a corresponding-sized ETT). Being of a shape and size more similar to conventional ETTs, the Univent may be a good alternative to a DLT in patients with difficult airways.

(3) DLTs consist of two bonded catheters, each with its own lumen; one lumen is used for ventilating the trachea and the other for ventilating the bronchus. Several types of DLTs have been used in thoracic surgery. The Carlens tube is a left-sided DLT with a carinal hook to aid in stabilization of the tube. Insertion is difficult, and the hook can cause vocal cord damage. A White tube is a right-sided DLT with a carinal hook.

(4) The Robertshaw DLT is available as a right- or left-sided DLT without a carinal hook. Disposable polyvinyl chloride tubes are available in French sizes 26, 28, 35, 37, 39, and 41. These correspond to internal lumen diameters ranging from 3.4 to 5 mm, respectively. Although the presence of dual lumens limits the internal diameter of each, the external diameter of a DLT is very large. The 37 Fr-DLT has an outer diameter equivalent to that of a standard 11.0 mm ID ETT. For this reason, DLTs are not used for small children; the external diameter of the 26 Fr-DLT is 7.5 mm. Sizing of DLTs is determined by patient height, usually leading to use of 35- to 37-Fr tubes in female patients and 39- to 41-Fr tubes in male patients.

(5) Modifications have been made in right-sided tubes to allow ventilation through a slot in the endobronchial cuff. It is thought that a greater margin of safety is associated with the use of a left-sided DLT for all right and left thoracotomies unless a left-sided tube is contraindicated.

(6) Contraindications to the use of DLTs include internal lesions of the trachea or main bronchi; compression of the trachea or main bronchi by an external mass; or the presence of a descending thoracic aortic aneurysm, which can compress or erode the left main bronchus. In these circumstances, it may be possible to use a DLT with the bronchial lumen on the unaffected side. Another contraindication is a difficult airway in which direct laryngoscopy is impossible. Intubation with the

large DLT can pose a challenge even in patients with a normal airway; insertion in those with poor airway anatomy may require a creative approach.

b) Placement of DLTs
   (1) The DLT has two curves along its length to aid in its placement. A stylet aids placement through the larynx. Some practitioners prefer the Macintosh blade for intubation because it offers greater clearance for the tube and may decrease the chance of balloon rupture from the teeth.
   (2) For laryngoscopy, the lubricated DLT is advanced with the distal curve concave anteriorly until the vocal cords are passed. The stylet is usually removed at this point. The tube is then rotated 90 degrees toward the bronchus to be intubated and advanced to around 27 cm depth in female patients or 29 cm in male patients or until resistance is met.
   (3) Usually the stylet is removed after the tube has passed the glottis because of concern about the rigid tube causing mucosal damage. One study found that the success of initial placement was significantly improved by keeping the stylet in place until the tube was fully situated in the bronchus. This technique was not associated with increased tissue trauma.
   (4) The tracheal cuff requires 5 to 10 mL of air, and the bronchial cuff requires 1 to 2 mL of air.
   (5) Overinflation of the bronchial cuff can cause its lumen to be narrowed or occluded and increases the risk of tearing the bronchus. Unlike most tracheal high-volume, low-pressure cuffs, the bronchial cuff holds a small volume and can produce high pressures on the endobronchial mucosa. For that reason, the bronchial cuff should be deflated during the procedure once OLV is no longer needed.
   (6) After the tube is situated in the bronchus, adapters are attached to the two lumens for interface with the anesthesia circuit. Auscultation of breath sounds is a simple, although not highly reliable, method of determining the position of a DLT, as listed in the following section.

c) Auscultation of breath sounds after placement of a DLT
   (1) Inflate the tracheal cuff.
   (2) Verify bilaterally equal breath sounds. If breath sounds are present on only one side, both lumens are in the same bronchus. Deflate the cuff and withdraw the tube 1 to 2 cm at a time until breath sounds are equal bilaterally.
   (3) Inflate the endobronchial cuff.
   (4) Clamp the endobronchial lumen, and open its lumen cap proximal to the clamp.
   (5) Verify breath sounds in the correct lung and the absence of breath sounds in the opposite lung.
   (6) Verify that breath sounds are equal at the apex of the lung and at the lateral lung. If the apex is diminished, withdraw the tube until upper lung sounds return.
   (7) Verify the absence of air leakage through the opposite lumen cap.
   (8) Unclamp the endobronchial lumen and verify bilateral breath sounds.
   (9) Clamp the tracheal lumen and open its cap.

(10) Verify breath sounds on the side opposite the lung with the endobronchial lumen and the absence of breath sounds on the other.
(11) When absolute lung separation is needed, as in bronchopulmonary lavage, connecting a clamped lumen to an underwater drainage system will show air bubbles if a leak is present.
(12) Flexible fiberoptic bronchoscopy is essential to verify placement of the DLT. Placement of the tube should again be verified by bronchoscopy after the patient is positioned laterally because the DLT will commonly withdraw from the bronchus by 1 cm.

d) Complications of DLTs
(1) Placement of DLTs carries the same risks as laryngoscopy and intubation with ETTs. In addition, there exists a risk of hypoxemia with malpositioning of the tube.
(2) Rupture of a thoracic aneurysm is possible with a left DLT if the aneurysm compresses the left mainstem bronchus.
(3) Damage to the vocal cords or arytenoid cartilages is possible from a carinal hook. A carinal hook can also break off, requiring retrieval with a bronchoscope.
(4) Bronchial rupture, which was thought to be caused by overinflation of the bronchial cuff, has been reported. Because of the possibility of being inserted too deeply, a DLT can also cause the entire tidal volume to be delivered to a single lung lobe, creating the potential for barotrauma. Peak inspiratory pressures should be monitored closely to alert the anesthesia provider of possible migration of the DLT.
(5) The larger size of the DLT is probably also responsible for the slightly increased incidence of hoarseness and vocal cord lesions observed in patients after DLT versus using a bronchial blocker for lung separation. Vocal cord paralysis can represent a life-threatening complication of DLT placement.

e) Physiology of OLV
(1) During two-lung ventilation (TLV), blood flow to the dependent lung averages approximately 60%. When one lung is allowed to deflate and OLV is started, any blood flow to the deflated lung becomes shunt flow, causing the Pao_2 to decrease. Without autoregulation of pulmonary blood flow, a 40% shunt would be anticipated.
(2) The lungs have a compensatory mechanism of increasing vascular resistance in hypoxic areas of the lungs, and this diverts some blood flow to areas of better ventilation and oxygenation. This mechanism is termed *hypoxic pulmonary vasoconstriction (HPV)*. HPV is an intrapulmonary reflex–feedback mechanism in inhomogeneous lungs to improve gas exchange and arterial oxygenation.
(3) Although hypoxemia causes vasodilation in the general circulation, it has the opposite effect on pulmonary arteries. HPV is a unique mechanism, suited specifically to match pulmonary blood flow with well-oxygenated areas of lung.

f) Characteristics of hypoxic pulmonary vasoconstriction
(1) A local reaction occurring in hypoxic areas of the lung. It may be very localized because of regional atelectasis or OLV or may affect both lungs entirely in hypoxic situations.

(2) Opposite to systemic reaction, it causes vasoconstriction in response to hypoxia in all but very proximal pulmonary arteries.
(3) The onset and resolution are very fast after changes in tissue Po_2.
(4) Triggered by alveolar hypoxia, not arterial hypoxemia
(5) May be inhibited by calcium channel blockade, volatile anesthetics, or vasodilators (see the box below.) Augmented by chemoreceptor agonists, HPV during OLV is effective in decreasing the cardiac output to the nonventilated lung to 20% to 25%. Shunt flow changes from 10% during TLV to 27% during OLV. This increase in shunt decreases the mean Pao_2 from greater than 400 mmHg during TLV to slightly less than 200 mmHg during OLV when the fraction of inspired is 100%. Hypoxic pulmonary vasoconstriction can decrease the shunt fraction during OLV by 50%.

Factors That Reduce the Effectiveness of Hypoxic Pulmonary Vasoconstriction

Shunt fraction <20%, or >80%
Hypervolemia
Hypovolemia
Excessive tidal volume or PEEP
Hypocapnia
Acidosis
Hypothermia
Volatile agents >1.5 MAC
Vasoactive medications

MAC, Minimum alveolar concentration; *PEEP,* positive end-expiratory pressure.

(6) HPV occurs whether the lung is rendered hypoxic by atelectasis or by ventilation with a hypoxic mixture. HPV improves arterial oxygenation when the amount of hypoxic lung is between 20% and 80%, which is the condition during OLV. When less than 20% of the lung is hypoxic, the total amount of shunt is not significant. When more than 80% of the lung is hypoxic, HPV increases pulmonary vascular resistance (PVR), but the amount of well-perfused lung is not sufficient to accept shunt flow to maintain arterial oxygenation. This increase in PVR increases the work of the right side of the heart and can cause an increase in workload for the right ventricle.

3. **Anesthetic technique during OLV**
   a) The primary goal during OLV is maintenance of adequate arterial oxygenation while providing a surgical field favorable for visualization and manipulation of the operative lung.
   b) TLV should be maintained as long as possible and the time of OLV minimized. In the past, large V_Ts of 10 mL/kg (range, 8-15 mL/kg) were recommended to prevent atelectasis in the dependent lung and maintain an adequate functional residual capacity (FRC). Recent data suggest that most patients during OLV develop auto-positive end-expiratory pressure (auto-PEEP) and have an increased FRC. The use of a large V_T in that case may lead to trauma of the lung. Besides the direct physical effect, higher V_Ts are also associated with

increases in inflammatory mediators and in alveolar fibrin deposition and other markers of procoagulant effect, which characterize acute lung injury.

c) The understanding of the detrimental effects of high tidal volumes has led to the more contemporary approach of using more physiologic volumes (6 mL/kg), adding PEEP to those patients without auto-PEEP, and limiting plateau inspiratory pressures to below 25 cm H_2O. With this approach, patients maintain adequate or even improved oxygenation (compared with using higher V_T) and minimal elevations in $Paco_2$. In any case, the effects of hypercapnia (consider the use of "permissive hypercapnia" as a strategy in treating severe lung injury) is far less detrimental than the potential trauma from excessive ventilation.

d) An appropriate air–O_2 mixture, at times as high as an Fio_2 of 1, is necessary to maximize the Pao_2. However, after ascertaining that oxygenation will be stable after 30 minutes of OLV, the Fio_2 should be reduced to lessen the effects of absorptive atelectasis.

e) The respiratory rate can be adjusted to maintain an adequate $Paco_2$. Whereas a high Fio_2 should induce vasodilation in the dependent lung, improving blood flow, hypocapnia would cause vasoconstriction and should be avoided. The relationship between $Paco_2$ and end-tidal CO_2 is not altered by OLV.

f) If hypoxemia occurs during OLV, the anesthesia provider should assess for physiologic causes or tube malpositioning. Physiologic causes may include bronchospasm, decreased cardiac output, hypoventilation, a low Fio_2, or pneumothorax of the dependent lung. Tube malpositioning implies that movement of the DLT may have excluded a portion of dependent lung, usually the upper lobe. If physiologic causes have been ruled out and adequate lung separation and ventilation have been determined, one or more of the following interventions will help improve Pao_2.

(1) First, continuous positive airway pressure (CPAP) to the nondependent, nonventilated lung is almost 100% efficacious in increasing Pao_2. This can be accomplished with a compact breathing system, such as a Mapleson C with a manometer for pressure determination, attached to the lumen of the deflated lung.

(2) Alternatively, some DLTs can be purchased that include such a CPAP device with each tube. Application of CPAP should help to oxygenate the persistent blood flow through the nondependent lung, but too much pressure will cause the lung to inflate, reducing surgical exposure.

(3) The lowest level of effective CPAP (start at 2 cm H_2O) should be sought. A CPAP device that incorporates a reservoir bag is also useful for providing intermittent ventilation to the operative lung, if that intervention become necessary. Providing gentle ventilation with a separate system will minimize the diminution of surgical exposure, as opposed to ventilating the lung with the same vigor as that required for the dependent lung.

(4) If CPAP to the nondependent lung does not improve oxygenation, PEEP applied to the dependent, ventilated lung acts to increase Pao_2 by recruiting collapsed airways, increasing compliance of the lung, and increasing FRC. Excessive PEEP may also detrimentally reduce cardiac output. Combined with a fast

respiratory rate and/or high tidal volume, PEEP may impair adequate exhalation, leading to a net volume increase through "auto-PEEP" and lead to the potential for trauma to the dependent lung. The actual end-expiratory pressure should be monitored during OLV to assure that it does not significantly exceed the intended level of PEEP. Although the intention of PEEP is to recruit collapsed alveoli, overdistention of alveoli with excessive PEEP may increase the areas of zone 1 effect (alveolar pressure exceeding capillary pressure) and create more dead space ventilation.

(5) Other methods of improving oxygenation during OLV include combining PEEP and CPAP to the respective lungs and intermittent reinflation of the nondependent lung.

(6) The use of different modes of ventilation, such as pressure control, may provide a different distribution of ventilation and improve oxygenation as well. Emerging in this area is the use of innovative ventilatory approaches, such as high-frequency jet ventilation to the operative lung, and jet ventilation selectively to nonoperative lobes of the operative lung via a bronchial blocker with insufflation port.

(7) In the failure of CPAP and PEEP, early ligation of the pulmonary artery in pneumonectomy patients may be used to improve oxygenation. If the pulmonary artery is planned to be ligated during the procedure, clamping it will immediately stop all significant flow through the lung that is contributing to the shunt.

(8) If it becomes impossible to maintain adequate oxygenation with OLV despite CPAP and PEEP, manual TLV can be used, with pauses in ventilation coordinated with the surgeon's activities to facilitate exposure, suturing of the lung, or other needs.

g) Communication with the surgical team is vital throughout the procedure, especially during the evaluation and correction of hypoxia.

h) At the conclusion of the resection, the surgeon will commonly ask that the operative lung be reinflated using large tidal volumes, so that air leaks may be detected. At this time, the lung separator (DLT clamp, bronchial blocker) should be discontinued, and the lung inflated with slow breaths, achieving a peak inspiratory pressure of 30 to 40 cm H_2O. Reexpansion of the lung can be observed while performing this maneuver, which also helps to reverse atelectasis in the lungs. After lung reexpansion, the bronchial cuff should be deflated on the DLT to both reduce pressure on the bronchial mucosa and to obviate any detrimental effects of slight tube malpositioning. Deflated, the cuff does not pose the threat of herniating over the carina, obstructing the right upper lobe takeoff, and so on.

H. THORACOSCOPY

1. Introduction

Advances in videoscopic technology have led to the increased use of thoracoscopy. The procedure used most commonly involves placing the patient in the lateral decubitus position. A trocar is introduced at the fourth to fifth or fifth to sixth intercostal space to allow passage of the thoracoscope. Additional trocars and cannulas can be passed to insert suction, cautery, or other instruments. Drainage and examination of the pleural space lobectomy, debridement of an empyema, removal of foreign bodies, instillation of chemotherapeutic agents into the pleural space, pleurodesis with physical abrasion or talc, stapling of blebs, diagnostic biopsies and staging, and evaluation of bronchopleural fistulas are some of the procedures possible with thoracoscopy.

2. **Anesthetic technique**
   a) Thoracoscopy has been performed under epidural anesthesia alone, and this technique is associated with the typical advantages of regional over general anesthesia.
   b) General anesthesia with a double lumen ETT (DLT) is most common and offers several advantages for thoracoscopy. The airway is secured before lateral positioning. This avoids the need to change to general anesthesia under less-than-optimal conditions if regional anesthesia or sedation techniques fails. It allows for deflation of the lung before the introduction of the trocar.
   c) If desaturation occurs:
      (1) Administer 100% oxygen.
      (2) Perform manual ventilation.
      (3) Confirm DLT placement.
      (4) Apply CPAP to the nonventilated (operative) lung.
      (5) Apply PEEP to the ventilated lung.
      (6) Reinflate the operative lung.
      (7) Perform pulmonary artery clamping of the pulmonary artery segment that supplies the operative lung.
   d) Controlled ventilation helps prevent paradoxic respiration and mediastinal shift, and the lung can be actively reinflated at the end of the procedure.
   e) Regardless of the anesthetic used, the anesthesia provider should always be prepared for a switch to an open thoracotomy if the surgeon encounters complications or becomes unable to complete the procedure by thoracoscopy.
   f) An arterial line is generally placed for thoracoscopy except in selected healthy patients. Patients for thoracic procedures are generally at risk for cardiopulmonary morbidity. Because of the ventilation–perfusion mismatch that accompanies OLV, the anesthetic plan should account for the potential need for rapidly obtaining arterial blood gas samples.
   g) Thoracoscopic sympathectomy for hyperhidrosis is an outpatient procedure. A DLT is preferred over a bronchial blocker because the procedure is bilateral. Positioning the DLT once at the beginning of the case so that each lung can be deflated one at a time is much easier than repositioning a bronchial blocker into the opposite bronchus after one side has been completed. The patient is in the supine position, and no chest tubes are inserted. Air and O_2 are preferred carrier gases.
   h) Pain after a thoracoscopy is generally more easily managed than after an open thoracotomy. The incision length is smaller, and spreading of the ribs is avoided. Adequate pain relief is commonly obtained with the use of oral analgesics or nonsteroidal anti-inflammatory drugs. More extensive procedures such as decortication and

pleurodesis often require parenteral narcotics. An intercostal block may also be used to treat pain from manipulation of the thoracoscope in the camera port.

I. THORACOTOMY

1. **Introduction**

Thoracotomy is usually performed in an attempt to resect malignant lung tissue, but it may also be performed for trauma; infections; and parenchymal abnormalities, such as recurrent blebs. Because thoracotomy involves incising the pleura, all patients require a chest tube postoperatively. Most patients are older than 40 years and have a history of smoking. Many also have associated cardiovascular disease.

2. **Preoperative assessment**
    a) Preoperative evaluation of patients for pulmonary surgery (see the table below).

Initial Preanesthetic Assessment for Thoracic Surgery

Patient Type	Assessments
All patients	Assess exercise tolerance, estimate PPO FEV_1%,* discuss postoperative analgesia, consider discontinuation of smoking
Patients with PPO FEV_1 <40%	DLCO, $\dot{V}/\dot{Q}$ scan, $\dot{V}O_2$ max
Patients with cancer	Consider the "4 Ms": mass effects, metabolic effects, metastases, medications
Patients with COPD	ABG analysis, physiotherapy, bronchodilators
Patients with increased renal risk	Measure creatinine and BUN

*PPO FEV_1% = Preoperative FEV_1 % × (1% of functioning lung tissue removed/100). For values above 40%, postoperative complications are rare; for values between 30% and 40%, postoperative problems are possible; for values below 30%, postoperative ventilation is likely to be required.
ABG, Arterial blood gas; *BUN,* blood urea nitrogen; *COPD,* chronic obstructive pulmonary disease; *DLCO,* diffusing capacity for carbon monoxide; *FEV_1,* forced expiratory volume in 1 second; *PPO,* predicted postoperative; *$\dot{V}O_2$* max, maximum oxygen consumption; *V/Q,* ventilation–perfusion ratio.
Modified from Slinger PP, Johnston MR. Preoperative assessment and management. In Kaplan JA, Slinger PD, eds. *Thoracic Anesthesia.* 3rd ed. Philadelphia: Churchill Livingstone; 2003.

(1) Contraindications for lung resection surgery relate to preoperative testing (cardiovascular and pulmonary) and the patient's inability to tolerate the physiological stress of the procedure.
(2) Patients should undergo cardiologic evaluation. Unstable angina, myocardial infarction within 6 weeks, or significant arrhythmias predict a high risk of cardiac complications.
(3) Before lung resection, spirometry should be performed. Forced expiratory volume in 1 second (FEV_1) greater than 80% of predicted or greater than 2 L indicates minimal risk; further testing is not indicated. FEV_1 less than 40% of predicted indicates a high risk for complications or death.
(4) With evidence of interstitial lung disease or dyspnea, DLCO (diffusing capacity for carbon monoxide) should be measured.

DLCO below 60% predicts increased complications; below 40% equals high risk.

(5) If FEV_1 or DLCO is below 80% of predicted, postoperative lung function should be estimated.

(6) If preoperative or predicted postoperative FEV_1 or DLCO is below 40% of predicted normal, exercise testing should be performed. A VO_2 max (maximal oxygen consumption) above or below 15 mL/kg/min) will dispute or confirm the risk conferred by the low FEV_1. An inability to climb one flight of stairs, VO_2 max below 10 mL/kg/min, or desaturation greater than 4% during exercise, indicates a high risk for complications or mortality.

(7) Lung volume reduction surgery may be associated with improved outcomes beyond what preoperative measurements would suggest.

3. **Patient preparation**
   a) Laboratory tests include a complete blood count, electrolytes, blood urea nitrogen, creatinine, glucose, prothrombin time, partial thromboplastin time, arterial blood gases, and type and crossmatch for at least 2 units (depending on the type of surgery and the patient's hemoglobin).
   b) Digitalization is recommended prior to pneumonectomy to help prevent postoperative heart failure. It will also reduce tachyarrhythmias intraoperatively.
   c) Have inhaled bronchodilators readily available. Many practitioners administer them prophylactically.
   d) Administer an antisialagogue, such as glycopyrrolate, to ease placement and verification of the DLT.
4. **Room preparation**
   a) Monitoring: This is standard, with an arterial line. A central venous pressure (CVP) is placed in patients with preexisting heart disease. Keep in mind that CVP readings may be inaccurate while the chest is opened.
   b) Additional equipment includes DLTs (at least two). (Balloon rupture on insertion is common.) A fiberoptic endoscope is used to check tube placement. Equipment is needed to add CPAP and PEEP intraoperatively. Epidural catheter insertion and infusion supplies are indicated (if used). Warming devices are needed for the patient and fluids.
   c) Positioning: Lateral or supine with lateral tilt. A beanbag, arm "sled," and axillary rolls may be used. Check for lack of pressure on the downward arm, eye, and ear. Ensure that the patient's arms are not hyperextended.
   d) Drugs and fluids: It is preferable to err on the side of underhydrating because these patients are prone to pulmonary edema. Usually, one gives use of no more than 4 to 5 mL/kg/hr. Have ephedrine/phenylephrine available to treat hypotension.
5. **Perioperative management and anesthetic technique**
   a) Use standard induction techniques, keeping in mind that the positioning and placement of a DLT require more time than does standard tube placement.
   b) Preoxygenate these patients.
   c) Arterial blood gases are obtained after induction for baseline, so they may be compared with later results on OLV.

d) During OLV, maintain tidal volume between 6 to 8 mL/kg and place the patient on 100% oxygen. If hypoxemia is present (verify tube placement first), add 5 cm of CPAP to the "upward" (surgical) lung. If hypoxemia is still present, add 5 cm of PEEP to the "downward" (ventilated) lung.
e) Extubation at the end of the procedure is preferable unless the patient had a preoperative respiratory indication for remaining intubated (e.g., bronchospasm) or there were large fluid shifts. If the patient needs to remain intubated, the DLT should be replaced with a standard ETT.
f) For patients with oat cell (small cell) carcinoma, consider the possibility of Eaton-Lambert syndrome.

6. Postoperative implications

Epidural anesthesia, patient-controlled analgesia, or another type of pain control (e.g., nerve block) should be planned preoperatively. The patient must understand and be able to perform deep-breathing exercises. Institute intensive care unit monitoring for at least 24 hours.

J. THYMECTOMY

1. Introduction

The thymus gland is a bilobate mass of lymphoid tissue located deep into the sternum in the anterior region of the mediastinum. Thymectomy involves two surgical approaches: median sternotomy or transcervical.

The thymus gland is believed to play a role in myasthenia gravis. This is a neuromuscular disorder in which postsynaptic acetylcholine receptors are attacked, inducing rapid receptor destruction.

2. Preoperative assessment and patient preparation

a) History and physical examination
   (1) Respiratory (based on the patient with myasthenia gravis)
      (a) Weakness of pharyngeal and laryngeal muscles is associated with a high risk of aspiration. Assess the patient's ability to cough and handle secretions.
      (b) "Myasthenic crisis": This exacerbation involves the respiratory muscles to the point of inadequate ventilation.
   (2) Cardiac: Potential cardiomyopathy
   (3) Neurologic
      (a) Fatigability and fluctuating motor weakness of voluntary skeletal muscles worsen with repetitive use and improve with rest.
      (b) Ptosis and diplopia are initial symptoms.
   (4) Endocrine: Potential hypothyroidism
b) Diagnostic tests
   (1) Pulmonary function studies are obtained as indicated.
   (2) Laboratory tests include electrolytes, complete blood count, type and screen, and others as indicated by the patient's medical condition.
c) Preoperative medications and IV therapy
   (1) Cholinesterase inhibitors retard the enzymatic hydrolysis of acetylcholine at cholinergic synapses and cause acetylcholine to accumulate at the neuromuscular junction. Continue up to the morning of scheduled surgery.

(2) Immunosuppressive drugs
   (a) These drugs interfere with production of antibodies that are responsible for degradation of cholinergic receptors.
   (b) Patients who have been receiving steroids for more than 1 month in the past 6 to 12 months need supplementary steroids.
(3) Antisialagogues and H_2 (histamine$_2$-receptor) blockers: Patients with bulbar involvement should be evaluated to determine the safety of these drugs.
(4) Sedatives and narcotics: Use with caution in patients with poor respiratory reserve.
(5) Antibiotics are used.
(6) An 18-gauge IV catheter with moderate fluid replacement is used.

3. Room preparation

a) Monitoring equipment: Standard
   (1) An arterial line is placed if blood gas monitoring is necessary.
   (2) Some suggest placing the arterial catheter in the left radial artery for continuous monitoring in case the innominate artery is damaged.
b) Pharmacologic agents
   (1) Standard agents are used.
   (2) Depolarizing muscle relaxants should be avoided if possible in patients with myasthenia gravis.
   (3) Nondepolarizing muscle relaxants: Patients with myasthenia gravis may be exquisitely sensitive.
c) Position: Supine

4. Anesthetic technique and perioperative management

General anesthesia is used, and endotracheal intubation is required.

a) Induction
   (1) When anesthetizing patients with myasthenia gravis, avoidance of all muscle relaxants is preferred.
   (2) An inhaled anesthetic by itself should provide sufficient relaxation of skeletal muscle for intubation of the trachea.
b) Maintenance
   (1) The ability to dissipate the effects of inhaled drugs at the conclusion of anesthesia is important for evaluation of muscle strength.
   (2) The prolonged effects of narcotics, especially on ventilation, detract from the use of these drugs for maintenance.
c) Emergence
   (1) Before extubating the patient, it is important to know that respiratory ability is adequate.
   (2) Minimal extubation criteria must be met.
   (3) Reversal of neuromuscular blockade is controversial; the additional anticholinesterase may increase weakness and precipitate a cholinergic crisis.

5. Postoperative implications

a) Patients may need to be observed in an intensive care unit.
b) Anesthesia and surgery often decrease the need for anticholinesterase drugs in the postoperative period.
c) Discuss postoperative ventilation possibilities with the patient.

Neurologic System

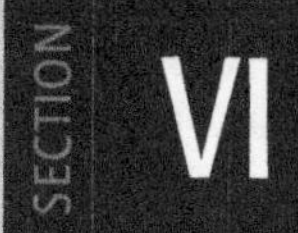

A. ARTERIOVENOUS MALFORMATION NEUROSURGERY

1. Introduction

Arteriovenous malformations (AVMs) are congenital, intracerebral networks in which arteries flow directly into veins. Patients with these malformations generally are younger than those with aneurysms. Patients may have bleeding or seizures or, less commonly, ischemia resulting from "steal" from normal areas or occurring with high-output congestive heart failure.

2. Anesthetic technique

The anesthetic problems parallel those associated with patients undergoing aneurysm surgery. Notably, AVMs do not autoregulate their blood flow. The operation is likely to be longer and bloodier than that of aneurysm clipping. Surgery may be preceded by an attempt at embolization by the neuroradiologist to diminish the risk of surgery. The neurologic examination should be repeated after embolization to document new deficits that otherwise might be attributed to anesthesia and surgery.

B. AWAKE CRANIOTOMY

1. Introduction

In a small percentage of patients (those in whom a seizure focus may be suppressed during general anesthesia or may be adjacent to an area of eloquent cortical function), awake craniotomy may be necessary. Awake craniotomy is the most reliable method to ensure neurologic integrity in cerebral gliomas that infiltrate or come close to the eloquent areas of the brain. It allows for the localization of eloquent cortical areas by electrical stimulation and epileptic foci through cortical recordings. Continuous monitoring of the functional integrity of the brain in awake patients is inherently protective while surgical removal of the gliomatous tissue is performed.

2. Patient preparation

a) Patient selection: To minimize the risk of intraoperative complications, contraindications for awake craniotomy include developmental delay, lack of maturity, an exaggerated or unacceptable response to pain, a significant communication barrier, and a failure to obtain patient consent. Only patients who have the ability to clearly understand risks and benefits and, in the opinion of the neurosurgeon, will cooperate during surgery should be considered as candidates for an awake craniotomy. Seizure management should be optimized with acceptable levels of antiepileptic medications verified.

b) Patient teaching: The single most important element in successful awake craniotomy is a highly motivated, well-informed patient. Each step of the procedure is discussed with the patient and family. Special emphasis is paid to prolonged surgical procedure, positioning, head immobility, pain anxiety, monitoring, noise, seizure management, and any individual considerations.

3. **Anesthetic technique**
   a) Upon arrival to the holding area, an intravenous (IV) line is established.
   b) Preanesthesia medications (antibiotics, steroids, antiemetic prophylaxis, and anticonvulsants as indicated) are administered.
   c) In the operating room suite, the application of noninvasive monitoring is completed.
   d) The patient is induced with propofol. Some sources use either dexmedetomidine singly or in combination with propofol.
   e) After satisfactory general anesthesia is established, a laryngeal mask airway (LMA) is placed with patient ventilation controlled using a continuous propofol infusion.
   f) Invasive monitoring is established (arterial line, central line), and a urinary catheter is placed.
   g) The scalp is anesthetized with 0.5% bupivacaine, and the head is placed in a pinion head holder.
   h) The patient is carefully positioned with all bony surfaces padded.
   i) The patient is carefully secured to the table to minimize a sense of falling when the table is moved during the awake phase of the surgery. Frameless stereotaxis registration is accomplished.
   j) Depending on the preoperative radiographic edema findings, hypertonic saline or mannitol is given.
   k) During the draping, an area is constructed around the patient's face such that the face may be clearly seen and accessed.
   l) A light is introduced under the drapes to keep the patient from darkness.
   m) During the scalp opening, spontaneous ventilation is established. Before bone flap removal, the LMA is removed and verbal contact established.

4. **Perioperative management**
   a) Awake phase
      (1) All sedation is stopped. All issues regarding patient comfort and concerns are addressed before the incision of the dura.
      (2) Conversation with the patient is confined to the surgeon and one member of the anesthesia team.
      (3) Stimulation of eloquent areas is carried out with results noted.
      (4) Any seizures are controlled with propofol. After the stimulation and mapping, volumetric surgical removal of the tumor or seizure focus is accomplished with interval monitoring.
      (5) Upon completion of the surgical removal and requisite monitoring, propofol sedation may be restarted and titrated to patient preference. Sedation is discontinued upon conclusion of surgery.
      (6) The most common complications associated with awake craniotomy are pain, seizures, nausea, and confusion.

C. CEREBRAL ANEURYSM

1. **Introduction**

Cerebral aneurysms are abnormal, localized dilations of the intracranial arteries. They are classified as berry or saccular, mycotic, traumatic, fusiform, neoplastic, or atherosclerotic. Rupture of a saccular aneurysm is a leading cause of subarachnoid hemorrhage (SAH).

a) Incidence

Approximately 5 million people in North America have cerebral aneurysms, with approximately 30,000 new cases of SAH occurring annually. The peak age for rupture of a cerebral aneurysm is 55 to 60 years. Aneurysmal ruptures are more common in women, occurring in three women for every two men.

More than one-third of patients with SAH die or develop significant and lasting neurologic disabilities before they receive any treatment. A small bleed occurs in approximately 50% of patients and is often tragically ignored or misdiagnosed. Even in patients who receive prompt care, only half remain functional survivors; the other half of patients die or develop serious neurologic deficits.

Aneurysms may arise at any point in the circle of Willis. The most common locations of aneurysms are shown in the following table. Most aneurysms are broad based and located in the middle cerebral system. Traumatic aneurysms develop as a result of direct trauma to an artery with injury to the wall.

Mirror aneurysms of the internal carotid system are common, and other combinations of locations occur (see table below). The site of the bleeding aneurysm is best located by computed tomography (CT) studies, evidence of vasospasm in the immediate vicinity, and lobulation of the aneurysm wall on angiographic studies.

Location and Occurrence of Cerebral Aneurysms

Location	Occurrence (%)
Internal carotid	38
Anterior cerebral system	36
Anterior communicating junction	30
Internal carotid at posterior communicating junction	25
Middle cerebral system	21
Vertebrobasilar system	5

From Frost AEM: Management of neurosurgical anesthesia: aneurysms. *Curr Rev Clin Anesth* 1991; 11:125-132.

b) Diagnosis of subarachnoid hemorrhage: Subarachnoid hemorrhage produces an abrupt intense headache in 85% of patients, and transient loss of consciousness may be seen in up to 45% of patients. Nausea and vomiting, photophobia, fever, meningismus, and focal neurologic deficits are common. The severity of an SAH can be graded clinically with the use of classifications listed in the table on pg. 372. Although surgical mortality rates vary somewhat among institutions, patients with a neurologic grade I SAH generally undergo surgical clipping with a low mortality rate (less than 5%), but grade V patients generally do not survive.

Hunt's Classification of Patients with Intracranial Aneurysms According to Surgical Risk

Grade	Perioperative Criterion	Mortality Rate (%)
I	Asymptomatic or minimal headache and slight nuchal rigidity	0-5
II	Moderate to severe headache, nuchal rigidity, no neurologic deficit, possible cranial nerve palsy	2-10
III	Drowsiness, confusion, or mild focal deficit	10-15
IV	Stupor, moderate to severe hemiparesis, possibly early decerebrate rigidity and vegetative disturbances	60-70
V	Deep coma, decerebrate rigidity, moribund appearance	70-100

From Hunt WE, Hess RM: Surgical risk as related to time of intervention in the repair of intracranial aneurysms. *J Neurosurg* 1968; 28:14.

c) General considerations

Hypertension often accompanies acute SAH and is postulated to develop secondary to autonomic hyperactivity, which may increase transmural pressure in the aneurysmal sac. Transmural pressure is defined as the differential pressure between mean arterial pressure (MAP) and intracranial pressure (ICP) and represents the stress applied to the aneurysm's wall.

Increases in blood pressure directly increase the transmural pressure and the likelihood of bleeding; conversely, reductions in blood pressure reduce transmural pressure. Caution should be exercised when purposefully reducing transmural pressure because cerebral autoregulation may be impaired after SAH, and a reduction in blood pressure may induce or aggravate cerebral ischemia, particularly if vasospasm is present. To balance these opposing concerns, many neurosurgeons attempt to maintain systolic blood pressure between 120 and 150 mmHg before clipping the aneurysm.

Electrocardiographic (ECG) changes are common after SAH and have been reported to occur in 50% to 80% of patients. The most common changes involve the T wave or the ST segment, but other changes such as the presence of a U wave, QTc-interval prolongation, and dysrhythmias may be present. Whether such changes in the ECG represent myocardial injury has long been debated. In the majority of patients, these changes do not appear to be associated with adverse neurologic or cardiac outcomes.

Rebleeding from a previously ruptured aneurysm is a life-threatening complication. The incidence of rebleeding is approximately 50% in the first days after SAH, and rebleeding is associated with an 80% mortality rate. The chance of rebleeding from an unsecured aneurysm declines over time, and by 6 months, the risk stabilizes at approximately 3% per year. Approaches used to decrease the risk of rebleeding include early surgical clipping, the use of antifibrinolytic agents, and blood pressure control.

(1) Vasospasm

(a) Vasospasm is reactive narrowing of cerebral arteries after SAH. Although arterial narrowing may be detected with angiography in 60% of patients, only half of these patients develop clinical symptoms. The accompanying neurologic deterioration, arising from impaired cerebral perfusion, ischemia, and secondary infarction of the brain, peaks between the fourth and ninth days after SAH and resolves over the following 2 to 3 weeks.

(b) Successful treatment of vasospasm depends on the maintenance of adequate cerebral perfusion pressure (CPP). This is accomplished with expansion of the intravascular volume, which augments blood pressure and cardiac output, avoidance of hyponatremia, and preservation of relative hemodilution (hematocrit approximately 32%). Because of the risk of rebleeding, both hypertension and hypervolemia are used with caution in the period preceding surgical correction.

(c) Pharmacologic vasodilatation of spastic vessels has been ineffective because vasospasm involves a structural alteration in the vessel wall rather than just a spastic contracture or failure of relaxation of the smooth muscle cells in the media of the vessels. Nimodipine and nicardipine (calcium channel blockers) are currently in wide use for prevention of delayed neurologic deficit after SAH. They diminish the level of myoplastic calcium in smooth muscle cells and impede the entry of extracellular calcium necessary for the contraction of the smooth muscle. Recent literature supports a role for magnesium as possible vasospasm prophylaxis.

(2) Timing of surgery

The presence or absence of vasospasm on angiographic studies has frequently determined the timing of aneurysmal surgery. Current neurosurgical practice suggests that a good outcome is achieved with early operation (within 24 to 48 hours) in patients who are neurologically intact (grade I or II) regardless of whether vasospasm has been demonstrated. Such emergency intervention decreases the likelihood of rebleeding. Only 53% of grade III patients achieve a good outcome after early surgery; this indicates that the gross neurologic condition preoperatively is the best prognostic indicator of intact survival. In the first few days after hemorrhage, the brain is swollen, soft, hyperemic, and prone to contusion and laceration. Impaired autoregulation may decrease cerebral tolerance to brain retraction. Although removal of a subarachnoid clot probably decreases the incidence and severity of delayed arterial narrowing, operative management may be hazardous. In more severely injured patients (grades III through V), surgery is often delayed in anticipation of resolution of vasospasm and improvement in neurologic status.

Endovascular coiling has been used increasingly as an alternative to neurosurgical clipping for treating SAH secondary to aneurysm rupture. The risk of late rebleeding is low. However, there is an increased risk of bleeding after endovascular coiling than after neurosurgical clipping.

2. Preoperative assessment

a) The baseline neurologic status must be ascertained. The level of consciousness may vary from perfect alertness to deep coma and is an important prognostic factor for the postoperative state. Evidence of increased ICP should be elicited preoperatively so that it can be managed appropriately intraoperatively. Focal motor and sensory signs may indicate intracerebral extension of SAH, vasospasm, or cerebral edema.

b) Pulmonary complications, such as pneumonia, neurogenic pulmonary edema, and atelectasis, are not uncommon and are potentially treatable. Patients often have an increased risk of aspiration because of their depressed level of consciousness, and measures should be taken to reduce gastric acidity and volume preoperatively. The use of prophylactic hypervolemia also increases the likelihood of pulmonary edema.
c) The hemodynamic status of the patient should be assessed, with particular attention paid to the relationship between neurologic deterioration and blood pressure changes. Continuous arterial blood pressure monitoring is essential. Serious dysrhythmias or evidence of ventricular dysfunction should be diagnosed preoperatively so that appropriate monitoring and management can be instituted.
d) The syndrome of inappropriate antidiuretic hormone (SIADH) and diabetes insipidus (DI) can occur in patients with SAH. Preoperative electrolyte studies should be examined to facilitate intraoperative management.
e) The presence of blood in the subarachnoid space may produce a 1° C to 2° C elevation of body temperature. Temperature elevation increases cerebral oxygen requirements and therefore should be treated to prevent an increase of cerebral ischemia.
f) Preoperative sedation is rarely necessary in these patients. Depression of ventilation associated with opioids, barbiturates, and benzodiazepines may result in hypercapnia with resultant increases in cerebral blood flow (CBF) and ICP. Additionally, the reduced level of consciousness preoperatively and postoperatively may make clinical assessment difficult. If preoperative sedation is considered necessary, a small dose of a benzodiazepine (midazolam) with continued observation after its administration is probably the best choice.
g) A type and cross with blood readily available to administer is necessary.

3. **Anesthetic technique**
   a) The maintenance of adequate intravascular volume requires two large-bore IV cannulas.
   b) Intraoperative monitoring includes continuous ECG (V5), arterial pressure monitoring, peripheral nerve stimulator, central venous pressure (CVP) monitoring, electroencephalogram (EEG), end-tidal CO_2 ($ETCO_2$) monitoring, pulse oximetry, and monitoring of temperature and fluid balance.
   c) The anesthetic induction should be slow and deliberate. The anesthetic depth should be sufficient to avoid the hypertensive responses that accompany laryngoscopy and endotracheal intubation.
   d) Anesthesia is induced with titrated doses of either thiopental or propofol. The addition of an opioid (5 to 10 mcg/kg of fentanyl or 1 to 2 mcg/kg of sufentanil) and IV lidocaine (1.5 mg/kg) further blunts the patient's response to sympathetic stimulation of laryngoscopy and intubation.
   e) An additional dose of opioid or propofol is required for the placement of the three-point pin head holder.
   f) Prior injection of local anesthetic minimizes the associated sympathetic stimulation. Isoflurane may be introduced after hyperventilation before laryngoscopy to increase the depth of anesthesia.

g) Ventilation is controlled with administration of 100% oxygen to achieve a $Paco_2$ of 35 to 40 mmHg with normal intracranial compliance.
h) Mild hyperventilation ($Paco_2$ of 25 to 30) is instituted when intracranial compliance is decreased and ICP is increased. Long-term maintenance of hypocarbia results in poor neurologic outcomes in patients with increased ICP.
i) Intubation can be accomplished with 1 mg/kg of rocuronium.
j) The patient is placed in one of several positions, depending on the site of the aneurysm.
   (1) Aneurysms that arise from the anterior part of the circle of Willis require that the patient be supine for a frontotemporal approach.
   (2) The lateral position for a temporal approach is required for aneurysms that arise from the posterior aspect of the basilar artery. Aneurysms that arise from the vertebral artery or from the lower basilar artery require a sitting or prone position for a suboccipital approach.
   (3) Aneurysms that arise from the anterior communicating artery are usually approached from the right; those from the middle cerebral and posterior communicating arteries are approached from the side on which the aneurysm is located.
k) Anesthesia is maintained with air and oxygen or N_2O and oxygen, with incremental titrated dosages of an opioid (fentanyl, alfentanil, or sufentanil) or an infusion of remifentanil and a muscle relaxant. Isoflurane may also be added in inspired concentrations not to exceed 1%.
l) Controlled hypotension is commonly used intraoperatively to make aneurysms softer and more pliable at the time of clipping, as well as to minimize blood loss should aneurysmal rupture occur at this time. Sodium nitroprusside and an inhalation anesthetic agent are the drugs most widely used for induction of hypotension.
m) The safe limit of controlled hypotension has not been definitively established. Because autoregulation is maintained to a MAP of 50 to 60 mmHg, some argue that this limit should not be exceeded. In addition, because patients with poor-grade aneurysms may not have intact autoregulation, some argue that a lower limit of 60 mmHg should be adopted. Limits of autoregulation are shifted to higher pressures in patients with preexisting hypertension, so MAP should probably be kept within 40% of baseline. Higher blood pressure maintenance is necessary to avoid cerebral hypoxia if the patients head is elevated.
n) Many neurosurgeons now routinely use temporary proximal occlusion of the parent vessel rather than induce hypotension to facilitate clip ligation of the neck of the aneurysm.
o) The use of mild intraoperative hypothermia has been advocated for cerebral protection during periods of temporary occlusion.
p) At the conclusion of the anesthetic procedure, patients with low-grade aneurysms may be extubated in the operating room, although care must be exercised so that coughing, straining, hypercarbia, and hypertension are avoided. Propofol, lidocaine, or small doses of fentanyl may be used for short-term anesthesia as the procedure is being finished and for reducing the hemodynamic responses to extubation.

q) Although the residual depressant effects of opioids may be reversed with judicious titrated dosages of naloxone, larger doses of naloxone can be hazardous because they may cause sudden, violent awakening of the patient and marked increases in systemic blood pressure.
r) Endotracheal tubes (ETTs) should be retained in patients with high-grade aneurysms and in those who have had intraoperative complications because these patients will probably require postoperative ventilation.

4. **Postoperative implications**
   a) Postoperative care is directed at the prevention of vasospasm via the maintenance of intravascular volume expansion and moderate hypertension (MAP of 80 to 120 mm Hg).
   b) Changes in the level of consciousness and development of focal neurologic deficits are usually early signs of vasospasm. These clinical signs should be aggressively managed with hypertension, hypervolemia, and hemodilution. Dopamine may be used for blood pressure support. CT should be used for ruling out other causes of neurologic deterioration, including rebleeding, infarction, and hydrocephalus.

5. **Aneurysmal rupture**

Intraoperative aneurysmal rupture can be catastrophic. An abrupt increase in blood pressure during or after induction of anesthesia may indicate that an aneurysm has bled.

a) The use of propofol or 0.5 to 1 mcg/kg of sodium nitroprusside decreases the transmural pressure of the aneurysm, although hypotension can be detrimental at this juncture.
b) Intraoperative aneurysmal rupture necessitates maintenance of the MAP between 40 to 50 mm Hg or lower to facilitate surgical control of the neck of the aneurysm or the parent vessel.
c) Alternatively, one or both carotid arteries may be compressed for up to 3 minutes to produce a bloodless field.
d) Blood that is lost should be continuously replaced with blood, blood products, or colloid solution so that intravascular volume is maintained.
e) A propofol drip or small bolus may be administered immediately before the aneurysm clipping to decrease the cerebral metabolic rate of oxygen consumption.

D. CRANIOPLASTY

1. **Introduction**

Cranioplasty can be performed for a bony tumor resulting from traumatic injury (e.g., depressed skull fracture) or, more rarely, from a condition resulting from a congenital malformation (e.g., fused suture lines). These defects may occur anywhere on the head, so the surgical procedure may take place with the patient in varying positions such as supine, sitting, prone, or supine with the head turned. Patients range widely in age from newborn to elderly.

2. **Preoperative assessment**

These are individualized according to the patient's need.

3. **Patient preparation**

Complete blood count (CBC), electrolytes, blood urea nitrogen, creatinine, glucose, prothrombin time, and partial thromboplastin time (D-dimer or fibrin split products if disseminated intravascular coagulation needs to be ruled out) are used. Type and crossmatch (for at least 2 units). Arterial blood gases are measured if the patient is being ventilated.

4. **Room preparation**
    a) Monitoring equipment: Standard. An arterial line and central line are used if suggested by the patient's history. Foley catheter is indicated if surgery is scheduled for more than 2 hours. Some patients may have an ICP monitor in place, and ICP monitoring should be continued intraoperatively.
    b) Additional equipment: Determine the patient's position during surgery. If the patient is supine or supine with the head turned, a foam support aids in positioning the head. Longer ventilation tubing is often needed because the table will be rotated 90 to 180 degrees. When the patient is in the sitting position, a Doppler device and a central line (with a 60-mL syringe attached) are needed to assess and treat venous air embolism (VAE). With the prone position, use prone foam rest shoulder rolls and multiple pads. In all cases, a nasal ETT assists in clearing the surgical field and in stabilizing the ETT. However, if traumatic injury to the facial structures or sinus has occurred, nasal instrumentation should be avoided.
    c) Drugs and tabletop: Thiopental and etomidate are useful in cranioplasty because of their cerebral protective properties. Propofol is known to decrease ICP. Most surgeons desire to administer antibiotics during surgery, and they may be helpful.
    d) Blood and fluid requirements: Glucose-containing solutions are best avoided in neurologic surgery. It is better to err on the side of underhydration. Fluid is usually replaced with normal saline or lactated Ringer solution at 2 to 4 mL/kg/hr. Blood loss may be substantial, and blood should be immediately available to avoid hypotension or crystalloid overload.
5. **Anesthetic technique**
    a) Induction is IV, with one of the agents known to decrease ICP. In severe trauma, one may wish to use only oxygen, narcotic, and muscle relaxant.
    b) For maintenance, keep the patient's mean arterial blood pressure slightly below the baseline and maintain normocarbia to slight hypocarbia.
    c) A constant infusion of thiopental, etomidate, or propofol with or without inhalation of isoflurane will help to maintain cerebral perfusion and will minimize the cerebral oxygen consumption.
    d) Muscle relaxation is not necessary if the procedure is confined to the skull, and the head is immobilized with tongs or some other type of fixator.
    e) Most practitioners leave the ETT in place until the neurologic status is certain to allow for regular respiration. Lidocaine is useful in minimizing cough.
6. **Postoperative implications**

Assess postoperative neurologic functions. Pain in patients with altered neurologic status is usually controlled with parenteral agents. Avoid hypercarbia in neurologic patients receiving opiates because it increases CBF and ICP.

E. CRANIOTOMY

1. Introduction

Intracranial masses may be congenital, neoplastic (benign, malignant, or metastatic), infectious (abscess or cyst), or vascular (hematoma or malformation). Most, but not all, anesthetics can be used safely in patients with cerebral lesions. The effects of the agent on ICP, CPP, CBF, $CMRo_2$ (cerebral metabolic rate of oxygen), promptness of return of consciousness, drug-related protection from cerebral ischemia or edema, blood pressure control, and compatibility with neurophysiologic monitoring techniques are important considerations.

Most craniotomy surgery in the United States today is performed after a propofol induction of anesthesia with intubation of the trachea after a nondepolarizing relaxant. Maintenance of anesthesia is commonly accomplished with a combination of an inhalation agent (usually isoflurane) and narcotic such as fentanyl, sufentanil, or alfentanil in various combinations during maintenance of low normocarbia.

2. Preoperative assessment

a) The clinical signs of a supratentorial mass include seizures, hemiplegia, and aphasia. The clinical signs of infratentorial masses include cerebellar dysfunction (ataxia, nystagmus, dysarthria) and brainstem compression (cranial nerve palsies, altered consciousness, abnormal respiration). When ICP increases, frank signs of intracranial hypertension can also develop.

b) Preanesthetic evaluation should attempt to establish the presence or absence of intracranial hypertension. CT or magnetic resonance imaging (MRI) data should be reviewed for evidence of brain edema, midline shift greater than 0.5 cm, and ventricular size. A neurologic assessment should evaluate the current mental status and any existing neurologic deficits.

c) Medications prescribed for the control of ICP (corticosteroids, diuretics) and anticonvulsant therapy should be reviewed. Laboratory evaluation should rule out corticosteroid-induced hyperglycemia and electrolyte disturbances (such as SIADH or DI) that may develop secondary to diuretic therapy. Anticonvulsants, dosage time of last dose, and blood levels should be noted.

d) The decision regarding the amount and timing of the premedication administration should be made only after a thorough patient evaluation. Benzodiazepines produce respiratory depression and hypercapnia. Premedication should be omitted in patients with a large mass lesion, a midline shift, and abnormal ventricular size. Opioids are universally avoided in the preoperative period. If premedication is desired in patients deemed appropriate, careful titration of IV midazolam may begin when the patient has been delivered to the preoperative holding area. In an attempt to help control ICP in patients with mass lesions, the head of the bed should be elevated 15 to 30 degrees during transport to the preoperative holding area and the operating room.

e) Due diligence to all existing hospital recommendations for prophylactic antibiotics given at the appropriate time and in the appropriate amount should be performed.

3. **Perioperative management**
   a) Intraoperative monitoring
      (1) Routine monitors for supratentorial procedures include continuous ECG, cuff measurement of blood pressure, precordial stethoscope, monitoring of the fraction of inspired oxygen, pulse oximetry, temperature, peripheral nerve stimulation, $ETCO_2$ monitoring, and indwelling urinary catheterization.
      (2) For patients with ischemic heart disease, use of a modified V_5 ECG lead is recommended. An arterial line placed either before or immediately after anesthetic induction provides for uninterrupted blood pressure monitoring and easy access for blood sampling for laboratory analysis.
      (3) Somatosensory evoked potentials (SSEPs) may be assessed and may warrant the need for half an alternative anesthetic of 0.5 minimum alveolar concentration (MAC) and propofol infusion.
   b) Fluid management
      (1) Preoperative fluid deficits and intraoperative blood and fluid losses must be adequately replaced during neurosurgical procedures. Judicious fluid administration minimizes the occurrence of cerebral edema and increased ICP, reduced CPP, and worsened cerebral ischemia.
      (2) In most neurosurgical patients, fluids that contain osmolarity similar to that of serum (e.g., lactated Ringer solution or 0.9% saline) are administered in a volume that is sufficient for the maintenance of peripheral perfusion but that avoids hypervolemia (0.5 to 1 mL/kg/hr).
      (3) Traditionally, less fluid is given than would be administered for nonneurologic surgery, although new recommendations indicate that patients should be kept isovolemic, isotonic, and iso-oncotic. No single IV solution is best suited for neurosurgical patients at risk for intracranial hypertension, but the use of iso-osmolar crystalloids is widely accepted and can be justified on a scientific basis.
      (4) Emerging evidence questions the rationale for routine administration of glucose. Hyperglycemia induces marked cerebrovascular changes during both ischemia and reperfusion. Multiple studies have demonstrated that hyperglycemia before and during an episode of global cerebral ischemia will exacerbate the neurologic injury.
      (5) Fluid therapy is most challenging during prolonged surgical procedures or in the surgical management of multiple traumas. If tissue trauma is severe or if hemorrhage has been prolonged, patients develop a marked reduction in functional extracellular volume as a result of the internal redistribution of fluids (third-space losses).
      (6) Although the extent of tissue manipulation in most routine neurosurgical procedures is small, third-space fluid losses during prolonged surgery and in patients with severe associated systemic trauma can be sufficient to decrease intravascular volume, reduce peripheral perfusion, and impair renal function. The sequestered extracellular fluid can be cautiously replaced with lactated Ringer solution or with 0.9% saline.

(7) In the absence of diuretic therapy, a urinary output of 0.5 to 1 mL/kg/hr suggests adequate replacement as do hemodynamic stability and cardiac filling pressures within the normal range. Although some clinicians prefer to use colloid-containing solutions in neurosurgical patients, such solutions appear to exert negligible effects on brain water and ICP.

4. **Anesthetic technique**
   a) Although induction of anesthesia for patients undergoing craniotomy can be performed with various agents, a smooth and gentle induction of general anesthesia is more important than the drug combination used. No evidence indicates that one technique or set of drugs is better than another.
   b) A reasonable induction sequence would combine preoxygenation, propofol (1-2 mg/kg), and a nondepolarizing muscle relaxant. No evidence suggests that any of the induction agents (midazolam, etomidate, propofol, and methohexital) is superior to thiopental.
   c) The hemodynamic response to intubation may be blunted with the administration of fentanyl (10-15 mcg/kg total dose) or lidocaine (1.5 mg/kg) administered 3 minutes before laryngoscopy. The dose of these induction agents may need to be adjusted according to the patient's age and physical status. Whatever agents are selected, the induction should be accomplished without the development of sudden hypertension or hypotension.
   d) The head typically is elevated from 15 to 30 degrees to facilitate venous and cerebrospinal fluid (CSF) drainage. The head may also be turned to the side to facilitate exposure. Excessive neck flexion may impede jugular venous drainage and increase ICP. Because of the flexion-extension-rotation of the head in combination with head fixation in a pinion headrest, the use of an armored or reinforced ETT is recommended to avoid kinking of the tube after positioning is accomplished.
   e) The anesthesia circuit connections must be firmly secured by simultaneously pushing and twisting to seat the plastic connectors. The risk of unrecognized disconnections may be increased because the operating table is usually turned 90 to 180 degrees away from the anesthesia provider, and both the patient and the breathing circuit are almost completely covered by surgical drapes.
   f) Maintenance of anesthesia may be accomplished with an oxygen–air–opioid technique, a selected potent inhalation agent, or oxygen–air and a continuous infusion of propofol.
   g) After endotracheal intubation, mechanical hyperventilation may be initiated, decreasing $ETCO_2$ to 30 to 35 mmHg, confirmed through arterial blood gas analysis. The patient should be covered with blankets or a forced air warming blanket to maintain core body temperature.
   h) An opioid-based anesthetic technique with air in oxygen with low-dose (less than 1%) isoflurane is a popular choice. Incremental administration of fentanyl, sufentanil, alfentanil, or an infusion of remifentanil is acceptable. Alternatively, sufentanil, 0.5 to 1 mcg/kg loading dose followed by either incremental boluses (not to exceed 0.5 mcg/kg/hr) or an IV infusion of 0.25 to 0.5 mcg/kg/hr in combination with less than 1% isoflurane in oxygen may be used. Sufentanil administration should be discontinued approximately

45 minutes before the end of surgery to ensure that the patient awakens promptly. The primary advantage of remifentanil is rapid awakening. If the patient experiences hypertension or tachycardia near the end of surgery, the anesthesia provider should consider giving either labetalol or esmolol, not additional opioids.

i) An inhalation agent (isoflurane, desflurane, or sevoflurane) with little or no opioid supplementation can also be used for maintenance of anesthesia. If isoflurane is used, the concentration should remain less than 1%. Hyperventilation in combination with less than 1% isoflurane generally results in stable intracranial dynamics.

j) N_2O may be used in an anesthetic regimen if it is deemed desirable. However, if the patient is suspected to have a pneumocephalus or if the potential for air embolism exists, N_2O use is contraindicated. N_2O expands both the pneumocephalus and the air embolus.

k) Hyperventilation is an important adjunct to any neuroanesthetic technique. Hypocapnia decreases ICP before opening of the dura and attenuates the vasodilatation produced by the volatile anesthetic agents. Optimal hyperventilation during surgery would yield a $Paco_2$ of 25 to 30 mmHg and is indicated for short periods when ICP is dramatically increased or brain compliance is decreased. Diuretics, when indicated, may be timed just before or after the cranial vault is opened to facilitate surgical exposure.

l) In choosing an agent for muscle relaxation, the length of the procedure and the impact of the drug on ICP should be considered.

m) Emergence

(1) Careful attention to appropriate planning for the emergence from anesthesia is important. Sudden emergence from anesthesia can result in uncontrolled hypertension. Delirium with coughing and straining on the endotracheal tube should be avoided. In a patient with a compromised blood-brain barrier, this stormy emergence can produce devastating consequences.

(2) Late emergence from anesthesia can result in a confusing diagnostic picture with possible intracranial hematoma, acute hydrocephalus, or other diagnoses masked by the residual anesthesia.

(3) The goal for emergence is control. A controlled emergence focuses on regulation of blood pressure, ICP, and CBF. Controlled emergence also accounts for the preexisting pathophysiology, the surgical trauma, the length of the procedure, and appropriate management of the airway.

(4) Emergence from anesthesia begins when the surgical pathology has been addressed. Collaboration with the surgeon is essential. The $Paco_2$ should be allowed to return to a normal level. At the surgeon's request, blood pressure can then be raised to 120% of the normal baseline level before closing of the dura. Hypertension is considered a frequent occurrence of the postoperative period. Tachycardia associated with hypertension "invariably" results from emergence excitement. By raising the blood pressure and the $Paco_2$ before dural closure, the surgeon can directly assess the ability of the brain to withstand such challenges.

(5) After the dura has been closed, the blood pressure is maintained at baseline levels throughout the remainder of the closure. There is strong support for the notion that sympatholytic

drugs should be used to decrease blood pressure during emergence. Studies have shown that during the first hour after craniotomy for supratentorial lesions, the arteriovenous oxygen content difference is low, suggesting a state of cerebral luxury perfusion. This event coincides with a high level of mean arterial blood pressure. Accordingly, it is supposed that this correlation is caused by changes in the mean blood pressure and impaired autoregulation. This may be deleterious because it enhances blood-brain barrier leakage, provoking edema and hemorrhage.

(6) A relationship between hypertension and postoperative hematoma formation exists. The parameters for these events for each individual patient are unknown. Normal autoregulation of CBF maintains adequate perfusion at mean blood pressures ranging from 50 to 150 mmHg. Labile hypertension and unstable blood pressure during the perisurgical period may be contributory to intracerebral hemorrhage remote from the site of the initial neurosurgical procedure.

(7) Judicious titration of antihypertensives (esmolol, labetalol) has great clinical utility in controlling the blood pressure during emergence. When access to the patient is regained, the use of anesthetic gases is discontinued and the muscle relaxant is reversed. IV lidocaine (1.5 mg/kg) can be given just before suctioning for cough suppression before extubation.

(8) Delayed awakening may result from residual opioid or remaining end-tidal concentrations of potent inhalation agent. After extubation, the patient is transported to the intensive care unit postoperatively for continued monitoring of neurologic function.

F. ELECTROCONVULSIVE THERAPY

1. Introduction

Electroconvulsive therapy (ECT) is the intentional inducement of a generalized seizure of the central nervous system (CNS) for an adequate duration of time to treat patients with certain severe neuropsychiatric disorders. Antidepressant medication administration, along with ECT, is well tolerated by patients, and both therapies can be beneficial to the patient. Most patients receive three treatments per week and can undergo a total of 6 to 12 treatments total. Clinical improvement is seen within the first three to five treatments, and positive response to treatment is seen in 50% to 90% of patients (even those who had been treatment resistant). ECT treatments exceed the total numbers of coronary revascularizations, herniorrhaphy, and appendectomy procedures performed in the United States. Death from ECT itself is possible but is rare. ECT also is used in certain patients who experience mania, catatonia, vegetative states, dysregulation, inanition, suicidal drive, and schizophrenia with affective disorders.

a) Procedures: Treatment involves placement of electrodes with a conducting gel either right-sided unilaterally or bitemporally bilaterally; an alternating current of electricity is passed through the electrodes. Theories for the mechanism of ECT are related to profound changes in brain chemistry, such as enhancement of dopaminergic, serotonergic, and adrenergic neurotransmission. Another theory postulates the release of hypothalamic or pituitary hormones, which have antidepressant effects. Finally, ECT produces anticonvulsant effects that raise the seizure threshold and decrease seizure duration, exerting a positive effect on the brain.

2. Anesthetic technique

Anesthesia for ECT involves the administration of an ultra-brief general anesthetic to provide lack of consciousness to the patient for the procedure (see table below).

Anesthetic Medications Used for Electroconvulsive Therapy

Drug	Dose
	Anticholinergics
Atropine	0.4-1 mg IV or IM
Glycopyrrolate	0.005 mg/kg IV or IM
Anesthetics	
Alfentanil	0.2-0.3 mcg/kg IV
Etomidate	0.1-0.3 mg/kg IV
Ketamine	0.5-1 mg/kg IV
Methohexital	0.5-1 mg/kg IV
Propofol	0.75-1.5 mg/kg IV
	Muscle Relaxant
Depolarizing	
Succinylcholine	0.75-1.5 mg/kg IV
Nondepolarizing	
Cisatracurium	0.15-0.25 mg/kg IV (onset 1-2 minutes)
Atracurium	0.3-0.4 mg/kg IV (onset 6 minutes)
Rocuronium	0.3-0.9 mg/kg IV (onset 1-2 minutes)

IM, Intramuscular; *IV,* intravenous.

Adapted from Ding Z, White PF. Anesthesia for electroconvulsive therapy. *Anesth Analg* 2002; 94:1351-1364; White PF. *Perioperative Drug Manual.* 2nd ed. Philadelphia: Saunders. 2005; Wagner KJ, Möllenberg O, Rentrop M, et al. Guide to anaesthetic selection for electroconvulsive therapy. *CNS Drugs* 2005;19:745-758.

a) A thorough preanesthetic assessment must be performed, with consideration given to the possible great physiologic hemodynamic responses generated by the induced seizure activity. The box on pg. 384 lists the possible physiologic effects as a result of ECT.
b) Adult patients about to undergo ECT should follow fasting guidelines of at least 6 hours for solids and 2 hours for liquids. Necessary bronchodilators may be taken. Oral medications, such as antihypertensives, cardiac medications, anticoagulants, and thyroid medications, may be taken with a sip of water up to 1 hour before the procedure.

Possible Physiologic Effects as a Result of Electroconvulsive Therapy

Cardiovascular	Cerebral
Parasympathetic Response During the Tonic Phase of Seizure	Increased cerebral blood flow (increase of 100% to 400% above baseline are possible)
Decreased heart rate	Increased intracranial pressure
Hypotension	
Bradydysrhythmias	**Other**
Sympathetic Response During the Clonic Phase of Seizure	Increased intraocular pressure
Tachycardia	Increased intragastric pressure
Hypertension	
Tachydysrhythmias	

Adapted from Lee M: Anesthesia for electroconvulsive therapy. In Atlee JL, editor: *Complications in Anesthesia.* 2nd ed. Philadelphia: Saunders; 2007:903-905.

c) Patients may have results of laboratory studies, a pharmacologic regimen, and ECG readily available because of their psychiatric hospitalization. Informed consent is obtained whenever possible from the patient or legal guardian. An IV catheter is inserted in a peripheral vein.
d) The patient is monitored with a pulse oximeter, ECG, noninvasive blood pressure monitor, temperature-monitoring device, and peripheral nerve stimulator. Use of $ETCO_2$ monitoring has been suggested because hypercarbia and hypoxia shorten seizure duration.
e) Suction, oxygen, a positive-pressure Ambu bag and face mask, and rubber bite protectors must be present, as well as necessary airway and cardiovascular resuscitation equipment (including a laryngoscope and ETT with stylet), medications, and supplies because ECT is usually performed in a dedicated psychiatric suite or special treatment room.
f) The patient is preoxygenated before induction. Anticholinergics may be administered as an antisialagogue or to prevent asystole.
g) The induction agent is administered intravenously. Propofol, etomidate, and ketamine have also been used, although an enhanced hemodynamic response and increased ICP is possible after using ketamine. Succinylcholine (0.25-0.5 mg/kg) is usually given and is the drug of choice because of its short duration.
h) Positive-pressure ventilation is applied to the patient via the positive pressure breathing bag and a face mask and is continued until after treatment is completed and spontaneous respirations resume.
i) To assess the duration of the induced convulsion, the psychiatrist usually applies a tourniquet or a manual blood pressure cuff (inflated to slightly greater than the systolic blood pressure) above a lower extremity so that the muscle relaxant cannot reach the skeletal muscle in the extremity.
j) A rubber bite block is gently placed in the patient's mouth to prevent biting down on the teeth, lips, and tongue at the end of the procedure.

k) A nerve stimulator must be used, and appropriate neuromuscular blockade reversal agents should be administered if necessary. The electrodes are applied, the proper waveform and current level are selected, and the electroconvulsive seizure is induced.

l) The seizure lasts from 30 to 90 seconds; the motor seizure is shorter than the seizure duration as seen on an EEG.

m) Use of an anesthesia awareness, level of consciousness, and depth of sedation monitor correlates with the EEG and can be a useful tool for the anesthesia provider and the psychiatrist.

n) The level of sedation displayed by this monitor correlates with the proper point to induce seizure, the duration of seizure, and the potential for awareness during the ECT procedure.

o) At the end of the seizure, spontaneous respirations resume, the patient is transferred to a recovery area, and vital signs are continually monitored until the patient is determined to be stable and able to be safely discharged.

p) Certain anesthetic medications and techniques such as hyperventilation can affect seizure duration.

3. Postoperative implications

a) Postanesthesia care

The intentional creation of CNS convulsions has profound effects on the patient's physiology. Patients usually experience temporary cognitive and memory impairment after ECT.

The first type of impairment that may be seen is postictal confusion, in which the patient is transiently restless, confused, and agitated immediately after the convulsive episode and for approximately 30 minutes. A second type of cognitive impairment that may be seen later is anterograde memory dysfunction, in which the patient may rapidly forget new information. A third cognitive dysfunction is retrograde memory dysfunction, which is the forgetting of memories from several weeks to several months before the ECT treatment. The cognitive effects described vary depending on the frequency and the number of ECT treatments the patient has received. The quantities of energy used to elicit the convulsions and the placement of the electrodes are also factors. Type of anesthetic drugs used may also be implicated.

Cardiovascular stimulation also occurs with ECT. The sympathetic and parasympathetic nervous systems are stimulated sequentially. Therefore, the patient may experience an increase in heart rate and blood pressure followed by a period of bradycardia or even asystole. Transient cardiac changes can be managed before ECT with anticholinergics, IV local anesthetics such as lidocaine, or IV narcotics such as remifentanil. Changes after ECT can be managed with β-blockers such as esmolol or labetalol, calcium channel blockers such as verapamil or nifedipine, or other antihypertensives such as nitroprusside or nitroglycerin.

Patients may also experience headache, muscle aches, or postoperative nausea and vomiting (PONV). Symptoms of headache or muscle ache respond well to acetaminophen, aspirin, or nonsteroidal antiinflammatory agents such as IV or intramuscular ketorolac or oral ibuprofen. Nausea can be caused by the stress and anxiety before the ECT treatment, the anesthetic agents used, the seizure itself, or air in the stomach from assisted ventilation. Nausea can be treated with agents such as ondansetron, dolasetron, or granisetron.

New Therapies for Major Depressive Disorders

Other therapies for severe major depressive disorders are now available, which require anesthetic treatment: repetitive transcranial magnetic stimulation (rTMS) and vagus nerve stimulation (VNS). Neuroanatomic studies have suggested that patients with major depressive disorder (MDD) have dysfunction within the frontal cortical–subcortical–brainstem neural network, specifically the dorsolateral prefrontal cortices (DLPFC). ECT and antidepressant medications do not act in these discrete areas of the brain, but new therapies stimulating these focal areas of the brain are now approved and in use in the United States.

Repetitive Transcranial Magnetic Stimulation or Magnetic Seizure Therapy

1. Introduction

rTMS uses electrical current passing through an electromagnetic coil that has been placed on the scalp. The coil delivers brief, rapidly changing magnetic field pulses to specific areas of the brain. These bursts of pulses are called a "train" of stimuli. Multiple trains of rTMS may be delivered in one session. The scalp and skull are transparent to magnetic fields, which is an advantage over ECT, where the scalp and skull are resistors to the electrical stimulation. A convulsion must be initiated by trains of rTMS in order to produce antidepressant effects because subconvulsive trains of rTMS are ineffective.

Convulsive magnetic energy levels are determined by the use of motor threshold (MT). MT is the point where a single pulse of magnetic energy begins to elicit an electromyographic response, (i.e., a twitch, usually of the abductor pollicis brevis muscle of the thumb or first dorsal interosseous muscle of the index finger). rTMS treatment is safe and well tolerated, with reduced cognitive side effects compared with ECT. Patients are found to recover much more rapidly from rTMS or MST therapy compared with ECT.

MST uses a higher intensity, more frequent, and longer duration magnetic seizure-inducing dose compared with the magnetic dose required for rTMS. MST can stimulate tonic-clonic seizures in more localized and focal regions of the prefrontal cerebral cortex when compared with ECT, as well as generalized tonic-clonic seizures that resemble ECT. MST does not produce the rigid bilateral masseter muscle contractions noted during ECT but can produce elevations in blood pressure and heart rate similar to those of ECT. After rTMS, some patients experience mild headache, disorientation, and inattention (although patients become reoriented much more quickly than with ECT), retrograde amnesia, some anterograde amnesia, transient auditory threshold increases caused by the high-frequency clicking sound heard during coil discharge (which can be alleviated with the use of foam earplugs), and rarely generalized seizure. A single TMS treatment may be all that is necessary for treating certain severe MDD nonpsychotic patients along with their medications, although rTMS may be necessary.

2. Anesthetic technique

a) Anesthesia for rTMS or MST may not be required, or a short general anesthetic may be required. The decision on type of anesthesia should be made based on the type of procedure, duration, and the patient's requirements or comorbidities.

b) A patent and secure IV catheter is established, and full monitors are applied.
c) Glycopyrrolate 2.5 to 5 mcg/kg is administered as an antisialagogue along with ketorolac 0.4 mg/kg 2 to 3 minutes before induction of ultra-brief general anesthesia.
d) Etomidate 0.15 to 0.2 mg/kg can be used for induction, as well as methohexital 1 to 2 mg/kg or propofol 1 to 2.5 mg/kg.
e) Succinylcholine 0.5 to 1 mg/kg can be used as the muscle relaxant after isolation of a lower extremity for observation of seizure duration.
f) Use the smallest amount of muscle relaxant necessary to enable recovery from paralysis before the return of consciousness.
g) The anesthesia provider can then manually hyperventilate the patient's lungs with a face mask to an $ETCO_2$ value of 30 to 34 torr.
h) At this point, the magnetic stimulus may be applied.

Vagus Nerve Stimulation

VNS requires surgical implantation of a programmable battery-powered electrical stimulator that connects with the patient's left vagus nerve (cranial nerve X). The stimulator is usually implanted in the patient's chest with minimal sedation, moderate sedation and analgesia, deep sedation and analgesia, or under general anesthesia. Patient movement should be limited because of the intricacy of the surgery and proximity of vital structures. Although originally approved for treatment-resistant epilepsy, the VNS is now approved for major depressive episodes that have not responded to four antidepressant medication trials.

G. EPILEPSY SURGERY

1. Introduction

Surgery is recommended for patients with epilepsy when seizure control is intractable to conventional medical treatment. The goal of epilepsy surgery is to remove a focal area of epileptogenesis without causing neurologic deficits. Epilepsy surgery consists of two types: intracranial electrode placement and surgical resection. Intracranial electrode placement and testing may be required to localize epileptogenic foci. After localization, surgical resection may be performed. Extensive testing is required to define the focal area and its physiologic activity.

2. Preoperative assessment and patient preparation

a) History and physical examination are required.
   (1) Neurologic: The patient should be assessed for history of uncontrollable focal or generalized seizures. Note the date of the last seizure. Obtain a description of seizure and prodromal symptoms. Obtain list of antiepileptic drugs. A Wada test (intracarotid injection of a barbiturate) may be performed to determine the dominance or speech function in the area of the surgery. A list of medications should be reviewed and the time of last antiepileptic drug noted.
b) Diagnostic tests
   (1) CBC: A low hematocrit can be found in patients taking phenytoin or phenobarbital. A low white blood cell count can be found in

patients taking carbamazepine or primidone. A low platelet count can be found in patients taking carbamazepine, valproate, ethosuximide, or primidone.

(2) Gastrointestinal: Antiepileptic drugs may cause liver damage.

(3) Obtain laboratory levels of antiepileptic drugs as necessary (e.g., phenytoin [Dilantin]).

3. **Room preparation**

a) Monitoring equipment: A standard monitors such as ECG, pulse oximeter, temperature, and noninvasive blood pressure cuff and required arterial line and a CVP catheter are used for general anesthesia. A Foley catheter is used to monitor urine output.

b) Additional equipment: Determine the position of the patient during surgery (supine, lateral, prone, semisitting, or table turned 90 or 180 degrees). A foam support aids in positioning the head. A long circuit, long IV tubing will be needed if the table is turned 90 to 180 degrees. Appropriate padding should be used according to the patient's position.

c) Drugs: Short-acting benzodiazepines, narcotics, or a propofol infusion are acceptable for providing conscious sedation. If intraoperative electrocorticography is used, benzodiazepines and anticonvulsants should be avoided. It is best to avoid anesthetics that may trigger seizure activity (e.g., ketamine). Higher drug doses (e.g., muscle relaxants and narcotics) may be needed because of enzyme induction by anticonvulsant therapy. If a semisitting position is used, the anesthesia provider should be prepared for VAE, and $N_2 0$ should be avoided.

4. **Perioperative management**

a) Induction: Local anesthesia with sedation and general anesthesia with an oral ETT are the anesthetic techniques of choice. Local anesthesia with sedation is used when the seizure focus is in the dominant hemisphere or if neurologic injury may be caused by temporal lobectomy. Screening is necessary to determine patients who will be able to tolerate the procedure. Standard induction is used for general anesthesia. If a stereotactic frame is used, fiberoptic awake intubation may be necessary.

b) Maintenance: If general anesthesia is used, low-dose isoflurane, nitrous oxide, and an opioid infusion are generally used. Isoflurane must be turned off during intraoperative electrocorticography and can be resumed if resection follows. The anesthesia provider may be asked to elicit a seizure by inducing hyperventilation or administering methohexital. Muscle relaxants generally are not readministered after induction to facilitate evaluation of motor response.

c) Emergence: The patient should be emerged smoothly and quickly from anesthesia to allow assessment for any neurologic deficits.

5. **Postoperative implications**

Seizure, bleeding, and cerebral edema are postoperative complications. The patient must be monitored carefully for altered mental status. If the patient shows any signs of delayed emergence or altered mental status, a CT scan should be performed.

H. POSTERIOR FOSSA PROCEDURES

1. Introduction

Neuropathology within the posterior fossa may impair control of the airway, respiratory function, cardiovascular function, autonomic function, and consciousness. The major motor and sensory pathways, primary cardiovascular and respiratory centers, reticular activating system, and nuclei of the lower cranial nerves are all concentrated in the brainstem. All of these vital structures are contained in a tight space with little room for accommodating edema, tumor, or blood.

2. Preoperative assessment and patient preparation

a) History and physical examination
   (1) Neurologic: The history and physical examination should include a thorough neurologic evaluation with documentation. Pay special attention to signs and symptoms of brainstem involvement, such as focal neurologic deficits, depressed respiration, and cranial nerve palsies. Changes in level of consciousness may be secondary to increased ICP resulting in headaches, nausea, vomiting, visual changes, and seizures from obstructive hydrocephalus of the fourth ventricle.
   (2) Cardiovascular: Evaluate for cardiovascular disease and hypertension. Increased ICP may result in brainstem herniation and manifest as Cushing triad (hypertension and irregular respirations).
   (3) Pulmonary: Assess for a coexisting disease process.
   (4) Renal: Correct fluid and electrolyte abnormalities, if present.
   (5) Gastrointestinal: Infratentorial tumors may involve the glossopharyngeal and vagus nerves. This may impair the gag reflex, increasing the chance for aspiration.
   (6) Endocrine: Patients maybe on high-dose steroid therapy to decrease cerebral edema. Preoperative steroid administration would therefore be warranted.

b) Laboratory tests: CBC, electrolytes, blood urea nitrogen, creatinine, glucose, prothrombin time, and partial thromboplastin time are obtained.

c) Diagnostic tests: CT and MRI are used.

d) Preoperative medications: Anxiolytics may be given to alert and anxious patients. Patients who are lethargic or have an altered level of consciousness should not receive premedication.

e) IV therapy: Central line is used if significant blood loss is anticipated or if there is a high risk for VAE; two 16- to 18-gauge IV catheters; consider placement of a pulmonary arterial catheter. Estimated blood loss is 25 to 500 mL.

3. Room preparation

a) Monitoring equipment: Standard monitors; arterial line; urinary catheter; with possible CVP; ICP monitoring; precordial Doppler; EEG; electromyography; and sensory, somatosensory, and brainstem auditory–evoked potential monitoring are used.

b) Additional equipment: Depending on the position of the patient, have appropriate padding available (i.e., prone pillow, doughnut, chest and axillary rolls); a fluid warmer is used.

c) Drugs
   (1) Miscellaneous pharmacologic agents: Vasoconstrictors, vasodilators, inotropes, adrenergic antagonists, steroids, osmotic and loop diuretics, thiopental, lidocaine, fentanyl, nondepolarizing muscle relaxants, and antibiotics are used.
   (2) IV fluids: Use isotonic crystalloid solutions. Avoid glucose-containing solutions. Limit normal saline to less than or equal to 10 mL/kg/hr plus replacement of urinary output. If volume is required, administer 5% albumin or hetastarch and limit to less than or equal to 20 mL/kg. Maintain hematocrit at 30 to 35. Transfuse to keep hematocrit greater than 30.
   (3) Blood: Type and cross match for 2 units of packed red blood cells.

4. **Surgical positioning**
   a) Although most posterior fossa explorations may be performed with the patient in either the lateral or the prone position, the sitting position is occasionally preferred because the enhanced CSF and venous drainage facilitates surgical exposure. The use of this position, however, has declined dramatically because of the potential for serious complications.
   b) The patient is semirecumbent in the standard sitting position with the back elevated to 60 degrees and the legs elevated (with the knees flexed) to the level of the heart. The latter is important for prevention of venous pooling and to decrease the risk of venous thrombosis.
   c) The head is fixed in a three-point head holder with the neck in flexion, and the arms remain at the sides with the hands resting on the lap.
   d) Pressure points such as the elbows, ischial spines, and forehead must be protected with foam padding.
   e) Excessive neck flexion has been associated with swelling of the upper airway (venous obstruction) and, rarely, quadriplegia resulting from compression of the cervical spinal cord and decreased cervical cord perfusion with elevation of the neck above the heart. Preexisting cervical spinal stenosis probably predisposes to the latter injury.

5. **Anesthetic technique**
   a) Increased ICP, although common in patients with supratentorial lesions, is less common in patients with posterior fossa lesions. Obstructive hydrocephalus is more typical because CSF outflow is occluded at the level of the aqueduct of Sylvius or fourth ventricle. This can be readily identified preoperatively by MRI or CT. This may be corrected before definitive surgical intervention with the placement of a ventricular catheter.
   b) Sedation is contraindicated in patients with obstructive hydrocephalus.
   c) Induction should be slow and deliberate to avoid changes in cerebral perfusion and increased ICP. Because the head is generally flexed and fixed in this position, a wire-reinforced ETT may prevent intraoperative kinking. These tubes may become permanently kinked if the patient is lightly anesthetized and bites the tube.
   d) Intravenous fluid administration during posterior fossa surgery should be limited to the infusion of deficit and maintenance quantities of a balanced salt solution. Major volume resuscitation can be accomplished with the infusion of blood, colloid, or crystalloid solutions.

e) Emergence from anesthesia should be as smooth and gentle as possible. The intraoperative use of opioids facilitates a smooth emergence without significant coughing and bucking. The administration of lidocaine 1.5 mg/kg intravenously decreases the airway irritation of the ETT.
f) The decision to remove the ETT should be made after the anesthetic course and the surgical procedure are reviewed.
g) Intraoperative air embolism may be followed by the development of pulmonary edema. Although this condition is self-limiting, continued mechanical ventilation is the treatment of choice.
h) Consideration should also be given to the possibility of cranial nerve damage during the operative procedure. Provided the patient is safely extubated, continued vigilant observation is essential because airway compromise may develop after injury to cranial nerves IX, X, and XI.

I. STEREOTACTIC SURGERY

1. Introduction

Stereotactic surgery is a neurosurgical technique that makes detailed use of the relationship between the three-dimensional space occupied by intracranial structures or lesions and an extracranial reference system to guide instruments to such targets accurately and precisely. This type of technique is used when the lesion is small and located deep within brain tissue or as a means of obtaining a biopsy of a lesion for diagnosis.

Stereotactic procedures can be frame based or image guided (frameless). If the frame-based procedure is used, the frame is anchored to the skull with either four pins or four screws. Application typically takes place outside the operating room using a local anesthetic. In a cooperative adult, frame application takes only 5 to 10 minutes. For children, general anesthesia is used. If the image-guided procedure is used, small markers called *fiducials* are placed on the head with adhesive. An imaging study is then performed to provide a system of reference.

2. Preoperative assessment

a) History and physical examination: Neurologic symptoms vary, depending on the site and size of the lesion; they should be carefully documented. In addition to the routine test, CT is performed preoperatively with the frame in place to determine stereotactic coordinates. After the coordinates are established, airway access is restricted because the frame should not be moved on the head until the operation is complete unless an emergency occurs.
b) Laboratory tests: CBC and other tests are as indicated by the history and physical examination.
c) Diagnostic tests: CT of the head and other tests are as indicated by the history and physical examination.
d) Medication: Usually, medication is not required.

3. Room preparation

a) Monitoring equipment: Standard
b) Additional equipment
   (1) Stereotactic instruments
   (2) Monitoring, ventilation, and oxygenation equipment during transport
c) Drugs
   (1) Standard emergency drugs

(2) Standard tabletop drugs
(3) IV fluids: 16 to 18 gauge × 2 (adults); 20 to 22 gauge (children) IV line with standard replacement therapy

4. **Anesthetic technique**
   a) General endotracheal anesthesia or monitored anesthesia care is used.
   b) In adults, the stereotactic frame or fiducials are placed the morning of the operation, and the patient is taken to the radiologic suite for CT to determine stereotactic coordinates. The patient is then brought to the operating room with the frame or fiducials still in place. If the operation is to be a biopsy, it is generally done using monitored anesthesia care.
   c) If a complete resection is planned, such as in the removal of an AVM, general endotracheal anesthesia is used. In children, it is usually necessary to induce general anesthesia before placing the frame, thus necessitating the maintenance of general anesthesia during the CT. The child is then moved to the operating room still anesthetized, and the operation is completed.
5. **Perioperative management**
   a) Induction
      (1) If monitored anesthesia care is planned, oxygen is administered by nasal prongs, and the patient is lightly sedated with combinations of propofol 25 to 50 mg/kg/min, midazolam to provide amnesia, and remifentanil 0.02 to 0.05 mg/kg/min or fentanyl to provide analgesia. The patient must be able to communicate with the surgeon as needed throughout the operation.
      (2) Stereotactic neurosurgery for movement disorders such as Parkinson's disease requires the anesthesia provider to limit sedation to ensure that the patient will be able to cooperate with the surgeon. If general endotracheal anesthesia is needed with frame-based stereotaxy, fiberoptic laryngoscopy is necessary before inducing anesthesia because the frame precludes intubation by direct laryngoscopy. After endotracheal intubation is established, anesthesia may be induced with propofol, followed by a nondepolarizing blocking drug to facilitate positioning of the patient.
   b) Maintenance
      (1) If general anesthesia is used, the ideal drug is one that decreases ICP and the cerebral metabolic rate of oxygen, maintains cerebral autoregulation, redistributes flow to the potentially ischemic areas, and provides protection of the brain from focal ischemia.
      (2) If children are to be transported from the site of placement of the stereotactic frame to the radiologic suite and then the operating room, it is best to use inhalational anesthesia with isoflurane and 100% oxygen with spontaneous ventilation to ensure adequate ventilation during transport and study. Opiates and neuromuscular blocking drugs should not be administered until the child is in the operating suite.
      (3) Hyperventilation and diuresis should be avoided in image-guided stereotaxy because they may cause the brain to shift. If a frame is used, emergent removal from the patient's head must always be available.

c) Emergence: No special consideration is reported. The patient is extubated awake and after the return of airway reflexes. If the surgeon suspects that the patient may have a slow recovery or a neurologic injury or if the anesthesia provider believes that recovery from the anesthesia may be delayed, it is advisable to leave the ETT in place at least overnight.

6. Postoperative implications

Focal bleeding may occur postoperatively, causing the onset of a neurologic deficit.

J. TRANSSPHENOIDAL TUMOR RESECTIONS

1. Introduction

Approximately 10% of intracranial neoplasms are found in the pituitary gland and are diagnosed because of their mass effects or the hypersecretion of pituitary hormones. These tumors are rarely metastatic and produce local symptoms via bone invasion, hydrocephalus, and compression of a cranial nerve (most often the optic nerve). Frontal-temporal headache and bitemporal hemianopsia are the most common nonendocrine symptoms of enlarging pituitary lesions. Nonsecreting pituitary tumors account for approximately 20% to 50% of lesions in this area and are classified as chromophobe adenomas.

Tumors that secrete excess growth hormone produce acromegaly. Increased growth hormone increases the size of the skeleton, particularly the bones and soft tissues of the hands, feet, and face. The enlarged facial structures may increase the likelihood of difficult intubation. Excess growth hormone may also contribute to the development of coronary artery disease, hypertension, and cardiomyopathy. Hyperglycemia is also a common finding, reflecting growth hormone–induced glucose intolerance.

a) Surgical approach: Medical and surgical therapies exist for both functional and nonfunctional pituitary tumors. Transsphenoidal surgery offers several advantages over the intracranial approach. Statistically, morbidity and mortality rates are reduced because of a decrease in blood loss and less manipulation of brain tissue. In addition, the risk of inducing panhypopituitarism and the incidence of permanent DI are both reduced. For patients with large tumors (>10 mm), tumors of uncertain type, and tumors that have substantial extrasellar extension, the transsphenoidal approach is inadequate and a bifrontal intracranial approach is required for successful removal. Current trends are moving toward endoscopic approaches to the pituitary tumor. Less invasive approaches, such as the transnasal approach combined with endoscopic resection of tumor, have been performed. The endoscopic technique has less morbidity and a shorter hospital stay than the traditional approach.

2. Preoperative assessment

a) Patients undergo transsphenoidal operations for the treatment of hypersecreting pituitary tumors or nonsecretory tumors that cause visual complications because of their size and location. Clinical symptoms of secretory pituitary tumors include amenorrhea, galactorrhea, Cushing disease, and acromegaly.

b) Each preoperative condition has its own constellation of systemic disorders and accompanying effects on intracranial dynamics that should be considered when an anesthetic technique is selected.

c) Pituitary tumors can damage decussating optic fibers, producing blindness in the temporal half of the visual field of both eyes (bitemporal heteronymous hemianopsia).
d) Occasionally, an aneurysm of one of the internal carotid arteries may produce nasal hemianopsia on the affected side.
e) Patients who have Cushing disease may also be affected by hypertension, diabetes, osteoporosis, obesity, and friability of skin and connective tissue.
f) Patients who have acromegaly may have hypertension, cardiomyopathy, diabetes, and osteoporosis, as well as cartilaginous and soft tissue hypertrophy of the larynx and enlargement of the tongue, complicating intubation of the trachea.
g) Patients who have panhypopituitarism may exhibit hypothyroidism, requiring preoperative thyroid supplementation.
h) Laboratory tests: CBC, electrolytes, BUN, creatinine, as indicated from history and physical. Hyponatremia may indicate DI; hypercalcemia may indicate multiple endocrine neoplasia type 1.

3. **Anesthetic technique**
   a) The transsphenoidal approach usually necessitates the head and back to be elevated 10 to 20 degrees. The patient's head is supported by a three-point pin head holder and centered within a C-arm fluoroscopy unit for radiographic control during surgery. The patient's arms are placed at the sides and padded so that injury to the ulnar nerves is avoided.
   b) The patient's airway is shared with the surgeon; therefore, great attention must be directed to the proper securing of the ETT and anesthesia circuit to prevent unintended extubation and anesthesia circuit disconnection.
   c) Hyperventilation is avoided after anesthetic induction because reductions in ICP result in retraction of the pituitary into the sella, making surgical access difficult.
   d) The anesthesia provider should also consider the potential for massive hemorrhage because the carotid arteries lie adjacent to the suprasellar area and may be inadvertently injured.
   e) Postoperative endocrine dysfunction may occur, namely DI, when the resection involves the suprasellar area.
      (1) DI that occurs after most transsphenoidal procedures is usually self-limited and resolves within 1 week to 10 days.
      (2) Although the onset is usually on the first or second postoperative day, DI may develop during the perioperative period or in the immediate recovery period.
      (3) Intraoperative diagnosis is made with the sudden onset of diuresis. The diagnosis may be confirmed with concurrent urine and serum osmolalities.
      (4) If DI persists or if it becomes difficult to match urinary losses, the patient may receive aqueous vasopressin (Pitressin) or desmopressin (DDAVP).
      (5) IV DDAVP is longer acting and is not associated with the coronary vasoconstriction that follows administration of aqueous vasopressin.

f) Anesthetic induction, maintenance, and emergence
   (1) After anesthetic induction and intubation, the ETT is typically moved to the left corner of the patient's mouth and secured to the chin with tape to maximize exposure to the surgical field. A right-angled ETT may be effective because such tubes are prebent and curve along the mandible when exiting the mouth.
   (2) The esophageal stethoscope and temperature probe are inserted and secured on the lower left as well, leaving the upper lip totally exposed. An orogastric tube is placed, aspirated, and then put to gravity drainage during the procedure.
   (3) The oropharynx is then packed with moist cotton gauze.
   (4) The eyes are first taped closed and then covered with cotton-padded adhesive patches or Tegaderm or to prevent corneal abrasion and seepage of cleansing solution and blood into the eyes.
   (5) Propofol, an opioid (fentanyl, sufentanil, alfentanil, or remifentanil), and a neuromuscular relaxant (either succinylcholine or a nondepolarizing neuromuscular relaxant for intubation followed by a selected nondepolarizing agent) with a combination of air and oxygen is a commonly used anesthetic combination for this procedure. Isoflurane may be added in low concentrations for blood pressure control; alternatively, it may be used as the primary anesthetic drug.
   (6) The topical use of cocaine and the oral and nasal submucosal injection of local anesthetic solutions containing epinephrine help constrict gingival and mucosal vessels and dissect the nasal mucosa away from the cartilaginous septum.
      (a) Epinephrine use may produce hypertension of dysrhythmias or both; cocaine interferes with the intraneuronal uptake of catecholamine and can augment both the hypertensive and dysrhythmogenic properties of epinephrine.
      (b) The use of epinephrine is relatively safe if concentrations of 1:100,000 to 1:200,000 are used and the total dose does not exceed 10 mL of 1:100,000 solution in 10 minutes for a 70 kg adult.
      (c) A total dose of 200 mg of cocaine should not be exceeded. Persistent dysrhythmias may require treatment with lidocaine or possibly a β-blocker. Hypertension may be controlled with an increased concentration of the selected inhalation agent or with small IV doses of hydralazine, labetalol, or esmolol.

g) In some cases, it may be necessary to insert a catheter into the lumbar subarachnoid space to facilitate the injection of preservative-free saline to delineate the suprasellar margins or for prevention of CSF leak postoperatively. If air is injected, N_2O must be discontinued from the anesthetic mixture because of rapid diffusion into the air present in the closed cranial vault.

h) Emergence from anesthesia should be conducted as described for craniotomy procedures.
   (1) IV lidocaine, 1,5 mg/kg given approximately 3 minutes before suctioning and extubation, decreases coughing, straining, and hypertension.

(2) Postoperatively, patients should be responsive to commands in the recovery room.
(3) Steroid therapy is continued throughout this period and is tapered over time, if appropriate.

K. VENOUS AIR EMBOLISM

1. Introduction

In addition to the previously mentioned monitoring modalities, monitoring during posterior fossa surgery requires consideration of patient position and the potential for VAE. Air may also be entrained from the cranial pin sites of the Mayfield head holder from improperly connected vascular lines (arterial, central, and IV and high-pressure mechanical ventilation).

The occurrence of VAE depends on the development of a negative pressure gradient between the operative site and the right side of the heart. As the gradient between the cerebral veins and the right atrium increases, the potential for air entry increases. The estimated incidence of VAE during neurosurgical procedures ranges from 5% to 50%, with an increased incidence in the sitting position. The physiologic consequences of VAE depend on both the volume and the rate of air entrainment.

a) Paradoxical air embolism
   (1) Paradoxical air embolism (PAE) develops with the entry of air into the systemic circulation. Individuals with an existing anatomic connection between the right and left sides of the heart (atrial or ventricular septal defect, probe-patent foramen ovale) are at risk.
   (2) If right-sided heart pressures exceed left-sided pressures (a situation that may occur in fluid-restricted neurosurgical patients), systemic air may embolize and enter the arterial circulation through a probe-patent foramen ovale.
   (3) Patients who require the sitting position should be carefully evaluated with echocardiograms if the history suggests the presence of an intracardiac defect (presence of heart murmur) or probe-patent foramen ovale. It is estimated that or many as 20% of adults and 50% of children have a probe-patent foramen ovale.
   (4) The presence of a probe-patent foramen ovale may be elicited with the injection of contrast material before, during, and after the patient produces a Valsalva maneuver. If a probe-patent foramen ovale is identified, the surgical procedure should be accomplished in an alternative position.

2. Preoperative assessment

a) Detection
   (1) The entrainment of air into the vascular system is usually of little consequence because the lungs serve as effective blood filters. Small bubbles of air are absorbed into the blood or enter the alveoli, where they are eliminated.
   (2) The efficient filtering capacity of the lung may be breached by a large bolus of air or after the administration of a pulmonary vasodilator (e.g., aminophylline), which acts to widen the

venous-arterial barrier. Air enters the venous circulation as small bubbles that pass through the right side of the heart, entering the pulmonary arterioles.

(3) A reflexive sympathetic pulmonary vasoconstriction is produced after the release of endothelial mediators, which are ultimately responsible for the clinical manifestations (pulmonary hypertension, hypoxemia, CO_2 retention, increased dead-space ventilation, and decreased $ETCO_2$).
(4) The continued entry of air produces an airlock within the right ventricle, producing right ventricular failure and decreased cardiac output.
(5) Altered ventilation-perfusion relationships parallel the hemodynamic changes.
(6) Obstructed pulmonary blood flow increases dead-space ventilation, resulting in decreased $ETCO_2$. The entry of a large volume of air in the alveoli may be detected by the sudden appearance of end-tidal nitrogen. However, detection of nitrogen requires use of a mass spectrometer.
(7) The selection of appropriate monitoring for the detection of VAE is based on the various sensitivities of the available monitoring modalities.
(8) Precordial Doppler monitoring can detect air entrainment at rates as small as 0.0021 mL/kg/min.
  (a) The Doppler probe is affixed over the right side of the heart along the right sternal border between the third and sixth intercostal spaces.
  (b) Proper positioning over the right atrium is confirmed if a change in Doppler signal is elicited when a 10-mL bolus of saline is injected rapidly into a previously placed right central venous catheter.
  (c) The placement of a right atrial catheter affords the means for diagnosis and recovery of IV air and also reflects cardiac preload.
  (d) When a right atrial catheter is placed, it is recommended that either radiographic confirmation or ECG confirmation of proper placement of the catheter tip be obtained.
(9) Capnography complements the capabilities of the Doppler device because small, hemodynamically insignificant air emboli detected with the Doppler device can be differentiated from emboli that may produce arterial hypotension.
(10) Transesophageal echocardiography (TEE) is the most sensitive method of air embolism detection, but it is also the most expensive. With TEE, it is possible to observe both cardiac contractility and air bubbles as they pass through the heart. TEE is also capable of detecting PAE in the heart.
(11) The detection of a "mill-wheel" murmur via precordial or esophageal stethoscope is a late sign of air entrainment.
(12) The use of nitrous oxide is contraindicated when developing a venous embolism is a possibility.

Advantages and disadvantages of selected monitors for detection of VAE are noted in the following table.

Monitors for Detection of Venous Air Embolism

Monitor	Advantages	Disadvantages
Precordial Doppler	Noninvasive Most sensitive noninvasive monitor Earliest detector (before air enters pulmonary circulation)	Nonquantitative May be difficult to place in obese patients, patients with chest wall deformity, or patients in the prone or lateral position False-negative result if air does not pass beneath ultrasonic beam (approximately 10% of cases) Useless during electrocautery IV mannitol may mimic intravascular air
Pulmonary artery (PA) catheter	Quantitative slightly more sensitive than $ETCO_2$ Widely available Placed with minimum difficulty in experienced hands Can detect right atrial pressure more easily than PCWP	Small lumen, less air aspiration than with right atrial catheter Placement for optimal air aspiration may not allow PCWP measurement Nonspecific for air
Capnography ($ETCO_2$)	Noninvasive Sensitive Quantitative Widely available	Nonspecific for air Less sensitive than Doppler, PA catheter Accuracy affected by tachypnea, low cardiac output, COPD
End-tidal nitrogen (ETN_2)	Specific for air Detects air earlier than $ETCO_2$	May not detect subclinical air embolism May indicate air clearance from pulmonary circulation prematurely Accuracy affected by hypotension
Transesophageal echocardiography (TEE)	Most sensitive detector of air Can detect air in left side of heart and aorta	Invasive, cumbersome Expensive Monitor must be observed continuously Not quantitative May interfere with Doppler

COPD, Chronic obstructive pulmonary disease; *$ETCo_2$,* end-tidal carbon dioxide; *IV,* intravenous; *PA,* pulmonary artery; *PCWP,* pulmonary capillary wedge pressure.
Modified from Smith DS, Osborne I. Posterior fossa: anesthetic considerations. In Cottrell JE, Smith DS. *Anesthesia and Neurosurgery.* 4th ed. St. Louis: Mosby; 2001:343.

3. **Perioperative management**
   a) Treatment of venous air embolus: Detection of VAE should prompt the steps listed in the box on pg. 399.
      (1) Supportive therapy is required for hemodynamic compromise.
      (2) Administration of ephedrine, 10 to 20 mg intravenously, and an IV fluid bolus improves the blood pressure.
      (3) If these measures do not restore blood pressure, additional vasopressors (epinephrine) may be required.

Therapy for Venous Air Embolism

- Notify surgeon on detection (flood surgical field with saline, and wax bone edges).
- Discontinue nitrous oxide administration. Administer 100% oxygen.
- Perform a Valsalva maneuver or compression of jugular veins.
- Aspirate air from the atrial catheter.
- Support blood pressure with volume and vasopressors.
- Reposition the patient in the left lateral decubitus position (Durant maneuver) with a 15-degree head-down tilt if blood pressure continues to decrease.
- Modify the anesthetic as needed to optimize hemodynamics.

L. VENTRICULOPERITONEAL SHUNT

1. Introduction

A ventriculoperitoneal shunt is placed to relieve increased CSF pressure. The hydrocephalus may be caused by a congenital defect, cyst, tumor, trauma, infection, or CBF absorption abnormality. Therefore, patients undergoing this procedure range in age from newborn to elderly. Besides a conduit to the peritoneum, the ventricle can also be drained into the pleura or right atrium.

2. Preoperative assessment

a) Neurologic; ICP monitoring is routine.

b) Headaches are the most common symptom. Assess for level of consciousness, headaches, nuchal rigidity, seizures, nausea or vomiting, and papilledema as indications of severe hydrocephalus (ICP >15 mmHg). Presurgical neurologic defects such as stroke, spina bifida, and focal defects should also be assessed.

c) Review results of CT of the head. Review blood pressure and heart rate trends in relation to ICP. Cushing triad is present with increased ICP and includes increased blood pressure, and decreased heart rate, and irregular respirations.

3. Patient preparation

a) CBC, electrolytes (especially if the patient is receiving diuretics), glucose (especially if the patient is taking steroids such as dexamethasone), prothrombin time, partial thromboplastin time, and type and screen are obtained.

b) Other diagnostic tests are as indicated. Communicate with the neurologist if steroids and diuretic therapy are anticipated during surgery. Usually, preoperative medication is not given to patients with increased ICP.

4. Room preparation

a) Monitors: Standard. An ICP monitor is also used.

b) Position: Supine with the head turned to the contralateral side. A shoulder roll may be used. A foam headrest aids positioning.

c) Additional equipment: The table will probably be turned, thus requiring an adequate length of ventilation tubing. Because much of the patient will be exposed, it is helpful to have a fluid warmer and a higher room temperature.

d) Drugs and tabletop: Standard. Fluids can be administered at approximately 4 to 6 mL/kg/hr. Overzealous fluid administration can exacerbate increased ICP.

5. **Anesthetic technique and perioperative management**
   a) Use general anesthesia with endotracheal intubation. With exception of ketamine, all induction agents are good choices because of their cerebroprotective properties by depressing cerebral metabolism. Muscle relaxation is desirable. Succinylcholine is relatively contraindicated for patients with increased ICP.
   b) Normocarbia aids the surgeon in cannulating the ventricles. It is wise to have the propofol or etomidate immediately available during the "tunneling," which is the most stimulating part of this procedure. Extubation is performed at the end of the procedure. Prophylactic antiemetics should be administered 30 minutes before the conclusion of anesthesia.
6. **Postoperative implications**

Assess the patient's neurologic status. Pain can usually be managed with oral preparations.

A. ANTERIOR CERVICAL DISKECTOMY OR FUSION

1. Introduction

Anterior cervical diskectomy or fusion is most commonly performed for symptomatic nerve root or cord compression. Compression may occur from protrusion of an intervertebral disk or osteophytic bone into the spinal canal. An intervertebral disk usually herniates at the fifth or sixth cervical levels. A bone graft may be taken from the iliac crest or backbone may be used.

2. Preoperative assessment and patient preparation

a) Airway assessment should include thorough assessment of the range of motion of the neck. Neurologic deficits with limited neck movement may require intubation with the head in a neutral position. Intubation can be performed using passive immobilization or in-line traction with assistance of the GlideScope. Awake fiberoptic intubation with proper positioning is the safest option. Avoid flexion, extension, and lateral rotation of the head.

b) Neurologic deficits should be documented. Patients typically complain of neck pain radiating down one arm, which can progress to weakness and atrophy.

c) Diagnostic tests include type and screen, complete blood count, and other tests as the patient's condition indicates.

d) Preoperative medication and intravenous (IV) therapy: Patients may have considerable pain preoperatively and require a narcotic with premedication. If a difficult airway is anticipated, premedication should be used sparingly. Use a 16- or 18-gauge IV catheter with minimal fluid replacement.

3. Room preparation

a) A standard tabletop setup is used.

b) The patient is in the supine position with the arms tucked at the sides; a small roll may be placed under the shoulders. Pad elbows to avoid ulnar compression and use slight knee flexion because many patients also have lumbar disease. A doughnut or foam headrest may be used.

c) Use a single, 18-gauge nonpositional IV catheter (arms tucked) with minimal fluid replacement.

4. Perioperative management and anesthetic technique

a) Induction

(1) General anesthesia with endotracheal intubation is used.

(2) Tape the endotracheal tube (ETT) to the side opposite of where the surgeon stands. Keep tape out of the sterile field.

b) Maintenance

(1) The trachea and esophagus are retracted laterally while the common carotid is retracted medially. The temporal artery can be palpated to monitor for carotid artery occlusion. There is the potential risk of damage to the recurrent laryngeal nerve, major arteries, veins, esophageal perforation, or pneumothorax.

(2) Blood loss is usually not significant, but epidural venous oozing can occur.
(3) Patients with spinal cord compression have an increased risk for decreased spinal cord perfusion and may not tolerate intraoperative hypotension. An arterial line is beneficial in these patients for close blood pressure monitoring.
(4) Spinal cord monitoring with somatosensory evoked potentials (SSEPs) may be performed. If SSEP is used, maintain the anesthetic using less than 1 minimum alveolar concentration (MAC) of inhalation agent IV narcotics and neuromuscular blocking agents.
(5) The absence of muscle relaxation is required for intraoperative motor evoked potentials (MEPs) testing.
(6) If a nerve stimulator is used on the face, limit twitch application to when the surgeon is not operating because the face may move during stimulation.

c) Emergence
(1) Most patients are extubated in the operating room after the procedure.
(2) Coughing and bucking on the ETT should be avoided because they can dislodge the bone plug. IV lidocaine can be administered before extubation. The neck must remain in a neutral position. A neck brace may be applied.
(3) Extubate before application of the neck brace; a jaw lift may be required. The patient should be awake before leaving the operating room to allow the surgeon to assess neurologic function.
(4) Consider leaving the patient intubated if there is large blood loss or fluid replacement, difficult intubation, multilevel surgery, or difficult tracheal retraction that can lead to tracheal or airway edema.
(5) Assess the patient's voice for recurrent laryngeal nerve damage, which rarely causes airway obstruction and usually resolves in a few days to 6 weeks.
(6) Assess for hematoma postoperatively

B. LUMBAR LAMINECTOMY OR FUSION

1. Introduction

Lumbar laminectomy is most commonly performed for symptomatic nerve root or spinal cord compression. Compression may occur from protrusion of an intervertebral disk or osteophyte bone into the spinal canal. An intervertebral disk usually herniates at the L4 to L5 or L5 to S1 intervertebral space. A laminectomy procedure involves the complete removal of lamina.

Lumbar fusion is performed when there is instability of the spine. This instability often leads to lower back pain. Bone graft material can be obtained from the patient's iliac crest or from backbone. Back injuries account for a large percentage of work-related injuries and are a leading cause of work absences.

2. Preoperative assessment and patient preparation

a) History and physical examination: Assess and document neurologic deficits of the lower extremities.

b) Diagnostic tests: Type and screen blood and obtain a complete blood count.
c) Preoperative medication and IV therapy
 (1) Consider a narcotic with premedication if the patient experiences pain.
 (2) Consider an antisialagogue because most spinal surgery is performed with the patient in the prone position.
 (3) Use a 16- or 18-gauge IV catheter with minimal fluid replacement.

3. **Room preparation**
 a) Monitoring equipment: Standard
 b) Pharmacologic agents: Vasopressors, steroids, and antibiotics
 c) Position
  (1) Prone, lateral, and knee-chest positions are used.
  (2) Have a foam headrest, doughnut, axillary roll, and indicated padding available.
  (3) Specially designed frames may be used to aid in positioning.
4. **Anesthetic technique**
 a) General anesthesia is most commonly used; however, local infiltrations and regional blockade are other options.
 b) Regional blockade: This reduces blood loss and shrinks epidural veins; analgesia to T7 to T8 is required, and regional anesthesia cannot be used if nerve function will be tested.
 c) Spinal: Hypotension may be accentuated with position changes.
5. **Perioperative management**
 a) Induction
  (1) If the prone or knee-chest position is used, anesthesia is induced while the patient is on the stretcher.
  (2) Position changes may be done in stages to avoid hemodynamic compromise. It may be necessary to lighten the anesthetic and increase fluids before the position change. A vasopressor may be needed to treat hypotension.
  (3) Tape the ETT to the side of the mouth that will be positioned upward. Confirm ETT placement after positioning.
 b) Maintenance
  (1) Question the surgeon regarding the use of muscle relaxants. If nerve function is to be tested, a single dose of an intermediate nondepolarizing muscle relaxant may be used for intubation.
  (2) Pad all pressure points, and check for pressure on the face every 15 minutes during surgery.
  (3) Blood loss is rarely sufficient to necessitate deliberate hypotension. The wound may be infiltrated with an epinephrine solution to decrease intraoperative blood loss.
  (4) Sudden profound hypotension may indicate major intraabdominal vessel (iliac, aorta) damage with bleeding occurring in the retroperitoneal cavity, which may not be visible to the surgeon.
  (5) Infiltration of the wound with a local anesthetic will decrease postoperative pain.
  (6) If the patient is positioned prone, do not administer more than 40 mL/kg of crystalloid over the duration of the procedure. This helps decrease the incidence of the patient developing ischemic optic neuropathy.

c) Emergence: Extubation is performed when the patient is supine. The patient may need to be awake at the end of the procedure to allow the surgeon to assess for neurologic deficits. If the operation was long and airway edema is of concern, the patient may need to remain intubated.

6. Postoperative implications

The patient can usually be transported in any position because stability of the back is rarely compromised. Postoperative complications may include hemorrhage, neurologic deficits, and visual loss.

C. SPINAL CORD INJURIES

1. Introduction

Spinal cord transection is the description of spinal cord injury that is manifested as paralysis of the lower extremities (paraplegia) or of all extremities (quadriplegia). Spinal cord transection above the level of C2 to C4 is incompatible with survival because innervation to the diaphragm is likely to be destroyed.

The most common cause of spinal cord transection is the trauma associated with a motor vehicle or diving accident that results in fracture dislocation of cervical vertebrae. Occasionally, rheumatoid arthritis of the spine leads to spontaneous dislocation of the C1 vertebra on the C2 vertebra, producing progressive quadriparesis. These patients can suddenly become quadriplegic. The most frequent nontraumatic cause of spinal cord transection is multiple sclerosis. In addition, infections or vascular and developmental disorders may be responsible for permanent damage to the spinal cord.

2. Preoperative assessment

Spinal cord transection initially produces flaccid paralysis with total absence of sensation below the level of injury. Temperature regulation and spinal cord reflexes are lost below the level of injury. The phase after the acute transection of the spinal cord is known as spinal shock and typically lasts 1 to 3 weeks. Several weeks after acute transection of the spinal cord, the spinal cord reflexes gradually return, and patients enter a chronic stage characterized by overactivity of the sympathetic nervous system and involuntary skeletal muscle spasms. Mental depression and pain are pressing problems after spinal cord injury.

a) History and physical examination

(1) Cardiovascular: Electrocardiograph abnormalities are common during the acute phase of spinal cord transection and include ventricular premature beats and ST–T-wave changes suggestive of myocardial ischemia. Decreased systemic blood pressure and bradycardia are also common secondary to a loss of sympathetic tone. Generally, this condition can be treated effectively with crystalloid and colloid infusion vasopressor and atropine to increase the heart rate. Around 85% of patients with spinal cord transection above T6 exhibit autonomic hyperreflexia, a disorder that appears after the resolution of spinal shock and in association with the return of the spinal cord reflexes.

(2) Respiratory: A transection between the levels of C2 and C4 may result in apnea from denervation of the diaphragm. The ability to cough and clear secretions from the airway is often impaired because of decreased expiratory reserve volume. Vital capacity

also is significantly decreased if the transection of the spinal cord is at the cervical level. Furthermore, arterial hypoxemia is a consistent early finding during the period after cervical spinal cord injury. Tracheobronchial suctioning has been associated with bradycardia and cardiac arrest in these patients secondary to vasovagal reflex, a finding emphasizing the importance of establishing optimal arterial oxygenation before undertaking this maneuver. Acute respiratory insufficiency and the inability to handle oropharyngeal secretions necessitate immediate tracheal intubation. Before intubation is initiated, the neck must be stabilized.

(3) Neurologic: Whereas patients with spinal cord trauma at the T1 level are paraplegic, traumas above C5 may result in quadriplegia and loss of phrenic nerve function. Injuries between these two levels result in varying loss of motor and sensory functions in the upper extremities. Careful assessment and documentation of preoperative sensory and motor deficits are important.

(4) Musculoskeletal: Prolonged immobility leads to osteoporosis, skeletal muscle atrophy, and the development of decubitus ulcers. Pathologic fractures can occur when these patients are moved. Pressure points should be well protected and padded to minimize the likelihood of trauma to the skin and the development of ulcers.

(5) Renal: Renal failure is the leading cause of death in patients with chronic spinal cord transection. Chronic urinary tract infections and immobilization predispose to the development of renal calculi. Amyloidosis of the kidney can be manifested as proteinuria, leading to a decrease in the concentration of albumin in the plasma.

b) Patient preparation

(1) Laboratory tests: Arterial blood gas analysis substantiates the degree of respiratory impairment. Urinalysis, complete blood count, coagulation profile, electrolytes, type and crossmatch, and other tests are as indicated by the history and physical examination.

(2) Diagnostic tests: Computed tomography, magnetic resonance imaging, radiography of the injured parts, and other tests are as indicated by the history and physical examination.

(3) Medications: Premedication is useful in this patient population and is individualized based on patient need. Patients with acute spinal cord injury often receive methylprednisolone, 30 mcg/kg loading dose over 15 minutes and then 5.4 mg/hr for 23 hours. The efficacy of steroid administration after spinal cord injury is controversial.

3. Room preparation

a) Monitoring equipment

(1) Standard

(2) Foley catheter

(3) Arterial line

(4) Central venous pressure line as clinically indicated

b) Additional equipment

(1) Patient warming devices

(2) Regular operating table

(3) Cervical traction, tong traction, or pins; shoulder rolls as clinically indicated

c) Drugs

(1) Standard emergency drugs are used.

(2) A standard tabletop is used.

(3) IV fluids are infused through a 16- or 18-gauge IV line with normal saline at 4 to 6 mL/kg/hr with a fluid warmer.

(4) Regardless of the technique selected for anesthesia, a drug such as nitroprusside must be readily available to treat precipitous hypertension. Nitroprusside administration, 1 to 2 mcg/kg/min, is an effective method of treating sudden hypertension.

4. Anesthetic technique

Use general endotracheal anesthesia. Management of anesthesia in the patient with transection of the spinal cord is largely determined by the duration of the injury. Regardless of the duration of spinal cord transection, preoperative hydration helps to prevent hypotension during the induction and maintenance of anesthesia.

5. Perioperative management

a) Induction: All trauma patients are considered to have full stomachs, and rapid-sequence induction should be performed. Succinylcholine is avoided in patients with spinal cord injury after 24 hours because of the risk of hyperkalemia from potassium release from extrajunctional receptor sites. Furthermore, succinylcholine-induced fasciculations can exacerbate spinal cord injury. Ketamine can be used in hemodynamically unstable patients if head trauma is not suspected. The anesthesia provider should determine whether the cervical spine radiographs have been cleared before intubation. Avoid manipulating the head and neck during intubation and positioning, which can cause further injury. If the patient's neck is unstable or if difficult intubation is anticipated secondary to a halo device or a body jacket, an awake fiberoptic intubation should be performed. The awake intubation has the advantage of preserving muscle tone, which may protect the unstable spine, and the patient's neurologic status can be assessed after the procedure. Blind nasal, awake fiberoptic nasal, or oral intubations are possible options depending on the patient's condition. A rigid laryngoscopy can be performed with in-line axial stabilization.

b) Maintenance

(1) Standard: A single dose of neuromuscular blocking drug (vecuronium 10 mg) may be administered to relax the neck muscles. Additional doses of relaxants are rarely necessary.

(2) Position: For the anterior approach, the patient is positioned supine with a roll under the shoulders, and the head is moderately hyperextended. Check and pad pressure points. A cervical strap may be placed below the chin to apply continuous cervical traction; avoid pressure on ears and facial nerves. Accidental extubation can result if the chin strap slips off the chin. For the posterior approach, the patient is positioned either prone with horseshoe headrest or three-point stabilization using a special frame or bolsters that allow the abdomen to hang freely to prevent venous engorgement. Occasionally, the sitting position is used, and this increases the risk of venous air embolism.

(3) Hypotension: The loss of sympathetic compensation response makes these patients more susceptible to hypotension from positioning, blood loss, and positive-pressure ventilation. One may need to treat with fluids and pressors. The goal is to maintain a systolic blood pressure of 90 mmHg. An arterial line should be placed before induction.

(4) Autonomic hyperreflexia: Patients with chronic spinal cord injury should be monitored for autonomic hyperreflexia. This condition is associated with injuries above the level of T6. It may be precipitated by cutaneous or visceral stimuli below the spinal cord lesion. Bladder, bowel, or intestinal distention is known to produce autonomic overactivity. An adequate level of general or spinal anesthesia is paramount. Symptoms are hypertension, bradycardia, dysrhythmias, headache, sweating, piloerection below the lesion, vasodilation above the lesion, hyperreflexia, convulsions, cerebral hemorrhage, and pulmonary edema. Treatment consists of eliminating the stimulus; deepening the anesthetic; raising the head of the bed; and administering vasodilators, α-antagonists, or ganglionic blockers.

(5) Hypothermia: Warming devices are necessary because the patient's core temperature will approach room temperature because of the interruption in sympathetic pathways to the hypothalamus.

c) Emergence

After a cervical fusion has been performed, the patient may have a halo device or body jacket. The patient should be fully awake and able to manage his or her airway before extubation. Lidocaine can be administered down the ETT or intravenously to prevent coughing and bucking. The patient should have a tidal volume of greater than 5 mL/kg, a negative inspiratory force of 20 to 25 cm H_2O, and vital capacity of greater than 15 mL/kg. Airway patency can be tested by deflating the cuff to determine whether the patient can breathe around the tube before extubation. The patient should be assessed for airway obstruction secondary to soft tissue occlusion or superior laryngeal nerve damage after extubation.

6. Postoperative implications

a) Airway obstruction is usually caused by soft tissue against the posterior pharyngeal wall. The neck fusion or postoperative traction or stabilization device (halo or body jacket) may impair attempts to open the airway. An oral or nasal airway may be required.

b) Pneumonia may result postoperatively.

c) Respiratory insufficiency can result from the development of a tension pneumothorax from entrainment of air through the surgical wound; oropharyngeal laceration during tracheal intubation; or bleeding into the neck at the surgical site, with progressive compression and occlusion of the airway.

d) The patient should be assessed for the presence of neurologic deficits. Reversible causes such as a hematoma should be excluded.

e) Deep venous thrombosis can occur from decreased blood flow and venous stasis. Heparinization and sequential compression stockings should be instituted.

f) Urinary retention may require urinary catheterization.

g) Stress ulcers and gastric ileus can be treated with a nasogastric tube, antacids, and H_2-receptor antagonists.

D. THORACIC AND LUMBAR SPINAL INSTRUMENTATION AND FUSION

1. Introduction

Anterolateral, posterior, or combined anteroposterior approaches can be used to treat pathologic processes of the thoracic and lumbar spine. *Spinal instrumentation* refers to implanted metal rods affixed to the spine to correct and internally splint a deformed spine. Originally designed for scoliosis, posterior spinal instrumentation is commonly performed simultaneously with spinal fusion for a variety of diagnoses, including fracture, tumor, degenerative changes, and developmental spinal deformity. The original Harrington rod is the simplest and still considered by many to be the standard. Other procedures, such as segmental spinal instrumentation, can distribute correctional forces by sublaminar wiring (Luque) or by hook or screw (Cotrel-Dubousset) procedures that apply multilevel corrective forces on the rods. Bone chips from the posterior iliac crest are placed over the site of fusion. Harrington rodding or similar extensive spinal instrumentation procedures to correct spinal column deformities put the spinal cord at risk for ischemia secondary to mechanical compression of its blood supply. This complication has been mitigated with methods to assess spinal cord function intraoperatively. These include intraoperative testing of neurologic function (wake-up test) and SSEP monitoring. Wake-up testing requires an informed cooperative patient and a practice trial of patient responses.

The anterior approach may use the Dwyer screw and cable apparatus or Zielke rod. It offers a limited fusion area and less blood loss and can correct significant lordosis. There is a greater risk of damage to the spinal cord compared with the Harrington rod procedure. The spinal cord can be damaged from the vertebral body screw, especially in the smaller thoracic vertebral bodies and larger number of segmental spinal arteries that require ligation. The patient is positioned laterally, and a transthoracic or retroperitoneal approach is used. The potential for respiratory compromise is significant when using the thoracoabdominal approach. Surgery above the level of T8 requires a double-lumen ETT to collapse the lung on the operative side. The procedure may require the removal of the tenth or sixth rib (or both) and diaphragmatic manipulation.

An anteroposterior fusion may be required for patients with unstable spines. Usually, the anterior procedure is performed first followed by posterior instrumentation after 1 to 2 weeks. Immediate posterior fusion is possible when the area to be fused is small and the primary curvature is below the diaphragm. The anteroposterior approach necessitates an intraoperative position change. Anesthetic considerations are similar to those required for posterior instrumentation. Anesthetic concerns for thoracic and lumbar spine procedures are positioning, replacing blood and fluid losses, maintaining spinal cord integrity, preventing venous air embolism, and avoiding hypothermia. The wake-up test and SSEPs are frequently used.

2. Preoperative assessment

Patients requiring spinal reconstruction usually have either idiopathic or acquired scoliosis. Scoliosis is a deformity of the spine resulting in curvature and rotation of the vertebrae, as well as an associated deformity of the rib cage. Scoliosis can be classified as idiopathic, neuromuscular, myopathic, congenital, or trauma or tumor related or as part of mesenchymal disorders. Most cases are idiopathic, with a male-to-female ratio of 1:4. Surgery is indicated when the curvature is severe (the Cobb angle is greater than 50 degrees or rapidly progressing). Spinal instability requiring surgery may also result from trauma, cancer, or infection. Patients with scoliosis need careful preoperative evaluation of their cardiac, pulmonary, neuromuscular, and renal systems because associated anomalies occur frequently.

a) History and physical examination
   (1) Cardiovascular: Patients have an increased incidence of congestive heart disease mitral valve prolapse, right ventricular hypertrophy, pulmonary hypertension, and cor pulmonale. Pulmonary vascular resistance is increased independent of the severity of scoliosis.
   (2) Respiratory: Respiratory impairment is proportional to the angle of lateral curvature. Respiratory involvement is more likely when the Cobb angle is greater than 65 degrees. There may be a decreased total lung capacity and vital capacity (restrictive pattern). Ventilation–perfusion mismatch and alveolar hypoventilation may result in hypoxemia. If vital capacity is less than 40% of predicted, postoperative ventilation usually is required. Patients with neuromuscular disease may also have impaired protective airway mechanisms and weakness of respiratory musculature, making them prone to aspiration and respiratory failure.
   (3) Neurologic: If an intraoperative wake-up test is planned, the patient should be informed preoperatively and assured that the procedure will involve minimal pain. A practice wake-up test helps to establish a baseline assessment and teaches the patient what to expect. Careful preoperative assessment and documentation of the patient's neurologic status are essential.
   (4) Musculoskeletal: Cardiomyopathy is a common finding in patients with muscular dystrophy. These patients are more sensitive to myocardial depression from anesthetic agents, changes in sympathetic tone, and hypercapnia. Patients with muscular dystrophy may require postoperative ventilation secondary to muscle weakness, impaired secretion removal, and atelectasis. The use of succinylcholine is contraindicated in patients with muscular dystrophy because it may lead to hyperkalemia and cardiac arrest. These patients may be at risk for developing malignant hyperthermia. The use of nontriggering anesthetic agents and careful observation for signs of malignant hyperthermia are essential.
   (5) Hematologic: Discontinue platelet inhibitors for 2 to 3 weeks before surgery. Autologous blood donation is recommended. Consider the use of intraoperative hemodilution, controlled hypotension, and cell-saver devices.

b) Patient preparation
   (1) Laboratory tests: Complete blood count, international normalized ratio, prothrombin time, partial thromboplastin time, arterial blood gases, electrolytes, type and crossmatch, and other tests as indicated by the history and physical examination
   (2) Diagnostic tests: Chest radiographs, pulmonary function test, spine studies, electrocardiography, and other tests as indicated by the history and physical examination
   (3) Medication: Standard premedication, if appropriate

3. **Room preparation**
   a) Monitoring equipment
      (1) Standard
      (2) Arterial line
      (3) Foley catheter
      (4) Central venous pressure line (if indicated)
   b) Additional equipment
      (1) Patient warming devices
      (2) Cell saver
      (3) SSEP monitor (if indicated)
      (4) Regular operating table with spinal frame or bolster
   c) Drugs
      (1) Antibiotics, vasodilators if hypotensive technique
      (2) Standard emergency drugs, tabletop
      (3) IV fluids through one to two large-bore IV catheters with normal saline at 8 to 10 mL/kg/hr with a fluid warmer
      (4) Blood loss possibly significant; at least 2 units of packed red blood cells need to be immediately available.

4. **Anesthetic technique**

General endotracheal anesthesia is used. For pediatric cases, preheat the room to 72° F to 78° F.

5. **Perioperative management**
   a) Induction: Standard; for prone cases, induction is performed while the patient is on the stretcher.
   b) Maintenance
      (1) Standard: If SSEPs are monitored, a constant state of anesthesia is used; stable hemodynamics and normothermia are essential. Question the SSEP technician regarding the use of nitrous oxide. The concentration of inhalation agents should be kept below 1 MAC. A sufentanil infusion of 0.25 to 1 mcg/kg/hr provides a continuous state of anesthesia and lowers the MAC of volatile agents. Muscle relaxation is acceptable and should be kept constant (1 twitch).
      (2) Position: The patient is prone on a spinal frame or bolster. Avoid abdominal compression, which impairs cardiac and pulmonary function and increases bleeding through epidural engorgement. Pressure points must be carefully padded and routinely assessed, especially during controlled hypotension. Anterior procedures are often performed with the patient in the lateral position; the dependent limb, ear, and eye should be checked frequently.
      (3) Wake-up test: Performed after completion of spinal instrumentation and requires 40 to 60 minutes of advance notice from the surgeon. Avoid narcotic or muscle relaxant boluses; decrease inhalation agent; hand ventilate; reverse muscle relaxants and narcotics (naloxone [Narcan], 20-mcg increments) if necessary; monitor train-of-four; and request hand squeeze followed by bilateral foot movement. Uncontrolled patient movement during a wake-up test can result in accidental extubation or dislodgment of the spinal instrumentation. Forceful inspiratory efforts may provoke venous air embolism. If the patient moves the hands and not the feet, the surgeon will decrease the spinal distraction. If

movement still does not occur, be prepared to increase the blood pressure and transfuse to increase spinal cord perfusion. The possibility of a hematoma should also be considered. After completion of the wake-up test, the anesthesia provider must be prepared to anesthetize the patient rapidly (have propofol ready). Intraoperative wake-up tests are infrequently performed if SSEP and MEP monitoring occurs.

(4) SSEP indications of spinal cord ischemia should be treated by notifying the surgeon, restoring normal blood pressure, and decreasing cord traction. Discontinue inhalation agents and ensure adequate oxygenation. Immediate transfusion may be necessary.

(5) Controlled hypotension may be used to decrease blood loss. Inhalation agents, vasodilators, nitroprusside, or nitroglycerin (or a combination) are usually used to achieve a mean arterial pressure of 65 mmHg in normotensive patients or lower the systolic blood pressure 20 mmHg from baseline in hypertensive patients. A major concern with hypotensive technique is compromising spinal cord blood supply. Blood pressure should be reduced slowly before the incision and allowed to gradually return to normal after surgery.

(6) Ischemic optic neuropathy can lead to blindness and is associated with deliberate hypotension, an increased length of surgery, pressure on the eyes, excessive fluid administration, and anemia. Consider the importance of early blood transfusion in patients undergoing hypotensive technique.

(7) Hypotensive technique requires an arterial line and Foley catheter to monitor urine output (0.5-1 mL/kg/hr).

(8) If a venous air embolism is suspected, the wound is packed, and nitrous oxide is discontinued if in use. Attempt to aspirate air using the central venous pressure catheter, use fluids and pressors, turn the patient supine, and institute cardiopulmonary resuscitation if necessary.

c) Emergence

(1) Emergence usually occurs after the patient is positioned supine. Most patients can be extubated in the operating room if the preoperative respiratory status was acceptable. Persistent narcotic or muscle relaxation may delay extubation. Assess neurologic function.

6. Postoperative implications

a) Pulmonary insufficiency: Postoperative ventilation may be required in patients with severe respiratory impairment. A patient with a preoperative vital capacity of less than 40% of predicted usually requires postoperative mechanical ventilation. Aggressive postoperative pulmonary care should be emphasized.

b) Neurologic sequelae are the most feared complications, and it is important to assess and document the postoperative neurologic examination.

c) Postoperative pain management allows for early ambulation and compliance with the pulmonary care regimen. Opioids can be administered by the intrathecal, epidural, or parenteral route.

d) Hypothermia may occur.

e) Pneumothorax may occur.

f) Dislodgment of internal fixation is possible.

g) Assess hemoglobin and hematocrit.

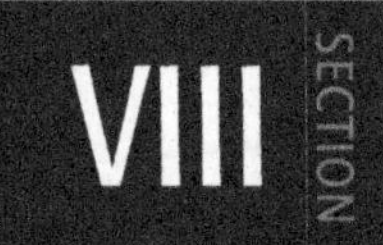

SECTION VIII Obstetrics and Gynecology

A. ASSISTED REPRODUCTIVE TECHNOLOGIES

1. Introduction

a) Procedure overview

Assisted reproductive technologies (ARTs) refers to all techniques used to retrieve and fertilize human oocytes. In vitro fertilization (IVF) is the most common technique used to artificially fertilize human oocytes.

The procedure is performed by initially stimulating maturation of the follicle with a gonadotropin-releasing hormone agonist that induces pituitary gland suppression and creates quiescent ovaries to prevent the production of a single dominant follicle. Follicle-stimulating hormone (FSH) and human menopausal gonadotropin are then administered, which induces 10 to 15 ovarian follicles. The patient is then given human chorionic gonadotropin (hCG), which induces the follicle to then mature and move into the follicular fluid. The oocyte is retrieved transvaginally, transabdominally, or via laparoscopy with an ultrasonically guided probe 34 to 36 hours after hCG administration. All visible follicles are collected, washed, incubated for 4 to 6 hours in a culture medium, and examined microscopically. Most follicles contain only one oocyte. Fertilization occurs in the IVF laboratory. The oocyte is identified and has minimal exposure to ambient room temperature, room air, and especially any chemical odors. Sperm are washed and centrifuged. Fresh media is added next to the centrifuged sperm, and those sperm that swim to the media, which can number 50,000, are placed with the oocyte. Timing must be coordinated with proper maturation of the uterine endometrium. ART is found to increase the risk of multiple gestations. Also, it has been reported that atypical implantations of the fertilized ovum or zygote, such as abdominal, cervical, ovarian, or tubal pregnancy, occur more frequently with ART. Common ART techniques are listed in the table on pg. 413.

Patients are assessed for antibodies to human immunodeficiency virus types 1 and 2 (HIV-1, HIV-2) and human T-cell lymphotropic virus type 1 (HTLV-1), hepatitis B antigen, and antibodies to hepatitis B and C. Patients are also tested for *Chlamydia*, syphilis, gonorrhea, and cytomegalovirus. Smokers require twice as many attempts at successful IVF than nonsmokers, so smoking is extremely discouraged.

2. Anesthetic technique

a) IVF is generally performed on patients who are American Society of Anesthesiologists (ASA) class 1 or 2 in their third or fourth decade of life.

b) Although IVF is a relatively simple procedure for the reproductive endocrinologist to perform, especially outside the operating room, IVF is an uncomfortable procedure and requires that patients do not move for the probe to be guided for retrieval and later reimplantation.

c) The vaginal wall must be pierced for the desired ovary to be accessed. Also, major blood vessels are present in the proximity of the ovaries, and their injury could lead to complications.

Common Assisted Reproductive Technology Techniques

In vitro fertilization (IVF)	Oocytes are removed, fertilization occurs in the laboratory, and the embryo is placed transcervically into the uterus or into the distal portion of the fallopian tube(s).
Gamete intrafallopian transfer (GIFT)	Oocytes and sperm are transferred into one or both fallopian tubes for fertilization. Advantage: oocyte retrieval and gamete transfer occur with a single procedure. Disadvantages: Requires at least one patent fallopian tube and laparoscopic surgery. Fertilization cannot be confirmed.
Zygote intrafallopian transfer (ZIFT)	Fertilized embryos are placed into the fallopian tube. Advantages: Fertilization is confirmed. Laparoscopic surgery can be avoided if fertilization has not occurred. The embryos can be transferred at an appropriate developmental stage. Disadvantage: Requires a two-stage procedure, with added risks and costs. Requires at least one patent fallopian tube.
Tubal embryo transfer (TET)	Cleaving embryos are placed into the fallopian tube.
Peritoneal oocyte and sperm transfer (POST)	Oocytes and sperm are placed into the pelvic cavity.

Modified from Speroff L. Clinical *gynecologic endocrinology and infertility.* 6th ed. Baltimore: Lippincott Williams & Wilkins; 1999: 1133-1148; Tsen LC. Anesthesia for assisted reproductive technologies. *Int Anesthesiol Clin* 2007;45:99-113.

d) Anesthesia requirements vary with the individual needs of the patient and the reproductive endocrinologist. Multiple ART procedures may need to be performed until one of them is successful, so safe yet inexpensive anesthetic techniques are desirable.
e) Minimal sedation, moderate sedation and analgesia, regional intrathecal anesthesia, paracervical block, or general anesthesia can be administered to assist in making the procedure as comfortable and successful as possible.
f) Moderate sedation with analgesia is usually sufficient for most patients. None of the anesthetic procedures caused differences in reproductive outcome.
g) Anesthetic medications generally considered safe for use in anesthesia for ART are listed in the box on pg. 414. Anesthesia providers should consider using safe anesthetic techniques with quick onset and a short duration.
h) It should be noted that propofol, lidocaine, thiopental, thiamylal, and alfentanil have been shown to accumulate in the follicular fluid.
i) Midazolam, when titrated in small doses to provide mild to moderated sedation and anxiolysis, has been shown to be safe, with no accumulation in follicular fluid or teratogenicity.
j) Ketamine (0.75 mg/kg) with midazolam (0.06 mg/kg) moderate sedation and analgesia has been safely used as an alternative to general anesthesia with isoflurane.

Anesthetic Medications Used for Assisted Reproductive Technologies

Intrathecal
Bupivacaine
Lidocaine
Fentanyl
Morphine

Paracervical Block
Bupivacaine
Lidocaine
Mepivacaine

Intravenous Sedation or Total Intravenous Anesthesia
Fentanyl
Alfentanil
Remifentanil
Meperidine
Ketamine
Midazolam
Propofol

Inhalational Agents
Nitrous oxide

k) The literature has suggested the use of caution when using a potent inhaled agent (especially sevoflurane and desflurane) because of possible negative effects to ART outcomes.

l) Nonsteroidal anti-inflammatory drugs (NSAIDs) such as ibuprofen, indomethacin, ketoprofen, ketorolac, meloxicam, naproxen, or oxaprozin are avoided because of inhibition of prostaglandin synthesis and possible effects on embryo implantation.

m) Droperidol and metoclopramide have both been shown to induce rapid hyperprolactinemia and should be avoided. Low plasma prolactin levels are associated with higher incidences of pregnancy.

n) The common anesthetic agents that could cause potential problems with ART are listed in the box below. The necessity for any medication given to the patient should be carefully considered, and the anesthetic technique should be kept simple and basic.

Common Anesthetic Agents That Could Cause Potential Problems with Assisted Reproductive Technologies

Morphine
Sevoflurane
Desflurane
NSAIDs (e.g., ibuprofen, indomethacin, ketoprofen, ketorolac, meloxicam, naproxen, oxaprozin)
Droperidol
Metoclopramide

NSAID, nonsteroidal anti-inflammatory drug.

B. CESAREAN SECTION

1. Introduction

A cesarean section (C-section) is the surgical removal of a fetus through an abdominal and uterine incision. A low transverse incision is the most common; in an emergency, a rapid vertical midline incision may be used. Indications for a C-section are failure of labor to progress, previous C-section, fetal distress, malpresentation of the fetus or umbilical cord, placenta previa, and genital herpes or other local infections.

2. **Preoperative assessment**
   a) A focused assessment should include obstetric and anesthetic history, maternal health, airway, allergies, and baseline vital signs. In emergency cases, the time for assessment will be brief. Special attention should be paid to airway assessment because failed intubation is a major cause of maternal morbidity and mortality.
   b) Key points regarding physiological changes in pregnancy
      (1) Cardiac output increases mostly because of the increase in stroke volume but also because of increase in heart rate.
      (2) The greatest demand on the heart is immediately after delivery when cardiac output increases 180%.
      (3) Blood volume is markedly increased and prepares the parturient for the blood loss associated with delivery.
      (4) Plasma volume is increased to a greater extent than red blood cell volume, resulting in a dilutional anemia.
      (5) Minute ventilation increases 45%, and this change is mostly caused by the large increase in tidal volume.
      (6) Oxygen consumption is markedly increased. Carbon dioxide production is similarly increased.
      (7) Pregnant women have an increased sensitivity to local anesthetics and a decreased minimum alveolar concentration (MAC) for all general anesthetics.
      (8) Platelets, factor VII, and fibrinogen are increased.
      (9) Intragastric pressure is increased in the last trimester, which, in combination with increased acid volume, often results in heartburn.
      (10) All pregnant women are at increased risk of aspiration because of the physiologic changes to the gastrointestinal system.
3. **Patient preparation**
   a) A nonparticulate antacid (e.g., sodium citrate, 30 mL) and metoclopramide 10 mg IV are routinely administered at most institutions regardless of the anesthetic technique chosen. Sedation is best avoided. Benzodiazepines have been implicated as possible teratogens, and it is best to avoid maternal amnesia during childbirth.
   b) Laboratory tests should include a type and screen, complete blood count (CBC), electrolytes, blood urea nitrogen, creatinine, glucose, prothrombin time, and partial thromboplastin time. In emergency C-sections, there may not be time to complete these tests.
   c) The parturient should have at least one large-bore intravenous (IV) lines in place before induction of anesthesia.
   d) An IV antibiotic should be administered either before abdominal incision or immediately after clamping of umbilical cord.
4. **Room preparation**
   a) Monitoring
      (1) Standard
      (2) If there is a history of pregnancy-induced hypertension, an arterial line is recommended.
      (3) If there is severe preeclampsia, a central line is also recommended, with a pulmonary catheter in cases of hemodynamic instability.

b) Positioning: Supine with left lateral uterine displacement. This is accomplished by placing a wedge under the right hip. Failure to use left lateral uterine displacement can result in aortocaval compression.
c) Drugs and tabletop
    (1) The tabletop should be set up for a general anesthetic.
    (2) Set out a smaller endotracheal tube (6-6.5) as well (because of airway edema).
    (3) Have ephedrine, phenylephrine, and oxytocin drawn up. Ensure immediate availability of Methergine and Hemabate.
    (4) Have difficult airway equipment available.
    (5) Unless there is maternal hypoglycemia, avoid giving IV solutions with glucose because they may lead to neonatal hypoglycemia.

5. Perioperative management and anesthetic techniques

The guidelines for general, spinal, and epidural anesthesia are listed below.

a) General anesthesia for C-section
    (1) Histamine$_2$-receptor antagonist or proton pump inhibitor or metoclopramide intravenously
    (2) Clear antacid orally
    (3) Left uterine displacement
        (a) Application of monitors
        (b) Denitrogenation (administration of 100% oxygen)
        (c) Traditional 3 to 5 minutes versus 4 vital capacity breaths
    (4) Cricoid pressure
    (5) Rapid-sequence IV induction
        (a) Propofol, ketamine, or etomidate
        (b) Succinylcholine (rocuronium or vecuronium if succinylcholine is contraindicated)
    (6) Intubation with a 6.0- to 7.0-mm cuffed endotracheal tube
    (7) Administration of a low concentration (e.g., MAC) of an inhalation agent with nitrous oxide
    (8) After delivery
        (a) Increased concentration of nitrous oxide with or without a low concentration of a volatile inhalation agent
        (b) Opioid titrated as needed
        (c) IV hypnotic agent (e.g., benzodiazepine, propofol), if needed
        (d) Muscle relaxant (e.g., succinylcholine boluses or infusion, vecuronium)
    (9) Extubation awake with intact airway reflexes
b) Epidural anesthesia for C-section
    (1) Metoclopramide 10 mg IV
    (2) Clear antacid orally
    (3) Intravascular volume replacement with Ringer's lactate or normal saline (10-20 mL/kg)
    (4) Application of monitors
    (5) Supplemental oxygen by face mask or nasal prongs
    (6) Epidural catheter at L2 to L3 or L3 to L4
    (7) Left uterine displacement
    (8) Test dose
    (9) Therapeutic dose: 5-mL boluses of 2% lidocaine + 1:400,000 epinephrine. Alternatively, 5-mL boluses of 0.5% bupivacaine, 0.5% ropivacaine, or 3% 2-chloroprocaine (boluses of lidocaine or 2-chloroprocaine every 1 to 2 minutes; boluses of bupivacaine or ropivacaine every 2 to 5 minutes)

(10) Aggressive treatment of hypotension: Exaggerated left uterine displacement; IV fluids; ephedrine or low-dose phenylephrine (or both)

c) Spinal anesthesia for C-section
   (1) Metoclopramide 10 mg IV
   (2) Clear antacid orally
   (3) Intravascular volume
   (4) Replacement with Ringer's lactate or normal saline (15-20 mL/kg)
   (5) Application of monitors
   (6) Supplemental oxygen by face mask or nasal prongs
   (7) Prophylactic intramuscular (IM) ephedrine (25-50 mg) in patients with a baseline systolic blood pressure of less than 105 mmHg
   (8) Lumbar puncture at L3 to L4 or below
      (a) Right lateral or sitting position
      (b) 24- or 25-gauge Sprotte needle or 25- or 27-gauge Whitacre needle
      (c) Bupivacaine 7.5 to 15 mg in 8.25% dextrose
      (d) Intrathecal morphine 0.1 to 0.2 mg or fentanyl 10 to 25 mcg for postoperative analgesia
      (e) Left uterine displacement
      (f) Aggressive treatment of hypotension
         (i) Exaggerated left uterine displacement
         (ii) IV fluids
         (iii) Ephedrine or low-dose phenylephrine (or both)

d) Tasks at delivery and postdelivery maintenance
   (1) The length of time from uterine incision to delivery has been shown to correlate with the degree of neonatal acidosis. The interval should be recorded. An interval of 3 minutes seems to be the critical value; neonates delivered later than 3 minutes after uterine incision are more likely to be depressed.
   (2) After the umbilical cord has been clamped, the anesthesia provider's options for anesthetic maintenance increase because the administered drugs will no longer reach the baby. If adequate uterine contraction is achieved with oxytocin, there is no reason why the use of an inhalation anesthetic cannot be continued.
   (3) A low-dose inhalation agent (up to 1 MAC), with or without nitrous oxide, and either fentanyl or sufentanil may be used. If uterine tone does not allow the use of an inhalation agent, an opioid and nitrous oxide technique is useful.
   (4) When opioids are used, nitrous oxide is usually needed. If nitrous oxide is not used, the anesthesia provider may consider giving a small dose of midazolam for amnesia. Opioid administration should be customized to the circumstances. One option is giving up to 5 mcg of fentanyl per kilogram, adjusting the dose according to the expected duration of the case and the patient's response. Another opioid choice is morphine 10 mg IV and 10 mg IM.
   (5) After the placenta has been delivered, oxytocin should be given immediately unless the obstetrician's plan for uterine contraction calls for the use of another agent.
      (a) The half-life of oxytocin varies from 4 to 17 minutes. It is metabolized by the liver, kidney, and plasma enzyme pathways in the parturient.

(b) Commercially available preparations of oxytocin contain a preservative that causes systolic and especially diastolic hypotension, flushing, and tachycardia when infused at high doses.
(c) The amount of oxytocin added to the IV solution should be tailored to the volume of solution remaining in the bag, the flow rate of the IV, and the patient's condition. If the IV bag is nearly empty or if IV solution is being administered rapidly, less oxytocin should be added to the bag.
(d) In general, the obstetrician is likely to desire the administration of 20 to 40 units of oxytocin over the first hour postpartum.
(e) If an unusually large blood loss results in hypotension and if fluid resuscitation is needed, it may be helpful to infuse the oxytocin at an appropriate rate and to start a second IV line for administering fluid volume at a rapid rate.
(f) If the solution with the added oxytocin is infused fast enough to replace volume, then it is likely that the high dose of oxytocin may cause further hypotension.

(6) If oxytocin does not adequately stimulate uterine contraction, the next drug used is usually an ergot alkaloid (Methergine, Ergotrate).
(a) Because of their potent vascular effects, ergot alkaloids are not administered intravenously. Ergot alkaloids normally cause an increase in blood pressure, central venous pressure, and pulmonary capillary wedge pressure.
(b) IV administration may result in arterial and venous constriction, coronary artery constriction, severe hypertension, cerebral bleeding, headache, nausea, and vomiting.
(c) An IM dose of 0.2 mg is commonly administered for stimulating uterine contractions.
(d) In some cases, the obstetrician may choose to administer oxytocin or ergotamine directly into the uterine muscle to maximize effect.
(e) Ergot alkaloids are metabolized and eliminated chiefly by the liver. The plasma half-life is approximately 2 hours, but uterine effects last much longer.
(f) Ergot alkaloids potentiate sympathomimetics, especially α-agonists (including ephedrine). Severe hypertension, cerebrovascular accidents, and retinal detachment have occurred when the two drugs were used simultaneously. These effects may persist even when the vasopressor is given well after the last dose of methylergonovine maleate.

(7) When the uterus does not contract well despite the use of oxytocin and ergot alkaloids, prostaglandin F_{2a} (Hemabate, 250 mcg) is administered either IM or directly into the uterine muscle.
(a) Prostaglandins are potent stimulators of uterine contractions. The contractions induced by prostaglandins are strong and painful.
(b) Nausea, vomiting, and diarrhea are frequent side effects. In addition to causing uterine contractions, prostaglandins may cause hypotension by relaxing vascular smooth muscle; however, cases of severe hypertension after prostaglandin administration have also been reported.

(c) Prostaglandins may cause a recalcitrant uterus to contract and stop bleeding. If they do not, the surgeon is likely to extend the procedure and include hysterectomy, for which the anesthesia provider must be prepared.

e) Emergence from anesthesia

(1) Even with the administration of metoclopramide, the parturient often has a large volume of gastric contents. Suctioning of the stomach with an orogastric tube while the patient is anesthetized decreases the incidence of vomiting after awake extubation.

(2) Before extubation, the anesthesia provider should verify full recovery of neuromuscular function. Because C-section is usually a brief procedure involving fairly limited exposure to anesthetic, emergence is often quick. Advance preparation limits patient discomfort before extubation.

C. DILATATION AND CURETTAGE

1. Introduction

Dilatation and curettage (D & C) involves dilation of the cervix and scraping of the endometrial lining of the uterus. The procedure is done to diagnose and treat uterine bleeding, cervical lesions, or stenosis. D & Cs are also used to complete an incomplete or missed abortion and are then referred to as suction D & Cs with the gestational week.

2. Preoperative assessment and patient preparation

a) History and physical examination: Assess for any cardiac, respiratory, neurologic, or renal abnormalities. Assess for a history of hiatal hernia or reflux; if a suction D & C, assess the gestational week; if greater than 16 weeks, consider the patient to have a full stomach.

b) Patient preparation

(1) Laboratory tests: Human chorionic gonadotropin, urinalysis, CBC

(2) Medications: Evaluation of any medications the patient is taking

(3) IV therapy: One 18-gauge peripheral IV line

3. Room preparation

a) Monitoring equipment: Standard

b) Additional equipment: Bair Hugger

4. Perioperative management and anesthetic technique

a) Drugs: Anxiolytic agents (midazolam [Versed], 0.01-0.02 mg/kg), narcotics (fentanyl, 1-2 mcg/kg), oxytocin (Pitocin) for suction D & Cs, and induction agents (propofol) can be used.

b) This procedure can be done either with a short-acting spinal or saddle block as a general anesthetic by mask, laryngeal mask airway, or with an endotracheal tube with inhalation agent or nitrous oxide or with heavy sedation (midazolam [Versed], fentanyl, and propofol).

c) Postoperatively, assess for bleeding, nausea, and cramping. Treat with narcotics, NSAIDs, and antiemetics.

d) Volume depletion and anemia can occur rapidly or slowly over time. IV rehydration and assessment of hemoglobin and hematocrit values are imperative.

D. GYNECOLOGIC LAPAROSCOPY

1. Introduction
Laparoscopy is a common endoscopic technique in gynecologic procedures. It is frequently used to diagnose or treat pelvic conditions that may include sterilization, adhesions, pain, endometriosis, ectopic pregnancies, ovarian cysts and tumors, infertility, and vaginal hysterectomy. A pneumoperitoneum is achieved by insertion of a trocar and insufflation of carbon dioxide.

2. Preoperative assessment and patient preparation
- a) History and physical examination: As indicated by the patient's history and medical condition
- b) Patient preparation
  - (1) Laboratory tests: CBC and other tests as indicated
  - (2) Diagnostic tests: Pregnancy testing and as indicated
  - (3) Preoperative medications: As indicated
  - (4) IV therapy: One or two 16- to 18-gauge IV catheters

3. Room preparation
- a) Monitoring equipment: Standard
- b) Additional equipment: Fluid warmer and Bair Hugger; other equipment as needed
- c) Drugs
  - (1) Anesthetic and adjunct agents and antibiotics are used.
  - (2) IV fluids: Depends on the procedure performed; calculate as indicated. Estimated blood loss is less than 50 to 100 mL.
  - (3) Blood: Type and screen
  - (4) The tabletop is standard.

4. Perioperative management and anesthetic technique
General anesthesia is preferred.
- a) Induction: Standard, as indicated
- b) Maintenance: Inhalational agent, oxygen, and opioid and nondepolarizing agent as indicated; antiemetics possible
- c) Position: Lithotomy; Trendelenburg to improve pelvic exposure
- d) Emergence: Standard

5. Postoperative implications
Complications include nausea, vomiting, and anemia.

E. HYSTERECTOMY: VAGINAL OR TOTAL ABDOMINAL

1. Introduction
Hysterectomy is commonly performed to treat uncontrolled uterine bleeding, dysmenorrhea, uterine myoma, gynecologic cancer, adhesions, endometriosis, and pelvic relaxation syndrome. Frequently, laparoscopy is used; for ovarian cancer prophylaxis, a bilateral salpingo-oophorectomy may be performed as well.

2. Preoperative assessment
- a) History and physical examination: As indicated by the patient's history and medical condition
- b) Patient preparation
  - (1) Laboratory tests: As indicated by the patient's history and medical condition

(2) Diagnostic tests: As indicated by the patient's history and medical condition

(3) Preoperative medications: Anxiolytics are given as indicated; consider prophylaxis for postoperative nausea and vomiting.

(4) IV therapy: Two 16- to 18-gauge IV lines are used; consider a central line or an arterial line (or both) if the procedure is radical.

(5) An epidural catheter may be placed for intraoperative or postoperative pain relief.

3. **Room preparation**
   a) Monitoring equipment is standard.
   b) Consider an arterial line and central venous pressure catheter if large blood loss is expected.
   c) Additional equipment includes a fluid warmer and Bair Hugger.
   d) Drugs
      (1) Anesthetic and adjunct agents and antibiotics are used.
      (2) IV fluids: For vaginal hysterectomy, calculate for moderate blood loss; crystalloids at 4 to 6 mL/kg/hr. Estimated blood loss is 750 to 1000 mL. For abdominal hysterectomy, calculate for a moderate to large blood loss; crystalloids at 6 to 10 mL/kg/hr. Estimated blood loss is 1000 to 1500 mL.
      (3) Blood: Type and crossmatch for 2 to 4 units of packed red blood cells if significant blood loss is expected.
      (4) The tabletop is standard.

4. **Perioperative management and anesthetic technique**

General or regional anesthesia is used, with a subarachnoid block or epidural with a sensory level of anesthesia of T4 to T6.
   a) Induction: Standard, with the choice as indicated
   b) Maintenance
      (1) General anesthesia: Inhalational agent, oxygen, opioid, anxiolytic, and nondepolarizing muscle relaxant
      (2) Regional: Local anesthetic of choice; supplemental anxiolytic and sedation
      (3) Position: Abdominal, supine; vaginal, lithotomy
   c) Emergence: Standard

5. **Postoperative implications**
   a) Complications: Nausea, vomiting, anemia
   b) Pain management: Patient-controlled analgesia; epidural opiates or an epidural local anesthetic such as 0.125% or 0.25% bupivacaine with fentanyl, 1 mcg/mL at an infusion of 8 to 10 mL/hr. Ketorolac 15 to 30 mg IV or IM every 6 hours may also be used for pain relief.

F. LOOP ELECTROSURGICAL EXCISION PROCEDURE

1. **Introduction**

The loop electrosurgical excision procedure is performed for the diagnosis and treatment of cervical intraepithelial neoplasia. This form of electrosurgery uses a loop electrode for excision and fulguration to prevent cervical bleeding. Other types of therapies that may be used to ablate cervical lesions are cryosurgery and carbon dioxide laser surgery.

2. **Preoperative assessment and patient preparation**
   a) History and physical examination: As indicated by the patient's history and medical condition
   b) Patient preparation
      (1) Laboratory tests: Pregnancy test, hemoglobin and hematocrit, urinalysis
      (2) Preoperative medications: Anxiolytics possible if the patient is not pregnant (e.g., midazolam, 0.01-0.02 mg/kg)
      (3) IV therapy: One 18-gauge IV catheter
3. **Room preparation**
   a) Monitoring equipment: Standard. If a pregnancy is more than 16 weeks' gestation, fetal monitoring may be used.
   b) Drugs: Standard tabletop agents are used.
   c) IV fluids: Calculate for minimal blood loss, 2 to 4 mL/kg/hr. Estimated blood loss is 50 to 200 mL.
4. **Perioperative management and anesthetic technique**
   a) Local, monitored anesthesia care, or regional or general anesthesia is used.
   b) Induction: Standard induction is indicated.
   c) In pregnant patients, rapid-sequence induction is used.
   d) In nonpregnant patients, mask ventilation may be appropriate.
   e) Maintenance: Standard, inhalational agent, oxygen, and opioid. Muscle relaxation is not required.
   f) Position is lithotomy.
   g) Emergence is standard.
5. **Postoperative implications**
   a) Complications include peroneal nerve injury from the lithotomy position, nausea and vomiting, bleeding, postdural puncture headache (PDPH), and premature labor.
   b) Pain management: Oral analgesics are used if the patient is not pregnant.

G. PELVIC EXENTERATION

1. **Introduction**

Pelvic exenteration is performed for the treatment of advanced, recurrent, radioresistant cervical carcinoma. It is considered a radical surgical approach because all pelvic tissues, including the cervix, bladder, lymph nodes, rectum, uterus, and vagina, are resected. Vaginal reconstruction and appropriate colon and urinary diversions are also performed.

2. **Preoperative assessment and patient preparation**
   a) History and physical examination: As indicated by the patient's history and medical condition
   b) Patient preparation
      (1) Laboratory tests: CBC, electrolytes, blood urea nitrogen, creatinine, calcium, magnesium, phosphate, prothrombin time, partial thromboplastin time, urinalysis, and renal function tests
      (2) Diagnostic tests: As indicated by the patient's history and physical examination
      (3) Premedication: Anxiolytics as indicated
      (4) IV therapy: Two 14- to 16-gauge IV catheters

(5) Central and arterial line; pulmonary arterial catheter considered if the patient has a significant cardiac history
(6) An epidural catheter possible for postoperative pain relief
(7) Patients should have IV hydration if given bowel prep

3. **Room preparation**
   a) Monitoring equipment: Standard; arterial line and central venous pressure useful because of major fluid shift, potential for major bleeding, obtaining laboratory values for a long duration, and possible need for vasoactive infusion. Foley catheter to monitor fluid status.
   b) Additional equipment: Fluid warmer; forced air warmer
   c) Drugs: Standard
      (1) Miscellaneous pharmacologic agents include opioid, anxiolytic, nondepolarizing muscle relaxant, local anesthetic, and antibiotics.
      (2) IV fluids: Calculate for major blood loss normal saline or lactated Ringer's solution at 10 to 15 mg/kg/hr. Estimated blood loss is 1000 to 4000 mL.
4. **Perioperative management and anesthetic technique**
   a) General anesthesia with an epidural block is used.
   b) Induction is standard, as indicated. Keep in mind that the surgery may be brief if metastatic tumor is found to be inoperable during initial exploration
   c) Maintenance is with inhalational agent, oxygen, and opioid anesthesia.
   d) Consider a local anesthetic through an epidural catheter.
   e) Use intermediate- or long-acting nondepolarizing muscle relaxants.
   f) Maintain normocarbia, mean arterial pressure of 60 to 88 mmHg, and urinary output at 0.5 to 1 mL/kg/hr; transfuse as indicated.
   g) Position: Both lithotomy and supine positions are used throughout the procedure.
   h) Emergence: The patient generally is transported to the intensive care unit for 2 to 3 days; postoperative ventilation may be necessary. If the patient is hemodynamically stable, extubation may be considered.
5. **Postoperative implications**
   a) Complications: Bleeding, fluid maintenance from large fluid shifts and mobilizations, and peroneal nerve damage from the lithotomy position (foot drop)
   b) Pain management: Epidural, opiates, or both

H. VAGINAL DELIVERY

1. **Preoperative assessment**

See the discussion of C-section earlier in this section.

2. **Patient preparation**
   a) All patients should have an IV catheter 18 gauge or larger placed and should receive a 500- to 1000-mL bolus before an epidural placement.
   b) Lumbar epidural analgesia provides segmental levels of analgesia that block pain impulses from the uterus but maintain sensation in the perineum and avoid motor blockade.
      (1) Generally, this is only administered when labor is well established, and the cervix is dilated 5 to 6 cm in primiparas and 3 to 4 cm in multiparas, with regular contractions.

(2) Bupivacaine is frequently used because it has little effect on the fetus and a longer duration of action. Solutions commonly used are 1/8% or 1/16% with fentanyl, 1 to 2 mcg/mL, with an infusion at 8 to 12 mL/hr and a bolus of 5 to 10 mL.
(3) Monitor blood pressure frequently for the first half hour and treat any blood pressure less than 100 mmHg with ephedrine, fluids, and left uterine displacement.
(4) Epidural topoffs may be used for forceps delivery or an extensive episiotomy repair with 5 to 10 mL of the infusion or 3% chloroprocaine (Nesacaine).
(5) Fetal heart tone needs to be assessed before and after placement of lumbar epidural.
(6) Monitor for signs of high level neuraxial block.
(7) Imperative to have emergency airway equipment available in situations where airway management is required.

c) A saddle block may be used for forceps delivery to block the perineum and inner thigh; 7.5 to 10 mg of lidocaine may be given while the patient is in the sitting position.
d) Pudendal nerve block: This blocks the pudendal nerves of S2 to S4 during the second stage of labor and results in low forceps delivery and episiotomy. It is administered transvaginally, with the local anesthetic injected posterior to the ischial spines beneath the sacrospinous ligaments. There is risk of puncture of the fetal scalp.
e) Paracervical block: This is injected into the fornix of the vagina lateral to the cervix. Nerve fibers from the uterus, cervix, and upper vagina are anesthetized; fibers from the perineum are not blocked. There is a high frequency of fetal bradycardia, so it is generally avoided.
f) Normal blood loss for a vaginal delivery is 400 to 600 mL.

I. OBSTETRIC COMPLICATIONS

From 1990 to 2005, the maternal mortality rate in the United States was 15 per 100,000 live births. The most common causes of maternal death include hemorrhage, embolic disorders, preeclampsia, infection, and cardiomyopathy.

1. Abnormal placental implantation

a) Introduction

(1) The placenta normally implants into the endometrium. A placenta implanted on or in the myometrium, the underlying muscular layer of the uterus, is termed *placenta accreta* (on the myometrium), *placenta increta* (into the myometrium), or *placenta percreta* (completely through the myometrium).
(2) Any of these abnormal placental implantations means that separation of the placenta from the uterine wall will be difficult and may be accompanied by severe bleeding.
(3) Placenta accreta, placenta increta, and placenta percreta are commonly associated with placenta previa and are more common in women who have had a previous C-section than in those who have not.
(4) The anesthetic implications are the same as those for other causes of increased blood loss.

2. **Blood loss**
   a) Introduction
      (1) Blood loss is difficult to estimate in obstetric patients. Often, lost blood is hidden inside the patient's body, soaked in laparotomy sponges, absorbed by drapes, or spilled onto the floor.
      (2) In general, approximately 500 mL is lost during a spontaneous vaginal delivery and approximately 700 mL during a C-section with general anesthesia; 1500 mL or more is lost if a hysterectomy is performed during C-section.
      (3) Because the term *parturient* has a 50% increase in blood volume, a great amount of blood can often be lost before the vital signs begin to change in response to the loss; 15% of the total blood volume may be lost without the occurrence of any compensatory tachycardia or vasoconstriction.
      (4) Hypotension may not occur until 30% of the total blood volume has been lost.
      (5) Approximately 4% of all parturients who deliver vaginally experience excessive postpartum bleeding.
3. **Breech presentation**
   a) Introduction
      (1) Many obstetricians now choose to deliver fetuses in breech presentations by C-section. In this case, C-section usually is elective, and either a regional or a general anesthetic can be used.
      (2) If the baby is to be delivered vaginally, an epidural anesthetic may be requested and is considered strongly indicated at some centers.
      (3) The muscle relaxation that it provides is helpful, and analgesia is required, at least for the forceps delivery of the fetal head.
      (4) Breech deliveries often result in laceration of the birth canal and therefore cause more bleeding than head-first deliveries.
4. **Cesarean hysterectomy**
   a) Introduction
      (1) After delivery, when hemostasis is unobtainable despite the use of some combination of oxytocin, ergot alkaloids, and prostaglandin, the surgeon performs a hysterectomy to stop uterine bleeding.
      (2) An atonic uterus, especially an incised uterus, can lose several liters of blood within a few minutes, outpacing the ability of even the most prepared anesthesia providers to replace intravascular volume.
      (3) Anesthesia at this point becomes trauma anesthesia, the primary purpose of which is the maintenance of vital signs, vital organ perfusion, and oxygenation; maternal analgesia and amnesia are important but secondary concerns. Etomidate, ketamine, benzodiazepines, and opioids are useful because they cause minimal hemodynamic depression.
      (4) If rapid blood loss begins during C-section with regional anesthesia, the anesthesia provider should consider the rapid induction of general anesthesia. It is difficult to manage volume resuscitation and to keep an awake patient both mentally and physically comfortable.

5. **Disseminated intravascular coagulation**
   a) Introduction
      (1) Disseminated intravascular coagulation (DIC) is frequently associated with three obstetric problems: retention of a dead fetus, placental abruption, and amniotic fluid embolism.
      (2) Circulatory shock, which often accompanies DIC, worsens the problem by decreasing peripheral and hepatic blood flow and causing further cell damage. Renal failure may result from the deposit of fibrin and cellular debris in the filtration system.
      (3) Clinically, patients with DIC have uncontrolled bleeding because of the consumption of clotting factors. Laboratory studies show decreased levels of fibrinogen and platelets, increased prothrombin and partial thromboplastin times, and excessive amounts of fibrin degradation products.
   b) Anesthetic technique
      (1) Patients with DIC need fluid resuscitation, and they almost always are hemorrhaging. Increasing intravascular volume dilutes activated clotting factors and slows the clotting process. Increased peripheral and hepatic perfusion limits cellular damage and improves clearance of activated clotting factors.
      (2) Because the patient is bleeding and many clotting factors are depleted, it appears as if repletion of clotting factors is necessary; however, administration of clotting factors fuels an already out-of-control coagulation process.
      (3) Definitive treatment of DIC first requires elimination of the cause. Replacement of clotting factors in obstetric patients should probably be postponed until the DIC has subsided.
6. **Embolism**
   a) Introduction
      (1) Thromboembolism
         (a) Thrombotic pulmonary embolism occurs in pregnant individuals fivefold more often than it does in nonpregnant individuals and is more likely to occur postpartum than antepartum.
         (b) It is associated with prolonged inactivity, cesarean delivery, obesity, and increasing age and parity.
         (c) Presentation varies from a few minor complaints to massive cardiovascular collapse. Pleuritic chest pain, dyspnea, hyperventilation, hypocapnia, coughing, hemoptysis, and distention of neck veins are associated with the disorder.
         (d) Thromboembolism is a major cause of maternal mortality, but while the parturient is in the delivery area, it is less likely to occur than either amniotic fluid or air embolism.
      (2) Venous air embolism
         (a) Venous air embolism can occur during labor, spontaneous vaginal delivery, and operative delivery and is frequently associated with placenta previa.
         (b) The overall incidence of subclinical venous air embolism in parturients has been reported to be as high as 29% during general anesthesia; the incidence in the parturient may be as high as 97%.

(c) Most venous air emboli are detected between delivery and uterine repair. The signs and symptoms of venous air embolism are as follows:
  (i) Mill-wheel murmur detected over the precordium
  (ii) Chest pain
  (iii) Dyspnea
  (iv) Decreased end-tidal CO_2
  (v) Elevated central venous pressure

(3) Amniotic fluid embolism
  (a) Although rare, amniotic fluid embolism is almost uniformly fatal. It may occur during labor, vaginal delivery, or operative delivery and is associated with placental abruption.
  (b) The pathogenesis is almost identical to that of venous air embolism except that patients who develop amniotic fluid embolism are prone to develop DIC if they survive the initial embolism.
  (c) Signs and symptoms of amniotic fluid embolism include a chill, shivering, anxiety, cough, dyspnea, cyanosis, tachypnea, pulmonary edema, and cardiovascular collapse. O_2 saturation has been reported to decrease quickly.
  (d) This cascade often leads to death within a few minutes.

b) Anesthetic technique
  (1) The incidence of postpartum thromboembolism can be affected by anesthetic interventions. C-sections performed with general anesthesia are associated with accelerated maternal coagulation compared with those performed with regional anesthesia, so the use of regional anesthesia may help reduce the incidence of postoperative thromboemboli.
  (2) The anesthesia provider can help prevent prolonged inactivity in those who have had a C-section by providing analgesia sufficient to allow comfortable ambulation. Use of epidural opioid analgesia is often an appropriate solution to this problem. It may be specifically indicated in those at risk for thromboembolism even if it must be administered after a general anesthetic has been given.
  (3) If embolism is suspected during spontaneous or operative delivery, the obstetrician should be informed immediately. The obstetrician can take steps to stop the entrainment of air or amniotic fluid, which include flooding the surgical field with saline, returning the uterus to within the abdomen, and stimulating uterine contractions.
  (4) One hundred percent O_2 should be administered by positive-pressure ventilation through a cuffed endotracheal tube.
    (a) Nitrous oxide administration should be discontinued because it rapidly expands the volume of an air embolus and prevents the delivery of 100% O_2.
  (5) An arterial line may be needed for monitoring of oxygenation and blood pressure. IV fluids are administered as needed to bolster central venous pressure.
  (6) A generous preload is necessary to enable the right side of the heart to pump volume forward against increased pulmonary vascular resistance.
  (7) If the fetus has not been delivered, left uterine displacement improves uterine blood flow and facilitates venous return to the

heart. Pharmacologic support of the cardiovascular system is likely to be needed.

(8) Patient position has been suggested to hinder the movement of the foreign substance into the pulmonary arteries. A slight anti-Trendelenburg (head-up) position with left lateral tilt of at least 15 degrees is designed to trap air in the right atrium, from which it can be aspirated via a central venous catheter. Unfortunately, it often is difficult to place the patient in this position and insert a central line in time to prevent pulmonary artery embolization.

(9) In the case of amniotic fluid embolism, prompt recognition and action are necessary to prevent maternal mortality. Immediate support of maternal circulation are necessary. Inotropic support should not be delayed (epinephrine, dopamine). Treatment for coagulopathy must also begin immediately and ideally with the consultation of a hematologist. Large-volume infusion devices may also be helpful for the resuscitation effort.

7. **Multiple gestation**

a) Introduction

(1) Multiple-gestation pregnancies carry higher risk for the both mother and fetuses than singleton pregnancies. Many of the risk factors affect anesthetic management.

(2) Multiple-gestation pregnancies, especially rare monoamniotic pregnancies, are associated with complications requiring emergent surgical intervention more often than singleton pregnancies.

(3) The anesthesia provider should constantly be prepared to provide anesthesia for an emergency C-section. The multiple fetuses are often small and premature.

(4) The large uterus compounds the problems of aortocaval compression; therefore left uterine displacement should be maintained at all times when the parturient is not lying on her side.

(5) If the fetuses are to be delivered vaginally, an epidural is valuable for maternal analgesia and neonatal safety. Because the neonate often is small and premature, a slow, controlled delivery through a well-relaxed birth canal makes birth trauma less likely.

(6) The epidural provides pelvic relaxation and reduces maternal discomfort, decreasing the likelihood that pain will induce a forceful reflexive expulsion of the fetus.

(7) Either regional or general anesthesia is appropriate for a C-section. After the babies have been delivered, the uterus may not contract well because it has been overstretched for many weeks.

(8) Larger-than-usual doses of oxytocin may be needed to induce the uterus to contract well and to stop bleeding. However, it is imperative that oxytocin administration not be started until after all the neonates have been delivered. Strong uterine contractions before the delivery of all neonates deprive any remaining fetuses of blood supply and oxygenation.

8. **Placental abruption**

a) Introduction

(1) Abruption occurs when the placenta begins to separate from the uterus before delivery; this allows bleeding behind the placenta and jeopardizes the fetal blood supply.

(2) Placental abruption results in bleeding (often hidden), uterine irritability (often hypertonic), abdominal pain, and fetal distress or death.
(3) Open venous sinuses in the uterine wall may allow products of hemostasis and amniotic fluid to enter the maternal circulation; this results in an incidence of DIC of up to 50%.
(4) The reported incidence of abruption in the general population varies widely but is much higher in women with hypertension (up to 23% among women with preeclampsia). When fetal death occurs, maternal mortality can exceed 10%.

b) Anesthetic technique
(1) In cases of placental abruption without fetal distress, vaginal delivery may still be possible. Because fetal distress can occur without warning, the anesthesia provider should be prepared to administer anesthesia for an emergency C-section.
(2) Taking an anesthetic history as soon as the diagnosis of placental abruption becomes known and checking for adequate IV access is recommended. If the mother is unstable or if fetal distress is present, operative delivery is necessary.
(3) Regional anesthesia usually is not indicated because of the potential for coagulopathy and because of the uncertainty of uteroplacental blood flow and therefore of fetal oxygenation.
(4) Generous venous access should be established as soon as possible. Although placental abruption does not usually result in sudden blood loss, a large volume of blood may be lost.
(5) When abruption results in fetal death, the volume of lost maternal blood can be as great as 5 L, all of which may be concealed. Volume resuscitation should begin as soon as IV access has been secured. Large volumes of crystalloid and colloid solutions and of red blood cells may be needed.
(6) General anesthesia can be induced with ketamine, up to 1 mg/kg. If the uterus is hypertonic, another drug should be chosen because the use of ketamine may further increase uterine tone, decreasing fetal O_2 supply.
(7) An alternate choice is etomidate, 0.3 mg/kg. If uterine tone is excessive, a volatile inhalation agent may be useful for maintenance of anesthesia and uterine relaxation.
(8) After the baby has been delivered, the uterus often becomes atonic; therefore, the use of inhalation agents should normally be discontinued. IV or intramyometrial oxytocin and intramyometrial ergotamine may be used with uterine massage to facilitate uterine contraction and to halt bleeding.

9. Placenta previa

a) Introduction
(1) When the placenta has implanted on the lower uterine segment and either partially or completely covers the opening of the cervix, placenta previa is present.
(2) Placenta previa has an incidence of up to 1%, and the mortality rate for those with it approaches 1%.
(3) Placenta previa is more common in women who have had it during a prior pregnancy.

(4) It most often results in painless vaginal bleeding before the onset of labor that may stop without intervention or hemodynamically significant blood loss. The potential exists, however, for *sudden* loss of large amounts of blood.

(5) The risk of bleeding increases if the placenta is disturbed by manual examination or cervical dilation. Postpartum bleeding is often increased as well because the lower uterine segment, where the placenta previa was implanted, does not contract as well as the rest of the uterus.

b) Anesthetic technique

(1) The diagnosis of placenta previa normally indicates an operative delivery. The anesthesia provider should prepare for heavy blood loss.

(2) The anesthesia provider may choose either a general or regional anesthetic technique, taking into consideration the parturient's current volume status and the potential for blood loss.

(3) Regional techniques should be performed only by an anesthesia provider who is very experienced with regional anesthesia and only after careful assessment and preparation.

10. Postpartum bleeding

a) Introduction

(1) Postpartum bleeding in moderate amounts is a normal event. Excessive bleeding may occur because of uterine atony (which accounts for 80% of all postpartum bleeding), placental retention, abnormalities of the uterus, lacerations of the delivery channel, uterine inversion, and abnormalities of coagulation.

(2) Uterine atony is associated with multiparity, prolonged infusions of oxytocin before delivery, polyhydramnios, and multiple gestation.

(3) A retained placenta or retained placental fragments must be removed manually to stop the bleeding. In the past, this has often required the administration of an inhalation agent for uterine relaxation.

(4) Nitroglycerin, a potent uterine relaxant with a relatively short duration of action, has been used successfully to provide uterine relaxation adequate for placental extraction. A dose of approximately 1 mcg/kg IV appears to be adequate.

(5) Sublingual nitroglycerin spray has also been used effectively and offers the added benefits of long shelf life and a ready-to-use preparation. Because nitroglycerin is a potent venodilator when given at low doses and is an arteriolar dilator when administered intravenously at a rate of 1 mcg/kg/min or higher, care should be taken to ensure that intravascular volume is adequate before this drug is administered.

(6) Analgesia for the procedure can be accomplished with a variety of methods, including the use of an already established epidural catheter or the administration of small IV doses of ketamine.

b) Anesthetic technique

(1) When postpartum bleeding is excessive, the anesthesia provider performs fluid resuscitation while simultaneously working with the obstetrician to eliminate the cause of the bleeding.

Fundal massage, IV oxytocin, IM methylergonovine maleate, or IM prostaglandin often is all that is needed. In some cases, anesthesia may be necessary for an additional procedure.

11. **Preeclampsia**
   a) Introduction: Preeclampsia is a vasospastic disease of pregnancy that affects 2.6% to 6% of parturients. The incidence of preeclampsia is highest in primigravidas younger than 20 years or older than 35 years of age and in women who have had preeclampsia during a previous pregnancy. The exact cause of preeclampsia is unknown but probably involves an abnormality in the ratio of thromboxanes to prostacyclins. Whereas thromboxanes are potent vasoconstrictors and platelet aggregators, prostacyclins have the opposite effect. Thromboxane A_2 and prostacyclin levels normally increase during pregnancy. An imbalance of prostacyclins and thromboxanes, both of which are produced by the placenta, has been demonstrated in preeclampsia.
   b) Clinical manifestations
      (1) Preeclampsia results in hypertension, 1+ to 2+ proteinuria, and edema after the 20th week of gestation. Generally, the diagnosis of preeclampsia is made when two of the three signs are present.
      (2) Hypertension is defined as a blood pressure greater than 140/90 mmHg or more than 30 mmHg above systolic baseline and more than 15 mmHg above diastolic baseline.
      (3) Severe preeclampsia is said to exist when the following conditions are present: maternal blood pressure greater than 160/110, 3+ or 4+ proteinuria, urine output less than 20 mL/hr, central nervous system (CNS) signs (blurred vision or changes in mentation), pulmonary edema, and epigastric pain. Blood pressure monitoring is a key indicator because it is technically easy to perform, and the severity of the hypertension frequently parallels the severity of the disease.
      (4) Preeclampsia results in maternal, fetal, and neonatal morbidity and mortality.
      (5) The chief cause of maternal mortality is cerebral hemorrhage caused by hypertension.
      (6) Pulmonary edema, renal failure, hepatic rupture, cerebral edema, and DIC also may cause maternal death.
      (7) Brain edema results in CNS irritability, seizures (a significant percentage of which occur postpartum), and an increase in sensitivity to depressant drugs. Fetal death results primarily from placental abruption or infarct. Delivery of the fetus is curative.
      (8) HELLP syndrome consists of hemolysis, elevated liver enzymes, and a low platelet count. From 5% to 10% of the sickest women with preeclampsia develop HELLP syndrome. Clinical signs of HELLP syndrome include epigastric pain, upper abdominal tenderness, proteinuria, hypertension, jaundice, nausea, and vomiting. Rarely, HELLP syndrome may result in liver rupture. Some experts believe that a degree of compensated DIC is present in all patients with HELLP syndrome.
   c) Pathophysiology

No uniform agreement exists with regard to the pathophysiology of preeclampsia. One view is that preeclampsia is a hyperdynamic state involving an early increase in cardiac output and elevated systemic vascular resistance (SVR). Another view is that preeclampsia is characterized by an increase in SVR and variable decrease in cardiac output. Thromboxane A_2 is found in increased levels during preeclampsia and has been correlated with disease severity.

(1) Increased vascular permeability results in extravasation of fluid and protein (proteinuria in the kidneys).
(2) Hypertension results in compensatory decreases in circulating blood volume and a loss of intravascular water and electrolytes via the kidney.
(3) Capillary injury stimulates platelet aggregation and fibrin deposition and may result in thrombocytopenia and, occasionally, DIC. It also results in multiple organ system dysfunction. Often, total body water is increased.
(4) Intravascular volume may decrease by as much as 40%.
(5) Marked peripheral and end-organ vasoconstriction is common, and it either causes or occurs in response to the decrease in vascular volume. An increased vascular sensitivity to vasopressin, angiotensin, and catecholamines has been demonstrated. Catecholamine levels often increase, and this results in decreased perfusion to the uterus, placenta, and fetus. Arteriolar constriction increases left ventricular work. When preeclampsia becomes severe, intravascular volume is either contracted or shifted centrally.
(6) Central venous pressure may be low because of a contracted blood volume, or it may be relatively normal because of a redistribution of vascular volume into the central circulation. Pulmonary capillary occlusion pressure may be normal or high because of left-sided heart failure and often does not correlate well with the central venous pressure.
(7) Uteroplacental insufficiency can result from a combination of decreased intravascular volume, vascular intimal deterioration, and increased vascular resistance. Placental perfusion in the preeclampsia patient may decrease by 70% compared with that in a healthy parturient. Decreased placental perfusion leads to intrauterine growth retardation and can cause fetal hypoxia and placental infarction.
(8) Platelet aggregation and fibrin deposition increase in preeclampsia. Platelet counts may drop as the platelets are consumed; however, even in the presence of a normal platelet count, platelet function may be below normal.

d) Perioperative management
(1) Magnesium sulfate is almost always administered to women with preeclampsia in the United States. Although it is not curative, it has been shown to reduce the likelihood of eclampsia by 58% and the risk of maternal death by 45%.
(2) Delivery presently is the only definitive way of ending the disease process of preeclampsia. When a fetus is at a gestational age of more than 37 weeks, obstetricians generally proceed with delivery. If the fetus is immature, delivery is delayed to allow the fetus time to mature.
(3) If preeclampsia is severe or fetal distress occurs, delivery is usually accomplished expeditiously. In any case, obstetric treatment

is aimed at preventing eclampsia (seizures), avoiding decreases in uteroplacental blood flow, and maximizing organ perfusion.

(4) Magnesium sulfate, which is also used as a tocolytic, causes venodilation, mild CNS depression, a decrease in the rate of fibrin deposition, and a reduction in uterine activity, if present.

(5) Decreasing fibrin deposition prevents further decay in organ perfusion and often greatly decreases liver pain in parturients with hemolysis, elevated liver enzymes, and a low platelet count (HELLP syndrome).

(6) Magnesium therapy is continued after delivery for the suppression of seizures.

(7) Regional anesthesia and preeclampsia
   (a) Epidural analgesia and anesthesia generally are preferred for both spontaneous vaginal delivery and C-section in the preeclampsia patient when they are not contraindicated.
   (b) A carefully initiated epidural infusion helps control maternal hypertension and may improve organ blood flow. Careful initiation of the block is necessary in women with preeclampsia because their mean blood pressure tends to decrease more than that of healthy parturients.
   (c) During a C-section, epidural anesthesia avoids stimulation of the airway, which can aggravate hypertension and possibly cause cerebral bleeding.
   (d) During a vaginal delivery, epidural analgesia allows a slower, more controlled expulsion of the premature infant and decreases the likelihood of trauma to the fetal head. Even these advantages, however, must be weighed against the risks of regional anesthesia, primarily hypotension and bleeding.
   (e) Because thrombocytopenia and other coagulation problems are associated with preeclampsia, careful consideration should be given to the patient's coagulation status before regional anesthesia is begun.
   (f) A careful history of bleeding should be taken and a platelet count evaluated before insertion of an epidural catheter in a patient with a diagnosis of preeclampsia. Coagulation problems are found almost exclusively in women with platelet counts below 100,000/mm^3.
   (g) Some evidence indicates that epidural analgesia can improve uteroplacental perfusion, and therefore fetal oxygenation, by decreasing plasma catecholamines. Epidural analgesia causes vascular dilation; this decreases blood pressure while maintaining—and, in some cases, improving—perfusion of the uterus and other organs, as long as hypotension is not allowed. Uterine artery systolic-to-diastolic ratios in women with preeclampsia decrease after the initiation of epidural analgesia, suggesting that resistance to blood flow is lowered.
   (h) Diastolic blood pressure should not be reduced to less than 90 mmHg in women with severe preeclampsia because such a reduction will probably result in inadequate uteroplacental blood flow.
   (i) Hypotension is a significant concern in parturients with severe preeclampsia because of the sometimes constricted

intravascular volume and the likelihood that the patient has already received an antihypertensive agent such as hydralazine or labetalol. When hypotension does occur, ephedrine and other vasopressors should be used cautiously because they may produce an exaggerated response in the preeclampsia patient.

(j) Epidural anesthesia can be accomplished safely in these patients if careful attention is devoted to volume status. Most but not all preeclampsia patients have a contracted blood volume.

(k) IV preloading may be necessary because of the constricted intravascular volume; however, some patients have a normal central venous pressure or left ventricular dysfunction. Preloading in these patients can result in pulmonary edema. Placement of a central venous pressure line or pulmonary catheter may be indicated in severe preeclampsia when the patient is oliguric or hypoxic.

(l) Bupivacaine is usually the local anesthetic of choice because of its long history of safe use in preeclampsia patients and because it has a slower onset than lidocaine and chloroprocaine. The slower onset allows time for the anesthesia provider to react to hemodynamic changes. Often, it is necessary to begin administering epidural anesthesia slowly with bupivacaine in these patients without any intravascular prehydration. Small incremental doses of bupivacaine can be administered and fluid given intravenously as needed when and if changes in blood pressure occur.

(m) After epidural analgesia or anesthesia has been instituted, the sympathectomy should not be allowed to wear off abruptly, because the increased intravascular volume could precipitate a hypertensive crisis or pulmonary edema. Instead, the block should be allowed to recede slowly, when the body is able to eliminate the intravascular fluid load and adequate monitoring is available.

(8) General anesthesia and preeclampsia

(a) Coagulopathy or decay in maternal or fetal condition is the most common indication for general anesthesia in the patient with preeclampsia. The maternal brain is edematous and more sensitive to CNS-depressant drugs.

(b) Induction of general anesthesia is hazardous in patients with preeclampsia. Their exaggerated hypertensive response to laryngoscopy and endotracheal intubation is potentially lethal. Compounding the problem, upper airway swelling may make identification of landmarks and intubation more difficult. Swelling may preclude the insertion of an endotracheal tube of normal size. Difficulty in intubation increases the duration of airway stimulation and worsens hypertension.

(c) The challenge during induction of general anesthesia is prevention of a further increase in blood pressure, which may result in intracranial hemorrhage. Control of blood pressure during induction of general anesthesia in these patients demands careful planning and skill in implementation.

(9) Muscle relaxants
   (a) Nondepolarizing relaxants are markedly potentiated in women with preeclampsia and therapeutic levels of magnesium. In these patients, half of an effective dose in 95% of the population dose produced 100% block for 35 minutes.
   (b) In healthy parturients not receiving magnesium sulfate, the same dose on average produced 42% blockade for approximately 9 minutes. Reduced doses of nondepolarizers can be used, if desired, but these drugs yield a longer-than-usual block.

12. Prematurity

a) Introduction
   (1) Premature delivery is estimated to occur in 12% to 13% of all pregnancies in the United States and is implicated in both maternal and neonatal death and considerable morbidity.
   (2) Premature labor is defined as regular uterine contractions that occur between 20 and 37 weeks of gestation and that result in dilation or effacement of the cervix. When labor begins prematurely, the ability to halt it can allow the fetus additional time to mature. Stopping labor is termed *tocolysis* (from the Greek *tokos,* meaning "childbirth," and *lysis,* meaning "breaking up").
   (3) The cause of preterm labor is not well understood; however, four pathways are supported by a considerable body of clinical and experimental evidence: excessive myometrial and fetal membrane overdistention, decidual hemorrhage, precocious fetal endocrine activation, and intrauterine infection or inflammation. The processes leading to preterm parturition may originate from one or more of these pathways.
   (4) Factors associated with preterm labor are listed in the box below.

Factors Associated with Preterm Labor

Demographic factors	Obstetric Factors
Nonwhite race	Multiple gestation
Age younger than 17 years or older than 35 years	Multiparity
	Abnormal uterine or cervical anatomy
Low socioeconomic status	Vaginal bleeding
Low pregnancy weight	Acute or chronic systemic disease
Drug use	Genetic fetal abnormalities
Tobacco use	

   (5) Methods of tocolysis
      (a) A variety of agents are used as tocolytics. These include β-adrenergic receptor agonists, nitric oxide donors, magnesium sulfate, calcium channel blockers, prostaglandin-synthesis inhibitors, and oxytocin antagonists. Labor-inhibiting drugs are only marginally effective.
      (b) Tocolytics act by two primary mechanisms: through generation or alteration of intracellular messengers or by inhibiting the synthesis or blocking the action of a known myometrial stimulant.

(c) Although more than 80% of women with preterm labor who are treated with tocolytics have their pregnancies maintained for 24 to 48 hours, few data suggest that tocolysis maintains pregnancy for a longer period.

(d) A critical goal of tocolysis is to delay delivery long enough to allow for the administration of corticosteroids, which reduces the risks of neonatal respiratory distress syndrome, intraventricular hemorrhage, necrotizing enterocolitis, and overall perinatal death. The initial benefit of corticosteroid therapy occurs approximately 18 hours after administration of the first dose with maximal effort at about 48 hours.

(e) Thus, treatment of acute preterm labor may allow time for the onset of the therapeutic effect of corticosteroids.

b) Magnesium sulfate

(1) Magnesium sulfate has been used for decades as a tocolytic; however, recently it has been noted that given its lack of benefit, possible harm, and expense, magnesium sulfate should not be used for tocolysis. Others believe it is still of some benefit when used properly.

(2) Magnesium causes relaxation of vascular, bronchial, and uterine smooth muscle by altering calcium transport and availability. Motor end-plate sensitivity and muscle membrane excitability also are depressed. Magnesium hyperpolarizes the plasma membrane and inhibits myosin light-chain kinase activity by competing with intracellular calcium, which in turn reduces myometrial contractility.

(3) The normal serum magnesium level during pregnancy is 1.8 to 3 mg/dL. A serum magnesium level of 4 to 8 mg/dL is therapeutic as a tocolytic, but even toxic levels do not eliminate uterine contractility. At 10 to 12 mg/dL, the patellar reflex is eliminated. Levels above 12 mg/dL cause respiratory depression; at approximately 18 mg/dL, respiratory depression progresses to apnea. The presence of higher levels (25 mg/dL) can cause cardiac arrest.

(4) Side effects

(a) The side effects of magnesium sulfate administration are dose dependent. As magnesium levels increase, skeletal muscle weakness increases, and CNS depression and vascular dilation occur. Magnesium sulfate infusion commonly results in a slight decrease in blood pressure during epidural anesthesia.

(b) Magnesium antagonizes the vasoconstrictive effect of α-agonists, so ephedrine and phenylephrine are less effective at increasing maternal blood pressure when administered concomitantly with magnesium.

(c) Cardiac muscle is not affected to a clinically evident degree when magnesium is administered at therapeutic levels, although magnesium can have profound myocardial effects during a gross overdose.

(d) Magnesium is eliminated unchanged by the kidneys. In a patient who is receiving a maintenance infusion of magnesium and who has decreasing urine output, blood levels of magnesium quickly increase, as do related side effects.

(e) Other side effects of magnesium sulfate include the following:
   (i) Cutaneous vasodilation with flushing
   (ii) Headache and dizziness
   (iii) Nausea
   (iv) Skeletal muscle weakness
   (v) Depression of deep tendon reflexes
   (vi) Respiratory depression
   (vii) Electrocardiographic (ECG) changes

(f) Patients on magnesium sulfate therapy have partial, if subclinical, neuromuscular blockade. Both depolarizing and nondepolarizing neuromuscular blocking drugs are potentiated by magnesium. Administration of priming or defasciculating doses of neuromuscular blocking drugs may cause significant paralysis when combined with magnesium therapy. The neuromuscular blocking effects of magnesium can be at least partially antagonized by calcium.

(g) Neonatal side effects after maternal magnesium administration are rare.

(h) Magnesium is also used in the treatment of preeclampsia, a vasospastic disease of pregnancy that can result in severe hypertension, coagulopathy, and seizure.

(i) Magnesium sulfate causes relaxation of vascular smooth muscle, a decrease in SVR, and a decrease in blood pressure. At serum levels of 7 to 9.5 mg/dL, it is an anticonvulsant. It also decreases fibrin deposition, improving circulation to visceral organs that are vulnerable to vasospasm and failure.

c) β-Agonists

(1) Stimulation of the β_2-receptor system causes smooth muscle relaxation, including relaxation of the uterus. The myometrium has β_2-receptors in cell membranes. Stimulation of these receptors triggers a cascade of biochemical effects, resulting in inhibition of myometrial contractility at the cellular level.

(2) β_2 stimulation also causes an increase in progesterone production. Progesterone, in turn, causes histologic changes in myometrial cells that limit the spread of contractile impulses. β-Adrenergic receptor agonists cause myometrial relaxation by binding to β_2-adrenergic receptors and subsequently increasing the levels of intracellular cyclic AMP, which activates protein kinase, inactivating myosin light-chain kinase, thus diminishing myometrial contractility.

(3) The administration of β-agonists results in downregulation of β-receptors over time. This results in a decreased tocolytic effect during long-term β-agonist therapy that has been demonstrated in animals after as few as 24 hours of ritodrine administration.

(4) Maternal side effects

   (a) Available β-agonists have both β_1 and β_2 effects, although some agents are fairly selective for one receptor subset over the other.

   (b) The side effects of β-agonist therapy can be predicted on the basis of a knowledge of systemic β effects. Cardiovascular effects are generally the most clinically important and troublesome. β_1 stimulation causes an increase in heart rate, myocardial contractility, and myocardial O_2 demand. Palpitations and premature ventricular contractions are common. β_2 stimulation causes vascular dilation, bronchial dilation, an increase in secretions, and various metabolic effects.

(c) Maternal side effects of β-agonists include the following:
  (i) Cerebral vasospasm
  (ii) Chest pain or tightness
  (iii) Glucose intolerance
  (iv) Hypokalemia
  (v) Ileus
  (vi) Myocardial ischemia
  (vii) Nausea
  (viii) Palpitations
  (ix) Pulmonary edema
  (x) Restlessness
  (xi) Tremor
  (xii) Ventricular arrhythmias

(d) β-Agonist therapy further increases the demand on the cardiovascular system. Complaints of palpitations and chest pain are common. ECG changes are sometimes seen, although myocardial ischemia is not always documented.

(e) Metabolic effects
  (i) β stimulation increases blood glucose and insulin levels. When a β-agonist infusion is started, the blood glucose level increases within a few hours and returns to baseline within 72 hours without treatment.
  (ii) Potassium is redistributed from the extracellular to intracellular compartments. This results in a decrease in serum potassium level, sometimes to less than 3 mEq/L. As with glucose levels, serum potassium levels return to normal within 72 hours after initiation of β-agonist therapy.

(5) Pulmonary edema
  (a) There is a small but notable incidence of pulmonary edema among healthy parturients receiving β-agonists. The mechanism for the development of pulmonary edema in these patients is unclear.
  (b) Fluid overload resulting from a physiologic increase in intravascular volume, antidiuresis, and IV fluid administration may have a role.
  (c) Myocardial fatigue caused by tachycardia also has been suggested as a possible cause. Pulmonary artery pressures are not uniformly elevated, however, and sometimes they are low; this finding can be used to argue against both of these hypotheses. However, it is clear that the danger of pulmonary edema increases when parturients receiving β-agonists are preloaded for regional anesthesia.
  (d) Risk factors associated with pulmonary edema during β-agonist tocolysis include anemia, fluid overload, magnesium, multiple gestation, and prolonged maternal tachycardia.

(6) Fetal and neonatal side effects
  (a) Clinically used β-agonists cross the placenta and have fetal and neonatal effects. Fetal tachycardia (fetal heart rate [FHR] >160 beats/min) is common.

(b) Ritodrine (Yutopar) is a selective β_2-agonist. Ritodrine therapy increases maternal heart rate by an average of 40 beats/min. Systolic blood pressure commonly increases, and diastolic pressure decreases. The manufacturer's literature recommends that patients on ritodrine therapy receive no more than 2 L of IV fluid over 24 hours.

(c) Before spinal or epidural anesthesia for C-section is initiated, it is common for a 2-L IV preload to be given in less than 30 minutes. However, even smaller IV preloads are not recommended in patients receiving ritodrine until use of the drug has been discontinued for at least 1 hour. Ritodrine is eliminated by the kidneys and has an elimination half-life of approximately 30 minutes.

(d) Terbutaline (Brethine, Bricanyl) is a synthetic, relatively β_2-receptor–selective, noncatecholamine sympathomimetic amine. When administered parenterally, terbutaline is less β_2-receptor–selective than ritodrine. Arrhythmias are more likely to occur with terbutaline use than during ritodrine administration, and tachycardia can be a problem. Terbutaline is approximately 50% eliminated by the kidneys and has a half-life of up to 16 hours. Similar to ritodrine, terbutaline has been associated with pulmonary edema when it is used for tocolysis.

d) Calcium channel blockers

(1) Nifedipine is the most commonly used agent because it can be administered orally. The calcium channel blockers inhibit the influx of calcium ions through the cell membrane and the release of intracellular calcium from the sarcoplasmic reticulum.

(2) This decreases intracellular free calcium leading to inhibition of calcium-dependent myosin light-chain kinase–mediated phosphorylation, resulting in myometrial relaxation.

e) Cyclooxygenase inhibitors

(1) Cyclooxygenase converts arachidonic acid to prostaglandin H_2. Prostaglandin H_2 serves as a substrate for tissue-specific enzymes, which is critical in parturition.

(2) Prostaglandins enhance the formation of myometrial gap junctions and increase available intracellular calcium by raising transmembrane influx and sarcolemmal release of calcium. Indomethacin is the most commonly used tocolytic agent in this class.

f) Therapy recommendations

(1) Nifedipine appears to be a reasonable choice for initial tocolysis, given the oral route of administration, low frequency of side effects, and efficacy in reducing neonatal complications. Nifedipine can be used at any gestational age when labor-inhibition therapy is being considered.

(2) For pregnancies of less than 32 weeks' gestation, an alternative to nifedipine is indomethacin. These agents have been shown to be more effective than the β-adrenergic receptor agonists in comparative studies.

(3) Indomethacin should be avoided in women with a platelet dysfunction or bleeding disorder, hepatic or renal dysfunction, gastrointestinal ulcerative disease, or asthma (in women with hypersensitivity to aspirin).

(4) The use of β-adrenergic receptor agonists is an alternative to therapy with nifedipine and indomethacin. The side effect profile of this class of drugs is less favorable than that of nifedipine, but their effectiveness in stopping contractions appears to be similar.

g) Anesthetic technique: When an anesthetic intervention is planned for a patient who is receiving a tocolytic agent, knowledge of maternal and fetal physiology and of the pharmacology of the tocolytic agent must be integrated.

(1) Regional anesthesia

(a) When tocolysis fails, preterm deliveries are often accomplished by C-section. In this situation, 1- and 5-minute Apgar scores have been shown to be higher in neonates delivered with epidural anesthesia than in those delivered with general anesthesia.

(b) Patients on magnesium therapy are often candidates for subarachnoid or epidural blocks as long as careful attention is devoted to volume status. Magnesium causes vasodilation, and maternal hemorrhage is tolerated poorly by both parturients on magnesium and their fetuses.

(c) Subarachnoid block has the advantage of involving very small amounts of local anesthetic, and this reduces the chance for fetal local anesthetic toxicity.

(d) Epidural anesthesia can be used throughout labor for analgesia and can be induced slowly; this minimizes the risk of sudden hypotension caused by sympathetic block.

(e) Even when volume status is accurately assessed, IV preloads before subarachnoid or epidural anesthesia are associated with an increased risk of pulmonary edema in parturients receiving β-agonist drugs.

(f) Use of ritodrine (and perhaps terbutaline) should almost always be discontinued, and enough time for the drug to be largely eliminated should be allowed to pass before regional anesthesia is induced.

(g) If time constraints do not permit the needed delay, induction of general anesthesia for an urgent or emergent procedure is almost always preferable.

(h) If the patient is already in pulmonary edema or has marginal to poor uterine artery blood flow because of vascular constriction, slowly induced epidural anesthesia may provide a beneficial vasodilation.

(i) Anesthesia-induced hypotension must be carefully avoided, however, because almost all therapies directed at restoration of blood pressure would be detrimental. Ephedrine could increase an already rapid heart rate, and IV fluid administration could precipitate or worsen pulmonary edema. A low dose of an α-agonist (e.g., 50-100 mcg of phenylephrine given intravenously) may be the least detrimental choice.

(2) General anesthesia

(a) Succinylcholine is the muscle relaxant of choice during the rapid-sequence induction of an obstetric patient.

In patients on magnesium therapy, defasciculation with a small dose of a nondepolarizing neuromuscular blocking agent is not recommended because significant paralysis may result, increasing the risk of aspiration of gastric contents.

(b) Magnesium potentiates depolarizing and, especially, nondepolarizing relaxants. The amount of potentiation is variable, and a peripheral nerve stimulator is invaluable. The duration of paralysis after administration of a standard dose of succinylcholine may give a clue as to how much longer than normal the effect of a nondepolarizer will last.

(c) Induction of general anesthesia in a patient receiving a β-agonist tocolytic can present a challenge. As with regional anesthesia, there are advantages to delaying induction of general anesthesia whenever possible until ritodrine has been largely eliminated (at least 1 hour).

(d) Thiopental has a long, safe history of use in obstetric anesthesia, and its cardiovascular depression may offset some of the cardiac stimulation caused by the β-agonist. Propofol may also be used. The use of a vagolytic, such as atropine, glycopyrrolate, or pancuronium bromide, is counterproductive.

(e) Induction of general anesthesia should usually be delayed until the patient has been prepared and the operating surgeon and assistants are ready for incision. Preterm neonates have a significantly higher incidence of low Apgar scores at 1 minute. Reducing the interval from the induction of anesthesia to the delivery of the infant minimizes the depressant effects of the anesthetic that the neonate must overcome.

(f) In pregnant patients, effective doses of fentanyl (5-8 mcg/kg) cross the placenta and result in significant neonatal depression. Fentanyl (1 mcg/kg) administered before the induction of general anesthesia for C-section does not affect the Apgar score or neurobehavioral test results of neonates significantly.

(g) β-Blockers may be used before the induction of anesthesia and instrumentation of the airway. Labetalol has been used successfully to decrease maternal blood pressure while uteroplacental blood flow is maintained. Neonatal side effects (hypotension, bradycardia) are apparently minimal. In women with preeclampsia, labetalol has been administered before the induction of general anesthesia to decrease mean blood pressure at induction and during the first 10 minutes of anesthesia.

(h) Anesthetic depth has important implications for fetal oxygenation. Light anesthesia results in maternal catecholamine outflow in response to surgical stimulation, which in turn results in uterine artery constriction and a decrease in uterine artery blood flow. Anything that decreases uterine artery blood flow decreases uteroplacental blood flow and therefore results in fetal hypoxia.

13. Prolapsed umbilical cord

A prolapsed umbilical cord is present when the cord protrudes through the cervix ahead of the fetus. Danger arises when compression of the cord against the wall of the cervix by the presenting part cuts off blood flow and oxygenation to the fetus.

The obstetrician attempts either to restore blood flow in the umbilical cord by pushing the presenting part back into the uterus or to deliver the fetus abdominally before asphyxia causes permanent injury. In the first situation, anesthesia is likely to be needed for uterine relaxation; in the second, it is necessary for emergent C-section.

14. Uterine rupture

a) Introduction

(1) Uterine rupture is most commonly associated with labor in the presence of a previous uterine incision (vaginal birth after C-section [VBAC]) but may occur in an unscarred uterus.

(2) The incidence of uterine rupture during attempted VBAC is approximately 0.6%. Uterine rupture has also been associated with cocaine abuse during pregnancy.

(3) The classic description of complete uterine rupture includes sudden, severe, tearing abdominal pain in a multiparous woman in hard labor. The pain may break through labor epidural anesthesia. Next, labor stops, and shock and fetal distress rapidly develop.

(4) Unfortunately, uterine rupture often does not present classically. For example, some ruptures occur during periods of mild labor. The clinical finding most commonly associated with uterine rupture is an abnormal FHR tracing.

(5) Whatever the presentation, bleeding is often severe. The uterus receives approximately 800 mL of blood per minute (≈10% of the cardiac output); therefore, a tear in this organ holds the potential for rapid exsanguination.

(6) Mortality from uterine rupture accounts for half of the maternal deaths attributed to blood loss each year. Fetal mortality rate after uterine rupture is nearly 80%.

b) Anesthetic technique: Uterine rupture requires surgery for hemostasis and often for delivery. Anesthesia providers should be prepared for heavy bleeding commensurate with any severe abdominal trauma. In the operating room, as much as 3500 mL of blood has been found in the abdomen at incision.

15. Postdural puncture headache

a) Introduction

Postdural puncture headache (PDPH) results from a loss of cerebrospinal fluid (CSF) from the subarachnoid space. The total volume of CSF present within this sac in an adult is approximately 150 mL. Approximately 500 mL of CSF is produced and reabsorbed each day.

PDPH occurs when CSF leaks out through a hole in the dura made during the performance of a subarachnoid block or accidentally during the attempted performance of an epidural block. Because the Tuohy needle used to place an epidural catheter has a large diameter, puncture of the dura with the needle results in the loss of a significant volume of CSF. Loss of CSF is not the only cause of headache after regional anesthesia in obstetric patients. Meningitis, although rare, can develop despite the adherence to aseptic technique, and this disease shares many of the signs and symptoms of PDPH (headache, nausea, and photophobia) in the initial stages.

b) Incidence: The incidence and severity of PDPH vary with factors thought to be related to the volume and rate of CSF leakage out of the subarachnoid space.
   (1) PDPH is infrequent in elderly adults and most frequent in young adults. Women may be slightly more susceptible than men.
   (2) Generally, the use of large needles is more likely to be associated with PDPH than use of small ones.
   (3) The configuration of the tip of the needle is also important. Other factors being equal, the use of beveled needles (e.g., the Quincke needle) results in headache more frequently than the use of pencil-point or bullet-tip needles (e.g., the Whitacre or Sprotte needle).
   (4) The orientation of the needle as it punctures the dural fibers also may be important. Spreading the fibers along their cephalad-to-caudad axis may result in less CSF leakage than cutting the fibers by inserting the bevel perpendicular to the axis of the dural fibers.
   (5) The angle at which the needle approaches the dura may also modify the amount of CSF leakage and therefore the incidence of PDPH; however, the angle of approach most often is dictated by anatomy and therefore is difficult for the anesthesia provider to modify effectively.

c) Clinical appearance
   (1) The hallmark of a PDPH is its postural nature. The headache is relieved by lying down and returns when sitting or standing up.
   (2) It is commonly fronto-occipital and sometimes is associated with neck and shoulder stiffness.
   (3) Photophobia may be present in patients with severe headaches; double vision occurs less frequently. Temporary deafness has occurred rarely. Nausea and vomiting may also occur.
   (4) The onset of the headache is usually not immediate, but it may take 1 to 2 days to become bothersome. It may be mild or severe, and it often becomes worse if the patient feels sick and does not consume liquids.

d) Treatment
   (1) Patients should be given a choice of treatments ranging from the most conservative to the most aggressive. PDPH may be a mild irritation for a few days, or it may be debilitating.
   (2) Patients with a mild PDPH may elect to rest in bed because the horizontal position often provides complete relief from the headache or to take over-the-counter analgesics if they are up and about. Adequate hydration should be encouraged. In hospitalized patients who are not taking fluids by mouth, IV hydration is warranted. Liberal hydration does not increase the production of CSF; however, it is important that the patient not be allowed to become dehydrated because dehydration decreases CSF production.
   (3) Caffeine is a cerebral vasoconstrictor and is effective in preventing or treating PDPH in some patients.

(4) The most effective treatment available for PDPH is an epidural blood patch. This treatment entails some risk because it is invasive; also, the headache is likely to become worse if another dural puncture is made in the course of placing the epidural (with a 17- or 18-gauge Tuohy needle). The usual contraindications to an epidural procedure also apply to this treatment.

(5) A blood patch is performed by placing a Tuohy needle in the epidural space, preferably at the same interspace as the dural puncture or one interspace below. After the Tuohy needle is in place, an assistant performs a peripheral venipuncture and draws 20 mL of the patient's blood using strict aseptic technique. The blood is slowly injected into the epidural space. The ideal volume for injection appears to be between 15 and 20 mL; the use of smaller volumes is associated with a significantly lower success rate, especially in the placement of prophylactic blood patches. If discomfort develops in the back or neck, the injection is temporarily stopped. After the discomfort has passed, injection of the target volume of 15 to 20 mL may continue (unless discomfort returns). After the desired volume is injected, the Tuohy needle is withdrawn, and the patient should lie quietly for at least 1 hour.

(6) For the next several hours, the patient should rest and not be overly active. This may need to be specifically discussed with the patient because she may feel quite well for the first time in days and therefore may want to be more active. Excessive activity before complete clot consolidation may result in the clot being dislodged from the dural puncture site, allowing CSF leakage to resume.

(7) The epidural blood patch is thought to plug the dural rent with a fibrin clot; the injected volume of blood applies pressure to the dura, in effect "autotransfusing" the cerebrum with CSF from around the spinal cord. An epidural blood patch is effective in more than 90% of patients when it is performed 24 hours after the dural puncture. A second patch is effective in approximately half of those who do not obtain relief from the first; this brings the total success rate to approximately 95%.

   (i) Epidurally administered fibrin glue has been shown to be an effective alternative to blood administration for the treatment of PDPH. Further study is needed to determine if it's a superior treatment compared with blood.

J. ANESTHESIA FOR THE PREGNANT PATIENT UNDERGOING A NONOBSTETRIC PROCEDURE

1. **Introduction**
   a) Surgery for nonobstetric procedures occurs in up to 2% of women.
   b) Approximately 42% of procedures occur in the first trimester, 35% during the second, and 23% during the third.
   c) Acute abdominal problems are most common, with appendectomy ranking first followed by cholecystectomy.
   d) Other common problems include adnexal disease (e.g., ovarian cysts, which may rupture or become torted) and trauma.

2. **Preoperative assessment**
   a) Aortocaval compression becomes clinically relevant from approximately 20 weeks of gestation. It can be relieved by a left lateral tilt of 15 degrees, which is therefore essential in all pregnant patients in the supine position after 20 weeks.
   b) There may be delay in the onset of the classical symptoms and signs of hypovolemia because of the increase in blood volume along with a resting tachycardia.
   c) Pregnancy is a hypercoagulable state with an increase in most clotting factors. The platelet count may fall, but there is actually an increase in production and consumption.
   d) Pregnancy is a significant risk factor for thromboembolism; therefore, thromboprophylaxis is essential in the postoperative period when the risk is further increased by immobility and the hypercatabolic state.
   e) Airway management may be challenging during pregnancy. Bag-mask ventilation may be more difficult because of increased soft tissue in the neck. Laryngoscopy can be hindered by weight gain and breast engorgement. Increased edema of the vocal cords because of increased capillary permeability can hinder intubation and increase the risk of bleeding.
   f) Increased maternal oxygen consumption and reduced functional residual capacity results in rapid oxygen desaturation during attempts at intubation.
   g) Smaller sized endotracheal tubes may be needed.
   h) Careful preoxygenation in a slightly head-up position is essential before induction.
   i) It is recommended that from 16 weeks' gestation, patients undergoing general anesthesia should be given prophylaxis against aspiration pneumonitis. This usually includes a nonparticulate antacid such as sodium citrate 0.3 M 30 mL and an H_2 receptor antagonist (e.g., ranitidine 150 mg orally or 50 mg intravenously).
   j) Induction of anesthesia should be by a rapid-sequence technique with cricoid pressure.
   k) At the end of the procedure, the patient should be extubated fully awake in the lateral position.
   l) Pharmacokinetic and pharmacodynamic profiles are altered in pregnancy, and drugs should be titrated accordingly.
3. **Perioperative management**
   a) Fetal safety
      (1) Prevention of fetal asphyxia
         (a) One of the most serious risks to the fetus during maternal surgery is intrauterine asphyxia. This must be avoided by maintaining maternal oxygenation and hemodynamic stability.
         (b) It is extremely important to avoid hypoxia, extreme hyper- and hypocarbia, hypotension, and uterine hypertonus.
         (c) Maternal hypoxemia causes uteroplacental vasoconstriction and decreased perfusion, causing fetal hypoxia, acidosis, and ultimately death.
         (d) Uteroplacental circulation is not autoregulated, and hence perfusion is entirely dependent on the maintenance of an adequate maternal blood pressure and cardiac output.

(e) Hypotension can be caused by anesthetic drugs, central neuraxial blockade, hypovolemia or aortocaval compression.
(f) Maternal hypotension needs to be treated aggressively by ensuring left lateral tilt and boluses of IV fluids. Additional vasopressors may be required, and currently it is believed that α-agonists such as phenylephrine and metaraminol produce a better fetal acid balance than indirect sympathomimetic agents such as ephedrine.

(2) Drugs and teratogenicity
(a) Teratogenicity is defined as the observation of any significant change in the function or form of a child secondary to prenatal treatment.
(b) During the first 2 weeks of human gestation, the teratogens have an all-or-none phenomenon; the fetus is lost or is preserved fully intact.
(c) The period from the third to the eighth weeks of gestation represents the most important time for organogenesis during which drugs can exert their most serious teratogenic effects.
(d) After this, drug exposure should not cause organ abnormalities, but fetal growth retardation may occur.
(e) Studies looking at the outcomes of women who underwent surgery during pregnancy suggest no increase in congenital anomalies in their offspring but an increase in fetal loss, growth restriction, and low birth weight attributed to the requirement for surgery (not anesthetic administration).
(f) Nitrous oxide inhibits methionine synthetase; therefore, there is concern that it could affect DNA synthesis in the developing fetus and should be avoided.
(g) Ketamine causes increased uterine tone and fetal asphyxia and should not be used in the first two trimesters. The effect is not seen in the third trimester.

(3) Prevention of preterm labor and fetal monitoring
(a) Surgery during pregnancy increases the risk of spontaneous abortion, preterm labor, and preterm delivery. This risk is increased with intra abdominal procedures.
(b) Uterine manipulation should be kept to a minimum, and drugs that increase uterine tone (e.g., ketamine) should be avoided.
(c) Prophylactic tocolytic therapy is controversial because there are associated maternal side effects, and efficacy during nonobstetric surgery has not been proven.
(d) Perioperative fetal monitoring is also an area of controversy. From 18 to 22 weeks, FHR monitoring is feasible, and from 25 weeks FHR variability can be observed.
(e) Continuous monitoring may be technically difficult during abdominal operations or in cases of maternal obesity.
(f) Anesthetic agents reduce both baseline FHR and FHR variability; therefore, interpretation is difficult and may lead to unnecessary interventions.
(g) Anesthetic agents do not cause decelerations or persistent fetal bradycardia, and these changes may indicate fetal distress.

(h) Monitoring may enable swift action to be taken such as the optimization of maternal hemodynamics, oxygenation, and ventilation.

4. **Postoperative implications**
   a) Attention to thromboprophylaxis is essential. This should include early mobilization, maintaining adequate hydration, thromboembolic deterrent (TED) stockings and other calf compression devices and consideration of pharmacological prophylaxis (e.g., subcutaneous low-molecular-weight heparin).
   b) Adequate analgesia is important because pain causes increased circulating catecholamines, impairing uteroplacental perfusion. Analgesia may mask the signs of early preterm labor, so tocometry is useful to detect contractions. This enables tocolysis to be administered without delay.
   c) If a pregnancy continues beyond the first postoperative week, the incidence of premature labor is no higher than in nonsurgical pregnant patients.
5. **Postpartum period**
   a) Covers the 6-week period after childbirth during which time the various changes that occurred during pregnancy revert to the nonpregnant state.
   b) The cardiovascular system and blood volume return to normal by the end of 2 weeks.
   c) After delivery of the placenta, the uterus is the size of a 20-week pregnancy and decreases by 1 finger breadth each day, so that by day 12, it is no longer palpable.
   d) Avoid elective surgery in the initial 6-week postpartum period to allow the body to return to its normal physiological function.
   e) If anesthesia is undertaken, explanation of the effects of the drugs on breastfeeding should occur. Administration of drugs to a breastfeeding mother can inhibit lactation or cause direct harmful effects to the infant because of excretion in breast milk. For many medications, there is insufficient evidence available to provide accurate guidance on drug safety during breastfeeding.
   f) Breast milk production is dependent on adequate maternal hydration and regular stimulation (either by the baby feeding or by the mother expressing). If scheduled for anesthesia or surgery, encourage the mother to breastfeed as near as possible to the procedure.
   g) General anesthesia
      (1) Propofol and thiopental are found in breast milk in insignificant amounts, as are levels of volatile agents. Because neuromuscular blocking agents are large, ionized, and water soluble, they are not excreted into breast milk.
      (2) After general anesthesia, women can be advised to express and discard the first sample of milk and to resume infant feeding after this.
      (3) All of the commonly used antiemetics are advised to be used with caution or only if essential by manufacturers.
   h) Regional anesthesia
      (1) Local anesthetics are not excreted into breast milk in amounts sufficient to be harmful.
      (2) Breastfeeding can continue as normal after regional anesthesia.

i) Analgesics
  (1) The American Academy of Pediatrics (AAP) published a statement on drug transfer into human milk and possible effects on the infant.
  (2) The AAP considers acetaminophen, most NSAIDs, and morphine compatible with breastfeeding.

j) When prescribing or administering drugs, consider:
  (1) Is the medication really needed?
  (2) Minimize drug exposure by administering just after breastfeeding.
  (3) Breastfeeding is the gold standard for infant nutrition. Balance the risk of drug excretion in milk with advantages of continued breastfeeding.

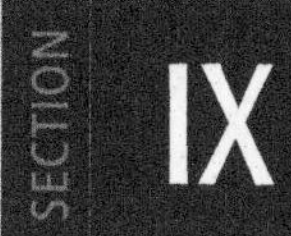

Orthopedics and Podiatry

SECTION IX

A. ARTHROSCOPY

1. Introduction

Arthroscopic surgery may be performed for diagnostic or therapeutic indications most often involving the ankle, knee, shoulder, hip, or wrist. Advances in arthroscopy permit many procedures to be performed primarily or adjunctively through the arthroscope. Arthroscopic surgery has replaced some procedures that previously were performed through open techniques. Most of these procedures are done in young, healthy patients. The advantages include minimal incisions, decreased postoperative morbidity, and potentially faster rehabilitation.

2. Preoperative assessment and patient preparation

a) Arthroscopic procedures may be anesthetically managed by almost any of the available anesthesia techniques (general anesthesia, regional anesthesia, combined regional and general anesthesia, local blockade, and sometimes monitored anesthesia care).

b) Patient selection for a given anesthetic technique is crucial with arthroscopic procedures, as with all operative procedures. Critical factors in the selection of the available anesthesia techniques appropriate for arthroscopic procedures are the patient positioning necessary to facilitate the proposed arthroscopic procedure and the overall state of health of the patient.

c) The choice of position is determined by the surgeon's operating requirements. Reviewing the patient's chart and, most important, personally interviewing the patient, along with understanding the physiologic changes associated with various positions, will assist the anesthesia provider in offering the best suggestion for anesthesia care for each patient.

d) The factors in the decision are listed in the following box.

Anesthetic Selection in Orthopedics

- What is the proposed surgical procedure?
- How long is the procedure estimated to take?
- What patient position will be necessary to accomplish the procedure?
- Is this patient's overall health status sufficient to remain in the required position for an extended period of time without general anesthesia?
- Is this patient receptive to an anesthesia technique (or techniques) other than general anesthesia?

3. Perioperative management

a) Complications: Complications from arthroscopic procedures represent a small percentage of the total number of procedures performed.

(1) The full range of potential anesthetic complications associated with patient positioning applies (e.g., inadvertent extubation, eye or corneal injury, and nerve injury from improper patient positioning).

(2) Because of the less invasive nature of arthroscopic procedures, concerns over blood loss are typically minimal. However, sudden sustained hypotension is a cause for immediate investigation.
(3) Perforation of a major blood vessel may occur during trocar insertion and may not be detected until the tourniquet is deflated. Such vascular injury may result from pressure exerted by excessive extravasated irrigation fluid during the procedure.
(4) Air and bone embolism

b) Other considerations
(1) To provide optimal visualization of joint structures during arthroscopic procedures, the irrigating fluid used to distend the operative joint is instilled under pressure.
(2) Take note of any deficits of inflow versus outflow of irrigating solution throughout the procedure.
(a) Depending on the complexity of the arthroscopic procedure, a large number of irrigation fluid bags may be required.
(b) Small individual inflow/outflow deficits may result in significant fluid absorption by the patient over the course of an extended procedure.
(c) Fluid absorption is of particular concern for shoulder or hip arthroscopic procedures in which fluid absorption is not relatively limited by the use of the pneumatic tourniquet.
(d) Absorption of excessive extravasated fluid may lead to the development of signs and symptoms of congestive heart failure, pulmonary edema, volume overload, or hyponatremia.
(e) If the patient experiences these symptoms, treatment with fluid restriction, supplemental oxygen, and diuresis should be instituted.
(3) Although the mechanism of occurrence has not been delineated, subcutaneous emphysema, tension pneumothorax, and pneumomediastinum have been reported during shoulder arthroscopy, specifically subacromial decompression.

4. Anesthetic technique

a) History and physical examination: Individualized

b) Diagnostic tests
(1) Radiographs of the affected extremity
(2) Chest radiography, electrocardiography (ECG), and laboratory tests as indicated

c) Preoperative medicines and intravenous (IV) therapy
(1) Anti-inflammatory medications: Stopped 5 to 7 days before surgery
(2) Antibiotics: Cefazolin, 1 g IV
(3) Sedatives and narcotics
(4) One peripheral large-bore IV line
(5) Epidural catheter placement: Test dose performed on an awake patient
(a) Choice of anesthetic method: Local, general, and regional anesthesia have all been used successfully.

5. **Room preparation**
   a) Standard monitoring equipment
   b) Standard drugs for general or regional anesthesia
   c) Special orthopedic tables
   d) Extra padding
   e) Circuit extension if table positioned away from anesthesia practitioner
6. **Perioperative management**
   a) Induction: Standard induction with routine medications are used.
   b) Positioning
      (1) Most often, the supine position is used for arthroscopic procedures of both the upper and lower extremities.
      (2) Arthroscopy on the knee requires the supine position with the foot of the operating room bed lowered. The nonoperative leg should either have a sequential compression device or some form of antiembolic stocking in place to reduce pooling of blood and reduce the potential for thrombus formation.
      (3) Patients undergoing elbow arthroscopy may be placed in the supine, lateral decubitus, or prone position; the position is dictated by operative necessity and surgeon preference. The prone position is more advantageous primarily because of the better limb stability during the procedure.
      (4) Shoulder arthroscopy is usually accomplished by either the modified Fowler position (beach chair position) or the lateral decubitus position, based on optimal access to the injury and surgeon preference. Because this procedure does not use a tourniquet, deliberate hypotension may be requested by surgeons. Blood pressure cuff measurements taken on the arm are not representative (underestimate) perfusion pressure in the brain when patients are in a sitting position. Therefore, it is recommended to maintain preoperative mean arterial pressures to avoid hypoxic brain injury.
      (5) Hip arthroscopy is also typically accomplished by the lateral decubitus position or the supine position, with the patient on a fracture table. The fracture table is used to provide greater stability while traction is applied using either weights and counterweights (lateral decubitus position) or mechanical traction attached to the leg-holding device of the fracture table (supine position).
   c) Tourniquet use: See the discussion of knee arthroscopy later in this section.
   d) Emergence: The patient is usually extubated in the operating room unless there was preoperative respiratory compromise.
7. **Postoperative implications**
   a) Pain is usually minimal to moderate, unless reconstruction was performed.
      (1) Intraarticular injections of local anesthetics or opioids are now widely used in an attempt to provide postoperative analgesia.
      (2) Inadequate pain control can lead to decreased mobility and an increased incidence of postoperative complications.
   b) Swelling or edema: Assess capillary refill in the affected extremity and avoid overhydration intraoperatively.
   c) Nerve damage: Assess neurologic function after surgery.

B. FOOT AND ANKLE SURGERY

1. Introduction

The feet and ankles are the basis of support on which the remainder of the body rests. Surgical correction of maladies and deformities of the feet and ankles falls under the scope of practice of two specialists: the orthopedic surgeon and the doctor of podiatric medicine, or podiatrist. Both these specialists are highly skilled in foot and ankle surgery to correct the multitude of maladies and deformities that occur with the feet and ankles.

The most commonly performed procedures on the ankle involve surgical repair of ankle fractures and fusion of the ankle joint. The Achilles tendon is also a frequent focus of surgery, particularly in more physically active persons. The most widely known surgical procedures on the feet are bunionectomy (with or without fusion), correction of hammertoe deformities (with or without fusion), and plantar fasciotomy (either open or endoscopic).

Open repair of ankle fractures is usually accomplished using plates and screws to hold the bone fragment in proper alignment until the fragments grow back together. Ankle fusion (arthrodesis) is performed for a multitude of medical reasons and may involve two or three bones fused together to provide pain relief and greater joint stability. Incisions are usually made on both the medial and lateral aspects of the ankle joint to allow for optimal surgical access to the involved bones. After the fracture is reduced, a plate is placed across the fracture site(s). Holes are drilled with the plate acting as the template, and screws are placed into these holes. For ankle fusions, the incisions are typically made across the medial and lateral aspects of the joint, and Kirschner wires or screws are used to fuse the appropriate bones in place. The incisions are closed, and some type of inflexible stabilizing device is applied (e.g., cast or plaster splints or ambulatory boot) while the patient is under anesthesia. Pneumatic tourniquets are almost always used to keep blood loss at a minimum and to provide a clear surgical field.

Bunion deformity usually involves the first or great toe. Incision is made along the anterior surface from about midtoe across the metatarsophalangeal joint. The bony deformity is excised. Depending on the variation of the bunionectomy procedure chosen, excision of the bony deformity may be the totality of the procedure, or the angular deformity may be corrected with a screw or Kirschner wire fusion.

Hammertoe deformity correction involves incision of the anterior surface of the malformed toe or toes. The incision crosses the joint containing the bony deformity. The surgeon dissects down to the joint and excises the bony deformity. Depending on the severity of the deformity, the interphalangeal joint may be fused by inserting a Kirschner wire.

Plantar fasciotomy is indicated for severe foot pain during or after ambulating or on arising after sleep, resulting from chronic plantar fasciitis that has not responded to conservative therapy. Open fasciotomy is accomplished through a small incision along the posterior surface of the calcaneus. The plantar fascia is incised to relieve the tension across the plantar arch. Endoscopic plantar fasciotomy is accomplished via two "miniature" incisions, one medial and one lateral, at the beginning of the plantar arch. A small trocar is inserted through these incisions. The sheath of the trocar is slotted to allow visualization of the plantar fascia with the endoscope. The full thickness of the plantar fascia is incised, and the skin incisions are closed.

2. **Anesthetic technique**
   a) Patients scheduled for foot or ankle surgery are excellent candidates for regional anesthesia.
   b) Most surgical procedures on the foot or ankle can be accomplished within a 2-hour time frame, often on an outpatient basis.
   c) Spinal anesthesia provides sufficient surgical anesthesia to allow completion of most procedures. However, the postanesthesia recovery phase may be unacceptably long and may require the patient to spend a night in the hospital or outpatient facility, which may be unacceptable to the patient.
   d) Nerve blocks are especially effective for surgical procedures on the foot or ankle. Posterior tibial nerve block, Mayo blockade, and Bier block are examples of blocks that are effective for foot and ankle procedures.
   e) One may provide IV sedation by either continuous infusion or intermittent bolus to provide amnesia and to minimize or eliminate any anxiety the patient may have. The surgeon can inject the surgical site with long-acting local anesthetic (e.g., bupivacaine) to maintain the patient's comfort immediately and for several hours postoperatively.

C. FOREARM AND HAND SURGERY

1. **Introduction**

Surgical procedures on the hand or forearm may be precipitated by violent trauma resulting in complex or dislocated fractures to the bones of the forearm, hand, or fingers, or they may be performed to alleviate numbness of the hand resulting from compression of the nerves of the forearm or wrist, such as carpal tunnel syndrome. Procedures on the fingers and hand are often relatively quick, requiring 1 hour or less to complete. Surgical correction of complex or dislocated fractures of the forearm may require considerable instrumentation and time to complete. For virtually all surgical procedures of the hand and forearm, a pneumatic tourniquet is used.

2. **Anesthetic technique**
   a) Patients scheduled for surgical procedures on the forearm or hand are excellent candidates for regional anesthesia.
   b) Axillary block and Bier block provide excellent surgical anesthesia for most surgical procedures of the forearm and hand that are anticipated to require 1 hour or less to accomplish.
   c) For procedures precipitated by traumatic injury, such as complex, comminuted fractures or reconstruction of the vascular and nerve structures of the hand or forearm (procedures that may require considerable amounts of time to accomplish), the better anesthetic choice may be general anesthesia.
   d) Tourniquet pain becomes an issue with such longer procedures if regional anesthesia is chosen.
   e) In addition, for a patient requiring surgery as the result of traumatic injury, the issue of the patient's nothing by mouth (NPO) status becomes important. Frequently, trauma patients have eaten or ingested liquids close to the time of the traumatic injury. Alcohol may be a precipitating factor in the traumatic injury as well. For these reasons, rapid-sequence induction of general anesthesia may be a more appropriate anesthetic course.

D. HIP ARTHROPLASTY

1. Introduction

The replacement of joint surfaces is required primarily for inflammatory or degenerative conditions within the joint, such as those accompanying rheumatoid arthritis or osteoarthritis from degeneration of the synovium or cartilage. As normal joint tissues deteriorate or degenerate, the bone ends are exposed, causing pain and limitation of joint movements. Joint stiffness and muscle atrophy follow, further increasing pain and limiting movement and mobility. Exposed bone surfaces lead to bone growth that may eventually adhere to the opposing bone ends, causing bony ankylosis and loss of joint movement. Therefore, replacement of the deteriorated or degenerated tissues and bones restores movement and relieves pain.

The hip joint is one of the most frequently replaced joints. Typically, the patient is placed in the lateral decubitus position, which offers greater range of motion and visibility throughout the surgical procedure. This procedure requires a large incision, extending from near the iliac crest across the joint to the midthigh level. Several large muscle groups must be incised and dissected through to gain access to the joint, after which the joint is disarticulated. The femoral head and neck are excised, leaving the femoral canal open. The femur is filled with rich marrow because it is one of the erythrocyte production areas for the body; therefore, it is also richly vascular. The acetabulum is a part of the pelvic girdle, also one of the erythrocyte production areas, and is richly vascular as well. After the femoral head and neck are removed, the femoral canal is reamed to the appropriate diameter to accommodate the prosthetic head and neck. The acetabulum is then reamed in a similar manner to accommodate its own prosthesis. During the reaming for both prosthetic components, bone is shaved from the canal and acetabulum to produce a smoother bony surface to achieve better adherence of the prosthetic device and cement. Also during the reaming process, venous sinuses within these bony structures are opened and often destroyed, and this can result in significant blood loss.

After the femoral canal has been satisfactorily prepared, the canal is cleaned out using pulse irrigation, which forces irrigation solution deep within the femoral canal under pressure in a high-frequency, pulsatile manner. The canal is further cleaned with a sponge, after which methylmethacrylate (MMA) cement may be instilled into the femoral canal. For some procedures, usually in younger or very physically active patients, MMA is not used to secure the femoral prosthesis, and the prosthesis is referred to as being "press-fit." After instillation of the MMA cement, the femoral prosthesis is inserted into the canal and is forcibly seated with a mallet. The acetabular component is secured in place with screws and bone grafting. The dislocated joint is reduced, and the soft tissues are returned to normal anatomic position during wound closure.

2. Preoperative assessment and patient preparation

a) History and physical examination

(1) With this elderly population, assess for coexisting medical diseases.

(2) Carefully assess blood volume, central venous pressure, and orthostatic hypotension because dehydration may mask hemoglobin changes resulting from hematoma formation.

b) Diagnostic tests
   (1) Radiographs: Hip and chest
   (2) Laboratory tests: Complete blood count, electrolytes, glucose, blood urea nitrogen, creatinine, urinalysis, prothrombin time, partial thromboplastin time, bleeding time of the patient on aspirin, and type and crossmatch
c) Preoperative medications and IV therapy
   (1) Anticoagulants: Heparin, low-molecular-weight heparin, oral anticoagulants
   (2) Antirheumatic or anti-inflammatory medications
   (3) Antibiotics
   (4) Sedatives and narcotics: Used with caution in the elderly population.
   (5) Two peripheral, large-bore (16- to 18-gauge) IV lines with moderate fluid replacement
   (6) Epidural catheter placement: Test dose performed on an awake patient

3. **Room preparation**
   a) Monitoring equipment
      (1) Standard
      (2) Indwelling urinary catheter: Controversial
         (a) Absence of bladder drainage can cause overdistention, affecting bladder function.
         (b) Insertion may cause urinary tract infection.
      (3) Central venous pressure: Trend of volume status.
      (4) Warming modalities are used.
      (5) ECG leads V_5 and II detect myocardial ischemia and diagnose tachyarrhythmias in the elderly population.
      (6) Transesophageal echocardiography: Assess fat and bone deposits when the acetabulum is reamed and curetted.
      (7) Use x-ray shields for self-protection.
      (8) Arterial line monitoring is indicated if hypotensive techniques are used.
   b) Pharmacologic agents: Vasopressors
   c) Position: Lateral; a special orthopedic table may be used.
4. **Anesthetic technique**
   a) Considerations: Regional blockade, general anesthesia, or a combination of both
   b) Technique of choice
      (1) Regional anesthesia
      (2) Reduced blood loss and postoperative deep venous thrombosis (DVT) or pulmonary embolism (PE)
   c) Regional blockade
      (1) Epidural catheter placement and preoperative test dose *or*
      (2) One-time spinal for analgesia to T8
   d) General anesthesia
      (1) An endotracheal tube must be inserted.
      (2) Combination with regional anesthetic allows reduced dosages of agents and control of airway.
   e) Induction
      (1) General anesthesia
         (a) Thorough airway assessment is done in an arthritic population.

(b) Induction is performed with the patient on the stretcher.
(c) Succinylcholine may be contraindicated with crush injuries if large amounts of muscle tissue are devitalized.

(2) Maintenance
(a) Monitor fluid and blood replacement therapy to minimize blood loss and transfusion that are applicable during hip arthroplasty (e.g., autologous donation and deliberate hypotension).
(b) Laminar flow is used to minimize infections and can increase evaporative fluid and heat losses from the operative site.
(c) Controlled hypotensive techniques facilitate surgical exposure and decrease blood loss.
(i) Individualize blood pressure parameters.
(ii) Maintain mean blood pressure of 50 to 70 mmHg if appropriate based on the patient's cardiac status.
(iii) Deepen anesthesia with an inhalation anesthetic
(iv) Initiate a vasoactive (nitroprusside) drip.

(3) The anesthesia provider must be particularly cognizant of the possible occurrence of hypotension, hypoxia, and potential cardiovascular collapse. These complications are observed most often during insertion of the femoral prosthesis during total hip arthroplasty.
(a) Possible causes of these complications include the MMA cement, fat embolism, air embolism, thromboembolism, and bone marrow embolism.
(b) MMA has been demonstrated to produce significant increases in both pulmonary vascular resistance and pulmonary wedge pressure while decreasing systemic vascular resistance, cardiac output, and arterial pressure.
(c) MMA cement is used to distribute the forces of the femoral and acetabular prosthetic components.
(i) Mixing the cement causes the monomer portion to polymerize (an exothermic reaction).
(ii) Problems with MMA relate to cementing the femoral prosthesis; unpolymerized monomer can be absorbed into the circulation.
(iii) It causes direct vasodilation, usually within the first minute; it can last as long as 10 minutes.
(iv) Venous embolism can occur when the femoral prosthesis is inserted into the femoral canal.
(v) Hypotension, hypoxia, and cardiovascular collapse after prosthesis insertion have been reported.
(vi) Prevent complications: Communicate with the surgeon regarding application.
(vii) Use 100% oxygen, decrease the vasodilating agent, maximize fluid status, and have vasopressor support available.

f) Emergence
(1) If a general anesthetic is implemented, patients are usually repositioned onto the stretcher before emergence.
(2) Extubation is based on the patient's status.
(3) Initiate regional blockade through the epidural catheter for postoperative analgesia before the end of the case.

5. **Postoperative implications**
   a) Obtain laboratory results: Hemoglobin and hematocrit; watch for hidden bleeding.
   b) Fat embolism typically appears 12 to 48 hours after a long bone fracture.
      (1) Signs and symptoms
         (a) Arterial hypoxemia
         (b) Adult respiratory distress syndrome
         (c) Central nervous system dysfunction (confusion, coma, and seizures)
         (d) Petechiae (neck, shoulders, and chest)
         (e) Coagulopathy
         (f) Fever
      (2) Treatment
         (a) Supportive
         (b) Oxygenation
         (c) Corticosteroids
         (d) Immobilization of long bone fractures
         (e) Other potential complications include DVT and PE. DVT is a precursor to PE development. DVT has been demonstrated in 40% to 60% of patients undergoing total hip arthroplasty and in approximately 80% of patients having total knee arthroplasty. From within the two patient populations, PE is believed to develop 1% to 5% of the time.

E. HIP PINNING (OPEN REDUCTION AND INTERNAL FIXATION)

1. **Introduction**

Hip pinning involves the open reduction of a hip fracture that is maintained by the application of plates and screws (internal fixation). Bone grafting may be used to repair any defects. Hip fractures may result from high-impact trauma, but most result from minor trauma in elderly persons. If the fracture is related to high-impact trauma, a coexisting trauma should be thoroughly evaluated.

2. **Preoperative assessment and patient preparation**
   a) History and physical examination: Obtain a verbal history from the patient or family member. Note any preexisting disease processes, social history, current medications, surgical history, and allergies.
   b) Laboratory tests: Hemoglobin, hematocrit, complete blood count, prothrombin time, partial thromboplastin time, and others are obtained as indicated by the history and physical examination.
   c) Diagnostic tests: 12-lead ECG, chest radiography, and others are obtained as indicated by the history and physical examination.
   d) Preoperative medications: These are individualized.
3. **Room preparation**
   a) Monitoring equipment: Standard, arterial line, central line as needed
   b) Additional equipment
      (1) Positioning devices and operating table: The patient is usually placed in a lateral position. Aging skin atrophies and is prone to trauma from adhesive tape, electrocautery pads, and ECG

electrodes. Arthritic joints may interfere with positioning; when possible, the elderly patient should be positioned for comfort. Meticulous padding of the axilla and all bony prominences decreases the risk of nerve injury and ischemia. Prevent pressure to the ears and eyes. Maintain the neck in neutral alignment.

(2) Because of the length of the procedure and surgical exposure, warming modalities should be implemented (fluid warmer, warming blankets).

c) Drugs

(1) Continuous infusion: Consider the use of a continuous epidural infusion intraoperatively or for postoperative pain control.

(2) IV fluids: Estimated blood loss may be greater than 1000 mL. Type and crossmatch for 2 units of packed red blood cells. Blood loss is replaced 1:1 with blood products or colloid solutions or 3:1 if crystalloid solutions are used. Maintain urine output at 0.5 mL/kg/hr. Keep in mind any preexisting disease processes that may easily place the elderly patient in a state of fluid overload. Consider the use of a cell saver intraoperatively. The insertion of 2 large bore IV's is warranted.

(3) Tabletop: Standard. All equipment needed to implement the anesthetic plan should be available.

4. Perioperative management and anesthetic technique

a) Regional and general anesthesia are both options for elderly patients.

b) Hip pinning may be performed using subarachnoid block or continuous epidural infusion extending to the T8 sensory level. Keep in mind the expected length of the procedure, the patient's history and physical examination findings, and the patient's level of cooperation and ability to lie still. Major advantages of regional anesthesia is a decreased incidence of postoperative thromboembolism and another is reduced blood loss. This is thought to be the result of peripheral vasodilation and maintenance of venous blood flow in the lower extremities. Local anesthetics also inhibit platelet aggregation and stabilize endothelial cells. Difficult patient positioning and altered landmarks related to degenerative changes of the spine may increase the technical difficulty of performing a regional block. Postdural puncture headaches are not as prevalent in the elderly population.

c) If a general anesthetic is the best choice for the patient, drugs for induction and maintenance should reflect findings from the patient's history and physical examination. One advantage of general anesthesia is that the anesthetic can be induced with the patient on the bed or stretcher before moving to the operating table, thus avoiding painful positioning. A disadvantage of general anesthesia is that the elderly patient cannot be positioned for maximal comfort. Consider the use of nondepolarizing muscle relaxants during induction if there are no airway concerns. Continued muscle relaxation is optional and is left to the discretion of the anesthesia provider or the request of the surgeon. The effects of nondepolarizing muscle relaxants that are renally excreted may be slightly prolonged in elderly persons because of reduced drug clearance.

d) Emergence: An epidural catheter may be placed for supplemental use with general anesthesia or for postoperative pain control.
e) Fat embolization: See the discussion of pelvic reconstruction later in this section.

5. **Postoperative implications**
a) Consider the use of a continuous epidural infusion for patient-controlled analgesia for postoperative pain control.
b) A marked decrease in blood pressure postoperatively may be related to hematoma formation.
c) DVT prophylaxis should be instituted postoperatively (support hose and deep venous thrombosis prophylaxis).

F. KNEE (TOTAL KNEE REPLACEMENT) ARTHROPLASTY

1. **Introduction**

Total knee arthroplasty is the other frequently performed joint replacement procedure. A pneumatic tourniquet is typically used to provide a relatively bloodless surgical field. Nevertheless, blood loss as a result of total knee arthroplasty can be significant. During the procedure, the articulating surfaces of the femur and tibia are excised by precise angular cuts, and the patellar articulating surface is shaved, all to conform the bones to the inner surfaces of the prostheses. Both the femoral and tibial surfaces are covered with MMA cement, and the individual prosthesis components are forcibly seated with a mallet. The high-density polyethylene patellar component is cemented and seated with a viselike clamp. The medial and lateral menisci are replaced with a conforming wedge of high-density polyethylene.

2. **Preoperative assessment**

Assessment is routine, including history and physical examination. These patients have been diagnosed with arthritis of the knee.

a) Respiratory: These patients may have rheumatoid arthritis and associated pulmonary conditions. Pulmonary effusions may be present. Rheumatoid arthritis involving the cricoarytenoid joints may exhibit itself by hoarseness. A narrow glottic opening may lead to a difficult intubation. Arthritic involvement of the cervical spine and temporomandibular joint may also complicate airway management.
b) Cardiovascular: Depending on the severity of the arthritis, the patient may have a lowered exercise tolerance. Rheumatoid arthritis is associated with pericardial effusion. Cardiac valve fibrosis and cardiac conduction abnormalities can occur with possible aortic regurgitation. Test with an ECG and, if possible, an echocardiogram and cardiac nuclear imaging.
c) Neurologic: A thorough preoperative neurologic examination may yield evidence of cervical nerve root compression. If indicated, obtain lateral neck radiographs for the determination of stability of the atlanto-occipital joint.
d) Musculoskeletal: Positioning may be difficult because of pain and the decreased mobility of the joints.
e) Hematologic and laboratory: Obtain hemoglobin and hematocrit and other tests related to the history and physical examination.
f) Premedication is individualized based on the patient's need.

3. **Room preparation**
   a) Standard monitoring equipment. A tourniquet may or may not be used.
   b) The patient should have one large-bore IV line.
   c) Fluid requirements include normal saline or lactated Ringer's solution at 4 to 6 mL/kg/hr.
   d) Standard drugs for general or regional anesthesia are used.
4. **Anesthetic technique**
   a) This procedure can be done using general or regional anesthesia.
   b) Regional anesthesia could be with a subarachnoid block or placement of an epidural catheter.
5. **Perioperative management**
   a) Induction: Standard induction with routine medications. Muscle relaxation is needed for the placement of the prosthesis.
   b) Monitor fluid and blood therapy.
   c) Requires the supine position with the foot of the operating room bed lowered. The nonoperative leg should either be wrapped with an elastic bandage or have some form of antiembolic stocking in place to reduce pooling of blood and reduce the potential for thrombus formation.
   d) Monitor for physiologic changes that are caused by tourniquets.
   e) Safety measures for preventing tourniquet complications are listed in the box below. Use of MMA can increase both pulmonary vascular resistance and pulmonary wedge pressure while decreasing systemic vascular resistance, cardiac output, and arterial pressure. MMA causes direct vasodilation, and these effects can last up to 10 minutes.

Physiologic Changes Caused by Limb Tourniquets

Neurologic Effects

Abolition of somatosensory evoked potentials and nerve conduction occurs within 30 minutes.

Application for more than 60 minutes causes tourniquet pain and hypertension.

Application for more than 2 hours may result in postoperative neurapraxia.

Evidence of nerve injury may occur at the skin level underlying the edge of the tourniquet.

Muscle Changes

Cellular hypoxia develops within 2 minutes.

Cellular creatinine value declines.

Progressive cellular acidosis occurs.

Endothelial capillary leak develops after 2 hours.

Systemic Effects of Tourniquet Inflation

Elevation in arterial and pulmonary artery pressures develops. This is usually slight to moderate if only one limb is occluded. The response is more severe in patients undergoing balanced anesthesia that does not include a potent anesthetic vapor.

Systemic Effects of Tourniquet Release

A transient fall in core temperature occurs.

Transient metabolic acidosis occurs.

A transient fall in central venous oxygen tension occurs, but systemic hypoxemia is unusual.

Acid metabolites (e.g., thromboxane) are released into the central circulation.

A transient fall in pulmonary and systemic arterial pressures occurs.

A transient increase in end-tidal carbon dioxide occurs.

(1) The tourniquet should be applied where the nerves are best protected in the underlying musculature. The pressure is frequently set at two times the systolic systolic blood pressure.
(2) Check the proper availability and functioning of the equipment before it is operated.
(3) The tourniquet should be used for no longer than 2 hours.
(4) Only the minimally effective pressure should be used for occluding blood flow to the extremity. For the lower extremity, twice the patient's systolic pressure should be used.
(5) The pressure display must accurately reflect the pressure in the tourniquet bladder.
(6) The cuff must properly fit the extremity.
(7) The limb must be padded, and the cuff must be properly applied to the limb with care and attention.

f) Emergence: These patients are usually extubated in the operating room unless there was preoperative respiratory compromise.

6. Postoperative implications

Watch for posterior tibial artery trauma, peroneal nerve palsy (foot drop), hemorrhage from the posterior tibial artery, thromboembolism, and tourniquet nerve injury, if indicated.

G. PELVIC RECONSTRUCTION

1. Introduction

Pelvic reconstruction is a surgical procedure that involves open reduction of pelvic fractures, which are then maintained by the application of plates and screws. Bone grafting may be used to repair any defects of the pelvis. The surgical time for the procedure is 3 to 6 hours. These fractures may be caused by minor trauma, especially in elderly persons, but most result from high-impact trauma (i.e., motor vehicle trauma). Evaluation of the patient for potential coexisting trauma should include a thorough neurologic, thoracic, and abdominal assessment. The extremities may also be involved.

2. Preoperative assessment

a) History and physical examination: Obtain a verbal history from the patient or family member. Note any preexisting disease processes, social history, current medications, surgical history, and allergies.
(1) Cardiac: Assess for cardiac contusion or aortic tear. Tests include 12-lead ECG, creatine phosphokinase isoenzymes, and chest radiography (wide mediastinal silhouette suggests aortic tear). Transesophageal echocardiography or angiography is indicated if an aortic tear is suspected. Consult with a cardiologist if indicated.
(2) Respiratory: Assess for possible hemothorax, pneumothorax, pulmonary contusion, fat embolism, and aspiration. The patient may require supplemental oxygen or mechanical ventilation to correct hypoxemia. Coexisting trauma to the head or cervical spine may require fiberoptic intubation. Tests include chest radiography and arterial blood gases.
(3) Neurologic: A thorough neurologic evaluation including mental status and peripheral sensory examination. Note any preexisting deficits. Consult with a neurologist if necessary. For tests, computed tomography of the head is indicated before anesthesia for patients who experience a loss of consciousness.

(4) Renal: Renal injury is possible with high-impact trauma. Rule out a urethral tear before placing the Foley catheter. A suprapubic catheter may be necessary. Intraoperative monitoring of urine output is mandatory to assess adequate renal perfusion. Consult a urologist if necessary. Tests include urinalysis, blood urea nitrogen, serum creatinine, hematuria, and myoglobinuria.

(5) Musculoskeletal: Cervical spine clearance may be required before neck manipulation (i.e., laryngoscopy). Consider evaluating thoracic and lumbar radiographs to rule out any deformity or instability before anesthesia. Tests include cervical spine radiography and others as indicated from the history and physical examination.

(6) Hematologic: Large blood loss associated with traumatic injury may occur. The patient's hematocrit should be restored to greater than 25% before induction of anesthesia. Type and crossmatch for 6 units of packed red blood cells. Consider the use of a cell saver intraoperatively.

(7) Gastrointestinal: Patients should be assessed for abdominal injury associated with trauma. The test used is diagnostic peritoneal lavage.

b) Patient preparation

(1) Laboratory tests: Hemoglobin, hematocrit, electrolytes, prothrombin time, partial thromboplastin time, and others are obtained as indicated from the history and physical examination.

(2) Medications: Anxiolytics, narcotics, antibiotics, and others as indicated from the history and physical examination. The patient may also be receiving anticoagulant therapy for the prevention of DVT. A broad-spectrum antibiotic should be administered preoperatively.

3. Room preparation

a) Monitoring equipment: Standard, arterial line, central venous pressure, two large peripheral IV catheters

b) Additional equipment

(1) Positioning devices and operating table: The patient may be placed in the supine, lateral, or prone position. A fracture table may be used. Meticulously pad the chest, axilla, pelvis, and extremities to prevent potential nerve injury and ischemia. Prevent pressure to the downward ear and eye if the patient is in the lateral position. Maintain the patient's neck in neutral alignment and support as necessary.

(2) Because of the length of the procedure and surgical exposure, warming devices should be implemented (i.e., fluid warmer, warming blanket).

(3) A nasogastric tube should be used to decompress the stomach if rapid-sequence induction is performed.

c) Drugs

(1) Continuous infusions: Consider the use of an IV narcotic infusion. If an epidural catheter is placed for postoperative pain control, consider an intraoperative continuous infusion to decrease anesthetic requirements.

(2) IV fluids and blood: Estimated blood loss is greater than 1000 mL. Type and crossmatch the patient for 6 units of packed red blood cells. Blood loss is replaced 1:1 with blood products or colloid

solutions or 3:1 if crystalloid solutions are used. Consider the intraoperative use of a cell saver. Maintain urine output at 0.5 to 1 mL/kg/hr. Consider the use of deliberate hypotension to control blood loss in patients without cardiovascular disease or carotid stenosis. Isoflurane, esmolol, sodium nitroprusside, or a combination thereof, titrated to decrease mean arterial pressure by 30% (but not less than 60 mmHg), is commonly used. Any fluid deficits must be replaced before the institution of deliberate hypotension.

(3) Tabletop is standard.

4. Perioperative management and anesthetic technique

a) Induction and maintenance

(1) Rapid-sequence induction must be used for trauma patients to decrease the risk of aspiration.

(2) A standard induction may be used if the procedure is performed electively. Severe hypotension can occur because of hypovolemia.

(3) Because of the painful nature of the injury, induction is best performed on the patient's bed or stretcher before moving to the operating table.

(4) Drugs for induction and maintenance should reflect the patient's history and physical examination and should account for any significant medical history, current physiologic states, and drug allergies.

(5) Consider the use of a nondepolarizing muscle relaxant during induction if there are no airway concerns.

(6) Anesthetic gases should be warmed and humidified. Continued muscle relaxation is optional and is left to the discretion of the anesthesia provider or the request of the surgeon.

b) Emergence

(1) An epidural catheter may be placed for supplemental use intraoperatively and for postoperative pain control.

(2) Trauma patients undergoing rapid-sequence induction should be fully awake and reflexive before extubation.

(3) Patients who have pulmonary complications related to trauma or the surgical procedure (i.e., fat embolism, pulmonary contusion, or aspiration) should not be extubated.

c) Fat embolization

(1) About 30% to 90% of patients with fractures are reported to experience fat embolization. Most patients remain asymptomatic. The incidence of fat embolization is higher in patients with long bone or pelvic fractures.

(2) Signs and symptoms include hypoxemia; tachycardia; tachypnea; respiratory alkalosis; mental status changes; petechiae on the chest, upper extremities, axillae, and conjunctivae; fat bodies in the urine; and diffuse pulmonary infiltrates.

(3) Treatment is supportive and prophylactic: Oxygen therapy and continuous positive airway pressure by mask or endotracheal tube, judicious fluid management to help decrease the severity of pulmonary capillary leaks, heparin, and high-dose corticosteroids may all be considered.

5. Postoperative implications

a) Consider the use of continuous epidural infusion or patient-controlled analgesia for postoperative pain control.

b) The L4 to S5 nerve roots may be damaged from the primary traumatic event or the operation. The result is hemiplegia with bladder and bowel dysfunction. Intraoperative pressure on the ilioinguinal ligament may cause neuropathy of the femoral genitofemoral or femoral cutaneous nerve.
c) A marked postoperative decrease in blood pressure may be related to retroperitoneal hematoma formation.
d) DVT prophylaxis should be instituted postoperatively (i.e., support hose and DVT prophylaxis).

H. UPPER EXTREMITY ARTHROPLASTY

1. Introduction

Arthroplasty in the upper extremity makes up a low percentage of the number of joint arthroplasties performed each year. Of the two more commonly replaced upper extremity joints (the shoulder and the elbow), shoulder arthroplasty accounts for approximately 5% of the total number of joint replacements performed each year. The primary goal of shoulder arthroplasty is to relieve pain, with the secondary goal being improvement in overall joint functioning. Indications for shoulder arthroplasty include glenohumeral joint destruction as a result of osteoarthritis, complex proximal humerus fractures, rheumatoid arthritis, avascular necrosis of the humeral head, and malunion or nonunion of the proximal humerus.

Shoulder arthroplasty is performed with the patient in either the lateral decubitus or modified Fowler (beach chair) position. Because a pneumatic tourniquet cannot be used, shoulder arthroplasty tends to result in significant intraoperative blood loss.

Elbow arthroplasty is performed less frequently than shoulder arthroplasty. The goals for elbow arthroplasty are much the same as for shoulder arthroplasty: pain relief and improvement in joint function. The indications for elbow arthroplasty include rheumatoid arthritis, traumatic arthritis, and ankylosis of the joint.

2. Preoperative assessment

a) Respiratory
 (1) Patients with rheumatoid arthritis may show signs of pleural effusion or pulmonary fibrosis. Hoarseness may result from cricoarytenoid joint involvement. Inflammation and destruction of laryngeal structures may make intubation difficult in these patients.
 (2) Tests: Chest radiography and pulmonary function tests (if indicated; arterial blood gases in compromised patients) are obtained.
b) Cardiovascular: Patients with rheumatoid arthritis may have chronic pericardial tamponade, valvular disease, and cardiac conduction defects. If indicated, a consult with cardiologist may be warranted.
c) Neurologic
 (1) Because of the modified Fowler position, blood pressure measurements taken on the arm underestimated cerebral artery autoregulation. Cerebral hypoxia has occurred. Maintenance of the preoperative mean arterial pressure may help to decrease the incidence of brain injury.

(2) Patients with arthritis may have cervical or lumbar radiculopathies. Preoperative documentation of these conditions is essential. Head flexion may cause cervical spinal cord compression.
(3) Patients with neck or upper extremity radiculopathy require cervical spine radiographs to rule out subluxation.

d) Musculoskeletal: With the possibility of limited neck and jaw mobility, special intubation may be indicated. Special attention must be paid to positioning in patients with bony deformities or contractures to prevent pressure ulcers and neuropathies.
e) Hematologic: Almost all nontrauma patients will be receiving some type of nonsteroidal anti-inflammatory drug, which should be stopped approximately 5 days before the procedure.
f) Endocrine: Patients with rheumatoid arthritis will most likely be receiving some type of corticosteroid; therefore, supplemental steroids should be given to treat adrenal suppression (e.g. IV hydrocortisone 100 mg) in patients on chronic corticosteroid therapy.
g) Laboratory tests: Hemoglobin and hematocrit are obtained from healthy patients; other tests are as indicated from the history and physical examination.
h) Premedication: If a peripheral nerve block is performed, moderate to heavy premedication is indicated.

3. **Room preparation**
   a) Standard monitoring equipment is required.
   b) The patient will be in a modified Fowler (beach chair) position. A precordial Doppler device may be used to detect venous air embolism.
   c) One large-bore IV line will be needed on the nonoperative side.
   d) If the patient is hemodynamically compromised, continuous hemodynamic monitoring may be indicated.
   e) Fluid replacement using normal saline or lactated Ringer's solution at 6 mL/kg/hr is indicated.
4. **Anesthetic technique: Shoulder**
   a) Patients undergoing total shoulder arthroplasty can be managed by general anesthesia, interscalene block, or supraclavicular block.
   b) If general anesthesia is chosen, caution is advised to observe for the ongoing potential for inadvertent extubation as a result of the surgical manipulations necessary while in close proximity to the patient's head and neck. The patient's neck may be subjected to excessive stretch during the surgical manipulations, and if the patient's head becomes dislodged from the supportive device used, there is the potential for cervical spine injury.
   c) For the patient undergoing shoulder arthroscopy, pulmonary function will more closely resemble "normal" function as a result of being in the modified Fowler position. This position puts the patients at increased risk for a venous air embolism.
   d) Recognize the risk of fat or bone marrow embolism and thromboembolism incumbent with the required reaming of the shaft of one of the body's long bones. The potential cardiovascular effects of MMA cement must also be considered if the humeral component is cemented in place.
   e) Blood loss during shoulder arthroplasty can be significant, just as it can with hip arthroplasty. Minimize blood loss and transfusion (e.g., autologous donation). Deliberate hypotension can be used if

the patient is positioned supine and the patient's cardiovascular and neurologic status are not compromised.

5. **Anesthetic technique: Elbow**
   a) Elbow arthroplasty can be performed in any of three positions: supine, lateral decubitus, or prone.
   b) The deciding factors on which position will be used for this procedure are based on surgeon preference and the health of the patient.
   c) Elbow arthroplasty can be managed by general anesthesia or supraclavicular, infraclavicular, interscalene, or axillary block.
   d) With the patient under general anesthesia, be mindful of the potential complications and physiologic changes associated with each position.
   e) During elbow arthroplasty, a pneumatic tourniquet may be used to minimize blood loss and to provide a clear surgical field. Tourniquet: For the upper extremity, the tourniquet is set 50 to 100 mmHg greater than the patient's systolic blood pressure.
   f) Be prepared to treat the patient's tourniquet pain whenever regional anesthesia is used.
   g) Be aware of the increased risk of thromboembolism development when the pneumatic tourniquet is used, particularly in patients with a history of DVT.
6. **Perioperative management**
   a) Induction: Standard. If the patient has a limited range of motion, awake fiberoptic intubation may be indicated.
   b) Maintenance: Standard maintenance with muscle relaxation
   c) Position: The patient is in the beach chair position or the lateral decubitus position.
   d) Considerations: If using nitrous oxide during placement of the humeral component, discontinue it because of the increased risk of a venous air embolism with moderate muscle relaxation at that time.
   e) After surgical completion the patient may be extubated in the operating room. The patient should be back to a supine position before reversing the muscle relaxant.
7. **Postoperative implications**

Consider a patient-controlled analgesia pump or a regional block technique for postoperative pain.

Other Procedures

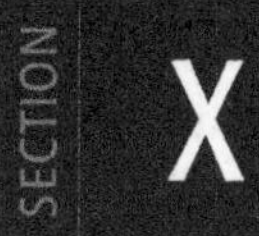

A. BURNS

1. Introduction

Burn injuries, regardless of their origin, are classified according to the depth and the extent of the skin and tissue destruction as well as the total body surface area (TBSA) involved. The degrees of burn injury with classification, tissue involvement, and appearance are shown in the following table.

Degrees of Burn Injury

Classification	Tissue Level Involvement	Appearance
Superficial, first-degree burn	Epidermis destroyed	Skin, red tone (sunburn); painful with erythema and blisters; heals spontaneously with no scarring
Partial-thickness, second-degree burn		
Superficial dermal	Epidermis and some (upper) dermis destroyed	Red or pale ivory with a moist, shiny surface; painful, immediate blisters with minimal scarring
Deep dermal	Epidermis and deep dermis	Mottled with white, waxy, dry surface; blisters may or may not appear; significant scarring
Full-thickness, third-degree burn	All epidermis and dermis	White, cherry red, or black; dry, tissue-paper skin; grafting necessary; decreased scarring with early excision
Fourth-degree burn	Muscle, fascia, bone	Complete excision required; limited function

Modified from Faldmo L, Kravitz M. Management of acute burns and burn shock resuscitation. *AACN Clin Issues Crit Care Nurs* 1993;4:351-366.

A major burn is defined as a second-degree burn involving more than 10% of the TBSA in adults or 20% at extremes of age, a third-degree burn involving more than 10% of the TBSA in adults, and any electrical burn or one complicated by smoke inhalation. A burn formula derived from the National Burn Registry estimating mortality is as follows: If the age of the patient plus the percentage of the TBSA burned exceeds 115, the mortality rate is greater than 80%. Additionally, from clinical observations, it is estimated that the mortality rate of a burn victim is approximately doubled if there is an inhalation injury sustained in conjunction with a thermal burn.

Patients who sustain full-thickness burns are seen in the operating room, often repeatedly, for débridement and grafting. The initial assessment of an emergency patient with a burn injury is initiated as for any trauma patient and begins with airway intubation. Keep in mind that airway edema occurs rapidly in a burn patient, and intubation after the edema occurs is difficult. Burn patients must have aggressive fluid resuscitation in the first 48 hours. Burns are described according to the rule of nines, which divides the body into areas of 9% or multiples thereof. For example, the head and neck combined, each arm, each leg, the posterior surface of the upper trunk, and the posterior surface of the lower trunk are each considered to be 9% of the surface area of the body. Survival is influenced by the percentage of the surface area involved and the age of the patient.

The pathophysiologic effects of major burns on each organ system are listed in the table below.

Pathophysiologic Effects of Major Burns

System	Considerations
Respiratory	
Upper airway	Thermal damage to soft tissue and respiratory tract requires early endotracheal intubation
Carbon monoxide poisoning	Considered in all victims of enclosed fires; treatment with 100% oxygen by mask or endotracheal tube
Cardiac	
Burn shock phase (0-48 hr)	Hypovolemia is a major concern; fluid resuscitation mandatory; expect impaired cardiac contractility
Hypermetabolic phase (after 48 hr)	Increased blood flow to organs and tissues; manifested by hyperthermia, tachypnea, tachycardia, increased oxygen consumption, and increased catabolism
Renal	
Early	
Reduced renal blood flow	Secondary to hypovolemia and decreased cardiac output; adequate fluid resuscitation and diuresis prevents renal failure
Electrical burns and muscle necrosis damage renal tubules	IV administration of sodium bicarbonate to alkalize the urine
Late	
Increased renal blood flow	Variable drug clearance
Nutrition	Nutritional requirements extreme because of hypermetabolism
Increased caloric requirements	Limited to no NPO status required
Ileus and duodenal ulcers	Treatment with H_2-blockers and antacids
Pharmacokinetics	
Decreased albumin	Benzodiazepines, phenytoin, and salicylic acid have an increase in the free fraction and thus a larger volume of distribution
Increased α_1-acid glycoprotein	Lidocaine, meperidine, and propranolol have the opposite effect
Denervation phenomenon with spreading of acetylcholine receptors	Succinylcholine avoided 24 hours after injury

Pathophysiologic Effects of Major Burns—cont'd

System	Considerations
Increased nicotinic acetylcholine receptors	Requires a two- to threefold increased concentration of nondepolarizer for paralysis
	Skin Integrity
Vulnerable to nosocomial infections	Strict adherence to aseptic individual patient rooms; wound care, including topical antimicrobial agents and early excision or grafting of the burn wound

IV, Intravenous; *NPO*, nothing by mouth.

2. **Preoperative assessment**
   a) Burn patients require a thorough and complete preoperative assessment. A complete medical history, including laboratory studies, and a brief physical examination with lung auscultation, assessment of chest compliance, and inspection of the neck and oral cavity to evaluate for difficulties with intubation or reintubation should be implemented.
   b) There are specific data unique to burn patients that anesthesia providers should know, including knowledge regarding the underlying trauma, the mechanism of burn (electrical, inhalation), the percentage of TBSA burned, the location of the burn sites, the area and the amount that the surgeon intends to débride, and whether the patient will undergo skin grafting during the perioperative course. The assimilation of this information affects the anesthetic plan in terms of anesthetic agents selected, appropriate monitoring, positioning, vascular access, and blood product requirements.
   c) A review of prior anesthetic records can be helpful in determining the anesthetic plan. Quite often, this is possible to do because, more often than not, these patients make several trips to the operating room.
3. **Pharmacologic considerations**
   a) Burn injury causes considerable changes in plasma protein levels, with significant consequences for the protein binding of drugs. In general, patients with burns exhibit decreased albumin and increased α_1-acid glycoprotein levels.
   b) Because the pharmacologic effect is often related to the unbound fraction of a drug, alterations in protein binding can also affect the efficacy and tolerability of drug treatment in patients with burns. This alteration causes the plasma binding of predominantly albumin-bound drugs, such as benzodiazepines, phenytoin, and salicylic acid, to be decreased, resulting in an increase in the free fraction and thus a larger volume of distribution (V_d) for the drug and possibly increased duration of action.
   c) Drugs primarily bound to α_1-acid glycoprotein (e.g., lidocaine, meperidine, propranolol) have the opposite effect.
   d) V_d may be increased or decreased in patients with burns. In general, two factors may cause alteration in V_d: changes in extracellular fluid volume and changes in protein binding.

e) Fluid loss to the burn wound and edema can decrease plasma concentrations of many drugs. After the initial resuscitation state, cardiac output increases as the hypermetabolic phase develops. This increases blood flow to the kidneys and liver with increased drug clearance. Dosage requirements may change if the drug has a small V_d and a narrow therapeutic range. Overall, there is significant patient variability based on fluid status and phase of recovery.

4. **Patient preparation**
   a) A successful anesthetic for the excision and grafting of a burn wound requires planning and preparing needed equipment. Specific anesthetic interventions should be done for these patients before their arrival into the operating room.
   b) Plan preoperative anesthesia for the burn patient.
      (1) Warm up the operating room ahead of time well before the patient arrives.
      (2) Check on the patient's blood status and order more blood and blood products if necessary based on the patient's preoperative hemoglobin and hematocrit values, the size of the burn, and the extent of the planned débridement.
      (3) Have the blood in the operating room and checked before surgical débridement is initiated. This is critical in pediatric patients.
      (4) Have at least one blood warmer primed, plugged in, and turned on. If the burn is large, have two available.
      (5) Make sure that you have adequate intravenous (IV) access before the surgeon begins débriding the burn.
      (6) Because of hypermetabolism and pharmacologic tolerance that occurs, narcotic requirements may be extreme.
      (7) Know whether invasive lines will need to be placed and plan ahead of time.
      (8) Have a plan but be willing to modify it if needed.
   c) Complete blood count, electrolytes, blood urea nitrogen, creatinine, glucose, urinalysis, prothrombin time, partial thromboplastin time (D-dimer or fibrin split products if disseminated intravascular coagulation is suspected), type and crossmatch (number of units depends on the area to be débrided or grafted), chest radiography, and arterial blood gases (with carboxyhemoglobin if indicated) are obtained. Other tests are done as suggested by the history and physical examination.
   d) Begin volume replacement with crystalloid or blood, or both, preoperatively. If the patient's condition permits, an anxiolytic (e.g., benzodiazepine) and a narcotic may be useful preoperatively.
5. **Equipment and room preperation**
   a) Burn patients require all the standard monitors intraoperatively. It can be challenging at times to adapt the standard monitors to the burn patient.
   b) Electrocardiogram (ECG) leads are often difficult to place secondary to a lack of intact skin. It may be necessary to staple the leads or use needle electrodes on the patient to obtain an acceptable ECG tracing.
   c) Ideally, blood pressure cuffs should be placed on an unaffected limb or, at times, at a nonsurgical site.

d) The placement of an arterial line for blood pressure monitoring may be warranted even in a healthy patient if the planned amount of surgical débridement is extensive or if manipulation of the patient's limbs intraoperatively limits the accuracy of noninvasive cuff readings. In large burns that are greater than 20% to 30%, TBSA invasive blood pressure monitoring should be instituted after induction, if not already in place preoperatively. Rapid blood losses, the potential for hemodynamic swings, and the need to check intraoperative laboratory values all validate this requirement.

e) The standard sites for pulse oximetry placement may not be available. Alternative sites include the nose, ear, and cheek.

f) Any preexisting invasive monitors such as arterial line catheters or central venous or pulmonary artery catheters should be continued in the operating room.

g) Accurate temperature monitoring is essential because burn patients can become very hypothermic intraoperatively. Temperature measurements should be obtained through an esophageal stethoscope. Skin temperature devices are highly inaccurate, and there may not be a suitable place to place one.

h) Patients with burns who are critically ill are usually transported directly to the operating room from the burn intensive care unit and vice versa postoperatively by the anesthesia provider. These patients are usually intubated, are receiving continuous infusions of pharmacologic agents, and have invasive lines in place. Astute monitoring of the patient's vital signs during transport is mandatory. Care must be taken while transporting the patient to not disrupt or dislodge any invasive or IV lines. A portable oxygen delivery system is another component of required transport equipment. Careful handling and vigilant guarding of the airway are vital. The anesthesia provider must also consider the patient's comfort and privacy during transport. Amnestic and analgesic drugs should be administered as needed.

i) Monitors: Standard. Needle electrodes may be needed for ECG. Blood pressure can be measured on the lower extremities; an arterial line or a cuff can be placed over the burned area with a sterile lubricated dressing after consultation with the burn specialist. Most patients with burns of more than 40% to 50% require an arterial line, a central line, and a pulmonary arterial catheter if they are hemodynamically unstable. Use caution in placement and avoid burned areas.

j) Additional equipment: Blood and fluid warmers. A heated circuit and warming blanket are used. Room temperature is increased. Burn patients are poikilothermic.

k) Positioning: Various positions may be required intraoperatively, depending on the area being treated. Assess limb contractures and stabilize fractures.

6. **Airway management**

a) Acute airway problems are frequently addressed upon admission to the burn unit. In a patient with a major burn or one who has an inhalation injury, preoperative intubation is likely.

b) Succinylcholine administration is contraindicated because of the potential for life-threatening hyperkalemia. Some practitioners believe that succinylcholine can be used safely up to 24 hours after an acute burn.

c) In a nonintubated patient without an inhalation injury and whose airway is normal, induction and intubation of the airway can proceed as during any other anesthetic regimen.

d) Preoperative airway evaluation is necessary as with any other patient. The anesthesia provider should exert good judgment in determining the degree of intubation difficulty. If the airway appears difficult, fiberoptic intubation should be considered or at least readily available.

e) In a severely burned patient who is intubated preoperatively, vigilance is required to protect the airway from accidental extubation. Loss of the airway in the patient may be impossible to regain because of edema of the airway structures. In this instance, cricothyrotomy or tracheotomy may be necessary.

f) Securing of such an airway can be problematic. Tape does not readily stick to burned skin. The use of soft beard straps to secure an endotracheal tube is a good option, especially if the plan is to extubate the patient at the end of the case. Cloth ties encircled around the head are frequently used in the burn unit to secure endotracheal tubes and should not be disrupted.

7. **Temperature regulation**

a) Depending on the percentage of TBSA affected by the burn, temperature regulation can be problematic in burn patients. These patients are at high risk of hypothermia development resulting from the loss of the skin's insulating mechanisms, radiation and evaporative heat losses, and the large amount of body surface area exposure intraoperatively.

b) The temperature in the operating room should be greater than 28° C. IV solutions and skin preparations should be warmed. All methods of heat conservation should be used while the patient is in the operating room.

c) The use of in-line Humidivents or low gas flows reduces evaporative respiratory tract heat loss.

d) Forced-air warming blankets are very effective, but their use can be limited. Over-body heating lamps can be used but need to be at a safe distance above the patient to prevent further skin burns. Plastic bags can also be used to insulate any exposed body parts not being treated surgically.

e) It is suggested that keeping a patient warm is more beneficial than rewarming. With hypothermia, vasoconstriction occurs that may curtail any later warming efforts. It has been shown that slow rewarming postoperatively in critically ill patients with burn injuries leads to an increase in mortality. If the patient becomes hypothermic even despite the best effort put forth, the surgeon needs to be advised to stop the procedure.

8. **Fluid and blood replacement**

a) Surgical burn débridements may result in excessive blood loss. Wound management involves removal of the burn eschar layer until brisk bleeding of the dermis is reached.

b) The surgical team may remove the eschar so rapidly that it becomes difficult to keep up with the massive blood loss, resulting in a suddenly hypovolemic patient. Some institutions stop the surgical procedure after 2 hours if more than two blood volumes have been lost or if the body temperature falls to 35° C or by greater than 1.5° C from baseline.

c) There are many formulas to approximate the amount of potential blood loss for a burn débridement. These vary from 200 to 400 mL of blood loss for each 1% of TBSA excised and grafted to as high as 4% to 15% of the patient's blood volume for every percent of skin débrided.

d) During and especially after the excision and débridement, gauze pads soaked in a vasoconstrictor (e.g., epinephrine, phenylephrine) are placed on the newly excised wound to control the bleeding. However, this may result in systemic absorption of vasoconstrictors, causing elevation of the patient's blood pressure even in the presence of hypovolemia. Thrombin-soaked sponges may be preferred for patients whose systemic absorption of epinephrine may cause myocardial ischemia or arrhythmias.

e) Adequate venous access is a must before the initiation of surgical débridement. The size and extent of the burn will mandate how much access is needed. It is optimal to have two large-bore peripheral IV lines in place to ensure the administration of fluids and blood products quickly.

f) Critically ill patients often have a central venous catheter in place, especially if the burn is extensive and access is difficult. Although a triple-lumen catheter is adequate in the intensive care unit setting, it may not be ideal in the operating room when fluid and blood replacement is needed quickly.

g) The readiness of blood and blood products should be ascertained before the patient is brought to the operating room. Ideally, the blood should be in the operating room, checked, and ready to use at the beginning of the surgical procedure. This is particularly necessary in pediatric patients. Some hospitals initiate blood transfusions before the beginning of the surgical débridement and apply compression dressings after excision and grafting.

h) Careful planning is necessary to manage the hemorrhage and potential complications associated with massive transfusion (citrate toxicity, loss of clotting factors) during the débridement. Visual estimation of the blood loss is subjective at best and is prone to be miscalculated. Suction is not used during débridements. Sponges may be accidentally thrown away or covered up during the procedure. Blood drips onto the floor, is covered up in the surgical drapes, or leaks under the patient, and it is possible to be lulled into a false sense of security immediately after the eschar incision. Proper monitoring of the patient's urinary output, hematocrit, and hemodynamic status is necessary for keeping the patient's volume within normal limits.

i) One IV catheter is adequate for the induction of anesthesia in most burn patients, but at least two large-bore IV catheters are necessary before beginning a major excision and grafting procedure. The use of central venous or pulmonary artery catheters is patient dependent. The risk of sepsis in immunosuppressed patients must be weighed against the benefit of information gained.

j) The guidelines for fluid resuscitation and urine output are listed in the box and table on pg. 474.

Fluid Resuscitation Formulas for Burn Patients

Formula	First 24 hr	Second 24 hr
	Brooke	
Crystalloid	2 mL LR/% burn per kg ½ in first 8 hr ½ in next 16 hr	D_5W maintenance
Colloid	None	0.5 mL/% burn per kg
	Parkland	
Crystalloid	4 mL LR/% burn per kg ½ in first 8 hr ½ in next 16 hr	D_5W maintenance
Colloid	None	0.5 mL/% burn per kg
	Massachusetts General Hospital	
Crystalloid	1.5 mL LR/% burn per kg ½ in first 8 hr ½ in next 16 hr	Not specified
Colloid	0.5 mL LR/% burn per kg None in first 4 hr ½ in second 4 hr ½ in next 16 hr	Not specified
	Evans	
Crystalloid	1 mL LR/% burn per kg ½ in first 8 hr ½ in next 16 hr	D_5W maintenance
Colloid	1 mL LR/% burn per kg ½ in first 8 hr ½ in next 16 hr	Not specified

D_5W, 5% Dextrose in water; *LR*, lactated Ringer's solution.

Consensus Formula for Fluid Resuscitation and Urine Output in Burn Patients (American Burn Association)

Adults: Ringer's lactate 2-4 mL × kg body weight × percent TBSA burned*
Children: Ringer's lactate 3-4 mL × kg body weight × percent TBSA burned*†

Minimum Urinary Output in Burn Patients
Adults: 0.5 mL/kg/hr
Children weighing less than 30 kg: 1 mL/kg/hr
Patients with high-voltage electrical injuries: 1-1.5 mL/kg/hr

*One half of the estimated volume of fluid should be administered in the first 8 hours after the burn. The remaining half should be administered over the subsequent 16 hours of the first postburn day.
†Infants and young children should receive fluid with 5% dextrose at a maintenance rate in addition to the resuscitation fluid noted above.
TBSA, Total body surface area.
From American Burn Association. *Advanced Burn Life Support Course Provider's Manual.* Chicago: American Burn Association; 2005.

9. **Perioperative management**
   a) Induction and management
      (1) There is no single best anesthetic agent to administer to burn patients. The anesthetic is individualized and should be based on the patient's preoperative status and medical history.

(2) The patient with an acute burn seldom comes to the operating room immediately after the injury. Patients are usually admitted and stabilized in the burn unit. If the patient requires surgery, the anesthesia provider must realize that the burn patient is quite "fragile" within the first 24 hours of the injury. Anesthetic agents can exert extreme depressant effects, especially if fluid resuscitation is not adequate or has not been fully completed. The loss of intravascular volume coupled with the potential for a depressed myocardium can result in a hemodynamically unstable patient under general anesthesia.

(3) Careful and slow titration of all anesthetic agents is vital. Premedicating stable patients with a benzodiazepine or a narcotic decreases anxiety and makes transfer to the operating room tolerable. Anxiety, depression, and pain are common in patients with burns.

(4) To minimize patient discomfort, induction can be performed on the patient's intensive care unit bed before moving the patient onto the operating room table.

(5) Regional anesthesia is sometimes considered for burn trauma limited to a small area or an extremity or for surgery during the reconstructive phase.

   (a) One advantage of this technique is prolonged postoperative analgesia. Regional anesthesia is generally limited for a variety of reasons.

   (b) The anesthesia provider must avoid performing any regional technique through burned tissue because of the potential for the spread of infection.

   (c) There is an almost universal presence of hypotension (hypovolemia) and vasodilation with or without sepsis, which is a relative contraindication to the use of spinal or epidural routes for pain control until the burn wound is closed.

   (d) Coagulopathy and cardiorespiratory instability are also reasons to avoid a regional anesthetic technique. The greatest limitation to the use of regional anesthesia is the extent of the surgical field. The anesthetized region must include both the area to be excised and the area to be harvested for donor skin.

   (e) In children, regional anesthesia blocks are sometimes a viable option for postoperative analgesia. A tried and true regional block to institute in children undergoing débridements in the lower extremities or skin harvesting from the buttocks or thighs is a single-shot caudal technique. This can be placed either after the induction of general anesthesia or at end of the case before emergence. Injection of bupivacaine 0.25% and levobupivacaine 0.25% with epinephrine 1:200,000 added are two options. The volume of local anesthetic injected into the caudal space is determined by the child's weight in kilograms and the analgesia level needed to be covered by the block. If the child is to be admitted postoperatively, the addition of morphine, at 30 to 50 mcg/kg, or clonidine, at 1 to 2 mcg/kg, can be added.

(6) Etomidate maintains hemodynamic stability during induction with less respiratory depression than barbiturates. However, repeated doses may inhibit adrenocortical function.

(7) Propofol has greater negative inotropic effects than does etomidate, which may lead to hypotension after induction. The high lipid content of propofol may limit its use during initial resuscitation and in septic patients.

(8) Another IV anesthetic is ketamine, a phencyclidine derivative that produces a dissociative anesthetic state of relatively short duration. Ketamine offers the advantage of stable hemodynamics and analgesia. Low doses produce adequate amnesia and analgesia for the débridement of superficial burns; higher doses may be administered for more extensive procedures, such as eschar excisions. Hallucinogenic episodes can be minimized with the administration of benzodiazepines in small doses, and an anticholinergic prevents excessive pharyngeal and tracheobronchial secretions.

(9) In the pediatric burn patient, inhalation induction with sevoflurane is certainly acceptable if the child does not have IV access before induction and if the airway appears normal.

(10) Anesthesia should be maintained with opioid or inhalational agents as the hemodynamic status of the patient permits. Inhalation agents have proved to be safe and effective, allowing rapid adjustment of anesthetic depth and the administration of high oxygen concentrations. The burn patient may be sensitive to the cardiovascular depressant effects of inhaled anesthetics, especially if acute fluid resuscitation is incomplete. Inhaled agents do not provide analgesia during the postsurgical period.

(11) Intubated burn patients frequently continued ventilation with specialized critical care ventilators (e.g., percussive ventilators) intraoperatively to maintain adequate oxygenation and ventilation. In this instance, a total IV anesthetic is indicated.

(12) The main group of anesthetic agents that can exert altered effects in the burn patient are the muscle relaxants. Within the first 24-hour window after the burn injury, the burn is considered stable. Succinylcholine is probably safe to use within this time frame. As stated previously, the postjunctional acetylcholine receptors begin to proliferate soon after a burn injury occurs. This phenomenon is thought to be fully complete by 7 days after the acute injury. Succinylcholine given after the initial first 24-hour window has produced significant hyperkalemia as a result of this upregulation of receptors.

(13) Nondepolarizing muscle relaxants are safe to use in burn patients. Anesthesia providers should realize that patients may demonstrate a resistance to their effects. Higher dosing or more frequent redosing may be necessary. The origin of the phenomenon again is thought to result from the increase in postjunctional acetylcholine receptors. Because responses to nondepolarizing muscle relaxants can vary significantly, neuromuscular blockade monitoring should always be used.

b) Emergence from anesthesia

(1) The postoperative anesthetic course should be planned in advance and is frequently intuitive. Critically ill and intubated

burn patients are kept intubated postoperatively and are directly transported to the burn unit.

(2) The anesthesia provider should safeguard the airway and be respectful of the patient's need for sedation and analgesia during this terminal phase of the anesthetic.

(3) If the patient is to be extubated, emergence from anesthesia should be planned in advance as well, similar to any other patient undergoing an anesthetic.

(4) Neuromuscular blockade should be adequately reversed and, if possible, the patient should be allowed to begin spontaneously breathing at an appropriate time.

(5) Narcotics for postoperative analgesia should be titrated according to the patient's respiratory status. Keep in mind that these are painful procedures, and patients' narcotic requirements can be tremendous.

B. TRAUMA

1. Introduction

Trauma is the fifth leading cause of death in the United States. Mortality is related to the age and prior condition of the patient, the type and severity of the trauma, and the response time for emergency treatment received.

2. Preoperative assessment

The time allowed for preoperative assessment is limited and is based on the severity of the trauma. A rapid assessment and review of pertinent patient data available are essential. Blood therapy and the establishment of multiple large bore IV lines are priorities. The preoperative considerations are listed in the following box.

Preoperative Anesthetic Considerations and Preparations for Trauma Patients

- Obtain initial radio or telephone report of patient's condition from field providers.
- Prepare the anesthesia machine, ventilator, anticipated drugs, equipment, and supplies.
- Establishment of a patent airway is the primary concern followed by adequate IV access without at least two large-bore catheters
- Prepare for standard endotracheal intubation and alternative airway interventions. (e.g., video laryngoscope, LMA, cricothyrotomy)
- Have proper monitoring equipment and supplies, as well as equipment for rapid infusion of blood and fluids.
- Use gloves, gowns, proper eyewear protection, and universal precautions for contact with patient during placement of invasive lines, endotracheal intubation, and surgical procedures.
- Conduct a sample history (sign and symptoms of injury, allergies, medications, medical history, last oral intake, events leading up to injury) on conscious patients.
- Obtain history from prehospital emergency team, family, or friends on unconscious patients.
- Evaluate airway and ventilation for adequacy of presenting status and need for immediate or delayed interventions.
- Evaluate airway to determine anticipated relative difficulty and plan for primary and possible secondary maneuvers for securing the airway.

Continued

Preoperative Anesthetic Considerations and Preparations for Trauma Patients—cont'd

- Determine the Glasgow Coma Score and Trauma Severity Score at the time of arrival.
- Obtain venous and arterial blood samples for typing and crossmatch, CBC, electrolyte levels, blood glucose levels, coagulation profile, toxicology screen, and blood gas analysis.
- Have appropriate crystalloids, colloids, and blood components available for use.
- Consider warming maneuvers (e.g., fluid warmer, forced-air warming, warm operating room)
- Formulate the plan for use of anesthetic agents and techniques appropriate for the patient.
- Provide airway and anesthesia support as necessary for diagnostic procedures (e.g., CT, MRI, angiography, ultrasonography, diagnostic peritoneal lavage, laparoscopy, examination during general anesthesia).
- Overall goals for trauma care are to establish a patent and secure airway, "provide" or "ensure"? adequate ventilation, protect the spine, provide fluid and blood resuscitation, and administer anesthesia according to the patient's condition.

CBC, Complete blood count; *CT*, computed tomography; *MRI*, magnetic resonance imaging.

a) Cardiac: Assess for symptoms of shock listed in the following table. Assess the chest wall for obvious contusion, or instability, and assess stability of vital signs.

Classification of Hemorrhagic Shock

	Class I	Class II	Class III	Class IV
Blood loss (mL)	=750	750-1500	1500-2000	>2000
Blood loss (% blood volume)	=15	15-30	30-40	>40
Pulse rate (beats/min)	<100	>100	>120	>140
Blood pressure	Normal	Normal	Decreased	Profound
Pulse pressure	Normal or increased	Decreased	Decreased	Decreased
Respiratory rate (breaths/min)	14-20	20-30	30-40	>35
Urine output (mL/hr)	=30	20-30	5-15	Negligible
Mental status	Slightly anxious	Mildly anxious	Anxious, confused	Confused, lethargic
Fluid replacement	Crystalloid	Crystalloid	Crystalloid + blood	Crystalloid + blood

Adapted from American College of Surgeons, Committee on Trauma. Shock. In American College of Surgeons, ed. *Advanced trauma life support course for physicians*. 7th ed. Chicago: American College of Surgeons; 2004:74:108.

b) Respiratory: Assess breath sounds and patterns of respiration.
c) Neurologic: Assess patient using the Glasgow Coma Scale (GCS). Assume a cervical spine injury until it is definitively ruled out by x-ray examination or computed tomography (CT). There are three categories of the GCS to which a value is assigned: eye opening, motor response, and verbal response. For eye opening: 4 = spontaneous,

3 = to speech, 2 = to pain, and 1 = none. For motor response: 6 = to verbal, 5 = localizes to pain, 4 = withdraws to pain, 3 = decorticate flexion to pain, 2 = extends to pain, and 1 = none. For verbal response: 5 = oriented, 4 = confused, 3 = inappropriate words, 2 = incomprehensible sounds, and 1 = none. A normal GCS score is 15. A score of 8 or less indicates a severe brain injury.

d) Renal: Assess the color and amount of urine.

e) Gastrointestinal: All trauma patients are considered to have a full stomach. Gastric emptying slows or stops at the time of the trauma. The presence of a nasogastric tube also provides a "wick" that may allow gastric fluid: to be aspirated.

f) Endocrine: The release of stress hormones transiently elevates blood glucose levels.

g) Hematologic: Severe physical stress can lead to coagulopathies, as can dilution of clotting factors during massive volume resuscitation.

h) Patient preparation

(1) Baseline laboratory tests are obtained as available: hemoglobin, hematocrit, and others as indicated by history and physical examination.

(2) Type and cross-match for at least 4 units.

(3) Other diagnostic tests are as indicated by history and physical examination.

(4) Premedication is usually avoided but can be individualized in trauma patients.

3. Room preparation

a) Standard monitoring equipment

b) Difficult airway equipment such as multiple laryngoscope blades, video laryngoscope, laryngeal mask airway (LMA) of various sizes, intubating LMA, bougie stylet, and emergency airway access kits.

c) Arterial line, arterial blood gas measurement, pulmonary artery catheters, blood warmers, rapid infuser, and patient warming equipment

d) Full range of standard and emergency resuscitative drugs immediately available

e) Transesophageal echocardiogram capabilities can aid in the assessment of heart function.

f) Position usually supine unless otherwise indicated.

4. Anesthetic technique

Immediate establishment of the airway is the priority. Anesthetics are introduced depending on the stability of the patient as assessed by vital signs and physical assessment. Muscle paralysis is provided to facilitate surgical procedures, which can lead to intraoperative awareness in the trauma patient.

5. Perioperative management

a) Induction

(1) This is individualized based on the patient's condition and the severity of trauma.

(2) Rapid-sequence induction and immediate establishment of the airway are necessary.

(3) Ketamine, propofol, and thiopental (Pentothal) may be administered depending on hemodynamic status. The specific anesthetic considerations for various trauma conditions are listed in the boxes on pg. 480.

Conditions Presented by Trauma Patients That Contraindicate the Use of Specific Anesthetic Agents

Shock
Most anesthetic agents cause dose-related cardiovascular depression. IV induction agents are used cautiously in small incremental doses. Inhalation agents are added slowly as cardiovascular stability improves. Use of histamine-releasing muscle relaxants (e.g., atracurium) and narcotics (e.g., morphine, codeine) that could aggravate shock are avoided.

Head Injury
Ketamine causes increases in ICP. N_2O causes increases in pneumocephalic tension. All inhalation agents tend to increase ICP as a result of increases in cerebral blood volume. However, inhalation agents decrease $CMRO_2$. The effects are temporarily attenuated by moderate hyperventilation of patients to $Paco_2$ levels of 30 to 35 mmHg. Succinylcholine causes rises in ICP that may be detrimental in certain situations of significant ICP elevation. Hyperventilation with a $Paco_2$ of 25 mmHg or less is not recommended.

Burns, Spinal Cord Injury, and Crush Injuries
In these categories, succinylcholine can produce dangerous rises in potassium levels if it is administered approximately 24 hours after the injury. This problem can occur indefinitely in patients with permanent spinal cord injuries (e.g., paraplegia, quadriplegia).

Pneumothorax, Pneumocephalus, and Pneumoperitoneum
N_2O causes a wide variety of problems in the trauma patient to the extent that it is not used in the acute anesthetic management of trauma patients. N_2O tends to accumulate in closed spaces, aggravating conditions such as pneumothorax, pneumocephalus, and bowel distention. N_2O exaggerates the effects of air embolism.

Malignant Hyperthermia
All potent inhalation agents are absolutely contraindicated. Succinylcholine is known to trigger malignant hyperthermia and is absolutely contraindicated.

$CMRO_2$, Cerebral metabolic rate of oxygen saturation; *ICP,* intracranial pressure; *IV,* intravenous; *N_2O,* nitrous oxide; *$Paco_2$,* partial pressure of arterial carbon dioxide.

Factors Considered When Securing the Airway of a Trauma Patient

- Need for rapid assessment and intervention in a limited time
- Decreased oxygen reserve or prolonged periods of hypoventilation may predispose patient to rapid desaturation
- Full stomach leads to frequent vomiting (high risk for aspiration)
- Monitor for signs and symptoms of hemorrhagic shock, cardiac instability, or respiratory failure
- Possible acute intoxication with alcohol or illicit drugs
- Patient may have a cervical spine injury with a cervical collar in place
- Trauma to airway may include:
  - Maxillofacial injuries
  - Inhalational injuries (e.g., burns, rear drowning, noxious gases)
  - Neck injuries
  - Thoracic injuries
- Soft tissue swelling, bleeding, gastric contents, or foreign bodies (teeth) in the airway can lead to difficulty during laryngoscopy and intubation (suction should be available).

Airway Evaluation and Interventions in Trauma Patients

- Administer oxygen immediately while the evaluation is being conducted.
- Evaluate the patency of the natural airway and the adequacy of ventilation.
- Evaluate the quality of gas exchange visually and with pulse oximetry and arterial blood gas analysis.
- When the patient's oxygenation and general condition appear adequate, one or more of the following imaging techniques are used before securing the airway: three-view cervical spine series, or thin-cut axial CT images with sagittal reconstruction.
- Evaluate the neurologic status (e.g., level of consciousness, ability to follow commands, presence of head and spinal cord injury).
- Evaluate blunt or penetrating facial and throat injuries that may complicate airway function or interventions.
- Evaluate for evolving edema that may compromise the airway.
- Evaluate complicated airway injuries with a surgeon who is prepared to establish an invasive primary or alternative "backup" airway (e.g., cricothyroidotomy, tracheostomy, or LMA) in the event that standard noninvasive attempts are ineffective.
- Perform oral endotracheal intubation after induction of anesthesia, and use an appropriate neuromuscular blocking agent with application of cricoid pressure and in-line axial immobilization of the cervical spine in most situations.
- Awake oral or nasal intubation can be attempted in cooperative patients who are adequately oxygenated and hemodynamically stable; nasal intubation is contraindicated in head-injured patients who may have cribriform plate injuries because of the potential for the endotracheal tube to enter the brain vault.
- Intubation over a flexible fiberoptic bronchoscope (if no active bleeding exists that can obscure visualization) using a flex-tip (Parker-Tube) is useful to increase initial success.
- Placement of chest tubes in the presence of a pneumothorax is completed before or simultaneously with intubation to avoid acceleration of the size of the pneumothorax, with the potential development of mediastinal shift and hemodynamic compromise.

CT, Computed tomography; *LMA,* laryngeal mask airway.

b) Maintenance
   (1) Oxygen and muscle relaxants are required in critically injured patients.
   (2) After assessment and stabilization, anesthetics are administered as appropriate and as tolerated by the patient.
   (3) Blood loss should be closely monitored and transfusions initiated with the type-specific blood products unless an emergency transfusion is required using O negative blood.
   (4) A 1:1:1 (packed red blood cells:fresh-frozen plasma:platelet) ratio should be considered during massive blood transfusions to limit the dilution of blood clotting factors.
   (5) Blood gas analysis and coagulation status should be frequently considered during resuscitative efforts.

c) Emergence: Continued ventilation and management of all major systems are required in the immediate postanesthesia period.

6. Postoperative implications

Continued ventilation and observation of cardiac, respiratory, renal, and coagulation status are required for at least the first 24 hours in severely injured patients. These patients are transferred to the critical care unit for long-term management of multiple sequelae. Pain control may include narcotics, patient-controlled analgesia, or regional block. Common problems in trauma are listed in the following boxes.

Assessment and Interventions for Common Problems in Trauma

Hypotension

The most common cause of hypotension is generally hypovolemia. Fluid resuscitation is initiated and continued as the underlying causes of the hypovolemia are investigated. Disruptions of major vessels in the chest, abdomen, and pelvis are the most common causes of hypovolemia. Cardiac tamponade is considered as a cause of persistent hypotension. Inotropes and vasopressors are seldom indicated in managing hypotension in trauma patients. Exceptions may include patients in spinal shock and patients who have sustained myocardial contusion.

Desaturation

Desaturation is usually noted first by pulse oximetry measurements or arterial blood gas determination. Check for adequate FiO_2, ventilation, and perfusion. Check breath sounds. Check for endobronchial intubation. Look for signs of pneumothorax (i.e., distended neck veins and increased resonance on affected side, tracheal deviation). Desaturation may be caused by pulmonary contusion, often treated with increasing levels of PEEP to open atelectatic areas. Copious secretions and mucous plugs are considered potential causes. A chest radiograph is helpful for ruling out many potential causes of desaturation. Aspiration of blood, stomach contents, or foreign bodies and postobstructive pulmonary edema are considered. Fiberoptic bronchoscopy can be both diagnostic and therapeutic. Consider the possibility of air embolism, especially in cases of penetrating injuries.

Hypertension

Trauma patients frequently become hyperdynamic after resuscitation; this problem is usually treated with adequate levels of anesthesia, including moderately large doses of potent narcotics such as fentanyl or sufentanil. Use of antihypertensive agents may need to be considered.

Tachyarrhythmias and Bradyarrhythmias

Hypoxemia and hypercarbia and hypovolemia must be considered first. Myocardial injury is also considered. 12-lead ECG is obtained. Consider performing echocardiography to assess cardiac motion and possible tamponade.

Sudden Cardiac Arrest

Check for obvious causes using ABCs (**a**irway patency, **b**reathing adequacy, and **c**irculatory adequacy). Sudden cardiac arrest is often a strong indication for open thoracotomy to inspect the heart for pericardial tamponade or other injuries or to perform open-chest cardiac massage; abdominal incision may also be indicated to look for other sources of bleeding; rapid blood and fluid resuscitation are continued as indicated, and ACLS protocols initiated.

ACLS, Advanced cardiac life support; *ECG*, electrocardiogram; FiO_2, fraction inspired concentration of oxygen; *PEEP*, positive end-expiratory pressure.

Preventing and Treating Hypothermia in Trauma Patients

- Remove all wet clothing and bedding and dry skin as soon as possible at the time of admission.
- Warm the admission, surgery, and recovery areas.
- Warm all fluids and blood products with an effective system (e.g., level I fluid warmer).
- Warm irrigating fluids and topical cleansers.
- Use in-line heat-moisture exchangers in the breathing circuit.
- Use convection warm-air devices
- During rewarming, use neuromuscular blocking agents to prevent shivering that may increase oxygen consumption by 200% to 400% without improving oxygen delivery.

XI SECTION Pediatrics

A. ANATOMY AND PHYSIOLOGY

1. **Cardiovascular physiology**
   a) During fetal development, oxygenation and carbon dioxide (CO_2) elimination are accomplished through the placenta. Oxygenated blood to the fetus travels from the placenta through the umbilical vein through the ductus venosus near the liver to the inferior vena cava. The foramen ovale, the opening between the right and left atria, allows the oxygenated blood direct access to the left heart circulation. From the left atrium, the blood is transferred to the left ventricle and then to the body. The blood returns to the placenta through two umbilical arteries. Deoxygenated blood from the superior vena cava flows into the right atrium. It is then ejected into the pulmonary artery. Because of high pulmonary vasculature pressure, the blood bypasses the lungs and is instead transferred through the ductus arteriosus to the aorta. The blood travels to the placenta through the umbilical arteries.
   b) Clamping of the umbilical cord increases systemic vascular resistance, increasing aortic and left-sided heart pressures and allowing the foramen ovale to close and the lungs to assume their role in oxygenation. Pulmonary vascular resistance decreases, and the ductus arteriosus closes as arterial oxygen pressure (Po_2) levels increase.
   c) Hypoxia, hypercarbia, and acidosis lead to persistent pulmonary hypertension and continued maintenance of fetal circulation. The diagnosis is made when right radial (preductal) and umbilical line (postductal) samples reveal a Po_2 difference of 20 mmHg. Shunting continues across a patent ductus arteriosus, resulting in hypoxemia and reversal of acidosis.
   d) Treatment of persistent pulmonary circulation includes hyperventilation, maintenance of adequate oxygenation, and alkalosis.
   e) Neonatal cardiac output is heart rate dependent because of a noncompliant left ventricle and fixed stroke volume.
   f) The pediatric basal heart rate is higher than that of adults, although parasympathetic stimulation, hypoxia, or deep anesthesia can cause profound bradycardia and decreased cardiac output.
   g) Sympathetic nervous system and baroreceptor reflexes are immature. Infants have low catecholamine stores and decreased responsiveness to exogenous catecholamines. Infants cannot respond to hypovolemia with vasoconstriction. Therefore, hypovolemia is suspected when there is hypotension in the absence of an increased heart rate.
   h) Normal parameters are given in the table on pg. 485.
   i) Physiologic anemia of the newborn: Hematocrit at birth is 50%, 80% of which is fetal hemoglobin. Fetal hemoglobin binds more strongly to O_2 than adult hemoglobin. This facilitates O_2 uptake in utero. After birth, the presence of fetal hemoglobin causes a shift in the oxyhemoglobin curve to the left and a decrease in O_2 delivery to the tissues. At age 1 to 3 months, hemoglobin levels

Normal Parameters

Age	Respiratory Rate (breaths/min)	Heart Rate (beats/min)	Systolic Blood Pressure (mmHg)	Diastolic Blood Pressure (mmHg)
Neonate	40	140	65	40
1 year	30	120	95	65
3 years	25	100	100	70
12 years	20	80	110	60

decrease, and levels of 2,3-diphosphoglycerate increase. This causes a shift of the oxyhemoglobin curve to the right and increased O_2 delivery to tissues.

2. **Respiratory physiology**
   a) Metabolic rate, CO_2 production, and O_2 consumption are increased.
   b) Functional residual capacity and O_2 reserves are decreased.
   c) Infants have a paradoxical response to hypoxia—initial hyperpnea followed by respiratory depression and depressed response to hypercarbia.
   d) The larynx is at C2 to C4 in children and at C3 to C6 in adults. This results in increased difficulty in alignment of the pharyngeal and laryngeal axes. A straight blade is useful for laryngoscopy in children.
   e) Children have a stiff, omega-shaped epiglottis. The vocal cords slant up and back.
   f) The narrowest part of the pediatric airway is the cricoid cartilage, as opposed to the adult glottis. The cricoid cartilage can form a seal around the endotracheal tube (ETT), eliminating the need for a cuffed tube. The cartilage is funnel shaped. Do not force fit the ETT. Properly fitted tubes allow a leak at 15 to 25 cm H_2O.
   g) Children have large occiputs that flex the head onto the chest, large tongues, and small chins. Tonsils and adenoids grow rapidly from ages 4 to 7 and may obstruct breathing.
   h) Infants are obligatory nasal breathers. The position of the epiglottis in relation to the soft palate allows simultaneous breathing and sucking or drinking.
   i) The neonatal trachea is 4 cm. Flexion of the head onto the chest forces the ETT to extend deeper into the right mainstem. Extension of the head may dislodge the tube.
   j) The number of alveoli increases until age 6 years. Mature levels of surfactant are reached at 35 weeks of gestation. Decreased amounts of alveoli and surfactant in the neonatal period increase the risk of infant respiratory distress syndrome.
   k) Increased work of breathing in the infant results from a decreased amount of type I muscle fibers in the diaphragm; this causes a predisposition to fatigue. Poor chest wall mechanics, lack of rib cage rigidity, horizontal orientation of the ribs, weak intercostal muscles, and increased fatigue result in paradoxical chest movements in the newborn.
3. **Nervous system**
   a) Cranial sutures are not fused in infants; the cranium is pliable. Fluid status is indicated by fullness of the fontanels.

b) Myelination of the nervous system continues until age 3 years. The spinal cord ends at L1 in adults and at L3 in pediatric patients. This is important to consider when using regional anesthesia techniques in the pediatric population.
c) Preterm and low birthweight infants are at risk for intracranial hemorrhage resulting from fragile cerebral vessels. Intracranial bleeding may result from hypoxia, hypercarbia, hyperglycemia or hypoglycemia, hypernatremia, or wide variations in blood pressure.

4. **Renal system**
a) The total body water in proportion to body weight is higher in neonates than in adults. Whereas the kidneys function in utero to eliminate urine into the amniotic fluid, the placenta eliminates waste.
b) Neonates have the complete number of nephrons at birth. Nephrons are immature in function until age 6 to 12 months.
c) The glomerular filtration rate (GFR) is decreased by renal vasoconstriction, low plasma flow in the renal system, and low blood pressure. GFR increases until age 1 year.
d) Infants are obligate sodium excretors because of their inability to conserve sodium. Renal tubules are not responsive to the renin–angiotensin–aldosterone system. Infants' kidneys cannot concentrate urine, leading to an increased risk of dehydration. The ability to reabsorb glucose is also impaired. If excessive glucose is given intravenously, the result is osmotic diuresis.
e) Pediatric patients have a tendency to develop acidosis because the metabolic rate and CO_2 production are double those of adults. There is a decreased ability to conserve bicarbonate and to excrete acids.

5. **Hepatic system**
a) Near birth, the fetal liver increases glycogen stores. Preterm infants are at increased risk for hypoglycemia because of a lack of glycogen stores.
b) Hepatic metabolism of drugs is decreased in the early weeks of life. The liver functions at the adult level by age 2 years.

6. **Impaired thermogenesis**
a) Infants are at risk for hypothermia from the following:
(1) Increased ratio of surface area to body weight
(2) Ineffective shivering mechanism
(3) Decreased amounts of subcutaneous fat present in preterm infants
b) Heat loss results from the following:
(1) Radiation: This is the transfer of heat between two objects of different temperatures not in direct contact. Reduce radiant loss by decreasing the temperature gradient (raise the room temperature closer to patient temperature). This factor is the major way that patients lose heat.
(2) Convection: This is the transfer of heat to moving molecules such as air or liquid. Cover exposed skin.
(3) Evaporation: This occurs through the skin and respiratory systems, including sweat, insensible water loss through skin, wounds, respiratory tract, and evaporation of liquids applied to the skin.
(4) Conduction: This is the transfer of heat from a warm infant to a cool object in direct contact.
c) Patients assume room temperature under anesthesia, a condition termed *poikilothermia.*

d) Nonshivering thermogenesis: Infants have impaired shivering capabilities. Autonomic nervous system activation during periods of cold results in metabolism of brown fat stores. Brown fat is located around the neck, kidneys, axilla, and adrenals in addition to spaces between shoulders, under the sternum, and along the spine. Fatty acids in the brown fat stores are oxidated in an exothermic reaction to produce heat. Nonshivering thermogenesis can occur. The consequence of hypothermia that initiates nonshivering thermogenesis is acidosis until age 1 to 2 years.

e) Hypothermia in neonates results in the release of norepinephrine, peripheral and pulmonary vasoconstriction, increasing acidosis, increased pulmonary pressures and right-to-left shunting, and eventually hypoxia, further perpetuating the cycle.

f) Avoid hypothermia by instituting the following: Increase room temperature, cover the patient's head and exposed extremities, and use overhead warming light. Beware of burns. Use recommended distances for safe use. Heat and humidify delivered gases.

B. PEDIATRIC PHARMACOLOGIC CONSIDERATIONS

1. **Introduction**
   a) Immature organ systems are responsible for existing pharmacologic differences between infants and children.
   b) Physiologic characteristics that modify the pharmacokinetic (what the body does to the drug) and pharmacodynamic (what the drug does to the body) activity include differences in total body water (TBW) composition, immaturity of metabolic degradation pathways, reduced protein binding, immaturity of the blood-brain barrier, greater proportion of blood flow to the vessel-rich organs (brain, heart, liver, and lungs), reductions in glomerular filtration, a smaller functional residual capacity, and increased minute ventilation.
   c) TBW, expressed in liters, is determined as a percentage of total body weight (1 L of water weighs 1 kg). The changes in TBW, intracellular fluid (ICF), and extracellular fluid (ECF) during maturation are listed in the following table.

Fluid Compartment Volumes

	Premature	Infant	Child	Adult
Total body water (%)	80-90	75	65-70	55-60
Extracellular fluid (%)	50-60	40	30	20
Intracellular fluid (%)	60	35	40	40

2. **Volume of drug distribution**
   a) Infants have a larger extracellular fluid compartment and greater TBW content.
   b) There is a greater adipose content and a higher ratio of water to lipid. Fat content is approximately 12% at birth, doubling by 6 months of age and reaching 30% at 12 months of age.

c) These factors lower plasma drug concentrations when water-soluble drugs are administered according to weight.
d) A larger drug loading dose is required to achieve the desired plasma concentration. The effect of immaturity on the volume of distribution is not as evident for lipophilic drugs that are transported across cell membranes.

3. **Protein binding**
a) Total plasma protein is decreased in infants, reaching equivalent adult concentrations by childhood.
b) Both albumin and alpha 1-acid glycoprotein (AAG) concentrations are diminished at birth but reach the adult equivalency by infancy (age 4 weeks).

4. **Metabolism**
a) Phase II reactions, which are immature at birth, consist of conjugation or synthesis. Conjugation couples the drug with an endogenous substrate (glucuronidation, methylation, acetylation, and sulfation) to facilitate excretion.
b) Newborns lack the capacity to efficiently conjugate bilirubin (decreased glucuronyl transferase activity), and metabolize acetaminophen, chloramphenicol, and sulfonamides.
c) Although the necessary enzyme systems are present at birth, enzyme activity is reduced, increasing drug elimination half-lives.

5. **Rectal and oral drug administration**
a) Drugs are usually formulated as liquids for oral administration in children.
b) Midazolam may be administered orally for premedication, and the rectal route may be selected for the administration of acetaminophen, opioids, barbiturates, and benzodiazepines.
c) Both routes rely on passive diffusion for drug absorption. The resulting plasma drug concentration depends on the molecular weight, degree of drug ionization, and lipid solubility.
d) Orally administered drugs are generally reserved for older children because gastric pH is elevated in neonates at birth (pH 6 to 8), and although decreased to a pH level of 1 to 3 within 24 hours, adult gastric pH values are not consistent until age 2 years.
e) Gastric absorption is reduced after oral administration of acidic drugs in infants. Gastric emptying time reaches adult values by 6 months of age. Although gastric emptying time does not affect drug absorption, it may alter peak drug concentration.
f) Acetaminophen, a metabolite of phenacetin, is a popular and safe analgesic and antipyretic commonly administered to children during the perioperative period.
g) The analgesic and antipyretic effects of acetaminophen are equivalent to those of aspirin when the drugs are administered in equipotent dosages.
h) Suppositories should not be divided in an attempt to provide the exact calculated dose because the suspended acetaminophen is distributed unevenly within the suppository. Recommended acetaminophen doses have been based on the age of the child, weight, body surface area calculations, and fractions of adult dosages.
i) Currently recommended oral and rectal doses of acetaminophen range from 10 to 15 mg/kg every 4 hours. Because of the variable absorption of acetaminophen suppositories, some practitioners

have advocated the administration of larger initial rectal dosages. It should be emphasized that subsequent rectal doses should be decreased (20 mg/kg), and the dosing interval should be extended to every 6 to 8 hours.

j) After acetaminophen administered during the perioperative period, the parents should be informed as to the time of administration and be advised of appropriate acetaminophen dosages (60-65 mg/kg/day).

k) The daily acetaminophen dosage administered either rectally or orally should be limited to 100 mg/kg/day for children and 75 mg/kg/day for infants.

l) Sedation with nasally administered midazolam (0.2 mg/kg) may be achieved in as little as 10 to 20 minutes and is explained in part through drug absorption via the olfactory mucosa. Nasal administration is unpleasant because midazolam produces a burning of the nasal mucosa.

m) Oral fentanyl, although effective in producing significant sedation, has been plagued by significant side effects, including facial pruritus (up to 80%) and postoperative nausea and vomiting, seven times greater than when a child receives an oral meperidine, midazolam, or atropine premedicant.

n) Water-soluble drugs (atropine, fentanyl, lidocaine, morphine) may be administered via inhalation; however, only 5% to 10% of the administered dose will reach the systemic circulation.

Inhalation Agents

1. Introduction

a) Although tidal volume is similar between children and adults (5-7 mL/kg), children have greater minute ventilation and a higher ratio of tidal volume to functional residual capacity (5:1) compared with adults (1.5:1).

b) The greater minute ventilation and higher cardiac output in infants and children are responsible for rapid inhalation anesthetic uptake and rapidly increasing alveolar anesthetic concentration. In addition, their decreased distribution of adipose tissue and decreased muscle mass affect the rate of equilibration among the alveoli, blood, and brain.

c) The percentage of blood flow to the vessel-rich organs is greater than in adults, and the blood-gas partition coefficients are lower in infants and children.

d) Anesthetic requirements are known to change with age. Neonates have a somewhat lower minimum alveolar concentration (MAC) than infants, which peaks at around 30 days of age.

e) MAC is higher in infants from age 1 to 6 months of age; thereafter, MAC values are known to decrease with increasing age.

f) Myocardial depression may be exaggerated when inhalation anesthetics are administered to pediatric patients. A more rapid rise F_A/F_I ratio, the greater percentage of blood flow to the vessel-rich organs, and higher administered anesthetic concentrations are central to the cause of myocardial depression.

g) Inhalation induction is more rapid in pediatric patients and is accompanied by a higher incidence of myocardial depression than in adults.

2. **Isoflurane**
   a) The MAC of isoflurane in oxygen is 1.6% in infants and children.
   b) Inhalation induction with isoflurane produces more adverse respiratory events (breath-holding, coughing, and laryngospasm with copious secretions) than sevoflurane.
   c) Administration of isoflurane to adults produces dose-dependent decreases in peripheral vascular resistance, but increases in heart rate maintain blood pressure. This touted advantage (e.g., increase in heart rate to maintain blood pressure) does not occur in infants.
   d) Anesthetic induction in infants with isoflurane produces significant decreases in heart rate, blood pressure, and mean arterial pressure that are not corrected with prior atropine administration.
3. **Desflurane**
   a) The MAC of desflurane in oxygen is 9% for infants and 6% to 10% for children.
   b) Desflurane has the lowest blood-gas partition coefficient of all the inhalation anesthetics (0.42), which facilitates a rapid induction, rapid alterations in anesthetic depth, and emergence.
   c) Similar to isoflurane, desflurane is pungent and is associated with more adverse respiratory events during inhalation induction, including breath-holding, laryngospasm, coughing, and increased secretions with accompanying hypoxia.
   d) After inhalation induction with sevoflurane, desflurane is appropriate for the maintenance of general anesthesia with face mask, ETT, or laryngeal mask airway (LMA).
   e) As in adults, dramatic increases in desflurane concentrations may induce sympathetic stimulation evidenced by tachycardia and hypertension.
4. **Sevoflurane**
   a) The MAC of sevoflurane in oxygen is 3% for infants up to 6 months of age, decreasing to 2.5% to 2.8% up to 1 year of age. The MAC of sevoflurane in oxygen is 2% to 3%.
   b) Sevoflurane produces a more rapid induction and emergence than halothane because of its low blood-gas partition coefficient.
   c) Sevoflurane is readily accepted for mask induction, and its safe cardiovascular profile (compared with halothane) is responsible for the increasing popularity of sevoflurane in pediatric anesthesia.
   d) Minute ventilation is significantly lower, and respiratory rate increases until apnea occurs.
   e) Sevoflurane metabolism may produce concentration-dependent elevations in serum fluoride levels that decline when sevoflurane is discontinued.
   f) Some clinicians, when performing longer procedures, use sevoflurane for anesthetic induction and subsequently introduce either desflurane or isoflurane for anesthetic maintenance. This clinical decision reduces patient cost and limits sevoflurane exposure.
   g) Sevoflurane does not sensitize the myocardium to the effects of endogenous and exogenous catecholamines, but concentration-dependent myocardial depression may occur.
5. **Emergence delirium**
   a) A variety of terms are used interchangeably when referring to postoperative agitation. These include *emergence delirium, emergence*

agitation, and *postanesthetic excitement.* These terms describe altered behavior in the immediate postoperative period manifesting as non-purposeful restlessness, crying, moaning, incoherence, and disorientation (known here as emergency delirium [ED]).

b) Case reports also suggest that ED occurs more frequently in preschool-aged children (younger than age 6 years).

c) The reported incidence of ED is between 25% and 80%, although the incidence has been difficult to pinpoint because previous studies are confounded by the previously mentioned varying definitions.

d) The Pediatric Anesthesia Emergence Delirium (PAED) scale for the assessment of ED is listed in the following box.

The Pediatric Anesthesia Emergence Delirium (PAED) Scale

1. The child makes eye contact with caregiver.
2. The child's actions are purposeful.
3. The child is aware of his or her surroundings.
4. The child is restless.
5. The child is inconsolable.

Items 1, 2, and 3 are reverse scored as follows: 4 = not at all, 3 = just a little, 2 = quite a bit, 1 = very much, and 0 = extremely. Items 4 and 5 are scored as follows: 0 = not at all, 1 = just a little, 2 = quite a bit, 3 = very much, and 4 = extremely. The scores are summed to obtain a total. The degree of emergence delirium increases directly with total score.

From Sikich N, Lerman J. Development and psychometric evaluation of the pediatric anesthesia emergence delirium scale. *Anesthesiology.* 2004;100(5):1138-1145.

e) Fortunately, ED is self-limiting but may manifest for as long as 45 minutes.

f) In a search for the causation of ED, several emerging themes have been examined. Proposed etiologies include rapid emergence in a strange environment, pain upon awakening, and preoperative behavior.

g) Several strategies have been advocated for the prevention of ED, although a scientific, clinically tested strategy for prevention has yet to be advanced. After inhalation induction with sevoflurane, propofol infusion for maintenance has been demonstrated to reduce ED.

h) Some anesthesia providers advocate the substitution of sevoflurane with isoflurane, yet no studies have detailed the effectiveness of this strategy.

i) The phenomenon of ED is clearly increased after the administration of sevoflurane (and likely desflurane).

Intravenous Anesthetics

1. Introduction

a) Infants and children have a higher proportion of cardiac output delivered to vascular-rich tissues (i.e., heart, brain, kidneys, and liver).

b) Intravenously administered drugs are readily taken up by these tissues and are subsequently redistributed to muscle and fat—tissues that are less well perfused.

c) Intravenously administered drugs may have a prolonged duration of action in infants and children because of decreased percentages of muscle and fat.
d) The central nervous system (CNS) effects of opioids and barbiturates may also be prolonged because of the immaturity of the blood-brain barrier.
e) Although this evidence suggests that intravenously administered anesthetic doses should be reduced, one must also recall the effect of increased body water. Increased doses of thiopental, propofol, and ketamine are required, presumably because of a greater volume of distribution.

2. **Propofol**
   a) Propofol has a rapid onset and a short duration of action and has been established as a sole agent for induction and maintenance of general anesthesia or may be combined with an opioid and nitrous oxide to provide total intravenous (IV) anesthesia.
   b) Propofol may be delivered as a continuous infusion for short diagnostic and radiologic procedures and is used as a primary sedative in chronically ventilated intensive care patients.
   c) Its antiemetic properties may reduce the incidence of postoperative nausea and vomiting in children undergoing strabismus correction.
   d) Infants require larger induction doses (2.5-3 mg/kg) than children (2-2.5 mg/kg). These induction doses produce moderate decreases in systolic blood pressure.
   e) The pain that accompanies IV administration may be reduced with the addition of as little as 0.2 mg/kg of lidocaine.
   f) Additional strategies suggested for decreasing the pain of injection include a slower injection of propofol into a rapid-running IV line or the injection into larger IV catheters placed in the antecubital space. Induction agents and analgesics are listed in the following tables.

Analgesics

Narcotics			
Drug	**Dose: Analgesic**	**Dose: Induction**	**Comments**
Morphine	0.05-0.2 mg/kg		
Meperidine (Demerol)	1-2 mg/kg		Causes less respiratory depression in neonates than morphine
Fentanyl (Sublimaze)	1-3 mcg/kg	10-100 mcg/kg	Can cause bradycardia and muscle rigidity*
Sufentanil (Sufenta)	0.5-2 mcg/kg		Can cause bradycardia*
Remifentanil (Ultiva)	Loading dose: 0.5-1 mcg/kg Continuous infusion: 0.25-0.5 mcg/kg/min		Bolus can cause bradycardia*
Naloxone (Narcan)	0.01 mg/kg		

*The use of pancuronium with fentanyl, sufentanil, and remifentanil can help to decrease the incidence of bradycardia.

IV, Intravenous; *PO,* oral; *PR,* per rectum.

Analgesics—cont'd

Nonnarcotic Analgesics	
Drug	**Dose**
Ketorolac (Toradol)	0.4-1 mg/kg IV
Acetaminophen (Tylenol)	10-20 mg/kg PO 30-40 mg/kg PR
Acetaminophen (Ofirmev)	IV: 1000 mg every 6 hr or 650 mg every 4 hr (maximum, 4000 mg/day)
Ibuprofen (Caldolor)	IV: 400-800 mg every 6 hr (maximum, 3200 mg/day)

Induction Agents

Drug	Induction Dose	Maintenance	Comments
Thiopental (Pentothal)	5-6 mg/kg IV	0.5-2 mg/kg	
Methohexital (Brevital)	1-2 mg/kg IV (1% solution) 5-10 mg/kg IM (3.5% solution) 20-30 mg/kg PR (10% aqueous solution)		
Propofol (Diprivan)	2.5-3.5 mg/kg IV	125-300 mcg/kg/min	May cause bradycardia; pretreat with atropine or glycopyrrolate
Ketamine	1-3 mg/kg IV	0.5-1 mg/kg IV	Provides cataleptic, dissociative state with analgesia
	5-10 mg/kg IM		Pretreat with benzodiazepine to prevent hallucinations
Dexmedetomidine (Precedex)	1 mcg/kg given over 10 min	0.5-0.8 mcg/kg bolus plus 0.4 mcg/kg/hr infusion	
Fospropofol (Lusedra)	Standard: Initial IV dose 6.5 mg/kg Supplemental dose: 1.6 mg/kg For patients age >65 years or with severe systemic disease: Modified dose 75% of standard dose		

IM, Intramuscular; *IV*, intravenous; *PR*, per rectum.

Neuromuscular Relaxants

1. Introduction

a) Increases in ECF volume and the ongoing maturation of neonatal skeletal muscle and acetylcholine receptors affect the pharmacokinetics and pharmacodynamics of neuromuscular relaxants.

b) The effective doses of clinical neuromuscular blocking drugs in various age groups are listed in the following table.

Effective Doses (ED_{95}) of Clinical Neuromuscular Blocking Drugs (mcg/kg)

	Neonate	Infant	Child	Adult
Succinylcholine*	620	729	423	290
Atracurium	120	156-175	170-350	110-280
Vecuronium	47	42-47	56-80	27-56
Rocuronium	600	600	600	300
Pancuronium	—	55	55-81	50-70

*Should be used for emergency airway stabilization in children younger than 12 years. Not for routine intubation.

c) The neuromuscular junction is incompletely developed at birth, maturing after 2 months of age. Skeletal muscle, acetylcholine receptors, and the accompanying biochemical processes essential in neuromuscular transmission mature during infancy into childhood.

d) The presynaptic release of acetylcholine is slowed compared with in adults, which explains the decreased margin of safety for neuromuscular transmission in neonates. The acetylcholine receptors of newborns are anatomically different from adult receptors, which may explain the sensitivity of neonates to the nondepolarizing class of neuromuscular relaxants.

e) This neuromuscular immaturity may be demonstrated with the appearance of fade after tetanic stimulation in the absence of neuromuscular blocking drugs.

2. Succinylcholine

a) Because succinylcholine contains acetylcholine moieties, its IV administration will reproduce the effects of acetylcholine when it interacts with nicotinic and muscarinic receptors, provoking both sympathetic and parasympathetic cardiovascular responses.

b) Stimulation of the parasympathetic ganglia or direct stimulation of cardiac muscarinic receptors produces sinus bradycardia, junctional rhythms, unifocal premature ventricular contractions, and ventricular fibrillation.

c) The prior administration of atropine 0.02 mg/kg will block cardiac muscarinic receptors and minimize the decreases in heart rate.

d) Dysrhythmia is more common in children, particularly after repeated doses in the presence of hypoxia or a concurrent electrolyte imbalance.

e) Myoglobinemia may occur in up to 20% of children who receive IV succinylcholine.

f) The prior administration of a small dose of a nondepolarizing neuromuscular blocking drug will modify the degree of myoglobinuria.
g) Myalgia is common after succinylcholine administration.
h) Succinylcholine is a known triggering agent for the development of malignant hyperthermia.
i) Neonates are more resistant to the effects of succinylcholine than children and adults. This sensitivity is illustrated by the effective dose in 95% of the population (ED_{95}) for neonates (620 mcg/kg), infants (729 mcg/kg), children (423 mcg/kg), and adults (290 mcg/kg).
j) The increase in dose requirement is in part a result of the increased volume of distribution within the large extracellular compartment.
k) Plasma cholinesterase activity is reduced in neonates; however, the duration of action after a single dose is of expected duration (6-10 minutes). A longer duration of action after a single bolus dose suggests the presence of an inherited deficiency of plasma cholinesterase activity.
l) IM succinylcholine may facilitate endotracheal intubation in children without suitable IV access. Because of the increased volume of distribution, a larger dose is required to achieve satisfactory relaxation. Although a dose of 3 mg/kg will produce satisfactory relaxation in 85% of patients, an IM dose of 4 mg/kg in the deltoid muscle will provide skeletal muscle relaxation in all, with a duration of action of up to 21 minutes.
m) To attenuate the effects of succinylcholine at both the nicotinic and muscarinic receptors, atropine at a dose of 0.02 mg/kg may be combined in the same syringe with the calculated dose of succinylcholine or in an additional syringe, which is administered in a selected muscle group before succinylcholine administration.
n) Unexpected cardiac arrest has been reported after the routine administration of succinylcholine, with fewer than 40% of patients successfully resuscitated.
o) Succinylcholine should not be routinely used for airway management in children younger than 8 years of age.

Nondepolarizing Neuromuscular Blocking Agents

1. **Introduction**
   a) Infants and children are more sensitive than adults to the effects of nondepolarizing neuromuscular blocking drugs.
   b) A lower plasma concentration of the selected neuromuscular relaxant is required to achieve the desired clinical level of neuromuscular blockade.
   c) This does not imply that the selected dosage should be decreased because infants have a greater volume of distribution.
   d) The larger volume of distribution and slower drug clearance result in longer half-life elimination, decreasing the need for repeated drug dosing (longer dosing intervals).
   e) Neuromuscular function monitoring must be used to guide repeated administration of these drugs in all pediatric patients.
   f) The selection of a nondepolarizing neuromuscular relaxant should take into consideration the desired degree and duration of skeletal muscle paralysis, the immaturity of organ systems, and the associated side effects of the selected relaxant.

2. **Atracurium**
   a) An intermediate-acting neuromuscular relaxant that is metabolized by nonspecific esterases and spontaneous breakdown of the parent compound by Hofmann elimination.
   b) Cisatracurium also uses Hofmann elimination and nonspecific ester hydrolysis for the metabolism of the parent compound.
   c) The duration of action of atracurium is relatively the same as in adults.
   d) The volume of distribution is greater in infants, yet the clearance is more rapid. Accordingly, an intubating dose (0.5 mg/kg) may be administered in infants and children with the same expected duration of action.
   e) Atracurium (intubating dose, 0.5 mg/kg; maintenance dose, 0.2-0.3 mg/kg) and cisatracurium (intubating dose, 0.1 mg/kg; maintenance, dose 0.08-0.1 mg/kg) may be the drugs of choice for the infant because these drugs are independent of mature organ function for elimination.
3. **Vecuronium**
   a) Vecuronium produces minimal alterations in cardiovascular function and stimulates the release of histamine.
   b) Infants are more sensitive to the effects of vecuronium than children (ED_{95} 0.047 vs. 0.081 mg/kg).
   c) Vecuronium may be administered as a continuous infusion at a rate of 0.8 to 1 mcg/kg/min.
4. **Rocuronium**
   a) An intermediate-acting neuromuscular blocker with a rapid to intermediate onset of 60 to 90 seconds after an intubating dose of 0.6 mg/kg.
   b) The potency of rocuronium is greater in infants than children; however, its onset is faster in children.
   c) Unlike vecuronium, rocuronium in intubating doses may produce transient increases in heart rate.
   d) Skeletal muscle relaxation can be maintained with repeat doses of 0.075 to 0.125 mg/kg.
   e) In clinical situations in which IV access is not available, rocuronium may be administered intramuscularly. Acceptable intubating conditions in lightly anesthetized infants occurs 2.5 to 3 minutes after a deltoid IM dose of 1000 mcg/kg and within 3 minutes after 1800 mcg/kg in children.
   f) The onset of action approximates the onset of succinylcholine after IM injection.
   g) Rocuronium injection into the deltoid provides a faster onset of twitch and ventilatory depression than does injection into the quadriceps muscle group.
   h) A disadvantage of this route of administration is the accompanying prolonged duration of relaxation—in excess of 60 minutes.
   i) Rocuronium may also be administered by continuous infusion at doses of 0.004 to 0.016 mg/kg/min.
5. **Antagonism of neuromuscular blockade**
   a) Residual neuromuscular blockade places infants and children at risk of hypoventilation and the inability to independently and continuously maintain a patent airway.
   b) Because of increased basal oxygen consumption, impaired respiratory function will lead to arterial oxygen desaturation and CO_2

retention. The resulting acidosis will potentiate residual neuromuscular blockade.

c) Accordingly, infants and children must have neuromuscular function restored at the conclusion of the surgical procedure. The detection of residual neuromuscular blockade requires the integration of clinical criteria and the assessment of neuromuscular blockade via a peripheral nerve stimulator.

d) Conventional doses of the anticholinesterase inhibitors (50-60 mcg/kg of neostigmine or 500-1000 mcg/kg of edrophonium) combined with appropriate doses of atropine or glycopyrrolate are acceptable for antagonism of nondepolarizing neuromuscular blockade.

e) Useful clinical signs of successful antagonism of neuromuscular blockade include the ability to flex the arms, lift of the legs, and flex the thighs upon the abdomen, providing evidence of the return of abdominal muscle tone, in addition to the return of a normal train-of-four response as assessed by the peripheral nerve stimulator.

f) Neonates are capable of generating a negative inspiratory force of -70 cm H_2O with the first few breaths after birth.

g) An negative inspiratory force of at least -32 cm H_2O has been found to correspond with leg lift, which is indicative of the adequacy of ventilatory reserve required before tracheal extubation.

h) Clinical investigation is ongoing in examining a novel antagonist of neuromuscular blockade. Sugammadex, a water-soluble, modified γ-cyclodextrin, is being investigated as a reversal of steroidal neuromuscular blocking agents.

i) The drug does not affect acetylcholinesterase, eliminating the need for the co-administration of an anticholinergic.

j) The application of Sugammadex for antagonism of neuromuscular blockade in the pediatric population is being studied.

k) Muscle relaxant reversal: See the following table.

Muscle Relaxant Reversal

Drug	Dose
Neostigmine	0.03-0.07 mg/kg
Pyridostigmine (Regonol)	0.2 mg/kg
Edrophonium	0.7-1.4 mg/kg
Atropine	0.01-0.02 mg/kg
Glycopyrrolate (Robinul)	0.01 mg/kg

C. PEDIATRIC ANESTHESIA EQUIPMENT

1. Introduction

The child's age, weight, and proposed surgical procedure guide the selection of essential pediatric anesthesia equipment. The anesthesia workroom should be appropriately stocked with a variety of sizes of masks, airways, LMAs, laryngoscope blades, ETTs, ETT stylets, blood pressure cuffs, pulse oximeter probes, calibrated pediatric fluid sets, syringe pumps for the delivery of both fluids and drugs, an assortment of IV catheters, tape, and arm boards.

2. **Airway equipment**
   a) The pediatric face mask is designed to fit the smaller facial features of children and eliminate mechanical dead space.
   b) Contemporary masks are manufactured from transparent plastics and have a soft, inflatable cuff that sits on the face.
   c) The transparent feature allows continuous observation of skin color, the presence of condensation from ventilation exhalation, and the appearance of gastric contents in case vomiting occurs.
3. **Oral and nasal airways**
   a) Appropriately sized oral airways must be readily available. Because of infants' relatively large tongues, the pediatric airway is predisposed to airway obstruction after the induction of general anesthesia.
   b) Oral airways that are too large may produce airway obstruction, inhibit venous and lymphatic drainage, and subsequently produce macroglossia, creating further airway compromise.
   c) The oral airway should be inserted with the aid of a tongue blade, displacing the tongue toward the floor of the mouth to allow smooth insertion of the airway.
   d) Insertion and rotation of an oral airway in children 5 to 10 years old should be performed with caution because the insertion or rotation may dislodge loose deciduous teeth.
   e) Nasal airways are infrequently used in children younger than 1 to 2 years of age. The internal diameter of the nasal airway may unnecessarily increase the work of breathing. Adenoid hypertrophy may make nasal airway placement difficult and produce severe epistaxis.
4. **Endotracheal tubes**
   a) The goal of ETT selection is the placement of an appropriately sized tube that allows controlled ventilation but minimizes laryngeal or tracheal injury.
   b) Because of patient variability, many formulas exist for the determination of the correct ETT size and for the depth of insertion. Despite countless practitioner recommendations, there is no agreed upon standard formula.
   c) In addition, many practitioners fail to appreciate the differences in the internal diameter of small ETTs. ETTs for neonates are sized by the internal diameter, yet the external diameters may differ by as much as 0.9 mm among manufacturers in tubes with identical internal diameters.
   d) The approximate size of ETT for children 2 years of age and older may be determined with the following formula: $16 + \text{Age} \div 4$.
   e) To accommodate the variability in patient airway size, ETTs one-half size larger and one-half size smaller should be immediately available.
   f) The depth of ETT insertion from the dental alveoli may be estimated using the "1, 2, 3, 4/7, 8, 9, 10" rule. For example, the ETT is inserted to a depth of 7 cm in a neonate weighing 1 kg and to a depth of 8 cm in a 2-kg neonate.
   g) Another approximate method is to insert the ETT to a depth in centimeters three times the internal diameter of the ETT in millimeters. For example, a 3-mm ETT should be inserted to a depth of 9 cm.
   h) Uncuffed ETTs are marked distally with a double black line that provides a visual indication of the depth of the ETT.

i) During intubation, the ETT is passed until the double black line has reached the level of the vocal cords.
j) Regardless of formula or technique used for assessing the depth of an ETT, the method for confirming placement is auscultation of bilateral breath sounds.
k) The table below provides approximate sizes of ETTs, suction catheters, and laryngoscope blades for preterm infants through 12-year-old children.

Estimation of Endotracheal Tube Size by Age

Endotracheal tube size	**28-34 Wk**	**Newborn**	**6 Mo**	**1 Yr**	**2 Yr**
	1.5-3	3	4	4	4.5-5
	4 Yr	6 Yr	8 Yr	10 Yr	12 Yr
	5-5.5	**5.5-6**	**6-6.5**	**6.5 cuffed**	**6.5-7 cuffed**
Suction catheter (Fr)	**28-34 Wk**	**Newborn**	**6 Mo**	**1 Yr**	**2 Yr**
	6-8	8	10	10	10
	4 Yr	6 Yr	8 Yr	10 Yr	12 Yr
	14	**14**	**14**	**14**	**14**
Laryngo-scope blade	**28-34 Wk**	**Newborn**	**6 Mo**	**1 Yr**	**2 Yr**
	0	0-1	1	1.5	1.5
	4 Yr	6 Yr	8 Yr	10 Yr	12 Yr
	2	**2**	**2**	**2-3**	**2-3**

l) If resistance is encountered with laryngeal advancement of the ETT, the ETT should be withdrawn and an ETT a half size smaller in internal diameter should be selected.
m) After proper placement is confirmed, the anesthesia provider should listen over the child's mouth (preferably with the aid of a stethoscope) while simultaneously squeezing the reservoir bag and noting the pressure at which an air leak is appreciated.
n) Positive-pressure ventilation may be ineffective when an air leak is detected at 8 to 10 cm H_2O.
o) A large or tight-fitting ETT that does not permit a detectable air leak until 25 to 30 cm H_2O may be too tight at the level of the cricoid cartilage and may result in postintubation laryngeal edema ("croup").
p) The selected uncuffed or cuffed ETT should have a demonstrable air leak detected at 20 to 25 cm H_2O.
q) Specialized uncuffed and cuffed oral and nasal ETTs may be chosen for otolaryngologic, ophthalmologic, and dental procedures.
r) The uncuffed ETT is a common choice in infants and neonates provided there is an accepted leak.
s) When an unacceptable leak occurs, for instance in a child about to undergo laparoscopy, a cuffed tube may be selected (a half size smaller than the previously selected tube) to minimize repeat laryngoscopies and the cuff inflated, allowing for a leak up to but no greater than to 25 cm H_2O.

t) Newer research has demonstrated that the use of cuffed ETTs (a half size smaller than a correctly calculated tube) has not resulted in an increased incidence in laryngotracheal edema or postextubation croup.

5. **Laryngeal mask airway**
   a) The LMA is used for short surgical procedures that do not require endotracheal intubation (herniorrhaphy, peripheral extremity surgical procedures) or resuscitation situations.
   b) The LMA is available in sizes specific for neonates, infants, children, and adolescents, as shown in the following table.

Laryngeal Mask Airway Sizes

Laryngeal Mask Airway Size	Suggested Inflation Volume	Patient Weight Guidelines (kg)
1	4 mL	Neonates: Up to 5 kg
1½	7 mL	Infants: 5-10
2	10 mL	Infants and children: 10-20
2½	14 mL	Children: 20-30
3	20 mL	30-50
4	30 mL	50-70
5	40 mL	70-100

From Brain AIJ, Denman WT, Goudsouzian NG. *LMA-Classic and LMA-Flexible Instruction Manual.* San Diego: LMA North America; 2011.

   c) The inflation of the pharyngeal cuff can produce undue pressure on pharyngeal structures. Similar to the case in an adult ETT cuff, the LMA cuff may be expanded during the course of the anesthetic procedure with the administration of nitrous oxide.
   d) The initial volume of air injected into the laryngeal cuff may be regulated by identifying the amount of air and airway pressure that produces an audible leak. This pressure is generally between 15 and 25 cm H_2O.
   e) Removal of the LMA in pediatric patients can be associated with biting, pulmonary edema, severe laryngospasm, and separation of the tube from the pharyngeal mask.

6. **Pediatric breathing circuits**
   a) The ideal pediatric breathing circuit should be lightweight, minimize dead space, consist of low resistance and a low compressible volume, be adaptable for both spontaneous and controlled ventilation, be capable of providing humidification and warming of inspired gases, and permit the collection and scavenging of exhaled anesthetic gases.
   b) For children with decreased minute ventilation (recent opioid administration or high concentrations of potent inhalation agent), fresh gas flow rates may need to be increased or ventilation controlled.
   c) The circle breathing system is the most common anesthetic gas delivery system, and technological advancements in anesthesia machine design have decreased the resistance imparted by the absorbent canisters and the one-way inspiratory and expiratory valves.

d) The breathing tubing for the pediatric circle systems is a smaller diameter than the adult tubing and has a lower compression volume, allowing accurate delivery of desired tidal volumes.
e) The circle breathing system is characterized by the presence of CO_2 absorbent canisters and a total of three valves (a one-way inspiratory valve, a one-way expiratory valve, and a pop-off or pressure-limiting [APL] valve) that directs exhaled gas to the scavenging system.
f) Advantages of the circle system include the conservation of potent inhalation agents, the ability to retain both heat and humidity, and the ease of collecting and scavenging waste gases.
g) The reservoir bag contains the anesthesia machine–delivered anesthetic mixture inspired by the patient and serves as a visual and tactile monitor of ventilation.
h) Reservoir bags range in size from 0.5 to 6 L. The selected reservoir bag must be appropriate for the patient's size (i.e., capable of containing a volume in excess of the child's inspiratory capacity).
i) The use of an inappropriately small reservoir bag may restrict respiratory efforts, and the use of a large reservoir bag inhibits the ability to use the reservoir bag as a monitor of ventilation.

D. PERIOPERATIVE CARE

Pediatric Preoperative Preparation

1. Introduction

The preoperative evaluation may take place during a scheduled clinic visit days or weeks before, but is typically accomplished the morning of, and occasionally within minutes before, the scheduled operative procedure. The current time constraints of preoperative evaluation may disrupt the surgical schedule with cancellations for the medically unprepared or for those who are acutely ill. Fortunately, the majority of pediatric surgical patients are in good health (American Society of Anesthesiologists classes I and II). Accordingly, the preoperative evaluation is generally straightforward.

2. Review of systems

a) Appropriate anesthetic evaluation and management depend on a thorough understanding of the surgical and anesthetic requirements for the proposed procedure. All possible sources of medical information, including the patient chart, physical examination of the child, and the parental or guardian interview are essential.
b) The review of the chart should focus on the medical history (beginning with the gestational history), previous hospitalizations, previous medical or surgical experiences, the presence of chronic illness or infectious disease, and any family history of anesthetic complications (e.g., family history of atypical pseudocholinesterase).
c) The child should also be evaluated for proper growth and development as determined by a review of norms and percentages for age and gender. Developmental delay may suggest a prenatal pathologic condition, the presence of a chronic illness, or the presence of a concurrent neurologic or neuromuscular disease.
d) The examination of any previous anesthetic records is invaluable in gleaning information regarding previous anesthetic encounters.

e) The parent or guardian verifies information obtained during the chart review during the face-to-face interview and physical examination of the child.
f) The physical examination allows the anesthesia provider to evaluate the child's general health. If not previously evaluated, the child's ears and nose should be examined.
g) Children between the ages of 5 and 9 years should be examined for the presence of loose teeth, and these should be noted on the evaluation. A loose deciduous tooth that is in danger of being dislodged during airway management should be removed after anesthetic induction with the consent of a parent.

3. **Preoperative laboratory testing**
   a) Preoperative laboratory tests should be ordered based on abnormal findings from the medical history and physical examination.
   b) Preoperative hemoglobin determination has characteristically been obtained to provide an assessment of "anesthetic fitness." An "adequate" hemoglobin concentration is essential for oxygen delivery and has been arbitrarily defined as a hemoglobin of 10 g/dL or a hematocrit of 30%. The determination of an acceptable value requires an understanding of the child's current medical history, the proposed surgical procedure, and an understanding of global oxygen transport and use. The value of a "routine" hemoglobin determination has been questioned for some time and rarely has been found to affect the anesthetic management of children.
   c) Children who benefit from preoperative hemoglobin determinations include premature infants less than 60 weeks of postconceptual age, children with concurrent cardiopulmonary disease, children with known hematologic dysfunction (sickle cell disease), and children in whom major blood loss is anticipated during the surgical procedure.
   d) The time constraints of preoperative evaluation hinder the child's psychological preparation, which has ostensibly become the responsibility of the parent or guardian and the surgeon. Children's exhibited behavior is age dependent and shaped by fears of parental separation, postoperative pain, the potential for disfigurement, and loss of control. Children during the first 6 months of age readily accept strangers and can be separated from their parents, but children from 6 months to 5 years of age become distressed when separated from their parents.
   e) Parental preparation is important. One of the most important tasks is allaying the fear of the parent and family members. The anesthesia provider will foster trust and confidence through a courteous and understandable explanation of the anesthetic experience. Parental anxiety may be driven by personal past anesthetic experiences, such as painful IV catheter placement; coerced mask induction; and postoperative pain, nausea, and vomiting.
   f) Parents offer invaluable information regarding their child's past anesthetic experiences. When the child appears for a repeat surgical procedure, the parents may have important information relative to "what works" and may be helpful in detailing a successful approach.
   g) Parental presence during anesthetic induction in preschool-aged and young children may allay the fears of separation for both the parent and child.

4. **Preoperative fasting**
   a) Guidelines for preoperative fasting are listed in the following table.

Preoperative Fasting Recommendations*

Ingested Materials	Minimum Fasting Period† (hr)
Clear liquids‡	2
Breast milk	4
Infant formula‡§	6
Nonhuman milk§	6
Light meal¶	6

*These recommendations apply to healthy patients who are undergoing elective procedures. They are not intended for women in labor. Following the guidelines does not guarantee complete gastric emptying.
†The fasting periods noted apply to all ages.
‡Examples of clear liquids include water, fruit juices without pulp, carbonated beverages, clear tea, and black coffee.
§Because nonhuman milk is similar to solids in gastric emptying time, the amount ingested must be considered when determining an appropriate fasting period.
¶A light meal typically consists of toast and clear liquids. Meals that include fried or fatty foods or meat may prolong gastric emptying time. Both the amount and type of foods ingested must be considered when determining an appropriate fasting period.
From American Society of Anesthesiologists Committee. Practice guidelines for preoperative fasting and the use of pharmacologic agents to reduce the risk of pulmonary aspiration: application to healthy patients undergoing elective procedures: an updated report by the ASAC on Standards and Practice Parameters. *Anesthesiology*. 2011; 114(3):495-511.

   b) Prolonged fasting may produce irritability as a result of thirst and hunger. Prolonged fasting may also alter fluid balance, producing preinduction hypovolemia and hypoglycemia.
   c) Hypoglycemia is especially problematic in premature infants. Preoperative access to clear fluids (e.g., apple juice, water) 2 hours before anesthetic induction has been shown to have a minimal impact on the resultant gastric volume and pH.

5. **Preoperative controversies**
   a) Upper respiratory infection
      (1) Upper respiratory infections (URIs) are common in the pediatric age group; are seasonal in occurrence; and may be accompanied by cough, pharyngitis, tonsillitis, and croup.
      (2) Children with an active or resolving URI have increased airway reactivity, a propensity for the development of atelectasis and mucous plugging of the airways, and the potential to experience postoperative arterial hypoxemia.
      (3) Bronchial reactivity may persist for 6 to 8 weeks after a viral lower respiratory tract infection, although this fact has been challenged by experts.
      (4) The presence of chronic respiratory disease (asthma or bronchopulmonary dysplasia) requires a thorough assessment to ensure that the disease is well controlled and the child is not currently experiencing an exacerbation.
      (5) The anesthesia provider must understand the child's routine pharmacologic management. A history of steroid use necessitates consideration of steroid supplementation throughout the perioperative period.

(6) Healthy children who are scheduled for the placement of tympanostomy tubes frequently have rhinitis. In deciding whether to proceed with anesthesia, additional patient history must be obtained to differentiate between a chronic allergic or an acute infectious presentation and to determine whether there is lower airway involvement.

(7) The assessment of the color and the duration of nasal drainage will assist in deciding whether rhinorrhea is chronic or acute. Purulent nasal discharge associated with pharyngitis, cough, or fever may indicate a bacterial or viral URI.

(8) Additional information may be obtained by questioning the parents regarding their assessment of the child's current health. Helpful questions include: Does your child appear sick? Is your child eating, sleeping, and playing normally? Is there anyone in the family (including siblings) who is currently ill? Children with chronic allergic rhinorrhea who exhibited a clear nasal drainage without accompanying signs of illness (no cough, pharyngitis, wheezing, or associated fever) are probably in satisfactory condition for elective general anesthesia with no imposed increased risk.

(9) Lower respiratory tract dysfunction typically accompanies viral or bacterial URI. This combination may be associated with a greater frequency of laryngospasm (fivefold greater incidence) and bronchospasm (10-fold greater incidence) during anesthetic management, particularly when endotracheal intubation is performed.

(10) Although mild URI may be inconsequential during the intraoperative period, significant problems may develop in the immediate postoperative period. Studies have noted an increase in the incidence of postintubation croup, hypoxemia, and bronchospasm in patients with URIs compared with asymptomatic children.

(11) Multiple factors must be considered when one is deciding whether to cancel an elective procedure. Children with signs and symptoms of acute airway dysfunction should have further medical evaluation by a pediatrician. A white blood cell count of 12,000 to 15,000/mm^3 suggests the presence of infection, and the surgery should be canceled. Clearly, elective surgery should be postponed for children who have a cough and pharyngitis accompanied by fever and wheezing.

(12) Current recommendations for patients with URI infections are listed in the box on pg. 505.

b) Heart murmur

(1) The parent may relay a previous history of a heart murmur, or a murmur may be discovered during the physical examination. A heart murmur may be detected in up to 50% of pediatric patients.

(2) It is important to properly classify the murmur as either innocent or pathologic before anesthetic intervention. The murmur may not impose a functional limitation; however, this may change with the physiologic stress associated with an anesthetic.

(3) Children with "functional" murmurs are generally asymptomatic without the presence of cyanosis and are growing appropriately. An example of a functional murmur is the Still

Recommendations for Patients with Upper Respiratory Tract Infections

These recommendations are neither clinical guidelines nor a consensus statement and should not replace clinical judgment, but they should serve as a guide to help make a rational decision with parents, surgeons, and patients. Efforts should make parents aware of the problems with respiratory tract infections and anesthesia, and parents should be encouraged to call before the day of surgery to discuss the symptoms and possible need for delay of surgery. There may be a role for pediatricians and other primary care practitioners to play in the process of perioperative evaluation and education.

- First, an emergency case mandates judicious airway management and logically must proceed regardless of the presence or absence of respiratory symptoms. In patients presenting for elective (nonurgent) surgery, initial consideration should be with respect to the severity of respiratory tract symptoms.
- Acute symptoms, such as runny nose and cough, must be differentiated from chronic symptoms related to underlying diseases such as allergic rhinitis (clear runny nose) and asthma (cough).
- Often careful questioning of parents can differentiate acute from chronic symptoms.
- Patients with severe symptoms such as fever (>38.4° C), malaise, productive cough, wheezing, or rhonchi should be considered for delay of elective surgery. A reasonable period of delay would be 4 to 6 weeks.
- If mild symptoms are present, such as nonproductive cough, sneezing, or mild nasal congestion, then surgery could proceed for those having regional or general anesthesia without endotracheal tube placement. However, patients who require endotracheal tube placement for anesthesia (especially children younger than 1 year of age) should be considered carefully for other risk factors such as passive smoke exposure and underlying conditions (e.g., asthma, chronic lung disease) because they may benefit from a slight delay of 2 to 4 weeks.

Modified From Easley RB, Maxwell LG. Should a child with a respiratory tract infection undergo elective surgery? In Fleisher LA, ed: *Evidence-based practice of anesthesiology.* Philadelphia: Saunders; 2004:424.

vibratory systolic murmur, which is common in children between the ages of 2 and 6 years.

(4) If the heart murmur has been previously detected and the child has undergone an evaluation, the parent may be able to provide the information as to the relevance of the murmur. Previous records may also contain information as to the significance and whether additional testing was performed to assess the physiologic significance.

(5) It is important that a pediatrician or cardiologist evaluate previously undiagnosed murmurs before the induction of anesthesia.

6. Premedication

a) The selection and administration of premedication for pediatric patients require an understanding of the desired goals, the planned surgical procedure (inpatient or outpatient procedure), the familiarity and previous experiences with the particular drug, and the availability of nursing staff to monitor the child after the drug's administration.

b) The ideal premedicant should be dependable with a rapid and reliable onset and offset and should be devoid of undesirable effects.
c) The commonly prescribed pediatric premedicants are listed in the following table.

Commonly Prescribed Pediatric Premedicants—Premedicant Dose and Route of Administration

Anticholinergics	
Atropine	0.02 mg/kg PO, IV, or IM
Glycopyrrolate	0.01 mg IV
Opioids	
Morphine sulfate	0.1-0.3 mg/kg IM
Meperidine	1.5-2 mg/kg PO
	1-2 mg/kg IM
Benzodiazepines	
Diazepam	0.1-0.5 mg/kg PO
Midazolam	0.05-0.1 mg/kg IM
	0.2 mg/kg nasally
	0.025-0.05 mg/kg IV
	0.25-0.5 mg/kg PO
	0.5-1 mg/kg PR
Barbiturates	
Methohexital (10%)	10 mg/kg IM
	20-30 mg/kg PR
Other	
Ketamine	3-6 mg/kg PO
	3 mg/kg nasally
	2-10 mg/kg IM

IM, Intramuscular; *IV,* intravenous; *PO,* oral; *PR,* rectal.

7. **Monitoring**
   a) Patient blood pressure and heart rate are monitored for the assessment of the cardiovascular system.
   b) Pulse oximetry and capnography are used for the assessment of the adequacy of oxygenation and ventilation, a temperature probe for intermittent or continuous assessment of core body temperature, and a neuromuscular function monitor for the evaluation of the child's response to the administration of neuromuscular blocking drugs.
   c) A precordial or esophageal stethoscope should be used for the continuous assessment of heart rate during anesthetic induction and throughout the perioperative period.
   d) Some circumstances require the application of arterial and central venous pressure monitoring. Small multilumen catheters are available for pediatric patients. These catheters are advantageous when large blood losses are expected (e.g., during burn débridement and skin grafting). However, these catheters have long, thin lumens that may severely limit the rate at which IV fluid or blood may be administered.

e) When rapid flow is required, a peripheral IV line may be used for maintenance and deficit fluid replacement, and a single-lumen venous catheter placed within the femoral vein may be reserved for colloid and blood administration.

8. **Anesthetic induction**
   a) Mask induction is the most popular and is easily accomplished in infants younger than 8 months of age, as well as in children.
   b) The essential monitoring modalities for inhalation induction include a precordial stethoscope and a pulse oximeter.
   c) Anesthetic induction is begun with a 70:30 mixture of nitrous oxide and oxygen via mask or a "cupped hand" that is placed on the child's chin with the anesthetic mixture directed toward the mouth and nose.
   d) A pacifier may quiet the infant during the induction, or the infant may suck on the end of the anesthesia provider's gloved finger. Sevoflurane is added to the nitrous oxide–oxygen mixture beginning with a 2% concentration, with a rapid increase to 8%.
   e) The mask may then be introduced as the inspired concentration is increased. The anesthesia provider should await the return of respiration and avoid the temptation to administer a breath because this may produce coughing and laryngospasm.
   f) Unconsciousness is produced with inspired sevoflurane concentrations 6% to 8%. After the loss of consciousness, nitrous oxide is discontinued, and sevoflurane is administered in 100% oxygen. Because of the low blood gas solubility coefficient and rapid uptake, the choice to use nitrous oxide is provider specific.
   g) At this time, the anesthesia provider should begin to assist respiration and promptly decrease the inspired anesthetic concentration of sevoflurane to 2% to 2.5%. Controlled ventilation with high-inspired concentrations of inhalation agent aggravates myocardial depression, precipitating the development of sudden cardiac arrest.
   h) During assisted ventilation, IV access should be established. The age of the child, proposed surgical procedure, and ease of airway management during induction are the determining factors for whether to proceed with IV access.
   i) For elective surgical procedures, neonates may be managed with a 24-gauge catheter, infants with a 22-gauge catheter, and children with a 20-gauge catheter.
   j) Surgical procedures with expected large third-space fluid loss or blood loss require an additional IV catheter. Preferred sites for IV access include the nondominant upper extremity (dorsum of the hand, antecubital fossa) and the lower extremity (dorsum of the foot, saphenous vein).
   k) After the establishment of IV access, preparations are made for endotracheal intubation. Intubation may be accomplished using the inhaled anesthetic agent without muscle relaxation or subsequent to the administration of a nondepolarizing neuromuscular relaxant.
   l) The administration of a neuromuscular relaxant decreases the potential for the cardiovascular depression that accompanies the administration of high concentrations of inhalation agents that may be required to facilitate laryngoscopy and intubation.

m) Whatever method is selected, the inhalation agent should be discontinued immediately before laryngoscopy. This practice minimizes the contamination of the operating room with free-flowing inhalation agent from the patient breathing circuit, and, more importantly, the delivery of high inspired anesthetic concentrations is avoided immediately after intubation during the confirmation of ETT placement. After confirmation, the ETT is secured and the position of the tube at the alveolar ridge or lip is noted on the anesthetic record.

9. **Parental presence during anesthetic induction**
   a) Children older than 1 year of age may have difficulty with parental separation and may require premedication to ease their anxiety.
   b) In addition to preoperative medication, a new strategy some anesthetic departments have adopted is to have one parent present for anesthetic induction. Parents prefer to stay with their children during diagnostic procedures such as bone marrow biopsy, immunization, dental rehabilitation, and the induction of anesthesia.
   c) Anesthesia departments may have age limitations, not allowing parental presence for children less than 12 to 18 months of age. Clearly, the parent should not be invited to participate in the induction of a child with a "full stomach" or compromised airway.

10. **Intravenous induction**
    a) IV induction is generally reserved for children with an existing IV line. An IV induction may be clinically indicated when a child has a full stomach or a history of gastroesophageal reflux.
    b) IV induction is quicker and more dependable, facilitating the rapid securing of the airway with endotracheal intubation.
    c) Venipuncture can be a frightening experience for needle-phobic child. Oral premedication with midazolam before the child enters the operating room may be beneficial to decrease the child's anxiety and gain his or her cooperation.
    d) The pain associated with preoperative IV access may be eased with the subcutaneous injection of local anesthetic via a 30-gauge needle. Additional analgesia may be provided by the administration of a 50:50 mixture of nitrous oxide and oxygen during venipuncture.
    e) The administration of concentrations in excess of 50% may produce significant disorientation and muscle rigidity, impeding the ability to obtain IV access.
    f) The timely application of a eutectic mixture of local anesthetic also minimizes the pain of venipuncture. Suitable IV sites are identified preoperatively and marked with an ink pen. The eutectic mixture of local anesthetic is applied well in advance (30-60 minutes) to ensure effectiveness and covered with a Tegaderm dressing.

11. **Intramuscular induction**
    a) On rare occasions, an intramuscularly administered drug may be required in uncooperative children or in children who refuse alternative routes (oral, nasal, or rectal) for premedication.
    b) Ketamine produces dose-dependent unconsciousness and analgesia, and the child may appear to be in a catatonic state.
    c) Parents who witness the administration of ketamine should be warned that their child might exhibit spontaneous involuntary movements and nystagmus.
    d) Ketamine is a cardiac stimulant that produces an increase in systemic blood pressure and heart rate. Additional undesirable effects

include bronchodilation, increases in intraocular and intracranial pressure, disorientation, unpleasant dreaming, and hallucinations.

e) The psychogenic effects may be decreased with the concomitant administration of a benzodiazepine. IM ketamine in a dose of 2 to 3 mg/kg facilitates inhalation induction in children who are reluctant to be subjected to inhalation induction or venipuncture.
f) Ketamine doses between 5 and 10 mg/kg are associated with a lengthy recovery period and the inability to accept oral fluids.
g) Ketamine may be injected in a small volume because a variety of formulated concentrations exist. Ketamine is particularly advantageous in children with cardiovascular instability because the cardiovascular system is stimulated via the CNS.
h) Intramuscular (IM) midazolam may be used to induce sleep. IM midazolam (0.1-0.15 mg/kg) may also be used as a premedicant. IM induction is less reliable and more uncomfortable for the child.

E. PEDIATRIC AIRWAY MANAGEMENT

1. The normal pediatric airway

There are important anatomic and physiologic differences between the adult and pediatric airway, as noted in the following table.

Differences Between the Adult and Pediatric Airway

	Pediatric	Adult
Laryngeal location	C2-C4	C4-C6
Narrowest location of airway	Cricoid	Glottis
Shape of epiglottis	Omega shaped	V-shaped
Right mainstem bronchus	Less vertical	More vertical
Tongue	Relatively larger	Relatively smaller
Cricoid	Conical shape	Cylindrical shape
Head	Pronounced occiput	Flatter occiput

a) These factors interact to maintain pharyngeal airway patency.
b) The infant larynx is located in a more cephalad position (C3-C4 interspace) achieving the adult position (C5) by 6 years of age. This position allows infants to swallow and breathe simultaneously.
c) The epiglottis is described as omega or U shaped, is short and stiff, and projects posteriorly at a 45-degree angle, which increases the difficulty of vocal cord visualization.
d) Because of these anatomic differences, the use of a straight laryngoscope blade placed into the vallecula improves visualization of the glottic opening.
e) The infant tongue is significantly larger in relation to the oral cavity, increasing the size and volume of soft tissue within the oral cavity.
f) There is a smaller submental space for displacement of the tongue during laryngoscopy.
g) Unlike neonates and infants, children have an increase in oropharyngeal tissue with the appearance and hypertrophy of the tonsil and adenoids between the ages of 2 and 7 years.

h) The size of the tongue and the position of the epiglottis increase the difficulty of mask ventilation.
i) Because of the more cephalad laryngeal position, the tongue lies closer to the palate and easily occludes it, producing upper airway obstruction. This explains why neonates and small infants are obligate nose breathers.
j) Attempted mask ventilation of an infant may be unsuccessful until the mouth is opened and the tongue is swept away from the palate.
k) These anatomic differences also make the airway appear more anterior during laryngoscopy. Various pediatric oral airways sizes should be immediately available before the administration of sedatives or the induction of general anesthesia.
l) The infant head and occiput are large relative to the shoulders and upper body. With slight head extension and a small towel placed under the shoulders, the alignment of the pharyngeal and laryngeal axis can be improved, and the infant will assume a proper intubating position.
m) The maintenance of a neutral head position is more helpful than an exaggerated head tilt.
n) Because of the higher position of the infant larynx and the larger occiput, the traditionally applied "sniffing" position may actually hinder glottic visualization.
o) A thorough dental evaluation should be conducted. Loose teeth should be suspected between 5 and 12 years of age.

2. Laryngospasm

Laryngospasm is a magnified glottic closure reflex in response to noxious stimuli of the superior laryngeal nerve and may persist despite the immediate removal of the stimuli. Laryngospasm precipitates a host of serious complications, including complete airway obstruction, gastric aspiration, postobstruction pulmonary edema, cardiac arrest, and death.

a) Etiology: The incidence of laryngospasm may be greater in the pediatric population because of specific practices in the anesthetic management of infants and children. Several factors generally associated with the development of laryngospasm are listed in the following box.

Risk Factors for Laryngospasm

Preoperative Factors

Exposure to secondhand tobacco smoke
Concurrent or recent upper respiratory tract infection
Gastroesophageal reflux
Mechanical irritants (oropharyngeal secretions)

Intraoperative Factors

Excitement phase of inhalation induction
Tracheal intubation or extubation during "light" anesthesia
Upper airway surgical procedures (tonsillectomy, adenoidectomy, nasal or sinus procedures, palatal procedures, laryngoscopy or bronchoscopy)

The risk of laryngospasm is increased on induction when airway instrumentation is attempted before an adequate depth of anesthesia has been achieved, without the benefit of neuromuscular blocking drugs, and in infants and children with residual effects of previous URIs.

b) Prevention of laryngospasm: The prevention of laryngospasm requires an understanding of the risk factors. Measures that may be undertaken for the prevention of laryngospasm are listed in the following box.

Preventive Measures for Laryngospasm

- Avoid noxious airway or surgical stimulation during "light" anesthesia.
- Ensure sufficient anesthesia before airway instrumentation.
- Apply topical lidocaine to suppress laryngeal sensory nerve activity.
- Administer intravenous lidocaine before extubation.
- Suction the oral pharynx before extubation.
- Perform tracheal extubation when fully awake.
- Administer 100% oxygen for 3 to 5 minutes before extubation.

c) Clinical management
  (1) Incomplete airway obstruction may be evident as "grunting" or audible inspiratory and expiratory sounds as heard through a precordial stethoscope accompanied by tracheal tug and thoracoabdominal asynchrony. A decrease in arterial oxygen saturation may also occur.
  (2) Management of laryngospasm on induction of anesthesia consists of three essential processes. First, the responsible noxious stimuli should be discontinued (surgical stimulation, attempted airway instrumentation during "light" anesthesia, removal of pharyngeal secretions with gentle suctioning). Next, anesthetic depth should be increased by the delivery of increased concentration of inhalation agent or the IV administration of a small dose of propofol. Third, gentle positive-pressure ventilation using 100% oxygen should be attempted using a properly applied face mask with concurrent airway opening maneuvers (slight head extension, chin lift and jaw thrust). On occasion, this may require two individuals, one to firmly apply the face mask and open the airway and one individual to attempt positive-pressure ventilation.
  (3) The transition to complete airway obstruction becomes evident with the absence of inspiratory and expiratory sounds, as well as the inability to deliver positive-pressure ventilation. Further deterioration of arterial oxygen saturation with accompanying bradycardia may occur despite the continued application of positive-pressure ventilation, which may not be effective. The administration of succinylcholine is then required to break the laryngospasm.
  (4) If complete airway obstruction continues unabated, the IV or IM administration of atropine and succinylcholine should be administered without delay.
  (5) In the absence of IV access, IM succinylcholine (4 mg/kg) and atropine (0.02 mg/kg) are administered in the deltoid or gluteus maximus muscle. After IM administration, the vocal

cords will begin to relax within 60 seconds, permitting positive-pressure ventilation and relaxation to facilitate endotracheal intubation.

(6) With continued deterioration in arterial oxygen saturation, intubation may be required before the onset of skeletal muscle relaxation. In an extreme situation, the application of lidocaine to the vocal cords may produce sufficient relaxation, allowing endotracheal intubation.

(7) The direct application of pressure to the laryngospasm notch, the space located immediately behind the ear, bounded anteriorly by the mandibular rami, posteriorly by the mastoid process, and cephalad by the base of the skull is advocated by some practitioners. Bilateral firm and direct application of pressure toward the skull base produces an anterior displacement of the mandible. In addition to producing a jaw thrust, the intense stimulation with postcondylar pressure in a lightly anesthetized patient often produces a ventilatory sigh. This maneuver may be successful for the treatment of laryngospasm.

3. **The difficult pediatric airway**
   a) A difficult airway may be defined as difficulty in accomplishing mask ventilation or endotracheal intubation. The identification of a difficult pediatric airway begins with a thorough history followed by physical examination of the mouth, head, and neck.
   b) A history of snoring, difficulty breathing with feeding, current or recent URI, and history of croup should be obtained.
   c) Previous anesthetic records are an invaluable resource in determining the history of difficult airway management. However, a prior uneventful anesthetic does not preclude the possibility of difficulty of airway management with succeeding anesthetics.
   d) The physical examination should focus on the assessment of craniofacial skeletal features, specifically the size and shape of the mandible

Pediatric Airway Pathologic Conditions

Nasopharynx
Choanal atresia
Foreign body or tumors
Adenoid hypertrophy

Tongue
Hemangioma
Angioedema
Down syndrome
Beckwith-Wiedemann syndrome
Mucopolysaccharidosis
Cystic hygroma
Lacerations

Skeletal Structure
Pierre Robin syndrome
Treacher Collins syndrome
Goldenhar syndrome
Fractures
Juvenile rheumatoid arthritis
Cervical spine injury
Mandibular ankylosis
Arnold-Chiari malformation

Pharynx and Larynx
Laryngeal web
Laryngeal stenosis
Laryngomalacia
Laryngeal papillomatosis
Foreign body
Postintubation croup (laryngotracheal edema)
Epiglottitis
Peritonsillar abscess
Retropharyngeal abscess

and maxilla, the size of the tongue in relation to the oral cavity, the absence of dentition, the presence of loose dentition, and the range of motion of the neck.

e) The pathologic conditions that affect pediatric airway management are listed in the box on pg. 512.

4. Classification

After the completion of the history and physical examination, the pediatric patient may be classified into one of four categories based on the noted airway pathology and degree of respiratory distress.

a) *Category I.* These individuals have a normal-appearing airway and minimal or no sternal retractions with an age-appropriate respiratory rate and normal arterial oxygen saturation.

b) *Category II.* These individuals presents with moderate airway distress or significant airway disease (e.g., laryngeal papillomatosis). The anesthetic history demonstrates previous successful airway management.

c) *Category III.* The delineating characteristic of this group is an abnormal airway identified by physical examination (micrognathia, macroglossia, palate deformities, or prominent dentition). Individuals with maxillary or mandibular pathology (e.g., Treacher Collins syndrome, Down syndrome) are grouped here. Included in this group are individuals with mediastinal mass.

d) *Category IV.* Individuals in this category have significant respiratory distress exemplified by marked sternal retractions, significantly decreased arterial oxygen saturations, and marked increases in respiratory rate that may ultimately lead to respiratory fatigue. An example is the pediatric patient presenting with an inhaled foreign body.

5. Anesthetic technique

a) This is often best accomplished in a controlled environment (operating suite) with general anesthesia and the presence of surgical expertise to obtain a surgical airway should there be an inability to provide mask ventilation.

b) For individuals who are category I and II, an inhalation induction with sevoflurane, with the application of continuous positive airway pressure (5-10 cm H_2O) minimizes soft tissue obstruction and pharyngeal collapse with increasing depths of anesthesia. After confirmation of the ease of positive-pressure ventilation and acceptable arterial oxygen concentration—then and only then—should a neuromuscular relaxant be administered to facilitate endotracheal intubation.

c) Individuals who are category III and IV require advanced preparation for airway management and require the immediate availability of surgical expertise during airway management.

d) Airway adjuncts, including size-appropriate LMAs, oral airways, various laryngoscope blades, video laryngoscopes, flexible fiberoptic bronchoscopes, or any other difficult airway adjunct requested, should be immediately available. A flexible fiberoptic bronchoscope with an external diameter of 2.2 to 4.0 mm will traverse a 2.5- to 4.5-mm internal diameter ETT. These individuals are best managed with spontaneous ventilation.

e) A slow and deliberate inhalation induction is accomplished with sevoflurane. The administration of a neuromuscular relaxant should be avoided because total airway obstruction may follow with the loss of pharyngeal and laryngeal tone.

F. PEDIATRIC INTRAVENOUS FLUID AND BLOOD THERAPY

1. Introduction

a) Intravascular fluid balance is influenced by a number of preoperative and perioperative circumstances. Preoperative IV fluid administration minimizes the degree of dehydration that accompanies the NPO (nothing by mouth) period. Unless there exists a compelling reason to place an IV catheter preoperatively, IV therapy is generally avoided in pediatric patients until general anesthesia has been induced via inhalation.

b) Perioperative fluid homeostasis is altered by a number of factors, including inhalation agent administration, surgical trauma, and preoperative fasting.

c) Potent inhalation agents produce peripheral vasodilation and varying degrees of myocardial depression, decreasing systemic blood pressure and end-organ perfusion.

d) Dehydration after prolonged preoperative oral fluid abstinence aggravates these decreases in systemic blood pressure.

e) The delivery of cold, dry anesthetic gases via an ETT bypasses normal anatomic humidification, increasing the loss of fluid from the respiratory tract. These insensible respiratory fluid losses can be minimized with the use of active or passive humidification systems during the intraoperative period.

f) General anesthesia modifies the neuroendocrine control of fluid balance. Surgical stress increases plasma glucose levels. Hyperglycemia induces an osmotic-induced renal loss of free water.

g) Anesthetic agents modify neuroendocrine regulation of fluids and electrolytes.

h) Surgical trauma modifies fluid balance, the degree of which depends on the invasiveness of the surgical procedure and potential blood loss.

i) IV fluids are used to replace intraoperative blood loss and fluid loss resulting from fluid shifts that develop from evaporative and third-space fluid losses. Physiologic parameters, such as heart rate, blood pressure, capillary refill time, urine output, and ongoing blood loss, are continually assessed. In addition, it is essential to monitor and accurate estimated blood loss because pediatric patients do not tolerate excessive loss well.

j) The rate of intraoperative fluid administration is continuously modified to maintain circulatory homeostasis. Peripheral surgical procedures (extremity procedures) have minimal evaporative or third-space fluid losses. However, intracavitary procedures (intraabdominal or intrathoracic procedures) are associated with greater blood loss, third-space fluid loss, and substantial evaporative fluid losses that approach 10 mL/kg of body weight per hour.

k) When administering fluids to pediatric patients younger than 2 years of age, one should consider use of a Buretrol and or IV fluid pump to avoid excess fluid administration.

2. Pediatric fluid compartments

a) The growth of newborns is accompanied by a decrease in the relative fluid compartment volumes of TBW and ECF volumes during the first year of life followed by additional decreases in ECF later in childhood.

b) Whereas the TBW of premature infants is as high as 80% of total body weight, the TBW of term infants is approximately 70% to 75% of total body weight. The adult value of TBW (55%-60%) is reached between 6 months and 1 year of age.

3. **Maintenance fluid calculation**

a) The most direct and widely accepted method for determining IV fluid requirements is based on body weight.

b) The hourly maintenance fluid level is determined by the "4-2-1" formula and is calculated as shown in the following tables.

Hourly Fluid Requirements: the "4-2-1" Formula

Weight (kg)	Fluid
0-10	4 mL/kg/hr for each kilogram of body weight
10-20	40 mL + 2 mL/kg/hr for each kilogram >10 kg
>20	60 mL + 1 mL/kg/hr for each kilogram >20 kg
Sample Calculated Fluid Requirements	**Maintenance Fluid per Hour**
4 kg	16 mL
9 kg	36 mL
15 kg	50 mL
30 kg	70 mL

Fluid Replacement

Weight = 8 kg	Hour 1	Hour 2	Hour 3
Maintenance fluid (mL/hr)	32	32	32
Deficit (mL/hr)	96	48	48
Hourly total (mL)	128	80	80

c) Preoperative fluid deficits develop during the period of time in which the child has not received oral or IV maintenance fluids.

d) The preoperative fluid deficit is calculated by determining the hourly maintenance fluid rate and multiplying this rate by the number of hours the child has been without IV or oral intake.

e) The calculated fluid deficit is replaced following the guidelines wherein half of the fluid deficit is replaced during the first hour with the remainder divided in half and replaced over the course of the subsequent 2 hours.

f) In addition to the calculated maintenance and deficit fluids necessary to replace insensible fluid losses, additional IV fluid is required to replace third-space fluid losses that occur with surgical trauma. Lactated Ringer's solution, 0.9% normal saline, and Plasmalyte are acceptable for the replacement of insensible and third-space fluid losses at the rate of 1 to 2 mL/kg/hr.

g) Expected third-space fluid losses can be categorized as minimal surgical trauma (an additional 3-4 mL/kg/hr), moderate surgical trauma (5-6 mL/kg/hr), and major surgical trauma (7-10 mL/kg/hr).

4. **Glucose-containing solutions**
   a) Most anesthesia providers administer a glucose-free IV solution (lactated Ringer's solution) for maintenance fluid administration in the replacement of third-space and intraoperative blood loss.
   b) If the child has had an extended NPO period, a plasma glucose level may be determined at the time of IV catheter insertion after inhalation induction.
   c) Hypoglycemia is likely to develop in a variety of clinical circumstances. Examples include infants who are premature, infants of mothers with diabetes, children with diabetes who have received a portion of daily insulin preoperatively, and children who receive glucose-based parenteral nutrition.
   d) A glucose-containing IV solution is administered to these patients as a controlled piggyback infusion with frequent plasma glucose determinations performed to avoid hyperglycemia.
   e) Infants born of mothers with diabetes and infants of mothers who receive glucose-containing solutions during labor may require a continuation of these solutions for the prevention of rebound hypoglycemia.
   f) Premature infants who have had less time to store glycogen in the liver than term infants are more susceptible to hypoglycemia. For this reason, premature infants may receive an infusion of 5% dextrose in 0.2% normal saline.
5. **Crystalloid intravenous fluids**
   a) Crystalloid IV solutions are advantageous for perioperative administration because they are the least expensive of the available IV solutions and are acceptable for the replacement of preoperative, intraoperative, and postoperative isotonic fluid deficits. Unlike colloid solutions, crystalloid solutions do not produce allergic reactions.
   b) Crystalloid IV solutions can be further subdivided by their tonicity in relation to plasma (hypotonic, isotonic, or hypertonic).
6. **Estimation of blood volume**
   a) The intravascular volume may be estimated by multiplying the child's weight by the estimated blood volume.
   b) The estimated blood volumes are as follows: premature infants, 90 to 100 mL/kg; full-term newborns, 80 to 90 mL/kg; infants age 3 months to 3 years, 75 to 80 mL/kg; and children older than 6 years, 65 to 70 mL/kg. For example, the estimated blood volume of a 6-month-old infant who weighs 7 kg is 525 mL (7 kg × 75 mL/kg = 525 mL).
   c) Ongoing surgical blood loss requires frequent reassessment of the child's physiologic responses. Moderate to severe decreases in intravascular volume produce tachycardia, hypotension, narrowed pulse pressure, low urine output, decreased central venous pressure, pallor, and slow capillary refill.
   d) A sudden decrease in blood pressure in neonates and infants with rate-dependent cardiac output is indicative of significant intravascular volume depletion.
7. **Allowable blood loss**
   a) Allowable blood loss must be defined individually for each patient based on current medical condition, surgical procedure, and cardiovascular and respiratory function.

b) Children with normal cardiovascular function may tolerate a lower hematocrit and may compensate with an increased cardiac output if a higher inspired oxygen concentration is provided to improve oxygen delivery. An exception is premature infants.
c) The incidence of apnea is higher in neonates and premature infants with hematocrit levels below 30%. The anesthesia provider, surgeon, and neonatologist should agree on a target hematocrit level, and this discussion should be documented in the medical record.
d) The allowable blood loss may be calculated by means of the following formula:

$$\text{MABL} = \frac{\text{EBV} \times (\text{Child's hematocrit} - \text{Minimum accepted hematocrit})}{\text{Child's hematocrit}}$$

An example for a 6-month-old infant who weighs 7 kg with a starting hematocrit of 35% and the selection of the lowest acceptable hematocrit of 25%, we calculate the following:

$$\text{MABL} = \text{maximum allowable blood loss}$$

$$H_5 = \text{starting hematocrit}$$

$$H_A = \text{allowable hematocrit}$$

$$\text{EBV} = \text{estimated blood volume}$$

$$\text{MABL} = (H_5 - H_A)(\text{EBV})$$

$$\text{EBV} = 7 \times 80 = 560\ H_5$$

$$\text{MABL} = (35 - 25)(560)$$

$$\text{MABL} = 35$$

$$\text{MABL} = 160\ \text{Ml}$$

e) Blood loss may be replaced with suitable crystalloid solutions (0.9% normal saline, lactated Ringer's solution) by administering 3 mL for each milliliter of blood loss.
f) Blood loss that is less than the calculated permissible blood loss may be replaced with colloid (1 mL for every milliliter of blood loss).
g) When the blood loss equals or exceeds the calculated allowable loss, transfusion should be considered. Before transfusion is performed, a current hemoglobin and hematocrit should be obtained. The surgeon should be included in the decision process. These discussions and the resultant hemoglobin and hematocrit are recorded in the anesthetic record.
h) The volume of packed red blood cells (PRBCs) to be infused may be determined by the following formula:

$$\text{PRBC} = \text{MABL} \times \text{Desired Hct}$$

$$\text{Hct of PRBC}_s \text{ (range, 60\%-80\%)}$$

i) Blood loss in excess of one blood volume can lead to coagulopathies and a reduction in clotting factors. Platelets, fresh-frozen plasma, and cryoprecipitate should be considered.

8. Blood transfusion

a) Before blood component therapy is initiated, the proper equipment (filters, infusion devices, blood warming devices) should be obtained and tested.

b) Standard blood transfusion sets contain a 170- to 200-μm filter. Microaggregate filters (20-40 μm) may be placed between the blood-dispensing bag and the filtered infusion set, although no studies prove these filters to be of benefit over the standard 170- to 200-μm filter.

c) Infusion pumps (syringe or piston driven) selected for the infusion of blood and blood products should be licensed for this function by the manufacturer. An excessive infusion rate can produce RBC lysis.

d) Blood should be warmed before infusion and used with an appropriate blood-warming device such as a Hotline fluid warmer. The selected blood component containers may be placed under the forced-air warming blanket or the measured aliquot of blood drawn into a syringe may be warmed with the hand. Syringes should not be placed into water baths because bacterial contamination may occur.

e) The blood bank can dispense small aliquots of blood into a calibrated syringe or provide 50- to 100-mL bags of the selected blood product transferred from an assigned donor unit.

f) Blood used for neonatal transfusion is preferably less than 1 week old to preserve 2,3-diphosphoglycerate levels and irradiated to prevent graft-versus-host disease. When PRBCs are transfused, the blood should not be diluted before transfusion because this may contribute to hypervolemia.

G. PEDIATRIC REGIONAL ANESTHESIA

1. Introduction

a) Regional anesthesia provides perioperative analgesia (minimizing the risk of respiratory depression), modifies the metabolic responses to anesthesia and surgery, and improves patient outcome.

b) Pediatric patients generally receive a peripheral or centrally administered regional anesthetic after the induction of general anesthesia. The inherent fear of needles and pain, the fear of neurologic injury in a combative child, and the difficulty in providing adequate sedation to ensure patient mobility during the introduction of the block often necessitates the safe execution of the regional anesthetic during general anesthesia.

c) Regional anesthetic procedures in children should be performed only by anesthesia providers with previous training, demonstrated skill in adult regional anesthetic procedures, and knowledge of the appropriate applications of each technique in the pediatric population.

d) Caudal anesthesia is a frequently used residual anesthetic technique that provides analgesia for lower abdominal, genital, urinary and lower extremity procedures.

e) The detection of intravascular injection in the child during the concurrent administration of inhalation agents has been the subject of several studies. Infants may have a greater risk of amide local anesthetic toxicity because of their decreased levels of AAG.

f) The routine administration of epinephrine-containing test doses of local anesthetics may be counterproductive during the concurrent administration of myocardial depressant drugs.

H. GENITOURINARY PROCEDURES

1. **Introduction**
   a) A cystoscopy is usually a brief procedure, allowing for administration of general anesthesia by a mask or LMA.
   b) Hypospadias repair, chordee release, and repair of undescended testicles are usually performed with the patient under general anesthesia with an ETT secured. If the testicle cannot be located directly, an intraabdominal approach with muscle relaxation may be required.
2. **Preoperative assessment and patient preparation**
   a) History and physical examination
      (1) Review systems to determine the presence of comorbidities.
      (2) Laboratory tests: As indicated by the history and physical examination
      (3) Diagnostic tests: As indicated by the history and physical examination
   b) Patient preparation: Administer midazolam, 0.5 mg/kg orally 30 minutes before the procedure, if desired.
3. **Room preparation**
   a) Monitoring equipment is standard.
   b) Additional equipment includes warming devices for prolonged procedures.
   c) Position: Supine for orchiopexy, chordee release, and hypospadias repair; lithotomy position for cystoscopy. Pad all pressure points and maintain proper body alignment to prevent nerve and soft tissue injuries.
   d) A standard pediatric tabletop is used.
   e) IV fluids: Depending on the patient's age and size, a 22- or 24-gauge catheter should be sufficient. Infuse 0.9% normal saline or lactated Ringer's solution at a rate of 2 to 4 mL/kg/hr. Additional fluid may be needed to replace fluid deficit and blood loss.
4. **Perioperative management and anesthetic technique**
   a) Mask induction with oxygen, nitrous oxide, and sevoflurane. If the patient has a preexisting IV line established, an IV induction is indicated. Muscle relaxation may be used if desired for intubation purposes, but it is not required for the procedure.
   b) Obtain a protected airway with an appropriately sized ETT. Ensure proper placement and secure with tape.
   c) Maintenance: Oxygen, nitrous oxide, and sevoflurane, halothane or isoflurane with an IV fluid rate as calculated. Maintain normothermia. Manipulation of the testicles or peritoneum may produce a profound vagal response. Pretreat with atropine or glycopyrrolate may be warranted. Caudal anesthesia prevents this response. If bradycardia occurs and is refractory to atropine, treat with a fluid bolus (10-20 mL) or epinephrine (10-20 mcg) intravenously.
   d) Emergence: Extubate when the patient is awake.

5. **Postoperative implications**
   a) Pain is a possible complication.
   b) Opioids may increase the incidence of nausea and vomiting.
   c) Caudal anesthesia is appropriate in children younger than 7 years old and may be performed after induction or before emergence to decrease volatile agent requirements or before emergence.

I. HERNIA REPAIR

1. **Introduction**

Inguinal hernia repair is the most common procedure performed in children. Premature infants are more likely to have incarcerations, mostly from failure of the processus vaginalis to obliterate. The procedure is performed through an inguinal crease incision. Complications of hernia repairs are rare. Umbilical hernias are more common in African Americans and may close spontaneously (95%-98% by age 5 years). Repair is performed through a transverse infraumbilical incision. Intraperitoneal exploration is rarely done.

2. **Preoperative assessment and patient preparation**
   a) History and physical examination
      (1) Cardiac: Routine assessment
      (2) Respiratory: Patients with prolonged ventilation or immature lungs are more susceptible to tracheomalacia, subglottic stenosis, and bronchopulmonary dysplasia.
      (3) Neurologic: Premature infants may display transient apneic and bradycardic episodes in response to hypoxemia. Premature infants are more prone to seizure disorders. Complications from general anesthesia may occur from effects on the immature CNS.
      (4) Renal: Routine assessment
      (5) Gastrointestinal: The patient may have abdominal compression if the umbilical hernia is large. Consider rapid-sequence induction for incarcerated hernia and bowel obstructions.
      (6) Endocrine: Premature infants are more prone to hypoglycemia. Check frequently blood glucose level.
   b) Patient preparation
      (1) Laboratory tests: As indicated by the history and physical examination
      (2) Diagnostic tests: None
      (3) Medications: Midazolam, 0.5 mg/kg orally 30 minutes before surgery for children older than 1 year of age
3. **Room preparation**
   a) Monitoring equipment is standard.
   b) Additional equipment: Use a pediatric circle or Bain circuit. Warm and humidify gases. A warming pad may be used on the table.
   c) Position: The patient is supine.
   d) Fluids: 0.9% normal saline or lactated Ringer's solution. Dextrose solutions may be used for infants younger than 1 month old.
   e) Blood loss is negligible.
4. **Perioperative management and anesthetic technique**
   a) General anesthesia with an ETT is required if laparoscopic hernia repair is to be accomplished.

b) General anesthesia, mask, or ETT. Caudal block may be performed after induction for postoperative pain and provides approximately 6 to 12 hours of pain relief postoperatively.

c) Induction: Mask or endotracheal intubation with halothane or sevoflurane, oxygen, or nitrous oxide. Obtain an IV line after induction. Administer atropine intravenously (0.02 mg/kg) before laryngoscopy, vecuronium (0.1 mg/kg), or cisatracurium (0.1 to 0.2 mg/kg). If applicable, perform a caudal block with bupivacaine (0.25%) 1 mL/kg after induction (onset of 15 minutes).

d) Maintenance: Caudal block will decrease the amount of volatile agent. Increase the MAC before incision to avoid laryngospasm.

e) Stretching or traction of the inguinal structures can cause mild, moderate, or severe bradycardia

f) Emergence: Extubate when the patient is fully awake. IV reversal is with neostigmine (0.07 mg/kg) and glycopyrrolate (0.01 mg/kg) is required.

5. Postoperative implications

Postoperative apnea can occur in infants at 50 to 60 weeks of gestational age, especially if they are premature. These patients should be admitted for postoperative observation for at least 24 hours.

J. MYRINGOTOMY

1. Introduction

Myringotomy is a common outpatient procedure in children. Myringotomy is usually associated with the insertion of ventilation tubes into the tympanic membrane as a treatment for recurrent otitis media.

Typically, a small incision is made with the use of a microscope in the tympanic membrane, and fluid is suctioned through a transcanal approach.

2. Preoperative assessment

Other than a history of frequent and recurrent otitis media, this patient population is generally healthy.

a) History and physical examination

(1) A careful family history should be obtained preoperatively, including any history of family problems with anesthesia.

(2) Respiratory: Many pediatric patients presenting for myringotomy have a history of frequent URIs. Each patient must be evaluated on an individual basis. Because the removal of middle ear fluid usually resolves the frequent URIs, surgery should not be delayed because of symptoms of URI. Instead, it is recommended to place the patient on supplemental oxygen in the postoperative period. It is controversial whether these patients have an increased increased risk of hyperactive airways and laryngospasm.

(3) Dental: Inspection of the airway and questioning of the parents should identify any loose teeth.

b) Patient preparation

(1) Laboratory tests: As indicated by the history and physical examination

(2) Diagnostic tests: As indicated by the history and physical examination

(3) Medications: Midazolam, 0.5 mg/kg orally, may be given with 20 to 30 mL of apple juice as a premedication. It is also available as an elixir.

3. Room preparation

a) Monitoring equipment is standard.

b) Additional equipment: None is needed.

c) Standard emergency drugs are used (including atropine, lidocaine, epinephrine, and succinylcholine).

d) Standard pediatric airway equipment.

e) IV fluids: Depending on the age of the patient, expected length of procedure, and history and physical findings, an IV catheter may be available for emergency use but is not started routinely. If necessary, use a 20- or 22-gauge peripheral catheter and normal saline or lactated Ringer's solution at 2 to 4 mL/kg/hr.

4. Perioperative management and anesthetic technique

a) Mask general anesthesia is usually adequate for uncomplicated myringotomy of otherwise healthy patients.

b) Induction: Mask inhalation induction with an inhalation anesthetic such as or sevoflurane, nitrous oxide, and oxygen. If an existing IV catheter is present, routine IV induction is appropriate. Routine IV induction is preferred in older children and adults.

c) Maintenance: Standard maintenance with halothane, sevoflurane or isoflurane, nitrous oxide, and oxygen. Muscle relaxation and opiates are not routinely used.

d) Emergence: The airway is maintained until the patient is fully awake. The patient should be placed in the lateral position while being transported to the recovery room. In older children and adults, antiemetics should be considered.

5. Postoperative implications

a) Nausea and vomiting can be treated with the following:

(1) Metoclopramide, 0.15 mg/kg/dose IV; maximum, 10 mg

(2) Ondansetron, 0.05 to 0.1 mg/kg/dose IV; maximum, 4 mg

b) These patients are often sensitive to sounds in the immediate postoperative period.

K. TONSILLECTOMY AND ADENOIDECTOMY

1. Introduction

Children may present for tonsillectomy or adenoidectomy with a history of recurrent infections (chronic tonsillitis) or a history of obstruction and sleep apnea.

2. Preoperative assessment and patient preparation

a) History and physical examination

(1) Cardiac: Echocardiography may be useful to determine the presence of right-sided heart failure from chronic airway obstruction. These patients are at increased risk for negative-pressure pulmonary edema and volume overload.

(2) Respiratory: Evaluate for potentially difficult airway management. If the child exhibits signs and symptoms of URI, there may be an increased risk of laryngospasm intraoperatively and postoperatively. The choice to cancel or proceed with surgery must be evaluated on an individual basis.

b) Patient preparation
   (1) Judicious use of preoperative medication in children with obstructive apnea
   (2) Midazolam, 0.5 mg/kg orally in children without obstruction
   (3) Antisialagogue is strongly recommended
   (4) Laboratory tests: As indicated by the history and physical examination
   (5) Diagnostic tests: As indicated by the history and physical examination

3. **Room preparation**
   a) Monitoring equipment: Standard
   b) Additional equipment: None
   c) Standard emergency drugs: Atropine, lidocaine, epinephrine, and succinylcholine
   d) Standard pediatric tabletop: ETTs (RAE or straight), laryngoscope blade and handle, oral airways, lubricant, gauze, and emergency drugs
   e) IV fluids: Depending on the age and size of the patient, a 22- or 24-gauge catheter is probably sufficient; infusion of normal saline or lactated Ringer's solution at 2 to 4 mL/kg/hr.
4. **Perioperative management and anesthetic technique**
   a) Mask induction is performed with oxygen, nitrous oxide, and sevoflurane.
   b) Obtain IV access; administer narcotic; give atropine as indicated; and administer muscle relaxant if desired (not necessary).
   c) Intubate with an appropriate-size ETT. Ensure correct placement by auscultation of breath sounds, movement of chest, and note the end-tidal CO_2 wave. Tape in the midline.
   d) An acetaminophen (Tylenol) suppository, 25 to 30 mg/kg, may be given at this point for postoperative pain control.
   e) A mouth gag will be inserted by the surgeon after the airway is secured. It is essential that a deep plane of anesthesia is achieved before insertion. Tube placement should be reconfirmed.
   f) Maintenance: Standard with a volatile agent, oxygen, and nitrous oxide. Muscle relaxation is not required. Opiates are given at induction.
   g) At the end of the case, reverse the remaining muscle relaxant if used. Carefully suction the stomach and oropharynx. Extubate when the patient is fully awake because of the increased risk of laryngospasm with the presence of blood in the airway. An alternative method is true deep extubation after patient initiates the first breath. Transfer the patient to the recovery unit in lateral-head down position so secretions do not pool in back of airway, thus increasing risk of laryngospasm.
5. **Postoperative implications**
   a) Nausea and vomiting can be treated with the following:
      (1) Metoclopramide, 0.15 mg/kg/dose; maximum, 10 mg.
      (2) Ondansetron, 0.01 to 0.5 mg/kg/dose; maximum, 4 mg, with or without dexamethasone.
   b) Pain
      (1) The severity of pain depends on the history of chronic infections and the surgical technique.
      (2) The site may be infiltrated with local anesthetic.

(3) Opioids may increase nausea and vomiting.
(4) Nonsteroidal anti-inflammatory agents are not recommended because of the increased risk of bleeding.
(5) Pain usually resolves in 7 to 10 days with sloughing of tissue.
(6) Admission to hospital may be required if pain prevents adequate oral intake.

c) Bleeding
(1) This occurs in first 6 hours postoperatively. Bleeding can occur immediately after surgery or can occur up to the sixth postoperative day.
(2) A bleeding tonsil that forces the patient to return to the operating room has several implications.
(a) The patient is hypovolemic: Establish IV access and infuse a balanced salt solution or lactated Ringer's solution.
(b) The airway may be compromised by the presence of blood and edema. Have an alternative plan for establishing a protected airway. The use of an ETT that is 0.5 mm smaller than the original tube is recommended because of the presence of edema.
(c) Plan rapid-sequence induction. The patient is considered to have a full stomach because of the presence of blood.

Neonatal Anesthetic Considerations

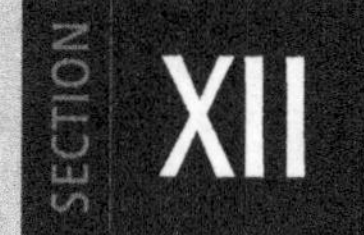

A. PREOPERATIVE ASSESSMENT

The perioperative management of any neonate is determined by the nature of the surgical procedure, the gestational age at birth, the postconceptual age at surgery, and associated medical conditions.

1. **Gestational age and postconceptual age at surgery**
   a) The gestational age and postconceptual age are critical to the determination of the physiologic development of the neonate. The history of the delivery and the immediate postdelivery course can influence the choice of anesthetic technique and assist in anticipating possible postoperative complications.
   b) Preterm neonates are classified as borderline preterm (36-37 weeks' gestation), moderately preterm (31-36 weeks' gestation), and severely preterm (24-30 weeks' gestation).
   c) Neonates can be classified according to their weight as well as their gestational age. Full term is considered to be 37 to 42 weeks' gestation.
   d) However, even full-term neonates who are small for gestational age (SGA) often present with conditions requiring surgical intervention. SGA neonates have different pathophysiologic problems from preterm infants (<37 weeks' gestation) of the same weight.
   e) Gestational age and neonatal problems are closely related. Maternal health problems also can have significant implications for preterm as well as full-term (even SGA) neonates.
   f) Several common maternal problems and the possible associated neonatal sequelae are listed in the following table.

Maternal History with Commonly Associated Neonatal Problems

Maternal History	Anticipated Neonatal Sequelae
Rh-ABO incompatibility	Hemolytic anemia Hyperbilirubinemia Kernicterus
Toxemia	Small birth weight and associated problems Muscle relaxant interaction after magnesium therapy
Hypertension	Small birth weight
Infection	Sepsis, thrombocytopenia, viral infection
Hemorrhage	Anemia, shock
Diabetes	Hypoglycemia, birth trauma, macrosomia, small birth weight
Polyhydramnios	TE fistula, anencephaly, multiple anomalies
Oligohydramnios	Renal hypoplasia, pulmonary hypoplasia
Cephalopelvic disproportion	Birth trauma, hyperbilirubinemia, fractures
Alcoholism	Hypoglycemia, congenital malformation, fetal alcohol syndrome, small birth weight

From Cote CJ, Ryan JF, Todres ID, ed. *A practice of anesthesia for infants and children.* Philadelphia: Saunders; 1993:41.

2. **Prematurity**
   a) Because of advances in neonatal medicine, many preterm babies born at exceptionally early gestational age and extremely low birth weights are surviving to be challenged with a plethora of unique diseases and pose many anesthetic challenges.
   b) Prematurity presents its own set of complications, which include anemia, intraventricular hemorrhage, periodic apnea accompanied by bradycardia, and chronic respiratory dysfunction.
   c) Postconceptual age (gestational age + postnatal age) should be determined at the time of the anesthetic evaluation. Premature infants of less than 60 weeks' postconceptual age have the greatest risk of experiencing postanesthetic complications.
   d) The manifestations of prematurity are thought to occur as a result of inadequate development of respiratory drive and immature cardiovascular responses to hypoxia and hypercapnia.
   e) Premature infants have a significant risk of postoperative apnea and bradycardia during the first 24 hours after general anesthesia.
   f) The contributing factors that may influence the occurrence of apnea in premature infants are listed in the following box.

Factors Contributing to the Incidence of Apnea in Premature Infants

Central Contributors
Inadequate development of respiratory centers
Incomplete myelination of central nervous system

Metabolic Contributors
Hypothermia
Hypoglycemia
Hypocalcemia
Acidosis

Anesthetic Contributors
Residual inhalation anesthesia
Residual opioid plasma concentrations
Residual neuromuscular blockade

From Aker J. Preoperative preparation of the pediatric patient: capsules and comments. *Nurse Anesth.* 1996;1:1.

3. **Apnea in premature infants**
   a) The incidence of apnea in the postoperative period is inversely related to postconceptual age and is most frequent in infants of less than 60 weeks of postconceptual age.
   b) Apnea may still occur when regional anesthetic techniques have been substituted for general anesthesia.
   c) Premature infants without a history of apnea or bradycardia may still experience postoperative apnea.
   d) Premature infants with histories of respiratory distress, concurrent respiratory disease, and periods of apnea are twice as likely to develop postoperative apnea.
   e) Concurrent anemia (hematocrit <30%) places additional risk for the occurrence of postoperative apnea.

f) Outpatient surgical care is usually not an acceptable venue for premature infants. Although the literature supports an increased risk for premature infants up to 60 weeks of postconceptual age, debate continues as to when this risk decreases.

g) Perioperative use of caffeine: The standard doses of caffeine and theophylline are 10 mg/kg and 6 mg/kg, respectively. Both have been shown to reduce the incidence of idiopathic apnea of prematurity and reduce the occurrence of apnea after surgery in premature infants.

4. **Preanesthetic assessment and neonatal anesthetic implications**
   a) Valuable information is obtained from those caring for the baby in the neonatal intensive care unit (NICU). It is often best to alter the infant's plan of therapy as little as possible (e.g., management of ventilation, acid-base status, and glucose). Consultation with the neonatologist is helpful.
   b) A maternal drug history is very important. In presence of illicit drugs, such as heroin and cocaine, the baby could be withdrawing from the drug at the time of surgery. Particularly with cocaine, there is an increased incidence of pulmonary hypertension and bowel perforation.
   c) Some mothers take large doses of aspirin or acetaminophen during pregnancy. Their infants could also exhibit pulmonary hypertension and persistent fetal circulation during the first few days of life.
   d) All of the information gathered during the assessment leads to the anesthetic plan based on the implications of all the transitioning body systems. The characteristics of the body system and the anesthetic implications are listed in the following table.

Preanesthetic Assessment and Neonatal Anesthetic Implications

System	Characteristics	Anesthetic Implications
CNS	Incomplete myelination	Judicious use of muscle relaxants
	Lack of cerebral autoregulation	Cerebral perfusion pressure control
	Cortical activity	Pain relief/adequate level of anesthesia
	ROP	Oxygen saturation (94%-98%)
	Respiratory	
Mechanical	↓ Lung compliance	Assist or control ventilation during G/A
	↓ Elastic recoil	
	↓ Rigidity of chest wall	
	↓ V̇/Q̇ caused by lung fluid	
	↑ Fatigue of respiratory muscles	
	↓ Coordination, nose or mouth breathing	Do not obstruct nasal passages

Continued

Preanesthetic Assessment and Neonatal Anesthetic Implications—cont'd

System	Characteristics	Anesthetic Implications
Anatomic	Breathing	
	Large tongue	At risk for obstruction
	Position of larynx, epiglottis, vocal folds, subglottic region	Anterior airway
Biochemical	Response to hypercapnia not potentiated by hypoxia	Avoid hypoxia Maintain normothermia
Reflex	Hering-Breuer reflex	Apnea or no desaturation
	Periodic breathing	Stimulation
	Apnea	Stimulation or airway support
Cardiovascular	↓ Myocardial contractility or ↓ myocardial compliance	Maintain adequate volume Maintain heart rate
	CO rate dependent	Use vagolytic agents
	Vagotonic	
	Limited sympathetic innervation	
	Reactive pulmonary vasculature	Avoid hypoxemia resulting in ↓ PBF and possible shunting
	PDA/FO shunting	
Renal	↓ GFR	Maintain vascular volume/CO
	↓ Tubular function	Avoid overhydration
	Low glucose threshold	Avoid excess glucose (0.5 to 1.0 g/kg)
Hepatic	Depressed hepatic enzymes	Judicious use of drugs metabolized by liver
	↓ Metabolism and clearance of drugs	
	Altered (decreased) protein binding	
	Hypoglycemia due to ↓ glycogen stores	
	Low prothrombin levels	Vitamin K (1 mg) before surgery
Hematologic	Fetal hemoglobin (does not readily release O_2 to tissues)	Avoid hypoxia
	Oxyhemoglobin curve shifted left	

CNS, central nervous system; *FO*, foramen ovale; *G/A*, general anesthesia; *PDA*, patent ductus arteriosus; *RPO*, retinopathy of prematurity; $\dot{V}/\dot{Q}$, ventilation/perfusion.

5. **System review and examination**
   a) When performing a physical assessment, one should look carefully for congenital anomalies. A rule of thumb is that if there is one anomaly present, there are probably more because many occur in clusters, labeled a syndrome.
   b) These problems can occur most often in SGA and large-for-gestational-age (LGA) neonates and should be analyzed and understood as listed in the box on pg. 529.

Common Metabolic and Structural Problems in Small- and Large-for-Gestational-Age Infants

Small for Gestational Age
- Congenital anomalies
- Chromosomal abnormalities
- Chronic intrauterine infection
- Heat loss
- Asphyxia
- Metabolic abnormalities (hypoglycemia, hypocalcemia)
- Polycythemia or hyperbilirubinemia

Large for Gestational Age
- Birth injury (brachial, phrenic nerve, fractured clavicle)
- Asphyxia
- Meconium aspiration
- Metabolic abnormalities (hypoglycemia, hypocalcemia)
- Polycythemia/hyperbilirubinemia

From Motoyama EK, Davis PJ, eds. *Smith's anesthesia for infants and children.* Philadelphia: Mosby; 2006:524.

6. **Head and neck abnormalities**
   a) Any abnormality of the head or neck should raise concerns regarding airway management. The shape and size of the head, with or without the presence of pathology, can make airway management difficult. A small mouth and large tongue can obstruct the airway during mask ventilation.
   b) Neonates have very small nares, and when obstructed by an anesthesia face mask, they do not convert to mouth breathing, particularly if the mouth is being held closed.
   c) A nasogastric tube can obstruct half of the neonate's airway and should be placed orally. A small or receding chin, as seen in Pierre Robin and Treacher Collins syndromes, may make direct laryngoscopy and visualization of the glottis impossible, requiring other types of airway management.
   d) Cleft lip, with or without cleft palate, may complicate intubation. Anomalies such as cystic hygroma or hemangioma of the neck can produce upper airway obstruction. In the case of a preterm neonate, it should also be determined if the patient has retinopathy of prematurity (ROP), cataracts, or glaucoma.
   e) Atropine administration could result in significant increases in intraocular pressure and further damage to the eye.
7. **Respiratory system abnormalities**
   a) Surfactant, which inhibits alveolar collapse, peaks between 35 and 36 of gestational age. Premature neonates are at dramatically increased risk for respiratory failure.
   b) The incidence of respiratory distress syndrome (RDS) and bronchopulmonary dysplasia (BPD) is inversely related to gestational age at birth.
   c) The onset of RDS can be as early as 6 hours after birth; symptoms include tachypnea, retractions, grunting, and oxygen desaturation.
   d) Bronchopulmonary dysplasia is a disease of newborns that manifests as a need for supplemental oxygen along with lower airway

obstruction and air trapping, carbon dioxide retention, atelectasis, bronchiolitis, and bronchopneumonia.

e) Oxygen toxicity, barotrauma of positive-pressure ventilation on immature lungs, and endotracheal intubation have been reported as causative factors. Management of the patient's oxygenation can be challenging.

f) Careful monitoring of the acid-base status and the use of increased peak inspiratory pressure and positive end-expiratory pressure (PEEP) may be needed to maintain oxygenation during surgery.

8. **Cardiovascular system abnormalities**

a) In evaluation of the neonate's cardiovascular system, several variables should be examined, including heart rate, blood pressure patterns, skin color, intensity of peripheral pulses, and capillary filling time.

b) The presence of a murmur or abnormal heart sound, low urine output, metabolic acidosis, dysrhythmias, or cardiomegaly, alone or in combination, raises the concern of some type of congenital heart lesion. These patients should be evaluated with chest radiography, electrocardiography (ECG), and echocardiography. The results of these diagnostic tests allow for effective planning of the anesthetic, decreasing the possibility of complications.

c) The common syndromes associated with cardiac defects are listed in the following table.

Syndromes Associated with Cardiac Defects

Syndrome or Malformation	Cardiac Defect	Other Associated Conditions
Beckwith-Wiedemann	Miscellaneous	Macroglossia, exomphalos, hypoglycemic
CHARGE syndrome	Tetralogy of Fallot, PDA, double outlet RV with AV canal, ASD, VSD	Choanal atresia, micrognathia, coloboma, cleft palate
Treacher Collins	Miscellaneous	Facial and pharyngeal hypoplasia, microsomia, cleft palate, choanal atresia
VACTERL	VSD	Vertebral anomalies, TEF, renal anomalies, imperforate anus, absent radius
Trisomy 21 (Down syndrome)	AV canal, ASD, VSD, PDA, TOF	Bowel atresia, large tongue, atlanto-axial instability
Trisomy 18 (Edwards syndrome)	VSD, PDA	Micrognathia, renal malformations
Trisomy 13 (Patau syndrome)	VSD, dextrocardia, ASD	Microcephaly, micrognathia, cleft lip and palate

ASD, atrial septal defect; *AV,* atrioventricular; *CHARGE,* coloboma of the eye or central nervous system anomalies, heart defects, atresia of the choanae, retardation of growth or development, genital or urinary defects, and ear anomalies or deafness; *PDA,* patent ductus arteriosus; *RV,* right ventricle; *TEF,* tracheoesophageal fistula; *TOF, Tetralogy of Fallot*; *VATERL,* vertebral anomalies, anal atresia, cardiac defects, tracheoesophageal fistula, renal abnormalities, and limb malformations; *VSD,* ventricular septal defect.

From Peutrell JM, Weir P. Basic principles of neonatal anesthesia. In Hughes DG, Mathes, S, Wolf A, eds. *Handbook of neonatal anesthesia.* London: Saunders; 1996:166.

d) Anesthetic implications of congenital heart disease in neonates include the following:
   (1) Direction and flow through any shunt
   (2) Baseline oxygenation
   (3) Dependence of the systemic or pulmonary circulation on flow through the ductus arteriosus also known as persistent fetal circulation.
   (4) The presence and size of any obstruction to blood flow
   (5) Heart failure (high output, low output, or hypoxic)
   (6) Drug therapy
   (7) Antibiotic prophylaxis against bacterial endocarditis

9. Central nervous system abnormalities

a) An assessment of the central nervous system (CNS) should include the status of the infant's intracranial pressure (ICP) and intracranial compliance.
b) Intraventricular hemorrhage (IVH) is almost exclusively seen in preterm babies; this occurs when there is spontaneous bleeding into and around the lateral ventricles of the brain.
c) The more preterm the neonate and the smaller the weight, the more likely one could find IVH.
d) The hemorrhage is usually the result of RDS, hypoxic-ischemic injury, or episodes of acute blood pressure fluctuation that rapidly increase or decrease cerebral blood flow. The classic example is laryngoscopy in the presence of inadequate anesthesia.
e) The symptoms of IVH include hypotonia, apnea, seizures, loss of sucking reflex, and a bulging anterior fontanel. Particular evaluation of a neonate with meningomyelocele (spina bifida) is discussed subsequently.

10. Preoperative laboratory studies

Neonates who are premature (<60 weeks of postconceptual age), those with concurrent cardiopulmonary disease, and babies in whom major blood loss is anticipated during the surgical procedure should have serial hematocrits, electrolytes, blood gases, glucose levels, and serum osmolality measured. The test values will assist in the fluid, electrolyte, and blood replacement during the surgical procedure.

11. Preoperative treatment of significance for anesthesia

Many of the preexisting conditions in neonates require medical treatment. Some of the preoperative drugs and their anesthetic implications are listed in the following table.

Preoperative Treatment of Significance for Anesthesia

Drug	Implication
Diuretics for heart failure, BPD	Hypokalemia
Digoxin for heart failure	ECG abnormalities
Steroids for BPD	Hyperglycemia
	Immunocompromised
Anticonvulsants	Cardiac arrhythmia
	Potent inducer of hepatic enzymes

Continued

Preoperative Treatment of Significance for Anesthesia—cont'd

Drug	Implication
Indomethacin	Increased risk of bleeding Displaced bilirubin from protein binding sites Transient hyponatremia Renal impairment
Theophylline or caffeine	Significant toxic side effects: convulsions, tachycardia, tremor
Prostaglandins E_1 or E_2	Ventilatory depression and apnea Hypotension Cerebral irritability Seizures Tachycardia Pyrexia
Tolazoline	Systemic hypotension Cardiac irritability Transient oliguria Increased gastric acid
Prostacyclin	Hypotension Inhibition of platelet aggregation Rebound PPHN with withdrawal

BPD, Bronchopulmonary dysplasia; *ECG,* electrocardiography; *PPHN,* persistent pulmonary hypertension of the newborn.

a) Parental preparation is important. In the case of institutions that do not have a NICU, the patient will have been transferred in from another institution, and the parents still may be in the institution where the baby was delivered.
b) It is imperative that the parents be prepared and the informed consent for anesthesia be obtained. Often this must be done via telephone or from the father, who may have accompanied the neonate to the NICU.
c) The anxiety of the parents of a newborn or neonate with a serious illness requiring surgical intervention is very high. The anesthesia provider fosters trust and confidence through a courteous and understandable explanation of the anesthetic experience.

B. REGIONAL ANESTHESIA IN NEONATES

1. **Introduction**
   a) Regional anesthesia in neonates is an acceptable option when the risks of complications during or after general anesthesia and endotracheal intubation are very high for anatomic or physiologic reasons.
   b) These techniques have allowed surgical procedures to be done on critically ill neonates under minimal general anesthesia, with considerable reduction in the need for CNS depressant drugs.
   c) An additional benefit to the use of regional anesthesia in this age group is postoperative pain control. The two most common techniques used in neonates are the spinal and caudal epidural blocks.

d) Anatomic differences in the neonate should be considered, particularly the location of the terminal end of the spinal cord, the dural sac, and the volume of cerebrospinal fluid (CSF).
e) The spinal cord extends as far as L3 in newborns and neonates and does not reach the adult position of L1 until 1 year of age. The dural sac extends to S3 to S4 in these babies and does not reach the adult position of S1 until approximately 1 year of age.
f) The volume of CSF is twice that of adults (4 mL/kg vs. 2mL /kg, respectively). This dilutes the local anesthetics injected and could explain the higher dose requirements and shorter duration of analgesia.
g) Bradycardia and hypotension are not often seen. It is thought that this could be because of the immature sympathetic nervous system or the proportionately small blood volume in the lower limbs, decreasing the amount of venous pooling.
h) The ventilatory response to the regional anesthetic is related to the level of the block. With a level as high as T2 to T4, there could be intercostal muscle weakness that requires the dependence on diaphragmatic movement for tidal breathing; however, tidal volume and respiratory rate are not usually affected.
i) There are pharmacologic considerations when regional anesthesia is used in neonates. The extracellular space is larger. This means the initial dose of local anesthetic is diluted into a larger volume of distribution, resulting in a lower initial plasma peak concentration.
j) Neonates have diminished concentrations of albumin and alpha acid glycoprotein, resulting in reduced protein binding of local anesthetics and significant increases in the concentration of free drug, which could increase the risk of CNS and cardiac toxicity.
k) Local anesthetics, particularly the amides, are broken down slower in newborns and neonates because of immature hepatic degradation. The major elimination pathway for ester local anesthetics is hydrolysis via plasma cholinesterases, and these levels are lower in neonates as well.
l) Demonstrations of the previous differences are shorter duration of blocks compared with adults and larger initial doses of local anesthetic per kilogram to achieve the same extent of blockade.
m) Most neonates have a regional technique performed after the induction of general anesthesia because of the age of the patient and the possibility of agitation and continuous movement affecting the placement and success of the block.
n) The possible complications of regional anesthesia in newborns and neonates that have been reported by several sources are neurologic injury caused by intraneural injection of local anesthetic and the decreased ability to detect intravascular injection of local anesthetic.
o) The use of ultrasonography has decreased the risk of complications associated with the placement of spinal and epidural needles and catheters as well as monitoring the spread of local anesthetics.
p) It is difficult to assess a dermatome level because these patients are nonverbal.

2. **Spinal anesthesia**
   a) Spinal anesthesia can be performed in the sitting or lateral position; however, the neck should be extended to prevent airway obstruction.
   b) The lumbar puncture is performed at the L3 to L4 or L4 to L5 interspace because the spinal cord ends at L3 in neonates.

c) A 1½-inch, 22-gauge needle is inserted and, even with this small needle, one should be able to feel resistance when the needle enters the ligamentum flavum and the characteristic "pop" when the needle enters the subarachnoid space. The distance is approximately 1 cm.
d) The most common local anesthetics are tetracaine 1% and bupivacaine 0.5% to 0.75% at doses of 0.4 to 1.0 mg/kg. When the local anesthetic is injected, the neonate should be immediately placed in the supine position, and the legs should be secured with tape to prevent them from being raised for any reason.

3. **Caudal anesthesia**
   a) Caudal anesthesia is the most commonly used regional block in pediatric anesthesia. It can be used for any procedure involving innervation from the sacral, lumbar, or lower thoracic dermatomes.
   b) In youngest patients, the caudal block can be used as an adjunct to general anesthesia or solely for postoperative analgesia.
   c) In neonates, it is most often placed after induction of general anesthesia before the beginning of the surgical procedure.
   d) The patient is placed in the lateral position with the upper knee flexed. The landmarks are identified: the tip of the coccyx to fix the midline and the sacral cornua on either side of the sacral hiatus.
   e) These landmarks form the points of an equilateral triangle with the tip resting over the sacral hiatus.
   f) A 22-gauge needle is placed, bevel up, at a 45-degree angle to the skin.
   g) When the sacrococcygeal membrane is punctured, a distinctive loss of resistance is felt, and the angle of the needle is reduced and advanced cephalad.
   h) The syringe is aspirated, and if there is no CSF or blood, the local anesthetic can be administered. Any local anesthetic can be used, and the volume of the local anesthetic determines the height of the block.
   i) Volumes of 1.2 to 1.5 mL/kg provide analgesia and anesthesia to the T4 to T6 dermatome.
   j) No matter which local anesthetic is used, the concentration is adjusted to deliver no more than 2.5 mg/kg.
   k) The addition of epinephrine (1:200,000) or clonidine (1 to 2 mcg/kg) will prolong the block significantly.
   l) Opioids such as morphine or fentanyl can be added to the caudal dose of local anesthesia to provide additional analgesia, however, when these medications are used, the patient should be monitored for respiratory depression up to 24 hours after injection.
   m) Any regional technique can theoretically be used in neonates, with careful attention to the potential for toxicity of local anesthetics and careful dosing parameters.

C. ANESTHETIC CONSIDERATIONS FOR SELECTED CASES

Pyloric Stenosis

1. **Introduction**

Pyloric stenosis is an obstructive lesion, characterized by the "olive-shaped" enlargement of the pylorus muscle. It is a common gastrointestinal anomaly, particularly in boys. It is usually diagnosed between 2 and 12 weeks of life. Clinical symptoms include nonbilious postprandial emesis, becoming more projectile with time; a palpable pylorus; and visible peristaltic waves. The procedure to correct the problem is a pyloromyotomy.

Historically, pyloric stenosis was considered a surgical emergency; however, as with medical progress on many fronts, the procedure is now treated as a medical emergency with the patient being optimized before elective surgery. Fluid, electrolyte, and acid-base balance should be corrected before anesthesia. Hypokalemia, hypochloremia, and metabolic alkalosis are the most common electrolyte abnormalities.

2. Anesthetic technique

a) Before induction, the neonate's stomach must be emptied via orogastric tube. Some anesthesia providers irrigate the stomach via the orogastric tube with warm normal saline until the aspirate is clear and minimal. Others tilt the baby in various directions to evacuate the remaining contents.
b) After preoxygenation, the induction should be a modified rapid sequence with properly applied cricoid pressure and gentle positive-pressure ventilation via mask. (Many practitioners still perform an awake oral or a true rapid sequence.)
c) Oral endotracheal intubation is mandated to protect the airway from any gastric contents that may be residual.
d) Maintenance can be with inhalation anesthetics or in combination with intravenous (IV) drugs.
e) These babies should be extubated awake.
f) Postoperatively these patients, particularly a preterm or SGA neonate, could exhibit drowsiness, lethargy, or apnea. This could be attributed to electrolyte abnormalities or postconceptual age.

Inguinal Hernia

1. Introduction

Inguinal hernias are particularly prevalent in preterm infants. The surgical problem presents the possibility of incarceration of the small bowel in the hernia defect, resulting in ischemia and tissue death. Also of concern is the potential injury to the ipsilateral testicle. These babies routinely have their hernia repair before discharge from the NICU, and the anesthesia provider is faced with all the usual problems of prematurity, such as BPD. The surgical approach can be the standard abdominal incision; in some centers, laparoscopy is the preferred technology. In most situations, the contralateral side is explored to rule out the presence of another defect because of the high incidence of bilateral involvement. When this procedure is performed by a urologist, the contralateral side is most often not explored.

2. Anesthetic technique

a) Because of the many possible patient issues, the anesthetic technique must be tailored for each patient.
b) Inhalation or IV induction is acceptable as well as airway management with a mask, laryngeal mask airway, or endotracheal tube (ETT).
c) The use of the laparoscopic approach necessitates the use of an ETT.
d) Maintenance can be with inhalation anesthetics or in combination with IV drugs.
e) Small neonates who are at risk for postoperative apnea and bradycardia may benefit from spinal anesthesia.

Congenital Diaphragmatic Hernia

1. Introduction

A congenital diaphragmatic hernia (CDH) is a defect of the diaphragm that allows extrusion of the abdominal contents into the thoracic cavity. This disorder has an incidence of one in 2500 live births. The herniated abdominal contents act as a space-occupying lesion and prevent normal lung growth and development. Most of these defects are left sided via the foramen of Bochdalek, and the lung affected to the greatest extent is on the ipsilateral side. However, the other lung can be affected as well. The lungs have reduced sized bronchi, less bronchial branching, decreased alveolar surface area, and abnormal pulmonary vasculature. There is a thickening of the arteriolar smooth muscle extending to the capillary level of the alveoli. This results in increased pulmonary artery pressure and causes right-to-left intrapulmonary shunting.

2. Clinical manifestations

Neonates with CDH present immediately after birth with a classic triad that includes cyanosis, dyspnea, and dextrocardia. Other symptoms include tachypnea, absence of breath sounds on the affected side, and severe retractions. Their physical appearance is a scaphoid abdomen and a barrel chest. Diagnosis is confirmed by chest radiographs documenting bowel in the thoracic cavity and a gasless abdominal cavity. Between 44% and 66% of neonates with CDH have other anomalies, particularly heart lesions.

The emergent nature of the repair has been recently reexamined, and more emphasis is now placed on the stabilization of the pulmonary hypertension and other medical issues. Extracorporeal membrane oxygenation (ECMO) is one method of bridging the gap between birth and surgical repair; however, it is not the mode of treatment for all patients.

3. Anesthetic technique

a) A thorough assessment of the baby, including laboratory, radiographic, and physical symptoms, is mandatory.
b) Listening to breath sounds will assist in evaluating the degree of ventilation on each side of the chest after intubation.
c) Because of the respiratory manifestations of the problem, the patient will be already intubated and have IV access and arterial lines in place when arriving in the operating room.
d) If the patient is not intubated, an ETT should be placed after a rapid-sequence induction. If a difficult airway is suspected, an awake intubation should be done.
e) It is important in these patients to administer an anticholinergic (atropine 0.02 mg/kg) IV just before induction to prevent the bradycardia during induction.
f) If an awake intubation is planned, some type of analgesia should be used to decrease the stress response of airway instrumentation.
g) Ventilation should be delivered gently to avoid inflating the stomach with air, further compromising the pressure in the chest. Volutrauma can be avoided by delivering small tidal volume and PEEP if necessary.
h) The patient's hemodynamic stability should determine the anesthetic drugs used. A high-dose narcotic technique is commonly used (fentanyl, 15-25 mcg/kg) if tolerated.
i) The use of inhalation agents must be judicious because they pose significant risk to the baby's cardiovascular stability.

j) Nitrous oxide should be avoided because it will increase the volume of gastrointestinal tissue and further impair ventilation.
k) Monitoring must include blood pressure, ECG, pulse oximetry, capnography, temperature, and heart rate.
l) To monitor for right-to-left cardiac shunting, oximeter probes should be placed preductal (right upper extremity) and postductal (lower extremity).
m) The use of arterial blood pressure monitoring not only allows beat-to-beat assessment of blood pressure but also provides an outlet for easier blood sampling.
n) All conditions that can increase pulmonary vascular resistance (hypoxia, hypothermia, or acidosis) should be avoided.
o) Carbon dioxide should be kept at normal or slightly elevated levels, and oxygen saturation should be maintained above 80 mmHg.
p) Any derangement of electrolytes should be corrected quickly, and any significant blood loss should be replaced.
q) In the event that cardiorespiratory instability prevents the neonate from being transported to the operating room, the anesthesia provider might be required to administer anesthesia in the NICU while the baby is still on ECMO.
r) Under these circumstances, the recommended anesthetic choice is an opioid and nondepolarizing muscle relaxant technique instead of an inhalation agent.
s) Postoperative ventilation is required with the goal of keeping the arterial oxygenation greater than 150 mmHg and slowing weaning to lower oxygen concentrations over a 48- to 72-hour period.

Omphalocele and Gastroschisis

1. Introduction

Omphalocele and gastroschisis present with similar physical findings, but they originate from distinct abnormalities that occur in utero. An omphalocele occurs from failure of portions of or the entire contents of the intestine to return to the abdominal cavity. In gastroschisis, the abdominal contents have already returned to the abdominal cavity, but ischemia from insufficient blood supply by the omphalomesenteric artery causes a defect at the base of the abdominal wall and thus extrusion of abdominal contents. It is more common to encounter omphalocele in term newborns and gastroschisis in preterm newborns. The primary difference in the two defects is the presence of a membrane (the peritoneum) covering the extruded abdominal contents in the baby with omphalocele and the lack of membrane in the baby with gastroschisis. They are often associated with other anomalies. These anomalies might be cardiac, genitourinary (bladder exstrophy), metabolic (e.g., Beckwith-Wiedemann syndrome, macroglossia, hypoglycemia, organomegaly, gigantism), malrotation, Meckel diverticulum, and intestinal atresia. When the omphalocele is in the epigastric region, cardiac and thoracic anomalies are more prevalent. If the omphalocele is located in the hypogastric area, cloacal anomalies and exstrophy of the bladder are seen more often. Both gastrointestinal anomalies, although very different in presentation, are almost identical in anesthetic management.

2. Anesthetic technique

a) A newborn with an omphalocele or gastroschisis is usually brought to the operating room very soon after birth to minimize the possibility of infection, the loss of fluid and heat, and the possible death of bowel tissue.

b) A thorough preoperative evaluation must be done to identify the presence of any of the previously mentioned associated anomalies.
c) Historically, the surgical approach was to immediately attempt primary closure of the defect. This entailed placing a large amount of abdominal contents into a cavity that was not usually large enough, and the result was a significant increase in intraabdominal pressure that impeded ventilation and profound hypotension secondary to aortocaval compression.
d) Over the past decade, surgeons have opted for a staged closure using a Silastic silo as a temporary housing for the bowel. This silo is sutured to the defect, and the silo is reduced over the next 3 to 7 days to allow for accommodation of the gastric contents and abdominal wall stretching. Then the neonate is usually brought for complete closure.
e) In the event primary closure is attempted, it should be noted that excessive intraabdominal pressure can increase the possibility of unsuccessful completion of the closure, as shown in the following box.

Criteria for Aborting Primary Closure

Intragastric pressure >20 mmHg
Intravesical pressure >20 mmHg
End-tidal carbon dioxide of 50 mmHg or greater
Maximum ventilatory pressure of 35 cm H_2O

f) The choice of anesthetic agent and technique is determined by several guiding principles: severe dehydration and massive fluid loss from exposed viscera and internal third spacing of fluid caused by bowel obstruction, hypothermia, the potential for sepsis and associated anomalies, and postoperative ventilation requirements.
g) It is common for the anesthesia provider to choose an opioid and nondepolarizing muscle relaxant technique; however, the abdominal wall may not allow primary closure even with the use of muscle relaxants.
h) Ventilatory compromise and decreased organ perfusion are major problems as intraabdominal pressure increases.
i) Adequate IV access is essential to infuse large amounts of fluid quickly and invasive monitoring guides the replacement.
j) A pulse oximeter probe on a lower extremity will indicate if there is compromise in the perfusion to the lower extremities caused by obstruction of venous return.
k) Postoperative ventilation will be mandatory on all of these babies requiring the continued use of paralytics and sedation with an opioid until their clinical status stabilizes.

Tracheoesophageal Fistula and Esophageal Atresia

1. Introduction

Esophageal atresia (EA), with or without tracheoesophageal fistula (TEF), is normally diagnosed immediately after birth when an orogastric tube cannot pass into the stomach, there is coughing and choking after the first feeding, or after recurrent pneumonia associated with feedings. In the past, this condition was often lethal; however, today there is an expectation of almost 100% survival.

2. **Clinical manifestations**
   a) There is a significant association of other serious congenital anomalies in these babies. Some sources report as high as 30% to 50% of newborns with EA and TEF have other anomalies, particularly VACTERL (vertebral anomalies, anal atresia, cardiac defects, TEF, renal abnormalities, and limb malformations) association.
   b) EA with a distal fistula is the most common presentation of TEF in approximately 80% to 90% of patients.
   c) The esophagus ends in a blind pouch, and the distal esophagus forms a fistula with the trachea, usually above the carina.
   d) There are five other configurations of this anomaly, varied by the location of the fistula and the presence or absence of EA.
   e) The morbidity and mortality of TEF are directly related to the resulting pulmonary complications from aspiration of feedings.
3. **Anesthetic technique**
   a) The focus of the preoperative preparation should be to minimize the pulmonary complications by discontinuing oral feedings, placement of a tube to suction nasopharyngeal secretions that accumulate in the blind esophageal pouch, maintain the infant in a semirecumbent position to minimize aspiration of secretions, and placement of a gastrostomy tube to prevent excess gastric distention from impairing ventilation, and to take measures to prevent dehydration.
   b) The surgical procedure is performed via a thoracotomy incision, usually on the right side. The sequence of the repair is the ligation of the fistula and then anastomosis of the two ends of the esophagus, if possible.
   c) Standard monitors should be used. The precordial stethoscope should be placed in the left axilla after induction to allow for monitoring of ventilation and heart sounds.
   d) The cardiorespiratory condition of the neonate should dictate the use of more invasive monitoring techniques such as an arterial line (umbilical or radial). In the youngest critically ill patients, preductal and postductal oximeter probes may be used.
   e) The technique of induction should be based on the clinician's evaluation of the airway. When there is concern of a difficult airway, an "awake intubation" should be performed. This technique minimizes the gastric distention from anesthetic gases passing through the fistula and allows proper placement of the ETT without positive-pressure ventilation.
   f) When airway management is determined to be "routine," an inhalation induction with gentle positive-pressure ventilation and intubation can be used.
   g) To further minimize stomach distention, spontaneous ventilation to an adequate depth of anesthesia followed by endotracheal intubation may be carried out.
   h) If this technique is used, care must be taken to avoid hypoxemia that will result from the respiratory depression produced by high concentrations of inhalation agents.
   i) Another accepted technique is the IV rapid-sequence induction with endotracheal intubation.

j) With any of the above-mentioned techniques, proper position must be verified after the ETT is placed. A common method of verifying the correct position is to actually intubate the right mainstem bronchus and then withdraw the ETT until breath sounds are heard on the left side of the chest. The tip of the tube is likely between the fistula and the carina.
k) If there is a gastrostomy in place, another method is to submerge the gastrostomy tube in water and, if there are bubbles on ventilation, the fistula is being ventilated and the tube must be repositioned.
l) The bevel of the ETT should be turned anteriorly to allow the posterior surface of the ETT to occlude the fistula.
m) In one configuration of TEF, the fistula is located very close to the carina. In this case, the ETT may need to be placed in the bronchus of the nonoperative lung until the fistula can be ligated. After ligation, the tube can be withdrawn to above the carina.
n) During the procedure, it is essential to monitor ventilation very carefully. Airway obstruction can occur if the trachea is compressed or if secretions or blood block the openings of the ETT. This must be corrected immediately.
o) The neonate without significant pulmonary complications, who is awake and moving vigorously, is most often extubated in the operating room.
p) Blood and secretions may be present in the ETT and should be suctioned gently before removal.
q) If there is any concern about airway obstruction or impaired ventilation, mechanical ventilation should be continued.
r) It is thought that if bag and mask ventilation or reintubation is required, undue stress could be placed on the suture lines of the repair with laryngoscopy and neck extension, resulting in damage to the esophagus and necessitating further surgical procedures.
s) Another problem that can occur with early extubation in smaller neonates is an inability to maintain the work of breathing because of preoperative lung disease.
t) If postoperative mechanical ventilation is needed, the ETT should be positioned 1 cm away from the fistula repair to allow for healing of the suture line.
u) A suction catheter should be clearly marked with a distance for insertion that approximates the distance just above the anastomotic repair.
v) Postoperative pain can be managed with opioids or a caudal epidural (or both) placed intraoperatively.

4. Complications

a) Complications may occur later that could influence anesthetic management.
b) Neonates who have had EA or TEF repair early in life can develop a diverticulum at the site of the old tracheal fistula. This could present problems in the future if inadvertent intubation of the diverticulum occurs.
c) Esophageal stricture could develop at the site of esophageal anastomosis, requiring repeated dilation or possible resection.

Malrotation and Midgut Volvulus

1. Introduction

As the intestine is moving from its extraabdominal location during the first trimester of gestation, it can become twisted. The result can be a compromised superior mesenteric artery and intestinal ischemia. This ischemia can cause bowel strangulation, bloody stools, peritonitis, and hypovolemic shock. When this occurs, it is termed *volvulus.* According to some sources, this is a true surgical emergency.

Many of these neonates are diagnosed in the first week of life when the neonate presents with bilious vomiting, a tender and distended abdomen, and increasing hemodynamic instability. The surgical procedure relieves the obstruction by reducing the volvulus, dividing the fixation bands between the cecum and the duodenum or jejunum, and widening the base of the mesentery.

2. Anesthetic technique

a) The major concerns in anesthetic management are airway management, fluid and electrolyte replacement, treatment of sepsis, and postoperative pain management.
b) Any baby with intestinal obstruction will likely have abdominal distention, which could impede diaphragmatic movement, and is at higher risk for aspiration of gastric or intestinal contents.
c) This necessitates the use of a rapid-sequence induction with the proper application of cricoid pressure.
d) If there is concern for a difficult airway, then awake intubation should be considered.
e) There is likely volume depletion caused by peritonitis, ileus, bowel manipulation, and sepsis. It is absolutely necessary to have adequate IV access, and it is desirable to have a central line and an arterial line.
f) The choice of anesthetic agents should depend on the neonate's condition. It is not advisable to use nitrous oxide, but other inhalation agents are acceptable.
g) As with other emergent abdominal procedures, postoperative mechanical ventilation may be required, making the intraoperative choice of an opioid and nondepolarizing muscle relaxant a good choice.
h) Although anesthetic agent choice is not critical, the maintenance of an adequate circulating volume and red blood cells is vital to ensure perfusion of vital organs.

Necrotizing Enterocolitis

1. Introduction

Necrotizing enterocolitis (NEC) is an intestinal inflammation that can become a life-threatening emergency situation. It occurs primarily in preterm babies with a gestational age of less than 32 weeks and with a weight of less than 1500 g. The etiology of the problem is reported to be secondary to bowel ischemia and immaturity, probable bacterial invasion, and premature oral feeding.

2. Clinical manifestations

a) Diagnosis is confirmed by abdominal radiography that shows fixed dilated intestinal loops, pneumatosis intestinalis, portal vein air, ascites, and pneumoperitoneum.

b) Accompanying laboratory values might show evidence of hyperkalemia, hyponatremia, metabolic acidosis, hyperglycemia, or hypoglycemia and, in the most serious cases, signs of disseminated intravascular coagulation.
c) The common symptoms of NEC are listed in the following box.

Common Symptoms of Necrotizing Enterocolitis

- Increased gastric residuals with feeding
- Abdominal distention
- Bilious vomiting
- Lethargy
- Occult or gross rectal bleeding
- Fever
- Hypothermia
- Abdominal mass
- Oliguria
- Jaundice
- Apnea and bradycardia
- Fever
- Acidosis
- Hypoxia

d) When an attempt at medical management is unsuccessful, surgical intervention consists of an exploratory laparotomy with resection of dead bowel, usually a colostomy, and peritoneal lavage.

3. **Anesthetic technique**
   a) These neonates are very sick and usually come to the operating room already intubated and with ventilator support.
   b) If they are not intubated, a rapid-sequence induction or awake intubation is indicated.
   c) The anesthetic drugs chosen should depend on the patient's condition, but a common choice is a narcotic and relaxant technique. These are thought to be the safest choice in the presence of cardiovascular instability because the inhalation agents may further depress the myocardium and lower the blood pressure to unacceptable levels.
   d) Nitrous oxide is avoided, and compressed air can be added to the gas mixture if there is concern over high oxygen concentrations.
   e) If cardiac output is low and renal perfusion is below normal, dopamine may be indicated.
   f) The amount of third space loss in these patients is very large and may require multiple blood volumes of crystalloid and colloid combinations to replace intravascular volume. Red blood cells, fresh-frozen plasma, and platelets also may be required to increase oxygen-carrying capacity or to treat factor deficiency.
   g) The postoperative care should focus on continuation of the fluid resuscitation and cardiorespiratory support and mechanical ventilation until the baby stabilizes.

Imperforate Anus

1. **Introduction**

During the first few days after birth, when there is no passage of meconium, the diagnosis of imperforate anus is considered. The degree of this anomaly can range from a mild stenosis to complete anal atresia that is associated with other anomalies. The VACTERL association (vertebral anomalies, anal atresia, cardiac defects, TEF, renal abnormalities, and limb malformations) contains all of the above-mentioned anomalies.

2. **Anesthetic technique**
   a) In male newborns, the operative procedure may be urgent to allow the passage of meconium via a colostomy.
   b) In female newborns, because of the usual presence of a rectovaginal fistula, the procedure can be delayed for a few weeks.
   c) The anesthetic considerations for the neonate are based on the existence of associated anomalies and fluid and electrolyte balance.

Other Intestinal Obstructive Lesions

Duodenal obstruction, jejunoileal atresia, and meconium ileus can all result in a complete intestinal obstruction. Although each of these pathologies is different in etiology and presentation, the anesthetic management is very similar to that for the previously mentioned midgut volvulus.

Neurosurgical Procedures

Neonatal Hydrocephalus

1. **Introduction**

Hydrocephalus is usually the result of some existing pathologic process. It is usually caused by an obstruction in the CSF system or an inability to absorb CSF. The standard treatment is the placement of a shunting catheter from the ventricle of the brain to another location to allow absorption of the fluid. Most often the shunt is placed from the cerebral ventricle to the peritoneal cavity. Occasionally, the catheter will be placed in the right atrium or pleural cavity. In newborns and neonates, if the hydrocephalus develops slowly, the cranial vault will expand to accommodate the increase in brain bulk. When there is no more ability to expand, ICP begins to increase, and the baby will start to exhibit signs and symptoms of increased ICP.

2. **Clinical manifestations**

The signs and symptoms of increasing ICP are a tense anterior fontanel, irritability, somnolence, or vomiting.

3. **Anesthetic technique**
   a) Anesthetic management is directed at controlling the ICP and relieving the obstruction.
   b) The urgency of the procedure will be determined by the preanesthetic assessment of the ICP.
   c) The major risk associated with delay is the possible herniation of the brain caused by increasing pressure in the cranial vault.
   d) Comorbidities such as prematurity and all associated problems must be addressed.
   e) Induction in the presence of increased ICP is usually a rapid-sequence induction and tracheal intubation.
   f) A variety of anesthetic agents are acceptable for maintenance with the goal being to extubate the patient at the end of the procedure.
   g) If the neonate is preterm, it is advisable to adjust the oxygen concentration to maintain oxygen saturation at 95% to 97%. This decreases the risk of retinopathy of prematurity.
   h) The neurologic status of the neonate could affect the decision to extubate immediately, and mechanical ventilation could be required.

Myelomeningocele

1. **Introduction**

Myelomeningocele is the most common CNS defect that occurs during the first month of gestation. Another common name for this defect is *spina bifida.* It is failure of the neural tube to close, resulting in herniation of the spinal cord and meninges through a defect in the spinal column and back. If the herniation only contains meninges, it is a meningocele. If the herniation contains meninges and neural elements, it is a myelomeningocele. These lesions mostly occur in the lumbosacral region but can occur at any level of the neuraxis. The repair of the defect is considered urgent and is usually undertaken within the first 24 hours of life to avoid the increasing risk of bacterial contamination of the spinal cord and further deterioration of neural and motor function.

2. **Clinical manifestations**
   a) Most newborns with myelomeningocele do not have other associated anomalies or congenital heart disease.
   b) These neonates, however, often have an Arnold-Chiari malformation. The Arnold-Chiari malformation is a result of the hindbrain being displaced downward into the foramen magnum, resulting in hydrocephalus.
   c) This will necessitate the placement of a ventriculoperitoneal shunt, usually during the myelomeningocele repair.
   d) There are usually significant neurologic deficits below the level of the lesion, and evaluation of the degree of deficit is important to anesthetic decision making.
3. **Anesthetic technique**
   a) Preoperative assessment should include a thorough review of all other organ systems to rule out additional congenital anomalies.
   b) Minimal laboratory work should include a complete blood count and a type and screen for blood.
   c) Routine neonatal monitoring is necessary, and the use of invasive monitoring techniques should be based on a risk-to-benefit analysis.
   d) Positioning and airway management are the biggest challenges for the anesthesia provider.
   e) Most of these babies can be induced and intubated in the supine position with the lumbosacral defect supported in a "donut" ring or with strategically placed towels to avoid direct pressure on the dural sac.
   f) If the defect is very large or if there is accompanying severe hydrocephalus, it may be necessary to place the neonate in the lateral position for induction and intubation.
   g) If there is a suspicion of a difficult airway, the ETT may be placed with the patient awake after administration of atropine and preoxygenation.
   h) Adequate IV access is essential because of the possibility of significant blood loss during the procedure.
   i) If the defect is large, the surgeon may be required to débride a large amount of tissue for closure, resulting in a large blood loss.
   j) Anesthesia can be induced with an inhalation or IV technique.
   k) After the ETT is placed, the procedure is performed in the prone position with appropriate protection of all body parts.
   l) In some institutions, the use of muscle relaxants is discouraged to allow for neurophysiologic monitoring.
   m) Anesthesia can be maintained with a variety of drugs, keeping in mind the goal of extubation at the end of the procedure and the possibility of postoperative apnea.

n) These patients are prone to hypothermia, and conservation of body heat should include warming the operating room to at least 80°F before the procedure and until the baby is draped.
o) Radiant heat lamps should be used during the preparation and positioning of the patient. A forced-air warmer should also be placed underneath the neonate to maintain body temperature.
p) Anesthetic gases should be humidified to prevent heat loss and minimize pulmonary complications.
q) An increased sensitivity to latex has been reported in these babies. As a precaution, they should be treated as latex allergic, avoiding all products that contain latex.

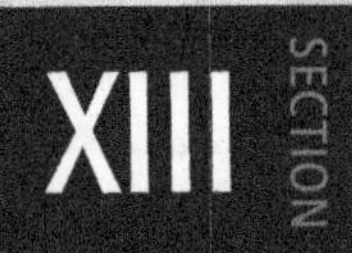

Anesthesia for Therapeutic and Diagnostic Procedures

A. BRACHYTHERAPY

1. Introduction

Palladium-103 prostate implants are being used for brachytherapy as an optional treatment for prostate cancer. The sources are permanently implanted directly into the tissue. The seeds are encased in a lead-lined cartridge that attaches to lead-lined placement needles. The seeds are placed by the radiation oncologist through these needles into the prostate through the perineum. Placement is guided by ultrasonography.

2. Preoperative assessment and patient preparation

a) The treatment is performed in the radiation oncology department.
b) Each patient is prescreened and admitted as an outpatient through the short stay unit.
c) The procedure lasts a maximum of 2 hours.
d) Patients may undergo a bowel preparation at home before the procedure.
e) An 18-gauge, 2-inch angiocatheter is placed before the procedure.
f) Each patient will require intravenous (IV) antibiotics before the procedure. One gram of cefazolin (Ancef) is required. If the patient has an allergy to penicillin, then clindamycin (Cleocin), 600 mg, is administered.

3. Room preparation

Required monitoring equipment, anesthesia, and airway supplies are provided.

4. Anesthetic technique

a) Anesthesia is usually maintained by spinal anesthesia. A minimal T8 level is desired. If the patient is required to have consecutive treatments, an epidural anesthetic may be placed.
b) Sedation is given as needed.
c) The patient is placed in a lithotomy position for the procedure. A Foley catheter is inserted with Hypaque in the balloon. An ultrasound probe and perineum template are placed before needle placement.
d) The time of treatment is the time of radiation. Everyone must leave the room. Visual contact is always present through monitors. Treatment time is usually 5 to 15 minutes.

5. Postoperative implications

a) Radiation precautions
   (1) Occasionally, seeds can become dislodged from the implanted tissue. Therefore, dressings and linens should not be removed from the room until they have been checked and cleared by the oncology physicist.
   (2) If a seed is discovered, do not touch it with your hands. Use long forceps to place it in a lead storage container.
   (3) Some seeds may pass in the urine for the first few days. Therefore, urine should be strained before being discarded.
   (4) Pregnant personnel are not to provide anesthesia for these patients.

(5) All personnel remaining in the room during the procedure should have proper badges. No person or material should leave the room without being surveyed with a Geiger counter.

B. COMPUTED TOMOGRAPHY

1. Introduction

Computed tomography (CT) uses x-rays generated from a rotating anode x-ray generator. The patient is placed supine on a flat, wheeled platform and moved inside the scanning gantry. X-rays are then projected through the patient at different angles. The X-rays penetrate tissues differently according to the atomic numbers of the atoms within the tissue. The diagnostic quality of a CT scan is enhanced with the injection of IV contrast media (ICM). Contrast media containing iodine may be administered to the patient enterally or parenterally to further attenuate the x-ray beam to enhance the images for CT vascular or gastrointestinal studies.

2. Anesthetic technique

a) CT scans require that the patient remain as motionless as possible for several minutes to an hour. Patient motion can produce artifacts in the diagnostic images to be read by the radiologist.
b) Patients should lie on a flat, lightly padded wheeled platform, which is rolled into the short bore scanning gantry of the CT scanner.
c) Although the majority of patients are able to cooperate and tolerate CT, others may not be able to cooperate because of extremes in age, concurrent medical conditions, or mental disability.
d) The CT scan is neither physically invasive nor painful. Patients enter the CT scanner without precautions for ferromagnetic objects as for a magnetic resonance imaging (MRI) scan. CT is more rapidly performed than an MRI scan, especially if a spiral CT scanner is used.
e) The patient may require anesthesia anywhere along the continuum from minimal sedation to general anesthesia.
f) Use of ferromagnetic anesthesia equipment and supplies around the CT scanner is not a concern.
g) A standard anesthesia machine, laryngoscope and blades, and IV infusion pumps can be used as if in the operating room.
h) A laryngeal mask airway (LMA) is an appropriate alternative choice as a minimally invasive and secure airway in the patient without contraindications to its use.
i) Attention should be paid to securing the airway, and the anesthesia breathing circuit, the leads for the electrocardiogram (ECG), the noninvasive blood pressure cuff, the IV line, and the pulse oximeter should extend into the scanning gantry. If the use of general anesthesia is used, it is important to verify the presence of a suction canister with tubing that will reach the patient's mouth in the event of an emergency. An Ambu bag with appropriately sized face mask should also be present.
j) The anesthesia provider should allow for extra anesthesia circuitry length and electrical monitoring leads lengths because of patient movement that will occur because of intermittent repositioning of the mechanized table that positions the patient within the scanning gantry.

k) Sedation can be performed with a variety of agents, including midazolam, chloral hydrate, diazepam, or propofol.
l) General anesthesia can be performed with total IV anesthesia (TIVA), such as with IV propofol, or with inhalation agents.
m) All personnel must be aware of the use of ionizing radiation during the CT scan and should take precautions to be shielded from any exposure to the radiation.
n) Radiation protection can be accomplished with the use of a lead glass barrier, a lead apron, a lead thyroid collar, and lead-glass safety glasses. Radiation dose badges that attach to the clothing are available.
o) ICM can cause an unexpected allergic reaction in some patients, varying from itching with hives to severe, life-threatening anaphylactoid and anaphylactic reactions that have led to patient death.
p) ICM can also cause renal toxicity as well as local tissue sloughing and necrosis if the ICM extravasates from the vein into the surrounding tissue.
q) The anesthesia provider will be involved with patient care related to ICM extravasation and should be familiar with treatment protocols to minimize patient morbidity, as shown in the following box.

Considerations and Treatment Protocols for Intravenous Contrast Media Extravasation Prevention

Considerations

- Use IV catheters (as opposed to metal needles or butterfly needles).
- Avoid use of the same vein if the first attempt at IV catheterization was missed.
- Ensure that the IV catheter is patent and is free flowing.

Treatments

- Attempt to aspirate as much ICM as possible.
- Elevate the affected limb.
- Apply ice packs for 20 minutes to 60 minutes until swelling resolves.
- A heating pad may be necessary in place of ice for swelling.
- Observe the patient for possible tissue damage related to continual contact with ice or heat.
- Observe the patient for 2 to 4 hours before discharge; consider medical or surgical consultation if necessary.

ICM, Intravenous contrast media; *IV,* intravenous.

C. GASTROENTEROLOGIC PROCEDURES: COLONOSCOPY, ESOPHAGOGASTRODUODENOSCOPY, AND ENDOSCOPIC RETROGRADE CHOLANGIOPANCREATOGRAPHY

1. Introduction

Endoscopy for gastrointestinal procedures is the use of a flexible fiberoptic endoscope that transmits brilliant, coherent, high-resolution, magnified, direct visual images to the operator. The operator can then examine, biopsy, dilate, or cauterize portions of the gastrointestinal tract. The endoscopist may pass accessory devices down the endoscope such as biopsy forceps, dilation devices, cytology brushes, measuring devices, needles for injection, Doppler probes, ultrasound probes, and probes to measure electrical activity and pH. Even foreign bodies may be removed with the aid of a snare passed through an endoscope.

2. **Procedures**
   a) A colonoscopy allows total diagnostic visualization of the mucosa of the tortuous colon from the anus to the cecum.
   b) An upper endoscopy, such as an esophagogastroduodenoscopy (EGD), is an accurate way for the operator to evaluate the mucosa of the esophagus, stomach, and duodenum.
   c) Endoscopic retrograde cholangiopancreatography (ERCP) is used for the diagnosis of obstructive, neoplastic, or inflammatory pancreatobiliary structures.
   d) Endoscopy for gastrointestinal procedures may be performed by a gastroenterologist, a general surgeon, a family practitioner, or a proctologist.
   e) The endoscope is passed into the gastrointestinal tract with the aid of lubricant.
   f) The endoscope has controls to change the direction of the flexible tip, allow flushing with water, apply suction, or insufflate air or carbon dioxide within the portion of the gastrointestinal tract being observed.
3. **Anesthetic technique for colonoscopy**
   a) Because of the expectations of patients, endoscopically caused discomfort, and the desirability for no patient movement, moderate sedation, deep sedation, and, in some cases, general endotracheal anesthesia are used.
   b) A proper preanesthetic assessment of the patient should be performed, focusing on the areas of age, ability to cooperate, level of anxiety, mental disability, allergies, fluid status, laboratory electrolyte values, cardiac history, hypertension, bleeding history, clotting status, respiratory status, obesity, drug and alcohol abuse, gastroesophageal reflux, and pregnancy.
   c) Patients should adhere to proper NPO (nothing by mouth) guidelines.
   d) Bacteremia is possible as a result of endoscopic procedures.
   e) Necessary medications may be given, such as cardiac medications, antihypertensives, and antibiotics.
   f) Preemptive analgesia with gargled flavored viscous Xylocaine helps patient acceptance of the procedure.
   g) Moderate sedation is usually accomplished with the short-acting sedatives midazolam or propofol and analgesics such as remifentanil, alfentanil, or fentanyl.
   h) Deep sedation can be achieved with titration of propofol until effective along with an analgesic medication. Upper endoscopy may necessitate the use of any antisialagogue such as glycopyrrolate.
   i) Colonoscopy requires thorough cleansing of the lumen of the colon of fecal material. The colon may be partly prepared with a cleansing enema. Full preparation of the colon is accomplished commonly with orally administered balanced electrolyte solutions in a volume of up to 4 L.

j) After the preparation, abdominal cramping, diarrhea, weakness, and nausea can occur. Patients who arrive for the procedure require reassessment and the insertion of an IV catheter with IV fluid, usually lactated Ringer's solution or normal saline.
k) Conventional monitors, including pulse oximeter, noninvasive blood pressure monitor, and ECG, are attached.
l) The patient is supplied with oxygen through a disposable nasal cannula or disposable face mask. The procedure is usually performed with the patient positioned in a lateral decubitus position with the body flexed, the head and back bent downward toward the knees, and the legs bent upward toward the abdomen.
m) Patient anxiety, distention because of insufflation, and acute discomfort during the maneuvering of the endoscope usually necessitate the administration of deep sedation or a general anesthetic in some cases.
n) Strong vagal nerve stimulation can occur as a result of distention of the colon. This may cause hypotension, bradydysrhythmia, and ECG changes.

4. **Anesthetic technique for EGD**
   a) EGD requires a general patient assessment with special emphasis on any cardiac history, hypertension, bleeding disorders, postoperative nausea and vomiting (PONV), dysphagia, and gastroesophageal reflux.
   b) The patient should be NPO according to guidelines. Most patients are able to have EGD performed with a spray or gargle of topical anesthetic such as Cetacaine, benzocaine, or 4% lidocaine liquid.
   c) Rapid absorption of highly concentrated local anesthetics, applied topically over highly vascular and absorptive mucosal tissues, can lead to possible toxicity reactions whose symptoms could be masked while the patient is receiving sedative anesthesia.
   d) Topical benzocaine can pose a small risk of methemoglobinemia if overused.
   e) An IV catheter is inserted, with fluids such as lactated Ringer's solution or normal saline attached.
   f) The patient is connected to standard monitors. Oxygen can be supplied through a disposable nasal cannula or a disposable face mask. EGD is generally performed with the patient positioned supine.
   g) After the patient is adequately sedated, the operator inserts a hollow oral airway gently into the patient's mouth, and the endoscope is advanced through this airway, allowing direct visualization of the larynx, hypopharynx, esophagus, and stomach, and through the pylorus into the duodenal bulb.
5. **Anesthetic technique for ERCP**
   a) ERCP requires thorough assessment of the patient, including a review of laboratory values of a complete blood count, serum liver chemistries and amylase or lipase levels to evaluate liver function, and clotting studies.
   b) Patients should also be evaluated for anticoagulant medications, bleeding history, and prosthetic heart valves.
   c) Allergies should be evaluated, especially those to iodinated contrast media.
   d) Patients who require ERCP are usually more ill than patients seen routinely for colonoscopy or EGD.

e) The patient should be NPO according to guidelines.
f) IV access is obtained, and fluid is administered.
g) Standard monitors are applied, and oxygen is supplied to the patient via a disposable face mask.
h) The procedure requires that the patient be in a prone or slightly left lateral decubitus position.
i) Deep sedation is generally required, although painful or complex ERCP may require general anesthesia.
j) Pediatric endoscopy has been performed with patients under deep IV sedation with agents such as propofol when the patient will allow placement of the IV catheter and under general endotracheal anesthesia.
k) These procedures can cause bowel rupture or duct rupture. One should be ready with immediate airway and hemodynamic support as necessary along with monitored emergency transport to the operating room for surgical intervention.

6. **Postoperative implications**
   a) Postprocedure morbidity differs with each of the described procedures. All patients should be monitored in a postanesthesia care area until they have recovered from the sedation or general anesthetic.
   b) Patients having colonoscopy frequently complain of intestinal or abdominal pain immediately after the procedure caused by insufflation during the examination. Rectal bleeding, PONV, and hypotension may also be seen. Administration of a bolus of IV fluids along with an IV antiemetic agent, such as ondansetron, dolasetron, or granisetron, is indicated.
   c) EGD morbidity relates to bleeding, PONV, aspiration, dysphagia, and hypotension. Treatments such as those used for colonoscopy may be indicated.
   d) ERCP morbidity relates to possible reactions to iodinated contrast media. Patient reactions can be mild (e.g., PONV, pruritus, diaphoresis, flushing, or mild urticaria), moderate (e.g., faintness, severe vomiting, profound urticaria, mild bronchospasm, mild hypotension, mild tachycardia, or bradycardia), or severe (e.g., hypotensive shock, angioedema, respiratory arrest, cardiac arrest, convulsions, or death). PONV can be treated as described previously.

D. INTERVENTIONAL RADIOLOGY, RADIOTHERAPY, STEREOTACTIC RADIOSURGERY, AND INTERVENTIONAL NEURORADIOLOGY

1. Introduction

Interventional radiology (IR) involves minimally invasive procedures and therapies performed by radiologists, especially in patients at high medical risk. Major IR therapies include angiography, embolization of blood vessels such as arteriovenous malformations or for epistaxis, delivery of chemical or physical vascular occlusive devices, removal of thrombi, ablation of aneurysms, and angioplasty of blood vessels with stent placement.

Gamma radiation is used for radiotherapy and radiosurgery. The gamma radiation is introduced to the patient by the use of either a Gamma Knife or a CyberKnife. The CyberKnife therapy delivers a sequence of many hundreds of gamma beams to the cancerous tumor from many different directions. Gamma Knife therapy delivers gamma radiation to the cancerous tumor simultaneously in a single dose.

Interventional neuroradiology (INR) is used for diagnosis and treatment of central nervous system (CNS) diseases endovascularly to deliver therapeutic medications or devices. Digital subtraction angiography first uses an original angiograph of the blood vessels to be studied. Then a contrast medium is injected into the same blood vessels, and opaque structures such as bone and tissues can be digitally subtracted or removed from the angiographic image, leaving a clear picture of the blood vessels.

Improvements in vascular access techniques, new thin and flexible catheters and guidewires, and the development of innovative coils and therapeutic medications have made new treatments possible. Conditions that once required extensive surgery with accompanying patient morbidity and mortality can now be performed less invasively. Some major procedures performed with INR are mechanical or chemical removal of emboli or thrombi that cause stroke, the physical occlusion of malformed vascular structures such as an arteriovenous malformations with chemicals or flow-directed balloons, dilation of stenotic blood vessels, and embolization (blocking blood flow) of cerebrovascular aneurysms using catheter-deployed coils.

2. **Anesthetic technique**
   a) As skills, techniques, and technology progress, more procedures will be performed with radiation or under radiological guidance.
   b) These procedures all require the absolute immobility of the patient, with periods of controlled apnea, which assist in the viewing or treatment of the targeted area of the patient, especially during whole-body therapeutic radiation treatment.
   c) These procedures are also time consuming, taking up to several hours to complete. Procedures may be necessary in patients within a wide range of ages (infant to geriatric) and with significant coexisting disease.
   d) A thorough preanesthetic assessment is imperative.
   e) With the exceptions of angiography or radiotherapy, procedures for IR are painful, are physically invasive to the patient, and may need to be accomplished over several treatment sessions.
   f) Treatment may be required electively or urgently.
   g) Patients may require anesthesia along the continuum from minimal or moderate sedation, local or regional anesthesia, and general anesthesia.
   h) Full monitors and IV access are required.
   i) Additional catheterization and monitoring of arterial pressure and central venous pressure may be necessary.
   j) Certain procedures require monitoring of the patient's neurophysiologic status for changes. The patient may also need to be assessed awake and then resedated at times during the procedure.
   k) Anesthetics that can be used are midazolam, propofol, ketamine, isoflurane, and the other potent inhaled general anesthetics.
   l) Rapid recovery from anesthesia at the end of the case is ideal to assess and monitor the patient's neurologic functioning.
   m) It may be necessary to manipulate or manage normal systemic blood flow, normal cerebral blood flow, or other regional blood

flow. The anesthesia provider may be called upon to control deliberate hypertension or deliberate hypotension, manage anticoagulation, and manage unexpected procedural complications.

n) Intraoperative radiation therapy (IORT) is the delivery of radiation to the patient via a linear accelerator, at times in conjunction with tumor surgery. If surgery is performed coincidental to the dose of radiation, normal tissues may be able to be moved away from the ionizing radiation beam. Normal tissues and organs can be shielded with lead beforehand.
o) Some facilities use a dedicated IORT suite, and others use an operating room with transport of the patient to the radiation oncology suite. General anesthesia is performed if the surgical and radiation procedures are concurrent.
p) All personnel should leave the room during IORT and stereotactically guided Gamma Knife or CyberKnife surgery so that high-dose radiation can be delivered to the patient and to protect personnel from the scattered radiation. The radiation oncology suite is heavily shielded and has a heavy lead or iron door that can take from 30 to 60 seconds to open.
q) The patient is monitored via closed-circuit video and hands-off anesthesia delivery during treatment.
r) Complications can occur rapidly and can be life threatening. Foremost is the possible complication of hemorrhage. A sedated patient experiencing hemorrhage may show sudden signs of headache, nausea and vomiting, and vascular pain.
s) A patient under general anesthesia may experience sudden bradycardia. The airway should be secured first if necessary followed by support of the cardiovascular system, discontinuation of heparin, and administration of protamine (1 mg/100 units of total heparin dose administered).
t) Other possible complications are radiocontrast reactions, embolization of particles or tissue, perforation of an aneurysm, and obliteration of unintended physiologically necessary arteries.
u) Patient safety necessitates skilled and competent staff assistance in treatment of complications.
v) Complications may necessitate the safe transfer of the patient to the operating room.

E. MAGNETIC RESONANCE IMAGING

1. Introduction

MRI uses the dipole moment (the ability of the atomic nucleus to behave as a magnet) of the hydrogen atom. The patient is placed supine within the scanning gantry or bore of the magnet. The magnet used for MRI can be a permanent magnet or a powerful superconducting electromagnet cooled with liquid helium to 4° Kelvin. The quality of the MRI image is directly related to the strength of the magnetic field. Contrast media are also used in MRI studies to enhance the patient's tissues and allow the scan to provide further diagnostic information. MRI contrast is most commonly gadopentetate dimeglumine (Magnevist) than CT scans, which contain the element gadolinium, bound as a chelated structure and administered primarily parenterally but rarely enterally.

2. **Anesthetic technique**
   a) MRI can take up to 1 hour or longer. During this time, the patient should remain extremely still to reduce motion artifacts. These artifacts can cause unfaithful representations of the tissues being studied. The motions of breathing, the heart, blood flow, swallowing, and even cerebrospinal fluid flow produce artifacts in a highly sensitive MRI scan.
   b) The patient is exposed to varying magnetic fields of up to 4 tesla (T), along with additional exposure to variable radiofrequency radiation. Blood flow is decreased by strong magnetic fields, and blood pressure compensates by rising. Patients also have reported symptoms of vertigo, nausea, headache, and visual sensations.
   c) The MRI machine produces loud vibratory and knocking noises as coils are switched on and off during the course of the study.
   d) Most patients are content with an explanation of what to expect during the procedure and with reassurance. Some patients need minimal or moderate sedation. Patients with claustrophobia and those who cannot or will not remain motionless during the study (children) as well as critically ill patients may require deep sedation or general endotracheal anesthesia.
   e) MRI is not painful, so opioids are not usually required. Sedation has been performed with oral and IV midazolam, ketamine, pentobarbital, chloral hydrate, and propofol.
   f) Minimal or deep sedation or general anesthesia requires IV access and full monitoring.
   g) The LMA serves as an excellent, relatively noninvasive airway for MRI. Some anesthesia providers prefer general endotracheal intubation.
   h) Because of the intense magnetic field always present in the MRI suite, anesthesia providers should be aware of every item on their persons and every item that is to be used in conjunction with anesthesia administered to the patient.
   i) Ferromagnetic (iron-containing) substances are attracted at astonishing rates of speed into the bore of the magnet. Personal items such as pens, certain types of eyeglasses, jewelry, watches, pagers, personal computers, calculators, name badges, coins, audiotapes, videotapes, and credit cards are some of the items that should never enter the MRI suite, as well as any ferromagnetic anesthesia equipment, medication vials, and supplies. If a patient were present within the bore of the MRI, injury or death could be possible from the missile created.
   j) Metals that are known to be safe within the proximity of the MRI bore are stainless steel, nonferrous alloys, nickel, and titanium. Materials and equipment constructed of plastic are safe.
   k) Patients possessing certain medical therapeutic devices may be prohibited from an MRI scan.
   l) Cardiac pacemakers may be affected several ways by the electromagnetic field: reprogramming may occur, the pacemaker may be inhibited, it may revert to an asynchronous mode, it may have the reed switch close, it may become dislodged, or it may become heated by the magnetic field.
   m) Any monitor leads and IV tubing should be kept in straight alignment because the intense magnetic fields in the MRI suite can

induce current flow in coiled leads or tubing, and severely burn the patient.

n) Flexible LMAs and endotracheal tubes (ETTs) that contain wire windings can also be sources of burns.

o) The American College of Radiology recommends strong attention to and the elimination of induced current that can be large tissue loops, such as the loop created by the hand touching the hip or thigh, or the loop created when the feet or calves of the legs touch.

p) Consideration should be given to the MRI contrast media administered to patients. The dyes used for MRI contrast are nonionic gadolinium chelates and have extremely low allergy rates. Nausea is a common side effect. Urticaria (hives) and anaphylactoid reactions occur in fewer than 1% of patients. The risk of a reaction to MRI dye is increased in patients with a history of asthma and other allergies or drug sensitivities, especially to iodinated contrast dyes.

q) Although MRI does not use ionizing radiation, patients and personnel are exposed to constant levels of magnetic force while in the MRI suite. Acute exposure to magnetic fields less than 2.5 T have not been shown to have adverse effects in humans. All care providers should make their own determinations regarding how much magnetic exposure they will accept during a patient's MRI scan. Doses both to the patient and to all personnel should be minimized.

r) If the anesthesia provider is away from the patient during the procedure, it should be ensured that all airway circuitry, monitoring leads, and IV connections are secure and tight.

s) Use monitors with both audible and visual alarms. Have a clear and continual view of the patient and the anesthesia monitors, in conjunction with recognized standards of safety. Consideration should be made for safe and rapid access to the patient, should the need exist.

t) Manufacturers have developed a host of MRI-compatible anesthesia equipment and supplies. This host of equipment and supplies allows performance of the anesthetic procedure directly within the MRI suite.

u) The following boxes list the equipment and supplies and the devices to be aware of for patient selection.

List of Available Magnetic Resonance Imaging–Compatible Equipment and Supplies

MRI-compatible anesthesia machine	ECG cable
Pulse oximeter	Capnograph
IV bag pole	Laryngoscope with lithium batteries and aluminum spacers
Liquid crystal temperature monitoring strip	Laryngoscope blades
Thermocouple temperature probe with RF filter	Nerve stimulator
Respiratory rate monitor	IV infusion pump
Noninvasive blood pressure monitor	Oxygen tanks
Pulse oximeter	Precordial stethoscope
ECG	Esophageal stethoscope
ECG patches	Patient carts
	Tables and trays

ECG, Electrocardiography; *IV*, intravenous; *MRI*, magnetic resonance imaging; *RF*, radiofrequency.

Devices or Metal Affected by Magnetic Resonance Imaging That Cause Patient Morbidity or Mortality

- AICDs
- Cardiac pacemakers
- Certain mechanical heart valves
- Cochlear implants
- Deep brain neurostimulators
- Dorsal column stimulators
- Pacing wires
- Penile implants
- Permanent eyeliner or tattoos
- Prostheses (including dental prostheses)
- Implanted pumps (e.g., baclofen, narcotic, or insulin pumps)
- Internal plates, wires, or screws
- Metallic aneurysm clips (clips manufactured after 1995 and certified MRI compatible can be scanned)
- Certain metallic implants (history or recent orthopedic implants inserted within three months, dental implants)
- Metallic sutures
- Shrapnel and metal fragments (especially intraocular metal shrapnel)
- Tissue expanders with metallic ports

AICD, Automatic implantable cardiac defibrillator; *MRI,* magnetic resonance imaging.

F. PEDIATRIC ANESTHESIA FOR THERAPEUTIC AND DIAGNOSTIC PROCEDURES

Radiation Therapy

1. Introduction

Radiation therapy uses ionizing photons to destroy lymphomas, pediatric acute leukemias, Wilms tumor, retinoblastomas, and tumors of the CNS. Repeat sessions are typical and require reliable motionlessness and remote monitoring with the child in isolation. As in many off-site locations, the key issue is maintaining an adequate airway because of limited access to the patient.

2. Preoperative assessment and patient preparation

a) The treatment is performed in the radiation oncology department.
b) Standard preoperative assessment is performed.
c) Check the previous anesthetic record for any potential problems and anesthetic requirements. Because several repeat sessions are common, it is likely that the patient will have a recent anesthetic record available for the anesthetist to review preoperatively.
d) Most children will have some type of medication access port. Flush the catheter with 0.9% normal saline using sterile technique. Give a bolus of propofol and start a propofol infusion in the preoperative area. Take the patient to the treatment room and maintain the airway.

3. Room preparation

a) Use standard monitoring equipment.
b) Bring portable oxygen if it is not in the treatment area.
c) Airway equipment is used.
d) Emergency medications are available.

e) Position the patient supine or prone.
f) Simulations: Use an offsite pediatric anesthesia machine.

4. **Anesthetic technique**
   a) The case may last up to 60 minutes. General anesthesia with an oral ETT usually is required. Many procedures are done with the patient in the prone position for brainstem or spinal cord tumors. The purpose of this is to have the child motionless, so the clinicians may design a mold to be used to hold the patient in a particular position for the upcoming treatments and for Groshong catheter insertion. Active scavenging through wall suction may be available, but TIVA is frequently used (after an IV line and an oral ETT are established) to expedite emergence and discharge.
   b) Treatments: Pediatric patients come for treatment series after the simulation-established mold and Groshong catheter insertion. Treatment may be as short as 10 minutes or as long as 40 minutes. Use a nasal cannula with end-tidal carbon dioxide tubing or two pediatric nasal cannulas.
5. **Postoperative implications**
   a) Ensure that all standard monitors and equipment are available for recovery of anesthesia.
   b) Have a means of providing 100% oxygen by positive-pressure ventilation.
   c) A resuscitation cart should be available.

Diagnostic Urology: Voiding Cystourethrogram

1. **Introduction**

Children requiring a voiding cystourethrogram (VCU) usually have had a failed previous attempt without anesthesia. The test requires placement of a urinary catheter followed by filling of the bladder and voiding. Children usually object to placement of the catheter.

2. **Room preparation**
   a) Pediatric gas machine
   b) IV medication tray
   c) Oxygen tank for transport (optional)
3. **Anesthetic technique**

Mask induction is a very quick procedure (less than 10 minutes), and an IV line is not usually started. The gas machine should be connected to scavenging through the wall suction pin index before induction.

4. **Postoperative considerations**

After the catheter is placed, start waking up the patient so he or she will be able to go to the bathroom to void. The age of the child is usually about 4 years.

Dimercaptosuccinic Acid Imaging

1. **Introduction**

Nuclear medicine imaging can be done with dimercaptosuccinic acid (DMSA) to identify renal function, scarring, and pyelonephritis. This requires the patient to remain still. Anesthesia is used for pediatric patients who are unable to cooperate. The procedure can take 1 to 2 hours.

2. **Room preparation**
   a) Pediatric gas machine
   b) IV medication tray
   c) Oxygen tank for transport optional

3. **Anesthetic technique**
   a) Standard mask ventilation followed by IV insertion
   b) Start propofol infusion at 25 to 50 mcg/kg/min, and adjust to maintain spontaneous breathing.
   c) Oxygen per nasal cannula

G. POSITRON EMISSION TOMOGRAPHY SCAN

1. Introduction

Positron emission tomography (PET) scan is used for the imaging and detection of malignant disease, neurologic function, and cardiovascular disease. The isotope fluorodeoxyglucose (FDG) is injected and is then absorbed into metabolically active cells. The absorbed isotope emits minute amounts of positron antimatter that are detected and produce high-resolution images of diseased tissue.

2. Anesthetic technique

The patient should remain still for about 1 hour after the injection of FDG to minimize the amount of the amount of muscle uptake of this glucose-like molecule. The patient should have fasted to minimize blood glucose levels. Any sedation medications containing sugar should also be avoided.

H. TRANSJUGULAR INTRAHEPATIC PORTOSYSTEMIC SHUNT

1. Introduction

Transjugular intrahepatic portosystemic shunt (TIPS) is an interventional radiologic procedure that creates a shunt between the hepatic and portal veins, created in the liver parenchyma and maintained by placing metallic stents across the tract. The aim is to decrease the portal venous pressure, thereby directing blood flow away from the portosystemic varices and decreasing the formation of ascitic fluid. Portal hypertension, most commonly from hepatic cirrhosis, leads to development of portosystemic varices and ascites. These varices can develop in a variety of sites, with gastroesophageal the most common. Rupture of gastroesophageal varices leads to massive hemorrhage.

2. Preoperative assessment

Refer to Section II of Part 2 for anesthetic implications related to hepatic cirrhosis.

3. **Patient preparation**
   a) Pretreat with H_2-blockers and nonparticulate antacid.
   b) Type and crossmatch 4 units because of the risk of hemorrhage.
   c) Use minimal sedation.
   d) Check laboratory values, including electrolytes, blood urea nitrogen, creatinine, complete blood count, coagulation studies, and liver function tests.
4. **Room preparation**
   a) Standard monitors
   b) Arterial line
   c) Pressure bags or rapid infuser
   d) Vasopressors ready to infuse if needed

5. **Perioperative management and anesthetic technique**
   a) Sedation with local anesthesia
   b) General anesthesia: Avoid nasogastric tube or esophageal stethoscope if esophageal varices are present.
      (1) Rapid-sequence induction
      (2) Standard maintenance
      (3) Maintain normocarbia to optimize portal blood flow
      (4) Awake extubation
      (5) Avoid nitrous oxide
   c) Complications
      (1) Portal vein rupture
      (2) Perforation of liver capsule
      (3) Complete heart block
      (4) Congestive heart failure

I. ADDITIONAL INFORMATION

The following boxes provide additional information relevant to anesthesia for therapeutic and diagnostic procedures.

Comprehensive List of Procedures That May Require Anesthesia Outside the Operating Room

Cardiologic and Vascular Procedures
Diagnostic angiography
AICD insertion
Cardiac catheterization—PCI
Cardioversion
Cryoablation
Electrophysiologic mapping
EVAR
Exclusion of thoracic or abdominal aortic aneurysms
Femoral arterial sheath removal
Pacemaker insertion
Percutaneous ventricular assist device insertion
RFCA for certain cardiac dysrhythmias
Transcatheter closure of atrial septal defects
Valvuloplasty
Venous filter insertion

Emergency Department Procedures
Diagnostic peritoneal lavage
Central venous catheter insertion
Emergency endotracheal intubation
Insertion of intracranial pressure monitor
Lumbar puncture
Orthopedic manipulations
Pericardiocentesis
Thoracocentesis
Tube thoracotomy
Vascular "cut down"

Gastroenterologic Procedures
Colonoscopy
ERCP
EGD
Liver biopsy
Percutaneous endoscopically placed gastrostomy
RF ablation of colorectal liver metastases
Upper endoscopy
Lower endoscopy

Gynecologic Procedures
Assisted reproductive technologies
Gamete intrafallopian transfer
In vitro fertilization
Ovular transvaginal withdrawal
Peritoneal oocyte and sperm transfer
Tubal embryo transfer
Zygote intrafallopian transfer

Hematologic and Oncologic Procedures
Bone marrow aspiration and biopsy
Infusion therapy
Lumbar puncture
Pediatric spinal tap for patients with blood dyscrasias

Continued

Comprehensive List of Procedures That May Require Anesthesia Outside the Operating Room—cont'd

RF procedures
Removal of indwelling central venous catheters

Intensive Care Procedures
Bronchoscopy
Cardioversion
Central venous catheter insertion
Diagnostic peritoneal lavage
Endotracheal intubation
Percutaneous endoscopic gastrostomy
Percutaneous tracheostomy
Thoracocentesis
Thoracotomy and tube thoracotomy
Vascular "cutdown"
Ventriculostomy

Office-Based Procedures
Neurophysiology laboratory
Brainstem auditory evoked responses

Office-Based Surgeries
Dental surgery
Pediatric dentistry (pedodontics)
Oral and maxillofacial surgery
Periodontics
Endodontics
Prosthodontics
General dentistry
Dental hygiene
Plastic surgery
Removal of superficial skin lesions
Rhizotomy
Liposuction
Ophthalmology suites
Electroretinography
Examination under anesthesia
Retinoscopy and tonometry
Various ocular surgical procedures

Orthopedic Procedures
Cast changes
Hardware removal
Joint aspiration

Psychiatric Procedures
ECT

Radiologic and Diagnostic Procedures
Biliary drainage and dilatation
Brachytherapy
CT
Embolization
Functional brain imaging
Interventional neuroradiology
IR (vascular and nonvascular)
Intraoperative radiotherapy
MRI
PET
Radiosurgery
Stereotactic radiosurgery
Radiotherapy and imaging procedures
Teletherapy
TIPS placement
Ultrasound-guided diagnostic and therapeutic procedures

Urologic Procedures
Cystoscopy procedures
Extracorporeal shock-wave lithotripsy
Percutaneous sclerotherapy and drainage of renal cysts
Prostate biopsies
Renal drainage and dilatation

Other Procedures
Anesthesia in military bases and war fields
Remote anesthetic monitoring using telecommunications technology
Veterinary anesthesia

AICD, Automatic implantable cardiac defibrillator; *CT*, computed tomography; *ECT*, electroconvulsive therapy; *EGD*, esophagogastroduodenoscopy; *ERCP*, endoscopic retrograde cholangiopancreatography; *EVAR*, endovascular aortic aneurysm repair; *IR*, interventional radiology; *MRI*, magnetic resonance imaging; *PCI*, percutaneous coronary intervention; *PET*, positron emission tomography; *RF*, radiofrequency; *RFCA*, radiofrequency catheter ablation; *TIPS*, transjugular intrahepatic portosystemic shunt.

Modified from Kotob F, Twersky RS. Anesthesia outside the operating room: general overview and monitoring standards. *Int Anesthesiology Clin.* 2003;41(2):1-15.

Specific Patient Conditions That Alert the Need for Special Attention and Care When Using Anesthetics for Therapeutic and Diagnostic Procedures

- Mental impairment with no possibility of cooperation
- Severe gastroesophageal reflux; delayed gastric emptying; aspiration risk
- Gastroparesis secondary to diabetes mellitus
- Orthopnea; obstructive sleep apnea
- Decreased level of consciousness; depression of airway protection reflexes
- Increased intracranial pressure
- Known difficult intubation; assessed oral, dental, craniofacial, cervical, or thoracic abnormalities that could preclude airway access and maintenance
- Respiratory tract infection; unexplained fever
- Morbid obesity
- Therapeutic or diagnostic procedures that impede airway access
- Therapeutic or diagnostic procedures that are complex, lengthy, painful, or invasive
- Positioning that is complex, atypical, or painful; prone positioning
- Acute trauma
- Extremes in age
- Prematurity
- Physical status 3 or 4

Requisites for Administration of Anesthesia in Remote Locations

- Utilities
- Adequate workspace
- Adequate overhead lighting
- Adequate numbers and current-carrying capacity of electrical outlets
- Electrical service with either isolated electric power or ground fault circuit interrupters
- Uncluttered floor space
- Two-way communication devices—telephone, intercom, Internet availability (instant messaging), PDA device, two-way radios; consider devices with power independent of the electrical service
- Backup power
- Suitable area for postprocedure recovery
- Compliance with all building codes, fire codes, safety codes, and facility standards
- Equipment
- Local infiltration, intravenous sedation, regional and general anesthesia
- Patient chair, cart, or operating surface that can be quickly placed into Trendelenburg position
- Regularly serviced and functioning equipment
- Patient monitors
- Pulse oximeter
- Electrocardiograph
- Blood pressure monitor with a selection of adequate-sized cuffs
- Capnograph
- BIS monitor
- Body temperature monitor
- Oxygen supplies
- Minimum of two oxygen sources should be available with regulators attached (compressed oxygen should be the equivalent of an E cylinder)

Continued

Requisites for Administration of Anesthesia in Remote Locations—cont'd

- Positive-pressure ventilation sources, including a self-inflating resuscitator bag capable of delivering at least 90% oxygen and a mouth-to-mask unit
- Defibrillator—manual biphasic or AED, charged, ready, and easily accessible
- Suction source or suction machine (electrical-powered suction, battery-powered suction, or foot-pump suction devices are available), tubing, suction catheters, and Yankauer suction instruments
- Lockable anesthesia cart to permit organization of supplies, including endotracheal equipment, LMAs, tube of water-soluble lubricating jelly, Combitubes, nasal cannulas, Connell airways, disposable face masks with oxygen tubing, oral and nasal airways, syringes (1 mL tuberculin syringe, 3 mL, 5 mL, 10 mL, 20 mL, 60 mL), needles, IV catheters, tourniquet, IV fluids and tubing, alcohol pads, adhesive tape, sterile IV site covers, disposable gloves, stethoscopes, precordial stethoscope with monaural earpiece and extension tubing, precordial stethoscope adhesive discs, and appropriate anesthetic medications
- Battery-powered flashlight for illumination of the patient, anesthesia machines, and monitors (along with spare batteries)
- Syringe pump, wall plug or transformer, and spare batteries
- Warm blankets, electric blanket (check with hospital policy before using an electric blanket), or forced-air warming devices with the appropriate blanket; towels or hat to cover the patient's head to preserve body warmth
- Blankets, towels, or foam for padding for protection of skin integrity, bony prominences, and body extremities
- Emergency medications to include at a minimum adenosine, aminophylline, amiodarone, atropine, dextrose 50%, diphenhydramine, ephedrine, epinephrine, flumazenil, hydrocortisone, lidocaine, naloxone, nitroglycerin, phenylephrine, succinylcholine, verapamil, and a bronchial dilator inhaler such as albuterol or nebulized epinephrine (e.g., Primatene mist)
- Preoperative anesthesia evaluation forms
- Anesthesia consent form
- Anesthesia charts, clipboard, black ink pens, indelible ink pens

AED, Automatic external defibrillator; *BIS,* bispectral index; *IV,* intravenous; *PDA,* personal digital assistant.

Additional Requirements for General Anesthesia

- Oxygen fail-safe system
- Oxygen analyzer
- Waste gas exhaust scavenging system
- $ETCO_2$ analyzer, extra $ETCO_2$ filter and extension sample tubing
- Vaporizers: calibration and exclusion system
- Respiratory monitoring apparatus (for the anesthesia circuit reservoir bag)
- Alarm system
- Anesthetic medications

In addition to the emergency medications listed above, consider the following:

- Premedication drugs: midazolam, pentobarbital, ketamine, nitrous oxide, diazepam, chloral hydrate
- Induction drugs: propofol, etomidate, methohexital, thiopental, ketamine
- Maintenance drugs: bottles of sevoflurane, isoflurane, desflurane, propofol, ketamine, dexmedetomidine
- Narcotics: midazolam, diazepam, fentanyl, alfentanil, sufentanil, remifentanil
- Muscle relaxants: succinylcholine, rocuronium, cis-atracurium, atracurium, vecuronium

Additional Requirements for General Anesthesia—cont'd

- Muscle relaxant reversal agents: edrophonium, neostigmine, atropine, glycopyrrolate
- Cardiovascular drugs: labetalol, esmolol, verapamil, hydralazine
- Narcotic reversal drugs—naloxone, flumazenil
- Antiemetic drugs: ondansetron, dolasetron, granisetron, metoclopramide, droperidol
- Emergency cart and equipment
- Basic airway equipment (adult and pediatric)
- Nasal and oral airways
- Face mask (appropriate for patient)
- Laryngoscope handle assortment with spare batteries
- Assortment of laryngoscope blades and spare light bulbs, endotracheal tubes (adult and pediatric), LMAs, and dental LMAs
- Combitube
- Self-inflating resuscitator bag (Ambu bag)
- Difficult airway equipment
- LMA
- Light wand
- Emergency cricothyrotomy kit
- Defibrillator: manual biphasic defibrillator or AED
- Supplemental oxygen and nitrous oxide tanks with attached and functional regulators; allow for safe transportation and storage of tanks
- Emergency medications
- CPR compression board
- Suction equipment (suction catheter, Yankauer type)
- Malignant hyperthermia emergency drugs, equipment, and the phone number for the Malignant Hyperthermia Association of the United States (MHAUS) (United States and Canada, 800-MH HYPER or 800-644-9737.

AED, Automatic external defibrillator; *CPR,* cardiopulmonary resuscitation; *$ETCO_2$,* end-tidal carbon dioxide; *LMA,* laryngeal mask airway

Remote Anesthetic Monitoring Using Telecommunications Technology

Communications technology and reliability in conjunction with reliable and accurate electronic monitoring have made it possible to perform anesthetic monitoring (telemonitoring) with the anesthesia provider in one location and the therapeutic or diagnostic procedure in a physically remote, geographically isolated, or environmentally extreme location.

The anesthesia provider may be involved with communication and monitoring involving landline telephone, cellular telephone, wireless walkie-talkies, amateur (ham) radio communications, satellite communications, real-time audio and video, computer and monitor interlinks, the Internet, and videoconferencing software.

The purposes of telemonitoring are the benefits to patients requiring therapeutic or diagnostic procedures with the added safety of available expert care to assist the anesthesia provider in performing anesthesia in a challenging environment. Anesthesia providers can collaborate and use their combined skills during the entire anesthetic procedure from preoperative planning to postprocedure care and eventual discharge. Telemonitoring also provides a tool for mentoring and teaching.

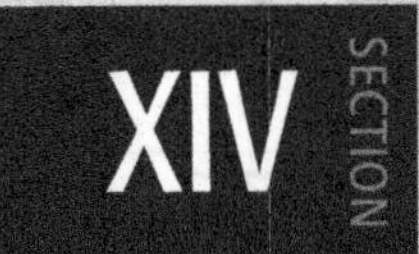

SECTION XIV Vascular Surgery

A. ABDOMINAL AORTIC ANEURYSM

1. Introduction

Surgical treatment of abdominal aortic aneurysm (AAA) may be required for atherosclerotic occlusive disease or aneurysmal dilation. These processes can involve the aorta and any of its major branches, leading to ischemia or rupture and exsanguination.

The primary event in aortic dissection is a tear in the intimal wall through which blood surges and creates a false lumen. The adventitia then separates up or down (or both) the aorta for various distances. Associated conditions include atherosclerosis and hypertension (which is present in 80% of these patients), Marfan syndrome, blunt chest trauma, pregnancy, and iatrogenic surgical injury (e.g., resulting from aortic cannulation during cardiopulmonary bypass [CPB]).

Aortic dissections involving the ascending aorta are considered type A. Surgical repair is through a median sternotomy using profound hypothermia and total circulatory arrest or CPB with moderate hypothermia. Aortic dissections involving the descending aorta (i.e., beyond the origin of the left subclavian artery) are considered type B. Aneurysms can also be classified as saccular, fusiform, or dissecting. Surgical repair involves proximal and distal clamping of the aorta, opening of the aneurysm, evacuation of the thrombus, and placement of a graft. A midline transabdominal surgical approach or retroperitoneal left thoracoabdominal approach may be used.

2. Incidence

The incidence of AAAs has increased over the last 5 decades from 12.2 to 36.2 per 100,000 surgical procedures. This increase may partially be the result of the detection of asymptomatic aneurysms by noninvasive diagnostic modalities, such as computed tomography (CT), magnetic resonance imaging (MRI), and ultrasonography. The occurrence of AAAs has increased because of the increased age of the general population and the vascular changes that occur as a result of aging. Aortic aneurysms can be identified in approximately 1% to 4% of the population older than 50 years and in approximately 5% of the population older than 60 years. Aneurysms are more common in men than in women and in whites than in African Americans.

The present mortality rate ranges from 1% to 11% (although most commonly estimated at 5%) compared with the mortality rates in the 1950s of 18% to 30%. Advanced detection capabilities, earlier surgical intervention, extensive preoperative preparation, refined surgical techniques, better hemodynamic monitoring, improved anesthetic techniques, and aggressive postoperative management have all contributed to this improvement in surgical outcomes. Surgical intervention is recommended for AAAs 5.5 cm or larger in diameter. Estimates of mortality resulting from ruptured AAAs vary from 35% to 94%. The 5-year mortality rate for individuals with untreated AAAs is 81%, and the 10-year mortality rate is 100% Early detection and elective surgical intervention are advisable because rupture leads to an increased incidence of mortality.

3. **Diagnosis**
   a) Frequently, asymptomatic aneurysms are detected incidentally during routine examination or abdominal radiography. Smaller aneurysms are often undetected on routine physical examination.
   b) Diagnostic techniques, such as ultrasonography, CT scan, and MRI, may identify vascular abnormalities in these patients. Such noninvasive techniques not only reveal the presence of aneurysms but also provide information about aneurysm size, vessel wall integrity, and adjacent anatomic definition.
   c) Invasive techniques, including contrast-enhanced CT scan, contrast angiography, and digital subtraction angiography (DSA), can provide additional information and more detailed representations of arterial anatomy. DSA is the best method of evaluating suprarenal aneurysms because this method provides superior definition of the aneurysmal relationship to the renal arteries.

Abdominal Aortic Reconstruction

1. **Patient selection**
   a) Most patients with abdominal aneurysms, including octogenarians, are considered surgical candidates. Although advancing age contributes to an increased incidence of morbidity and mortality, age alone is not a contraindication to elective aneurysmectomies.
   b) Physiologic age is more indicative than chronologic age of increased surgical risk.
   c) Contraindications to elective repair include intractable angina pectoris, recent myocardial infarction (MI), severe pulmonary dysfunction, and chronic renal insufficiency.
   d) Patients with stable coronary artery disease (CAD) with coronary artery stenosis of greater than 70% requiring nonemergent AAA repair do not benefit from revascularization if beta blockade has been established.
2. **Patient preparation**
   a) Preoperative fluid loading and restoration of intravascular volume are perhaps the most important techniques used to enhance cardiac function during abdominal aortic aneurysmectomies.
   b) Reliable venous access should be secured if volume replacement is to be accomplished. Large-bore intravenous (IV) lines and central lines can be used to infuse fluids or blood.
   c) Massive hemorrhage is an ever-present threat; therefore, the availability of blood and blood products should be ensured. Provisions for rapid transfusion and intraoperative blood salvage should be confirmed.
3. **Monitoring**
   a) Standard monitoring methods include electrocardiography (ECG) with display of lead II for detection of dysrhythmias and the precordial V_5 lead for analysis of ischemic ST segment changes, pulse oximetry, and capnography.
   b) An esophageal stethoscope allows for continuous auscultation of heart and breath sounds as well as temperature determination.
   c) Placement of an indwelling urinary catheter is necessary for the continuous measurement of urinary output and renal function. Neuromuscular function is also routinely monitored.
   d) Invasive blood pressure monitoring permits beat-to-beat analysis of the blood pressure, immediate identification of hemodynamic

alterations related to aortic clamping, and access for blood sampling.

e) Pulmonary artery catheters can be used in abdominal aortic reconstruction for monitoring left-sided filling pressures as a guide for fluid replacement.

f) Pulmonary artery catheterization not only provides clinical indexes that reflect intravascular volume but also facilitates calculations of stroke volume, cardiac index, and left ventricular stroke work index.

g) Myocardial ischemia can be detected by analysis of pulmonary artery catheter tracings. Some pulmonary artery catheters allow for measurement of mixed venous oxygen saturation.

h) By detecting changes in ventricular wall motion, two-dimensional transesophageal echocardiography provides a sensitive method for assessing regional myocardial perfusion. Wall motion abnormalities also occur much sooner than ECG changes during periods of reduced coronary blood flow.

i) Myocardial ischemia poses the greatest risk of mortality after abdominal aortic reconstruction. Intraoperative monitoring may enable earlier detection and intervention during ischemic cardiac events.

4. Application of aortic cross-clamp: Hemodynamic alterations

a) The hemodynamic effects of aortic cross-clamping depend on the application site along the aorta, the patient's preoperative cardiac reserve, and the patient's intravascular volume.

b) The most common site for cross-clamping is infrarenal because most aneurysms appear below the level of the renal arteries. Less common sites of aneurysm development are the juxtarenal and suprarenal areas.

c) When aortic cross-clamping is used, hypertension occurs above the cross-clamp, and hypotension occurs below the cross-clamp. Organs proximal to the aortic occlusion may experience a redistribution of blood volume.

d) There is an absence of blood flow distal to the clamp in the pelvis and lower extremities.

e) Increases in afterload cause myocardial wall tension to increase. Mean arterial pressure (MAP) and systemic vascular resistance (SVR) also increase.

f) Cardiac output may decrease or remain unchanged. Pulmonary artery occlusion pressure (PAOP) may increase or display no change.

g) The percentages of change in cardiovascular indexes at different levels of aortic occlusion are listed in the following table.

Change in Cardiovascular Variables at Different Levels of Aortic Occlusion as Assessed by Two-Dimensional Transesophageal Echocardiography

	Change After Occlusion at Different Levels (% Increase or Decrease)		
Variable	Infrarenal	Suprarenal-Infraceliac	Supraceliac
Mean arterial pressure	↑2	↑5	↑54
Pulmonary artery occlusion pressure	0	↑10	↑38

Change in Cardiovascular Variables at Different Levels of Aortic Occlusion as Assessed by Two-Dimensional Transesophageal Echocardiography—cont'd

	Change After Occlusion at Different Levels (% Increase or Decrease)		
Variable	**Infrarenal**	**Suprarenal-Infraceliac**	**Supraceliac**
End-diastolic area	↑9	↑2	↑28
End-systolic area	↑11	↑10	↑69
Ejection fraction	↓3	↓10	↓38
	Number of Patients Affected		
Patients with wall motion abnormality	0	33	92
New myocardial infarction	0	0	8

Modified from Roizen MF, Beaupre PN, Alpert RA, et al. Monitoring with two-dimensional transesophageal echocardiography: comparison of myocardial function in patients undergoing supraceliac, suprarenal-infraceliac, or infrarenal aortic occlusion. *J Vasc Surg* 1984;1(2):300-305.

h) Patients with ischemic heart disease or ventricular dysfunction are unable to fully compensate as a result of the hemodynamic alterations. The increased wall stress attributed to aortic cross-clamp application may contribute to decreased global ventricular function and myocardial ischemia. Clinically, these patients experience increases in PAOP in response to aortic cross-clamping. Aggressive pharmacologic intervention is required for restoration of cardiac function during this time.

5. **Metabolic alterations**
   a) After the application of an aortic cross-clamp, the lack of blood flow to distal structures makes these tissues prone to developing hypoxia. In response to hypoxia, metabolites (e.g., lactate) accumulate.
   b) The release of arachidonic acid derivatives may also contribute to the cardiac instability that is observed during aortic cross-clamping. Thromboxane A_2 synthesis, which is accelerated by the application of an aortic cross-clamp, may be responsible for the decrease in myocardial contractility and cardiac output that occurs.
   c) Traction on the mesentery is a surgical maneuver used for exposing the aorta. Decreases in blood pressure and SVR, tachycardia, increased cardiac output, and facial flushing are common responses to mesenteric traction.
   d) The neuroendocrine response to major surgical stress is believed to be mediated by cytokines such as interleukin 1-beta (IL-1β), interleukin-6 (IL-6), and tumor necrosis factor alpha (TNF-α), as well as plasma catecholamines and cortisol. These mediators are thought to be responsible for triggering the inflammatory response that results in increased body temperature, leukocytosis, tachycardia, tachypnea, and fluid sequestration.
6. **Effects on regional circulation**
   a) Structures distal to the aortic clamp are underperfused during aortic cross-clamping. Renal insufficiency and renal failure have been reported to occur after abdominal aortic reconstruction.
   b) Suprarenal and juxtarenal cross-clamping may be associated with a higher incidence of altered renal dynamics; however,

reductions in renal blood flow can occur with any level of clamp application.

c) Infrarenal aortic cross-clamping is associated with a 38% decrease in renal blood flow and a 75% increase in renal vascular resistance. These effects may lead to acute renal failure, which is fatal in 50% to 90% of patients who have undergone aneurysmectomies.

d) Preoperative evaluation of renal function is one of the most significant predictors of postoperative renal dysfunction. Therefore, a complete evaluation of renal function is required in the preoperative period.

e) Spinal cord damage is associated with aortic occlusion. Interruption of blood flow to the greater radicular artery (artery of Adamkiewicz) in the absence of collateral blood flow has been identified as a causative factor in paraplegia.

f) The incidence of neurologic complications increases as the aortic cross-clamp is positioned in a higher or more proximal area.

g) Ischemic colon injury is a well-documented complication that is associated with abdominal aortic resections. Ischemia of the colon is most frequently attributed to manipulation of the inferior mesenteric artery, which supplies the primary blood supply to the left colon. This vessel is often sacrificed during surgery, and blood flow to the descending and sigmoid colon depends on the presence and the adequacy of the collateral vessels. Mucosal ischemia occurs in 10% of patients who undergo AAA repair. In fewer than 1% of these patients, infarction of the left colon necessitates surgical intervention.

7. **Aortic cross-clamp release**

a) While the aorta is occluded, metabolites that are liberated as a result of anaerobic metabolism, such as serum lactate, accumulate below the aortic cross-clamp and induce vasodilation and vasomotor paralysis.

b) As the cross-clamp is released, SVR decreases, and blood is sequestered into previously dilated veins, which decreases venous return.

c) Reactive hyperemia causes transient vasodilation secondary to the presence of tissue hypoxia, the release of adenine nucleotides, and the liberation of an unnamed vasodepressor substance that acts as a myocardial depressant and a peripheral vasodilator.

d) This combination of events results in decreased preload and afterload. The hemodynamic instability that may ensue after the release of an aortic cross-clamp is called *declamping shock syndrome.*

e) Evidence demonstrates that venous endothelin (ET)-1 may be partially responsible for the hemodynamic alterations that accompany declamping shock syndrome. Venous ET-1 has a positive inotropic effect on the heart as well as a vasoconstricting and vasodilating action on blood vessels.

f) The most frequently observed hemodynamic responses to aortic declamping are listed in the table below.

Hemodynamic Responses to Aortic Declamping

Clinical Index	Response to Clamp Release
Mean arterial pressure	Decrease
Systemic vascular resistance	Decrease
Cardiac output	No change or increase
Pulmonary artery occlusion pressure	Decrease

g) The magnitude of the response to unclamping the aorta may be manipulated. Although SVR and MAP decrease, intravascular volume may influence the direction and the magnitude of change in cardiac output.
h) Restoration of circulating blood volume is paramount in the provision of circulatory stability before release of the aortic clamp.
i) The site and the duration of cross-clamp application, as well as the gradual release of the clamp, influence the magnitude of circulatory instability. Partial release of the aortic cross clamp over time frequently results in less severe hypotension.

8. **Surgical approach**
   a) The standard approach for elective abdominal aortic reconstruction is the transperitoneal incision. The advantages of this route include exposure of infrarenal and iliac vessels, ability to inspect intraabdominal organs, and rapid closure. Unfavorable consequences associated with this approach include increased fluid losses, prolonged ileus, postoperative incisional pain, and pulmonary complications.
   b) The retroperitoneal approach has gained popularity as an alternative to the standard route. Its advantages include excellent exposure (especially for juxtarenal and suprarenal aneurysms), decreased fluid losses, less incisional pain, and fewer postoperative pulmonary and intestinal complications. After implantation with a synthetic graft, the aortic adventitia is closed. In addition, the retroperitoneal approach does not elicit mesenteric traction syndrome. The reported limitations of this approach are unfamiliarity of surgeons with this technique, poor right distal renal artery exposure, and inability to inspect the integrity of the abdominal contents.
9. **Management of fluid and blood loss**
   a) Extreme loss of extracellular fluid and blood should be expected with abdominal aortic aneurysmectomies. Evaporative losses and third spacing occur, with the magnitude of loss depending on the surgical approach, the duration of the surgery, and the experience of the surgeon.
   b) Most blood loss occurs because of back bleeding from the lumbar and inferior mesenteric arteries after the vessels have been clamped and the aneurysm is opened.
   c) The use of heparin also contributes to blood loss. Excessive bleeding, however, can occur at any point during surgery, and blood replacement is commonly administered during abdominal aortic resections.
   d) Because of the heightened awareness of transfusion-related morbidity, the use of autologous blood has generated increasing interest. Presently, three options are available for the use of autologous transfusions: preoperative deposit, intraoperative phlebotomy and hemodilution, and intraoperative blood salvage.
10. **Preoperative assessment**
    a) The presence of underlying CAD in patients with vascular disease has been well documented. CAD is reported to occur in more than 50% of patients who require abdominal aortic reconstruction and is the single most significant risk factor influencing long-term survivability. MIs are responsible for 40% to 70% of all fatalities that

occur after aneurysm reconstruction. In the presence of such threatening mortality rates, the extent of CAD and the subsequent functional limitations should be clearly defined and cardiac function optimized preoperatively before elective aortic vascular reconstruction is performed.

b) Advanced age, cardiac history, aberrations on physical examination, ECG abnormalities, and previous surgical procedures are identifiable factors in the cardiac risk index that contribute to cardiac complications.

c) Patients with unremarkable medical histories and normal physical examinations, exercise testing, ECG, and laboratory studies have a decreased surgical risk. Currently, investigators advocate the use of coronary angiography in selected patients who have positive findings on the initial cardiac evaluation.

d) Patients with symptomatic CAD require more extensive cardiac evaluation. Dipyridamole thallium testing is perhaps one of the most reliable methods for evaluating the extent of myocardial dysfunction associated with CAD and for predicting coronary events after vascular surgery.

e) Techniques capable of evaluating left ventricular performance, such as echocardiography, are of some value in the prediction of adverse cardiac events. Ambulatory ECG monitoring has also been very successful in the identification of postoperative cardiac complications. Coronary angiography provides the most reliable definition of coronary anatomy and the extent of CAD.

f) The end point of any method of preoperative cardiac evaluation for aneurysmectomy is identification of functional cardiac limitations. Depending on the degree of cardiac dysfunction, preoperative optimization of cardiac function may range from simple pharmacologic manipulation to surgical intervention.

g) Hypertension, chronic obstructive pulmonary disease, diabetes mellitus, renal impairment, and carotid artery disease are frequently observed in patients with AAAs.

h) Measures should be taken to optimize organ function because each of these disease states contributes to postoperative complications. Preoperative renal dysfunction deserves special consideration because aortic cross-clamping produces alterations in renal dynamics. The degree of preoperative renal insufficiency contributes to the extent of any postoperative renal damage.

11. Intraoperative management

a) Anesthetic selection

(1) The anesthetic selection should be based on the following objectives: provision of analgesia and amnesia, facilitation of relaxation, maintenance of hemodynamic stability, preservation of renal blood flow, and minimization of morbidity and mortality.

(2) Inhalation agents

(a) All inhalation anesthetics may depress the myocardium and cause hemodynamic instability. Therefore, high concentrations of inhalation agents in patients with moderate to severe decreased ejection fraction should not be used.

(b) Potential organ toxicity and lack of postoperative analgesia may be additional limitations to the use of these agents.

(c) Beneficial effects attributed to the use of inhalation agents include the ability to alter autonomic responses, reversibility, rapid emergence, and potentially earlier extubation.

(3) Narcotic technique

(a) A balanced technique using a combination of high-dose narcotics with nitrous oxide can be used as the anesthetic for major vascular surgery.

(b) The cardiovascular stability provided by opioids has been well documented, and this feature is especially attractive for patients with ischemic heart disease and ventricular dysfunction.

(c) Provision of intense analgesia for the initial postoperative period after major abdominal vascular surgery, via the administration of a neuraxial opioid, does not alter the combined incidence of major cardiovascular, respiratory, and renal complications.

(4) Regional anesthesia

(a) The use of epidural anesthesia for abdominal aneurysmectomies has gained renewed interest. Several benefits of epidural use include decreased preload and afterload, preserved myocardial oxygenation, reduced stress response, excellent muscle relaxation, decreased incidence of postoperative thromboembolism, and increased graft flow to the lower extremities.

(b) Hypotension may also be a significant unfavorable result of an epidural technique. In fact, this technique requires the administration of approximately 1600 to 2000 mL more IV fluid than is usual with general anesthetic.

(c) The controversy regarding hematoma formation after heparinization during epidural techniques is still noteworthy. Studies have shown that the simultaneous use of epidural anesthesia and low-dose heparinization rarely produces complications.

(d) Postoperative pain control is vital to maintain hemodynamic stability and to alleviate patient suffering. Epidural narcotics have been shown to decrease pain after major surgery.

(e) Because of the high incidence of CAD in patients presenting for abdominal aortic reconstruction, severe postoperative pain can result in an increased heart rate and blood pressure, which may contribute to cardiac-related morbidity and mortality. Pain relief may decrease respiratory splinting and decrease the likelihood of hypoxemia.

(5) Combination techniques

(a) Combining anesthetic techniques for major vascular surgery is more popular than using them alone because the advantages of each technique contribute to a smoother anesthetic.

(b) A balanced technique supplemented by low-dose inhalation agents maintains cardiovascular hemodynamics and controls momentary autonomic responses to surgical stimulation.

(c) Another choice is to use epidural anesthesia combined with light general anesthesia. This provides the benefits of epidural anesthesia and the ability to provide amnesia and controlled ventilation.

b) Fluid management
   (1) The maintenance of intravascular volume may be an extreme challenge during abdominal aortic resections. Controversy exists regarding whether the administration of crystalloids or colloids affects the overall incidence of morbidity and mortality.
   (2) Crystalloids may be used for replacing basal and third-space losses at an approximate rate of 10 mL/kg/hr.
   (3) Blood losses initially can be replaced with crystalloids at a ratio of three to one. The combination of crystalloid and colloid administration is also acceptable.
   (4) Regardless of the choice of fluid, volume replacement should be dictated by physiologic parameters. Fluid replacement should be sufficient for the maintenance of normal cardiac filling pressures, cardiac output, and urine output of 1 mL/kg/hr.
   (5) Patients with limited cardiac reserve can develop congestive heart failure if hypervolemia occurs.

c) Hemodynamic alterations
   (1) Hemodynamic changes are likely to occur throughout the anesthesia process.
   (2) Momentary fluctuations in heart rate and blood pressure should be anticipated during induction and intubation.
   (3) Preoperative replacement of fluid deficits prevents exaggerated responses to vasodilating induction agents.
   (4) For patients with adequate left ventricular function, hemodynamic stability can be preserved with a "slow" induction using opioids and β-adrenergic blocking agents.
   (5) Etomidate has minimal myocardial depressant effects and may be most suitable for patients with limited cardiac reserve.
   (6) The response to mesenteric traction is also associated with momentary hemodynamic changes.
   (7) Application of the aortic cross-clamp produces various hemodynamic responses. Patients without underlying ischemic heart disease usually demonstrate slight changes in PAOP when the aorta is occluded, requiring minimal intervention. However, patients with a history of CAD may experience an increase in PAOP and a decrease in cardiac output, indicating left ventricular decompensation.
   (8) Although several different pharmacologic agents may be used, nitroglycerin appears to be the drug of choice because of its primary pharmacologic effect of decreasing preload and thereby decreasing myocardial oxygen demand.
   (9) Whereas inotropic agents, such as dopamine and dobutamine, may improve cardiac output, pharmacologic agents that decrease afterload, such as sodium nitroprusside and isoflurane, may decrease SVR.
   (10) The more proximal the application of the aortic cross-clamp, the greater the magnitude and the severity of these responses. Vasoactive medications should be readily available throughout the surgery.

(11) When the aortic cross-clamp is released, declamping shock syndrome may occur. Severe hypotension and reduction in cardiac output may ensue. These conditions can be prevented by volume loading and raising of the central venous pressure 3 to 5 mmHg or raising the PAOP 3 to 4 mmHg just before the clamp is released.

(12) If severe acidosis is present, sodium bicarbonate may be administered. Temporarily increasing minute ventilation may also be useful for the control of acidosis.

d) Renal preservation

(1) The incidence of acute renal failure after infrarenal cross-clamping is 5%, and this value increases to 13% after suprarenal cross-clamping.

(2) The mortality rate is four to five times greater in patients who develop acute renal failure postoperatively.

(3) Alterations in renal dynamics during intrarenal cross-clamping may continue up to 1 hour after the clamp is released. Such alterations can be profound and can extend into the postoperative period.

(4) Mechanisms for the preservation of renal function during aortic cross-clamping include improving renal and glomerular blood flow.

(5) Maintenance of cardiac output and intravascular volume is vital. Prevention of hypovolemia is the best prophylaxis against renal failure.

(6) Administration of mannitol 20 to 30 minutes before aortic clamping may help preserve renal function because of hydroxyl free-radical scavenging properties.

(7) Further intervention includes IV administration of low-dose dopamine at 3 to 5 mcg/kg/min, fenoldopam, and use of loop diuretics. Renal dose dopamine has not been proven to decrease the risk of postoperative renal dysfunction.

12. Postoperative implications

a) Cardiac, respiratory, and renal failure are the most common complications observed postoperatively in patients recovering from abdominal aortic reconstruction.

b) Cardiovascular function should be closely monitored in the intensive care unit for at least 24 hours after surgery. Maintenance of adequate blood pressure, intravascular fluid volume, and myocardial oxygenation is paramount during this period.

c) MI frequently contributes to postoperative morbidity and mortality. Serial cardiac enzyme analysis may be monitored.

d) Pharmacologic agents used in the treatment of hypertension should also be available.

e) Most patients require ventilatory assistance during the postoperative period. Vigilant monitoring of respiratory function is mandatory, especially when epidural catheters are used for postoperative analgesia.

f) Renal function should be continuously evaluated in the postoperative phase. Urine output should be maintained at 1 mL/kg/hr. Administration of fluid, maintenance of physiologic hemodynamics, and concurrent administration of pharmacologic agents should be considered to improve urine output.

Juxtarenal and Suprarenal Aortic Aneurysms

1. **Introduction**
   a) Although most AAAs occur below the level of the renal arteries, 2% extend proximally and involve the renal or visceral arteries.
   b) Juxtarenal aneurysms are located at the level of the renal arteries, but they spare the renal artery orifice. More proximal suprarenal aneurysms include at least one of the renal arteries and may involve visceral vessels.
   c) The effects of aortic cross-clamping for juxtarenal or suprarenal aneurysms are similar to those for infrarenal aortic occlusions; however, the magnitude of hemodynamic alterations increases as the aorta is clamped more proximally.
2. **Anesthetic technique**
   a) Preoperative preparation includes a thorough evaluation of coexisting disease, with an emphasis on cardiac function.
   b) As the aorta is clamped more proximally, left ventricular afterload increases; consequently, myocardial ischemia is more likely to occur.
   c) Diligent cardiac monitoring is necessary, and direct intraarterial blood pressure assessment, cardiac filling pressure monitoring, and transesophageal echocardiography are advocated to detect cardiac dysfunction and allow for immediate pharmacologic intervention.
   d) Renal failure, although possible during infrarenal aortic cross-clamping, occurs more frequently as a result of suprarenal aortic occlusion. Maintaining adequate intravascular volume and administering osmotic and loop diuretics may minimize renal ischemia and dysfunction.
   e) If the ischemic episode persists for longer than 45 minutes, renal cooling is suggested. Renal cooling consists of flushing the kidney with an iced electrolyte perfusate that contains heparin and glucose.
   f) Paraplegia is possible when the blood supply to the spinal cord is interrupted by aortic cross-clamping at or above the level of the diaphragm.
   g) Increasing the MAP or decreasing the cerebrospinal fluid (CSF) pressure may be used as a means to increase spinal cord perfusion pressure.

Ruptured Abdominal Aortic Aneurysm

1. **Introduction**
   a) A high mortality rate of up to 94% is associated with a ruptured AAA.
   b) The most common symptoms of ruptured AAAs are abdominal discomfort with a pulsatile mass, back pain, decreased peripheral pulses, and hypotension.
   c) Hypotension and a history of cardiac disease are two factors associated with the poorest prognosis.
   d) Patients with these symptoms should be immediately transferred to the operating room for surgical exploration. When hypotension is absent, more time is available for a comprehensive CT scan to search for other causes of abdominal discomfort.
   e) When the patient arrives in the operative suite, a brief preoperative evaluation, establishing of venous access, and provisions for fluid and blood product administration can be completed.

f) Induction of anesthesia should follow the principles of trauma anesthesia. Hemodynamic stability should be the primary objective, and anesthetic induction and maintenance agents should be selected on a case-by-case basis.
g) Cardiovascular resuscitation is the anesthesia provider's primary focus until blood loss from the proximal aorta is controlled by surgical intervention. Fluid resuscitation can begin with crystalloids, and blood products can be administered as they become available. Intraoperative blood salvage provisions should be secured.
h) If large amounts of blood products are given, coagulation studies and ionized calcium values should be calculated. The use of fresh-frozen plasma has been shown to decrease the total transfusion requirements and the incidence of coagulopathies. The ability to administer platelets may also be necessary.
i) After initial fluid resuscitation has been performed and hemodynamic stability has been ensured, direct arterial blood pressure monitoring should be instituted. A central venous or pulmonary artery catheter may be inserted.
j) The hemodynamic effects of aortic cross-clamping and release are similar to those for elective surgery; however, responses may be extreme, especially if hypotension exists when the clamp is released.
k) Measures for ensuring the adequacy of renal circulation, such as administering mannitol, should be incorporated. Because mannitol is an osmotic diuretic, decreased vascular volume resulting in hypotension can occur. Because most patients require large amounts of fluid and blood replacement, postoperative mechanical ventilation is recommended.

B. AORTOBIFEMORAL BYPASS GRAFTING

1. Introduction

Aortobifemoral bypass grafting is commonly performed to correct symptomatic unilateral iliac occlusive disease, which generally occurs in men older than 55 years.

2. Preoperative assessment and patient preparation

a) History and physical examination
  (1) Cardiovascular: 30% to 50% of patients have coexisting CAD. Other common risk factors are MI, hypertension, angina, valvular disease, congestive heart failure, and arrhythmias.
  (2) Respiratory: Most patients have a significant history of smoking and possibly chronic obstructive pulmonary disease.
  (3) Neurologic: Check for coexisting cerebrovascular disease.
  (4) Renal: Chronic renal insufficiency is common.
  (5) Endocrine: Many patients have diabetes and its associated complications.

b) Patient preparation
  (1) Laboratory tests: Complete blood count, prothrombin time, partial thromboplastin time, bleeding time, electrolytes, blood urea nitrogen, creatinine, creatinine clearance, and urinalysis are obtained.
  (2) Diagnostic tests: 12-lead ECG, pulmonary function tests, arterial blood gases, chest radiography, MRI, CT, and arteriography are obtained.

(3) Preoperative medications: Knowledge of daily medications is essential. Cardiac medications are continued, and anticoagulant therapy is sometimes held for 4 hours before surgery. Anxiolytics, sedatives, and analgesics are used as indicated.
(4) IV therapy: Have a central line with two 14- to 16-gauge IV lines. The estimated blood loss is 500 mL.

3. Room preparation

a) Monitoring equipment: Standard with arterial line and central venous pressure catheter, pulmonary arterial catheter, or both. ST segment analysis and transesophageal echocardiography are beneficial.
b) Additional equipment: This includes a fluid warmer; consider a cell saver.
c) Drugs
   (1) Miscellaneous pharmacologic agents: Osmotic and loop diuretics, local anesthetics, antibiotics, adrenergic antagonists, inotropic agents, vasodilators or constrictors, and heparin are used.
   (2) IV fluids: Calculate for major blood loss. Consider rapid infusion of crystalloids, colloids, or both to treat hypovolemic states.
   (3) Blood: Type and cross-match for 4 units of packed red blood cells.
   (4) Tabletop: Standard

4. Anesthetic technique

General anesthesia, epidural anesthesia, or a combination of general and regional anesthesia is used.

5. Perioperative management

a) Induction: Use smooth induction to preserve cerebral perfusion and to maintain hemodynamic stability. For general anesthesia, consider etomidate, fentanyl, lidocaine, and muscle relaxants to decrease episodes of tachycardia and hypotension. For regional anesthesia, consider placing an epidural catheter before beginning anticoagulation.
b) Maintenance: For general anesthesia, consider oxygen and a volatile agent or narcotic. For regional anesthesia, use a local anesthetic, narcotic, or anxiolytic. Maintain blood pressure within the high-normal range.
c) Emergence: Maintain hemodynamic stability; prevent hypertension and tachycardia. For general anesthesia, use full reversal of muscle relaxants and smooth extubation.

6. Postoperative implications

Complications include hemodynamic instability, myocardial ischemia, hemorrhage, respiratory failure, renal failure, and neurologic changes.

C. CAROTID ENDARTERECTOMY

1. Introduction

Cerebrovascular accidents, or strokes, are the third leading cause of death in the United States and account for a yearly cost of $14 billion in medical expenses and lost productivity. Most strokes are caused by cerebral ischemia. In carotid atherosclerotic disease, subintimal fatty plaques can increase in size over time and incrementally occlude the vascular lumen, which results in decreased cerebral blood flow (CBF). The plaque may rupture and release fibrin, calcium, cholesterol, and inflammatory cells. This phenomenon can lead to abrupt occlusion of the lumen from thrombosis from platelet activation, or an embolus may form and decrease CBF distal to the carotid artery. In each scenario, an abrupt decrease in CBF leads to transient ischemic attacks (TIAs) or strokes.

More than half of all strokes are preceded by a TIA. The Framingham study reported that the risk of a stroke was 30% 2 years after a TIA and approximately 55% 12 years after a TIA had occurred. It is this increased risk of stroke associated with TIA that provides the rationale for use of carotid endarterectomy (CEA), the surgical procedure in which the internal carotid artery is incised, the carotid arterial lumen is opened, and the plaque within the lumen is removed to improve CBF.

2. Indications

The initial indication for CEA is symptomatic stenosis but not complete occlusive carotid disease. This presentation occurs in most patients who undergo carotid surgery. Some centers have extended the indications to include evolved (nondense), nonhemorrhagic strokes and asymptomatic severe stenosis or lesser stenosis associated with contralateral occlusive disease.

3. Morbidity and mortality

The surgical outcomes reported for CEA remain inconclusive because of differences in patient populations and varying degrees of surgical expertise. Other variables that cannot be stratified in studies but that may affect outcome include the state of collateral flow through the circle of Willis, the presence of concurrent atherosclerotic disease in the cerebral vasculature, the size and morphology of the offending plaque, the specific presenting symptoms, and the presence of concurrent cardiovascular disease. The perioperative mortality rate for CEA is approximately 0.5% to 2.5%, and the long-term postoperative stroke incidence ranges from 1% to 3% per year.

4. Patient selection

Criteria for the best candidates for carotid artery surgery remain unclear. The risks associated with having surgery and the possibility of a stroke should be measured against the risks associated with not having surgery and undergoing medical management. Several conditions that can increase the risk of perioperative complications include severe preoperative hypertension, CEA performed in preparation for coronary artery bypass, angina, internal carotid artery stenosis near the carotid siphon, age older than 75 years, and diabetes mellitus. Because CEA is performed prophylactically, it would seem prudent that patient selection be based on the risks associated with the neurologic and myocardial ischemia of surgery as opposed to the risks associated with the neurologic sequelae of nonsurgical management.

5. Diagnosis

The neurologic symptoms of cerebrovascular dysfunction (e.g., TIAs and strokes) are most frequently related to a decrease in CBF. Asymptomatic carotid bruits may be a sign of the possibility of carotid artery disease. Amaurosis fugax or monocular blindness occurs in 25% of patients with high-grade carotid artery stenosis. This syndrome is believed to be caused by microthrombi that travel into the internal carotid artery and that decrease the blood supply of the optic nerve via the ophthalmic artery. Duplex ultrasonography, a noninvasive diagnostic modality that combines ultrasonography and Doppler analysis, is currently one of the most sensitive noninvasive techniques capable of evaluating extracranial occlusive disease. Arteriography may be performed if surgery is being contemplated and can provide anatomic details of arterial vessels. CT scan or MRI may be useful in patients with a neurologic deficit, in whom an alternative diagnosis may be discovered.

6. **Preoperative assessment**
   a) The presence of concurrent CAD and carotid stenosis is well documented. Although stroke is a devastating consequence of CEA, MI contributes more frequently to poor surgical outcomes than stroke. Although coronary angiography may not be justified in all patients undergoing CEA, a systematic approach to the identification of CAD and its subsequent risks should be performed before elective surgery.
   b) Patients with no significant medical history, normal physical examination, and normal ECG should proceed directly to surgery because these patients have low surgical risks.
   c) When abnormal cardiac information is obtained, further evaluation should be performed. Radionuclide imaging is highly sensitive in diagnosing CAD. Redistribution demonstrated on dipyridamole-thallium imaging is very suggestive of increased risk of adverse cardiac events. In these patients, coronary angiography is suggested as a means of quantifying CAD and selecting an appropriate therapeutic intervention.
   d) The progression of surgical intervention when CAD is present with carotid artery disease is controversial. Most agree that in cases of mild CAD, patients may undergo CEA with a low degree of risk. However, in cases of moderate to severe CAD, the direction of surgical intervention is unclear. One option is the simultaneous performance of CEA and coronary revascularization. Decisions should be guided by the patient's symptoms, the associated risk factors, and the center's experience.
7. **Perioperative considerations**
   a) Cerebral physiology
      (1) CBF can remain relatively constant at different cerebral perfusion pressures as a result of cerebrovascular autoregulation. Cerebral perfusion pressure can be expressed as the difference between MAP and intracranial pressure (ICP). During CEA, ICP is usually not elevated; therefore, MAP plays the predominant role in determining cerebral perfusion pressure.
      (2) When MAP is maintained between 60 and 160 mmHg, CBF remains constant. However, the adverse effects of chronic systemic hypertension shift the patient's cerebral autoregulatory curve to the right, and therefore a higher than normal MAP may be required to ensure adequate cerebral perfusion. CBF is also influenced by arterial carbon dioxide and oxygen levels as well as by inhalation agents.
      (3) Carotid occlusive disease jeopardizes the cerebral perfusion pressure in the ipsilateral artery. Ischemia leads to the disruption of autoregulation and compensatory vasodilation, and thus blood flow becomes pressure dependent. During CEA, the anesthetic goals should focus on improvement and protection of CBF and diligent monitoring of brain function.
   b) Cerebral monitoring
      (1) In addition to standard monitoring, direct intraarterial pressure is continuously assessed to evaluate near–real-time values. During the administration of anesthetic agents, blood pressure

fluctuation commonly occurs in patients who have a history of hypertension.

(2) Because of the high incidence of CAD and neurovascular disease in this patient population, prompt treatment of blood pressure values below 20% of the preoperative MAP value is imperative.

(3) Pulmonary artery catheterization is not warranted in most individuals unless the presence of concurrent cardiac disease justifies its use.

(4) Carbon dioxide has a potent effect on cerebrovascular tone. Both hypocapnia and hypercapnia directly affect CBF; therefore, maintenance of normocapnia is paramount.

(5) During repair, the carotid artery cross-clamp is applied.

(6) Various monitoring techniques have been proposed for the assessment of the adequacy of CBF during this maneuver.

(7) A summary of cerebral monitoring techniques is listed below. Each of these monitoring modalities has limitations, and the most sensitive and specific measure of adequate CBF is an awake patient.

(8) Electroencephalographic (EEG) monitoring constitutes the gold standard in the identification of neurologic deficits related to carotid artery cross-clamping. EEG has demonstrated reliability in the monitoring of cortical electrical function. Loss of β-wave activity, loss of amplitude, and emergence of slow-wave activity all are indicative of neurologic dysfunction.

(9) Cerebral monitoring modalities during general anesthesia during CEA are listed in the following box.

Cerebral Monitoring Modalities During General Anesthesia for Carotid Endarterectomy

Electroencephalography (EEG): Assesses cortical electrical function
Somatosensory evoked potential (SSEP): Assesses sensory evoked potentials
Carotid stump pressure (CSP): Assesses perfusion pressure in the operative carotid artery
Transcranial Doppler (TCD): Assesses blood flow velocity in the middle cerebral artery
Cerebral oximetry: Assesses cerebral regional oxygen saturation
Intraarterial xenon injection: Assesses arterial xenon concentrations

c) Cerebral protection: The major objective during carotid artery revascularization is to maintain CBF and decrease cerebral ischemia. Prevention of cerebral ischemia can be accomplished in one of two ways: by increasing the collateral flow (placement of intraluminal shunt) or by decreasing the cerebral metabolic requirements (pharmacologic adjunct).

(1) Temporary shunt placement

(a) When the carotid artery is clamped, CBF is compromised. Therefore, maintenance of coronary perfusion pressure (CPP) is dependent on collateral blood flow for adequate cerebral perfusion. The EEG changes that are associated with cerebral ischemia can be reversed when an intraluminal shunt is inserted.

(b) The shunt acts as a temporary conduit that allows for arterial blood flow during the time the surgeon is dissecting plaque from the intima of the carotid artery. Although some surgeons routinely insert shunts before plaque removal, others do not use shunts or use shunts only in a select group of patients.

(c) The application of a shunt imposes the risk of embolic complications and intimal dissections. Cerebral ischemic events are most often the result of embolic complications. Stump pressures and EEG measurements are the intraoperative monitoring modalities that can be used to determine the need for shunt placement.

d) Cerebral metabolism

(1) Barbiturates and propofol have the capability of decreasing cerebral metabolism to 40% below normal values.

(2) During transient focal ischemia, barbiturates and propofol decrease the cerebral metabolic rate of oxygen consumption, which results in cerebral protection.

(3) The disadvantages of administering barbiturates and propofol during CEA surgery include myocardial depression and delayed emergence.

(4) The surgeon may request that one of these cerebral depressants be administered before the carotid artery is cross-clamped.

(5) Hypothermia is also associated with decreases in cerebral metabolic rates and oxygen consumption. A decrease in core temperature of 1° C decreases cerebral metabolic rate for oxygen ($CMRO_2$) by 7%. When core temperature has been reduced to 12° to 20° C, the safe duration of ischemia is 30 to 60 minutes.

(6) Hypothermic techniques were initially advocated; however, the risks associated with these techniques outweigh the clinical usefulness.

e) Blood pressure control

(1) The presence of hypertension in patients with cerebrovascular disease is well known. Therefore, one of the most challenging aspects of care associated with anesthesia for CEA is blood pressure control. Patients with cerebral insufficiency are vulnerable to perioperative blood pressure instability.

(2) Hypotension occurs in 10% to 50% of patients who undergo CEA and is believed to be the result of carotid sinus baroreceptor stimulation. Conversely, 10% to 66% of patients experience hypertension, which is attributed to surgical manipulation of the carotid sinus.

(3) Preoperative blood pressure control, volume status, and depth of anesthesia can also contribute to intraoperative hemodynamic instability.

(4) All patients should continue taking their antihypertensive medications until the time of surgery.

(5) Additional pharmacologic adjuncts may be required in the preoperative period, especially during the insertion of IV and intraarterial catheters, to reduce increases in heart rate and blood pressure.

(6) The induction of anesthesia, initial incision, dissection, manipulation of the carotid sinus, and emergence from anesthesia are all events that precipitate blood pressure fluctuations. The use of pharmacologic adjuncts, such as short-acting β-adrenergic blockers, may stabilize blood pressure during induction and emergence.

(7) Continuous IV use of nitroglycerin or sodium nitroprusside should be available to treat hypertension. Patients with chronic hypertension are predisposed to dramatic decreases in blood pressure after the induction of general anesthesia. This condition should be treated promptly and can be successfully managed through provision of IV fluids or administration of a vasoconstrictor, such as phenylephrine hydrochloride.

(8) Hypotension and bradycardia, which result from carotid sinus baroreceptor manipulation, can be inhibited by infiltration with local anesthetic.

8. **Anesthetic technique**

a) The anesthetic objectives for vascular surgery are similar to those for any type of elective procedure; they are to provide analgesia and amnesia, facilitate surgical intervention, and minimize operative morbidity and mortality.

b) Specific objectives for CEA include maintaining cerebral and myocardial perfusion and oxygenation, minimizing the stress response, and facilitating a smooth and rapid emergence.

c) Overall the anesthetic goal is to optimize perfusion to the brain, minimize myocardial workload, ensure cardiovascular stability, and allow for rapid emergence.

d) Anesthetic selection

(1) There is no consensus that a particular technique is more effective in decreasing overall perioperative morbidity and mortality. Studies have shown that regional anesthesia is associated with improved postoperative outcomes such as lower mortality rate; lower perioperative stroke rate; less intraoperative hemodynamic variability; fewer major adverse cardiac events, including MI 30 days after endarterectomy; a 10% decreased rate of unnecessary shunting; and decreased length of hospital stay.

(2) Anesthetic selection should be based on the anesthesia provider's familiarity and competence with a specific technique as well as the patient's condition and the surgeon's preference.

(3) Regional anesthesia

(a) A regional anesthetic technique during CEA can be accomplished by local infiltration or by superficial and deep cervical plexus block.

(b) The greatest advantage of regional anesthesia is the anesthesia provider's ability to directly assess neurologic function in an awake patient. Assessing the level of consciousness is the most effective method assessing the adequacy of CBF and detecting cerebral ischemia.

(c) The use of regional anesthesia has been associated with shorter operative times, less frequent cardiopulmonary complications, and shorter postoperative hospitalization.

(d) The limiting factor for use of a regional technique is patient acceptance. Because these individuals are awake, preoperative patient education is essential, and their cooperation during surgery is vital.

(e) Anxiety, fear, and apprehension can initiate sympathetic stimulation and, as a result, extreme hemodynamic responses can occur. Deep sedation that can be required in an apprehensive patient may confound the neurologic assessment, which negates the advantages of a regional technique.

(f) Hypercarbia can result from hypoventilation, and dysphoria is most likely to occur. Converting to a general anesthetic technique after surgery has begun can be problematic.

(g) If adequate cerebral perfusion is compromised, symptoms include dizziness, contralateral weakness, decreased mentation, and loss of consciousness. In the event this scenario occurs, immediate shunt placement is warranted. Emergent airway management may be necessary.

(4) General anesthesia

(a) General anesthesia is commonly used during CEA. Perhaps the greatest benefit of this technique is that it counters the most cited disadvantage of regional anesthesia: lack of patient cooperation.

(b) General anesthesia promotes a motionless field during surgery. Inhalation agents may provide hemodynamic stability and may have beneficial effects on cerebral circulation.

(c) By decreasing cerebral and cardiac metabolism, inhalation agents provide a degree of protection against ischemia, an effect called *anesthetic preconditioning*.

(d) Comparison of inhaled agents with narcotic-based techniques yields no scientific evidence to suggest that patient outcome is improved.

(e) Remifentanil can be used and, because of rapid metabolism, neurologic recovery is improved.

(f) The inhalation agents may alter the monitoring methods used for detecting cerebral ischemia, such as EEG and somatosensory evoked potential (SSEP) monitoring.

(g) In these cases, general anesthetic techniques may require modification, and direct communication is required between the anesthesia provider and the surgical team.

(h) The use of nitrous oxide during CEA can potentially increase the incidence of a clinically significant pneumocephalus. During shunt placement and carotid artery cross-clamp release, microbubbles can be entrained into carotid artery blood flow. For this reason, if nitrous oxide is used, it should be discontinued before removal of the carotid artery cross-clamp.

9. Postoperative implications

a) The most common problem experienced in the postoperative period is hypertension. Although the specific cause remains unclear, postoperative hypertension may be related to events or conditions that alter cerebral autoregulation, such as use of halogenated hydrocarbons, diabetes mellitus, and cerebral hypoperfusion.

b) A systolic blood pressure greater than 180 mmHg is associated with an increased incidence of TIA, stroke, or MI.
c) Patients with systolic blood pressures of 145 mmHg or less have fewer postoperative complications.
d) Although an uncommon complication, carotid artery hemorrhage can occur in the postoperative phase. Hemorrhage is a devastating event that requires immediate surgical intervention. Initial manifestations of hemorrhage may be those of upper airway obstruction, which may make reintubation difficult or impossible because of tracheal deviation.
e) The complications associated with carotid artery stenting (CAS) are listed in the following box.

Complications Associated with Carotid Artery Stenting

- Stroke
- Myocardial ischemia or infarction
- Bradycardia
- Hypotension
- Deformation of expandable stent
- Stent thrombosis
- Horner's syndrome
- Cerebral hyperperfusion syndrome
- Carotid artery dissection

Carotid Artery Stenting

1. Introduction

A less invasive surgical approach for treatment of carotid artery stenosis is carotid artery angioplasty and stenting. The safety and efficacy of CAS have been in question. Early stents were not equipped with distal protection devices, and a high number of patients developed CVAs as a result of embolization. Controversy exists regarding the degree of success that this procedure affords as an alternative to CEA. The long-term results of CAS appear to be comparable to CEA in terms of prevention from stroke, freedom from new neurologic events, and patency rates.

Carotid artery stenting should be used instead of CEA in the presence of specific patient factors or severe vascular or cardiac comorbidities, which are listed in the following box.

Specific Factors and Severe Vascular and Cardiac Conditions

Specific Patient Factors

- Contralateral laryngeal nerve palsy
- Radiation therapy to neck
- Previous CEA with recurrent restenosis
- High cervical internal carotid
- Severe tandem lesions
- Age older than 80 years
- Severe pulmonary disease

Continued

Specific Factors and Severe Vascular and Cardiac Conditions—cont'd

Severe Vascular and Cardiac Comorbidities
• Congestive heart failure
• Severe left ventricular dysfunction
• Open heart surgery needed within 6 weeks
• Recent MI (>24 hours and <4 weeks)
• Unstable angina
• Contralateral carotid occlusion

CEA, Carotid endarterectomy; *MI*, myocardial infarction.
Modified from Cremonesi A, Setacci C, Bignamini A, et al. Carotid artery stenting: first consensus document of the ICCC-SPREAD Joint Committee. *Stroke* 2006; 37(9):2400-2409.

2. Procedure

Before CAS procedure, patients receive an aortic arch, carotid, and cerebral angiogram or a high-resolution MRI. This allows the physicians to evaluate the individual anatomy and angiopathology of the aortic arch, brachiocephalic artery (for right carotid artery stent), or left common carotid artery. Determination of the type of sheaths, stents, and cerebral embolic protection device can then be planned. Femoral artery access is obtained, and then a sheath is threaded through the aortic arch and into the operative carotid artery. The guidewire or embolic protection device is advanced through the sheath and positioned across the stenotic region. An embolic protection device sequesters emboli during angioplasty and stenting to avoid distal occlusion in cerebral arteries. In elderly patients, adjunctive distal embolic protection lowers the risk of intraoperative and postoperative adverse events. Angioplasty with a 5.0-mm balloon dilates the carotid artery, and then the stent is deployed. The guidewire or device wire is removed after angiographic confirmation that carotid artery dissection or occlusion has not occurred.

3. Anesthetic technique

a) The anesthesia that is routinely used for CAS is local anesthesia at the femoral insertion site and minimal sedation.
b) Fluoroscopy is used throughout the surgery; therefore, it is important that all operating room personnel are protected with lead.
c) Anticoagulation is attained with a heparin bolus 50 to 100 units/kg to maintain an activated clotting time (ACT) greater than 250 seconds.
d) Balloon inflation in the internal carotid artery can stimulate the baroreceptor response, resulting in prolonged bradycardia and hypotension. Glycopyrrolate or atropine can be administered before inflation to offset this vagal response.
e) The most common complication is stroke caused by thromboembolism. Interventions for a patient with an acute stroke include airway and hemodynamic management. Currently, the only treatment approved for acute ischemic stroke is IV recombinant tissue plasminogen activator (rt-PA). Mechanical devices such as snares and balloons are being developed so that the physician will be able to physically remove thromboembolic material and restore blood flow.
f) Patients typically remain in the postanesthesia care unit for 30 minutes after carotid stent placement and then are transferred to a monitored floor. A carotid duplex scan is performed before discharge, and scans are then routinely obtained at 6 weeks, 6 months, 1 year, and then yearly. Patients remain on aspirin therapy for anticoagulation for life.

D. ENDOVASCULAR AORTIC ANEURYSM REPAIR

1. Introduction

In 1991, the first endovascular stent was performed to repair an infrarenal aortic aneurysm. The development of this technique has created a less invasive approach to aortic aneurysm repair. Because of severe cardiac and respiratory pathology, it is believed that as many as 30% of patients with aortic aneurysms are not surgical candidates. Endovascular AAA repair (EVAR) was initially intended for patients with severe coexisting disease; however, its popularity has increased as the success of the procedure has improved. It is estimated that 20,000 EVAR procedures take place in the United States per year, which comprises 36% of aortic aneurysm repair.

Endovascular aortic aneurysm repair is also being used to treat patients with thoracic aortic aneurysms. The mortality rate for EVAR for elective descending thoracic aneurysm repairs range from 3.5% to 12.5% compared with an open approach, which is approximately 10%. There is a low incidence of spinal cord ischemia and paraplegia, which is reported from 0% to 6%. Potential reasons for the lack of spinal cord complications are no thoracic aortic cross-clamping and no prolonged periods of extreme hypotension. Perioperative hypotension (MAP <70 mmHg) was a significant predictor of spinal cord ischemia in patients having EVAR for thoracic aneurysm repair. Endograft therapy has also been used with success and may eventually become the treatment of choice in patients older than 75 years of age for thoracic aneurysm repair.

The mortality rate for patients with a ruptured AAA who are alive when diagnosed in emergency departments is 40% to 70%. The EVAR approach has been used successfully to repair ruptured AAAs. The number of patients treated and the quality of randomized controlled data on this subject are limited. Medical centers that consider EVAR for ruptured AAA repair should have emergent CT imaging capabilities, a trained endovascular team, adequate endovascular supplies available, and a surgical suite.

2. Procedure

Endovascular aortic aneurysm repair involves deployment of an endovascular stent graft within the aortic lumen. The graft restricts blood flow to the portion or the aorta where the aneurysm exists. This procedure can be performed for patients who have descending thoracic aortic aneurysms or AAAs. Cannulation of both femoral arteries is performed. A guidewire is threaded through the iliac artery to the level of the aneurysm. Next, a sheath is inserted over the guidewire and positioned at the aneurysm location through the use of fluoroscopy. The proximal end of the sheath should extend beyond the aneurysm. After the sheath is deployed, migration is prevented by the use of radial force or fixation mechanisms such as hooks, barbs on the stent become embedded into the aortic wall.

The procedure frequently takes place in an interventional radiology suite. Advantages of the endovascular approach compared with the conventional surgical method include improved hemodynamic stability, decreased incidence of embolic events, decreased blood loss, reduced stress response, decreased incidence of renal dysfunction, and decreased postoperative discomfort.

3. Anesthetic technique

a) Systemic anticoagulation with heparin 50 to 100 units/kg is administered before catheter manipulation.
b) A first-generation cephalosporin is recommended at the beginning of surgery.
c) The anesthetic techniques that can be used for EVAR include general anesthesia neuraxial blockade or local anesthesia with sedation.
d) There is presently a lack of data suggesting that one anesthetic technique is superior for patients having EVAR.
e) The goals for intraoperative management for EVAR include maintaining hemodynamic stability, providing analgesia and anxiolysis, and being prepared to rapidly convert to an open procedure.
f) With infrarenal or suprarenal EVAR, creatinine clearance values decrease by 10% in the first year. However, proximal endovascular graft migration can occur, causing renal artery occlusion and postoperative renal failure.
g) Other complications that can arise as a result of EVAR include endograft thrombosis, migration or rupture, graft infection, iliac artery rupture, and lower extremity ischemia. Fatal cerebral embolism resulting in sudden respiratory arrest has occurred during EVAR.
h) A serious complication that can occur as a result of this procedure is termed *endoleak,* defined as persistent blood flow and pressure *(endotension)* between the endovascular graft and the aortic aneurysm. This complication has been reported to occur in 15% to 52% of patients as diagnosed by postoperative CT scan. Most endoleaks are type II, and 70% spontaneously close within the first month postimplantation.
i) Type II endoleaks are caused by collateral retrograde perfusion. Type I and type III endoleaks are caused by device-related problems. The most frequent intervention used to correct these complications includes implantation of a second endograft or open repair.
j) Long-term results of endovascular aortic aneurysm repair have demonstrated that this procedure yields good results, but the overall durability of conventional surgical techniques is superior.

E. PERIPHERAL VASCULAR PROCEDURES

1. Introduction

Peripheral vascular procedures include femoral–femoral, femoral–popliteal, femoral–tibial, iliofemoral, axillofemoral, and embolectomies. Obstruction most often is in the superficial femoral artery followed by common iliac claudication in the gastrocnemius muscle, but pain and ischemic ulceration or gangrene occur with severe occlusion.

Procedures are classified as inflow or outflow vascular reconstruction. The inflow reconstruction procedures bypass the obstruction in the aortoiliac segment (aortoiliac endarterectomy or aortofemoral bypass). These are more stressful procedures requiring cross-clamping of the aorta. Outflow procedures are performed distal to the inguinal ligament to bypass the femoropopliteal or distal obstruction. The stages of aortic clamping and anesthetic considerations are shown in the table on pg. 587.

Stages of Aortic Cross-Clamping and Anesthetic Considerations

Clamping Stage	Goals	Drug to Prepare
Preclamping	Maintain blood pressure 20% baseline (low normal)	Volatile anesthetic Nitroglycerin, nitroprusside (Nipride) If PCWP is increased and cardiac output is decreased, inotropic support (dopamine, epinephrine) may be needed.
	Maximize urinary output	Mannitol, furosemide (Lasix)
	Minimize fluids	Monitor crystalloid administration
	Prevent thrombosis	Heparin: monitor activated clotting times
Cross-clamping	Prevent myocardial infarction	Decrease afterload (nitroglycerin and nitroprusside) Monitor electrocardiogram for ischemia Monitor cardiac output, and expect a decline
	Maintain oxygenation	Oxygen/air or 100% oxygen Monitor oxygen saturation and arterial blood gases
	Maintain urinary output (0.5 mL/kg/hr)	Anuria is rare Dopamine (1-5 mcg/kg)
Prerelease	Prevent MI from declamping, hypotension	Monitor ECG Ask surgeon for a 10-min warning before aortic clamp is removed Lighten anesthesia depth Discontinue vasodilating agents (nitroglycerin and nitroprusside) Increase CVP and PCWP 4 to 6 mmHg with fluids (and blood if needed) Have vasopressors ready
Postrelease	Maintain blood pressure and vital signs	Use vasopressors (dopamine, epinephrine, phenylephrine)
	Correct acidosis	Mechanical ventilation Bicarbonate administration (pH <7.25) Calcium chloride administration
	Correct coagulation profile	Protamine
	Maintain urine output	Volume: Crystalloids and colloids, dopamine

CVP, Central venous pressure; *ECG*, electrocardiography; *MI*, myocardial infarction; *PCWP*, pulmonary capillary wedge pressure.

2. **Preoperative assessment**
   a) History and physical examination
      (1) See the discussion of AAA earlier in this section.
      (2) Musculoskeletal: This includes decreased or absent popliteal and pedal pulses, delayed capillary refill, blanching on elevation of the leg followed by dependent edema after lowering it, and pain with walking relieved by rest.

PART 2 Common Procedures

b) Diagnostic tests
   (1) See the discussion of AAA earlier in this section.
   (2) Doppler studies
      (a) Determinations of systolic blood pressure at the level of the ankle are compared with brachial determinations.
      (b) Assess the severity of ischemia, urgency of revascularization, and baseline values for evaluation of operative results.
   (3) Angiography: Determine the precise site of the actual lesion.

c) Preoperative medications and IV therapy
   (1) For elderly patients with coexisting medical disease requiring pharmacologic support (i.e., antihypertensives, antianginals, antiarrhythmics, digoxin), these medications may be continued up to the day of the operation.
   (2) Sedatives and narcotics are used.
      (a) Use with caution in patients with poor respiratory reserve.
      (b) The onset of IV medications may be delayed because of potentially low cardiac output.
   (3) Two peripheral large-bore (16- to 18-gauge) IV lines with moderate fluid management are used.
   (4) Epidural catheter: Test the dose on the awake patient; there is a risk of epidural hematoma from anticoagulation during surgery.

3. Room preparation

a) Monitoring equipment
   (1) ECG leads V5 and II to detect myocardial ischemia and diagnose tachyarrhythmias.
   (2) Warming modalities
   (3) Foley catheter
   (4) Arterial line and central venous pressure monitoring is possibly necessary.

b) Pharmacologic agents
   (1) Have nitroglycerin and nitroprusside drugs within quick access.
   (2) Drugs include vasopressors, heparin, and β-blockers.

c) Position: Supine

4. Anesthetic technique

a) Regional block, general anesthesia, or a combination. The technique of choice is regional anesthesia; it avoids airway problems and sequelae, provides greater hemodynamic stability with coexisting diseases, provides sympathetic block that increases circulation in the lower extremity, reduces the incidence of intravascular clotting, facilitates postoperative pain relief, suppresses the endocrine stress response, and decreases blood loss in selected cases.

b) Regional block: Analgesia to T10; epidural or spinal
   (1) The elderly population is more sensitive to local anesthetics; reduce the dose by 50%.
   (2) Some practitioners administer ephedrine prophylactically to prevent hypotension.
   (3) The level is slightly above the skin dermatome necessary for the usual incisions (T12), but sympathetic innervation of lower extremities, which contain visceral afferent fibers, is believed to occur at T10 to L2.

5. **Perioperative management**
   a) Induction
      (1) General anesthesia
         (a) The goals are a smooth transition from awake state to surgical anesthesia and the maintenance of cardiovascular stability.
         (b) A slow, "controlled" induction is preferred with an opioid and nondepolarizing muscle relaxant.
         (c) Muscle relaxation may be chosen on the basis of cardiovascular effect.
            i. Pancuronium: If the heart rate is slowed during induction
            ii. Vecuronium: If the heart rate is in the desired range
         (d) The onset of drugs may be delayed with low cardiac output.
         (e) Omit thiopental and other cardiac depressors in patients with poor left ventricular function.
         (f) Anticipate exaggerated blood pressure changes; maintain within 20% of baseline.
         (g) Minimize pressor response during intubation of trachea by limiting the duration of laryngoscopy to less than 15 seconds.
      (2) Regional anesthesia
         (a) Review the principles of sympathetic block.
         (b) Consider administering block with the operative side down so that the onset of sympathetic and sensory blockade is faster on the dependent site. Theoretically, the level will be higher on the dependent side. The total volume of anesthetic requirements may be decreased.
   b) Maintenance
      (1) The surgeon will ask that heparin be administered by IV push; ensure the patency of the port before injection.
      (2) If intraoperative angiography is used:
         (a) Allergic reactions may occur with dye.
         (b) The degree of surgical stimulation changes; blood pressure decreases when surgical activity stops in preparation for angiography. Blood pressure and heart rate may increase when dye is injected.
         (c) Repeated injection of contrast dye during multiple attempts at angiography may cause osmotic diuresis.
      (3) Hyperkalemia and acidosis resulting from ischemic extremities are possible, and myoglobin can be released into the circulation.
      (4) Maintain the hematocrit at more than 30 to maximize oxygen-carrying capacity.
      (5) Unclamping of the femoral artery rarely affects hemodynamics significantly. The lower extremity receives arterial blood through collateral vessels, even when the femoral artery is occluded.
      (6) Regional anesthesia
         (a) Attention to patient comfort is important.
         (b) Sedation is aimed at reducing patient anxiety without producing respiratory depression or unresponsiveness.
   c) Emergence
      (1) Initiate regional block through the epidural catheter for postoperative analgesia before the end of the case.

(2) Base extubation on the patient's general health, amount of blood loss, and overall status after the procedure.

6. Postoperative implications

a) Obtain hemoglobin and hematocrit values.

b) Assess the musculoskeletal status of the operative extremity.

F. PORTOSYSTEMIC SHUNTS

1. Introduction

Portosystemic shunt procedures are performed to prevent or cease variceal hemorrhage resulting from portal hypertension in patients with liver disease, cirrhosis, ascites, and hypersplenism. The redistribution of blood from the portal vein to the inferior vena cava causes variations in flow and resistance of the liver, intestine, and spleen. This hemodynamic alteration aids portal perfusion and oxygenation with the net effects of increased venous return and cardiac output. Variations in procedures include portocaval, end-to-end, end-to-side, mesocaval, mesorenal, and splenorenal shunts.

2. Preoperative assessment and patient preparation

a) History and physical examination

(1) Cardiac: Associated conditions include increased heart rate, circulating blood volume, and intrathoracic pressure. Variations of cardiac output, cardiomyopathy, congestive heart failure, CAD, and decreased response to catecholamines and SVR may be present.

(2) Respiratory: Hypoxemia may be related to ventilation/perfusion mismatch, increased closing volume, decreased functional residual capacity, atelectasis, right-to-left pulmonary shunting, increased diphosphoglycerate, pulmonary infections, and impaired hypoxic pulmonary vasoconstriction.

(3) Neurologic: Manifestations may include hepatic encephalopathy with associated confusion and obtundation.

(4) Renal: Renal impairment and failure with electrolyte imbalance are frequently observed.

(5) Gastrointestinal: Gastric or esophageal varices with gastrointestinal bleeding are common.

(6) Endocrine: Abnormal glucose utilization, increased growth hormone, intolerance to carbohydrates, and irregular sex hormone metabolism may be observed.

b) Patient preparation

(1) Laboratory tests: Arterial blood gases, complete blood count, prothrombin time, partial thromboplastin time, bleeding time, electrolytes, blood urea nitrogen, creatinine, creatinine clearance, urinalysis, diffuse intravascular coagulation profile, albumin, bilirubin, serum glutamic-oxaloacetic transaminase, serum glutamic-pyruvic transaminase, ammonia, alkaline phosphatase, and lactate are obtained.

(2) Diagnostic tests: ECG, echocardiography, pulmonary function tests, and chest radiography are obtained.

(3) Preoperative medications: Avoid intramuscular injections. Anxiolytics are administered in small doses as indicated. Consider metoclopramide (10 mg) and ranitidine (50 mg).

(4) IV therapy: This involves a central line and two 14- to 16-gauge IV lines. Consider a pulmonary arterial catheter.

3. **Room preparation**
   a) Monitoring equipment: Standard with arterial line, central venous pressure catheter, and urinary catheter
   b) Additional equipment: Fluid warmer, cell saver, Bair Hugger, and rapid infuser
   c) Drugs
      (1) Miscellaneous pharmacologic agents: Opioid (fentanyl), midazolam, vasodilators and vasoconstrictors, inotropes, nondepolarizing muscle relaxants, and antibiotics are used.
      (2) IV fluids: Calculate for major blood loss. Estimated blood loss is 1000 to 2000 mL.
      (3) Blood: Type and cross-match for 8 to 10 units of packed red blood cells, platelets, fresh-frozen plasma, and cryoprecipitate.
      (4) Tabletop: Standard
4. **Perioperative management and anesthetic technique**
   a) General anesthesia, epidural anesthesia, or a combination of general and regional anesthesia is used.
   b) General anesthetic is the technique of choice.
   c) Induction: Use rapid-sequence induction with thiopental (3-5 mg/kg) and succinylcholine (1-2 mg/kg). Consider etomidate (0.2 mg/kg) or ketamine (1 mg/kg).
   d) Maintenance: Inhalational agent, oxygen, fentanyl, midazolam and nondepolarizing muscle relaxant. Position is supine.
   e) Emergence: The patient generally is transported to the intensive care unit. Patients may remain intubated while hemodynamic stability is achieved.
5. **Postoperative implications**
   a) Complications: Coagulopathy, renal failure, hypothermia, encephalopathy, jaundice, and anemia
   b) Postoperative pain management: Patient-controlled analgesia

G. THORACIC AORTIC ANEURYSM

1. Introduction

The mortality rate associated with thoracic aneurysms is well established. Patients with aortic dissections have only a 3-month survival time if they do not undergo surgical repair because the incidence of rupture is high. The refinement of synthetic grafts, surgical and perfusion techniques, and intraoperative management has contributed to improved surgical outcomes. Today the early mortality rate is thought to be less than 10%, demonstrating that elective surgical intervention is an acceptable means of treating thoracic aortic aneurysms.

2. Classification

Aneurysms of the thoracic aorta may be classified with respect to type, shape, and location. Typically, aneurysms involving all three layers of the arterial wall, tunica adventitia, tunica media, and tunica intima are considered to be true aneurysms. In comparison, aneurysms that solely involve the adventitia are termed *false aneurysms*. The shape of the lesion can also serve as a means of characterizing aneurysms. Fusiform aneurysms have a spindle shape and result in dilation of the aorta. Saccular aneurysms are spherical dilations and are generally limited to only one segment of the vessel wall. Aortic dissection is the result of a spontaneous tear within the intima that permits the flow of blood through a false passage along the longitudinal axis of the aorta. Aneurysms can also be classified according to their location within the aortic arch. In addition, thoracoabdominal aneurysms can be classified into four types on the basis of their location.

3. Etiology

Atherosclerosis is the most common cause of aneurysmal pathology. Atherosclerotic lesions occur most often in the descending and distal thoracic aorta and are most often classified as fusiform. Less common causes include the histologic contributions of cystic medial necrosis observed in patients with Marfan's syndrome, infective and inflammatory processes within the vessel wall, and Takayasu's arteritis. A genetic predisposition is thought to contribute to the development of aortic aneurysms.

4. Diagnosis

The symptomatology of thoracic aneurysms is often related to the site of the lesion and its compression on adjacent structures. Pain, stridor, and cough may result from compression of thoracic structures. Symptoms related to aortic insufficiency may be observed in aneurysms of the ascending aorta. An upper mediastinal mass may be an incidental finding on conventional chest radiography in an asymptomatic patient. Further investigation with noninvasive methods (e.g., CT and MRI) can show the configuration and location of the aneurysm. Invasive aortography, although associated with a higher risk of complications, provides the most information because it allows evaluation of the coronary vessels and branches of the aortic arch.

5. Treatment

Early detection and surgical intervention have made significant contributions to long-term survival. The surgical approach and mode of resection vary according to the location of the lesion within the thoracic aorta. Resection of the ascending aorta and graft replacement necessitate the use of CPB. The aortic valve may also require replacement. Surgical resection of lesions in the transverse arch compromises cerebral perfusion, although various bypass techniques combined with profound hypothermia and circulatory arrest have been used. Aneurysms of the descending aorta may be resected by application of an aortic cross-clamp. However, perfusion to distal organs can be compromised during this procedure. Endovascular thoracic aortic repair is also an option.

Aortic Dissection

1. Aortic dissection is characterized by a spontaneous tear of the vessel wall intima, which permits the passage of blood along a false lumen. Although the cause of the dissection is unclear, lesions that were thought to be related to cystic necrotic processes may actually be caused by variations in wall integrity.
2. Hypertension is the most common factor that contributes to the progression of the lesion. Manipulation of the ascending aorta during cardiac surgery may be associated with aortic dissection.
3. The symptoms of aortic dissection are the result of the interruption of blood supply to vital organs. The most serious complication is aneurysm rupture.
4. Diagnosis can be accomplished by the previously mentioned noninvasive techniques; however, aortography appears to be most reliable.

5. Treatment of dissecting aortic lesions depends on their location within the thoracic aorta. Type A lesions have the highest incidence of rupture and require immediate surgical intervention. Type B lesions may initially be managed medically, with the administration of arterial dilating and β-adrenergic blocking agents. Surgical intervention contributes to an improved long-term survival rate. Studies have shown a survival rate of 94% to 95% for repair of dissecting aortic aneurysm by investigators using the newer techniques.
6. The surgical method used is dependent on the location of the aortic lesion. Anesthesia for aneurysms of the ascending and transverse aorta requires CPB.

Descending Thoracic and Thoracoabdominal Aneurysms

1. **Preoperative assessment**

Patients who undergo major vascular surgery are frequently elderly and have varying degrees of concurrent disease. The incidence of thoracic aortic aneurysm is increasing, and the 5-year survival rate after diagnosis without intervention is 9% to 13%. The preoperative evaluation focuses on cardiac, renal, and neurologic function. Although most fatalities related to thoracic aortic surgery are cardiac in origin, renal and neurologic dysfunction contribute to poor surgical outcomes.

2. **Perioperative management**
   a) Monitoring
      (1) Intraoperative monitoring devices used for thoracoabdominal aneurysm resection are the same as those used for abdominal aneurysmectomies.
      (2) Direct intraarterial blood pressure and pulmonary artery pressure monitoring is mandatory. If the aneurysm involves the thoracic region or the distal aortic arch, right radial arterial line monitoring is preferred because left subclavian arterial blood flow may be compromised during surgery.
      (3) Use of two-dimensional transesophageal echocardiography is suggested for cardiac monitoring in patients with myocardial dysfunction.
      (4) An indwelling urinary catheter is used for assessing renal function.
      (5) To facilitate exposing the descending thoracic aorta, a double-lumen endotracheal tube (ETT) is inserted to allow for one-lung ventilation. As a result, careful monitoring of oxygenation is mandatory. Pulmonary artery catheters equipped with fiberoptics are useful for the measurement of mixed venous oxygen.
      (6) Routine use of pulse oximetry may be limited if the left subclavian artery is manipulated; therefore, the right hand, the ear, or the nasal passages should be used for monitoring oxygen saturation.
      (7) A lumbar intrathecal catheter is inserted to access CSF. SSEPs or motor evoked potentials (MEPs) may be used to detect neurologic dysfunction; however, their clinical usefulness remains uncertain.
   b) Aortic cross-clamping
      (1) Simple aortic cross-clamping and graft replacement is an acceptable method for surgical repair of descending thoracic or thoracoabdominal aortic aneurysms.

(2) Application of a simple cross-clamp has eliminated the need for shunts and extracorporeal circulation; however, the consequences of this maneuver include myocardial compromise and occlusion of blood flow to distal structures.
(3) The hemodynamic alterations produced by the application of an aortic clamp are discussed earlier in the aortic aneurysms section. Similar responses are observed during proximal aortic occlusion; however, the magnitude of these responses is extreme.
(4) When the aorta is occluded, afterload and therefore myocardial workload increase. As a result, increases occur in left ventricular end-diastolic pressure, left ventricular stroke work index, and myocardial oxygen consumption.
(5) When oxygen demands are not accompanied by an increase in oxygen supply, ischemia results, and myocardial failure can occur.
(6) Although methods have been instituted to decrease myocardial afterload (e.g., partial bypass and shunts), the use of sodium nitroprusside appears to be the most effective means of decreasing afterload during cross-clamp application. Administration of nitroglycerin may be required to decrease preload during aortic occlusion.

c) Hemodynamic alterations: Unclamping
(1) The hemodynamic consequences of releasing the aortic cross-clamp are similar to those of abdominal aortic occlusion, but they are of greater magnitude.
(2) Metabolites that have accumulated during aortic cross-clamping are released into circulation. The combination of reactive hyperemia and sequestration of blood volume within hypoperfused areas can lead to severe hypotension.
(3) Restoration of blood volume, guided by left-sided filling pressures, before the gradual release of the clamp can minimize hemodynamic alterations.
(4) Increasing ventilation and the administration of sodium bicarbonate may control carbon dioxide increases at the time of declamping.

d) Spinal cord ischemia
(1) Neurologic dysfunction is a serious complication of thoracic aortic reconstruction. The incidence of paraplegia is reported to be approximately 20% after elective surgery and as high as 40% after surgery for dissecting and ruptured aneurysms.
(2) Neurologic deficits are the result of hypoperfusion to the spinal cord during thoracic aortic reconstruction. The artery of Adamkiewicz, which is also known as the greater radicular artery, originates from the aorta branch between T8 and L2 and provides the majority of the blood flow to the anterior spinal artery. The anterior spinal artery perfuses the ventral aspect of the spinal cord, which is responsible for motor control.
(3) Although attempts have been made to reimplant the intercostal branches that contribute blood flow to the spinal cord, these efforts do not always decrease the incidence of paraplegia.
(4) The duration of aortic occlusion also contributes to spinal cord ischemia.

(5) Systemic hypothermia and selective cooling of the spinal cord may lengthen ischemic time intervals; however, the clinical benefits of these methods are unclear.
(6) The use of various bypass mechanisms and distal shunts may minimize the length of aortic occlusion time; however, the risks associated with the implementation of these techniques could be greater than the potential benefits.
(7) One method that has been successful is CSF drainage. CSF drainage involves manipulation of spinal cord perfusion pressure during aortic clamping. Spinal cord perfusion pressure can be defined as the arterial pressure minus the CSF pressure. During aortic clamping, CSF pressure increases, and arterial pressure decreases distal to the clamp. The spinal cord perfusion pressure can therefore be manipulated by alteration of arterial blood pressure and draining of CSF through the intrathecal catheter.
(8) The intraoperative use of SSEPs and MEPs can provide early identification of neurologic dysfunction; however, these monitoring modalities do not ensure spinal cord integrity.
(9) Factors that contribute to the development of neurologic deficit include level of aortic clamp application, ischemic time, embolization or thrombosis of a critical intercostal artery, failure to revascularize intercostal arteries, and urgency of surgical intervention.
(10) Neurologic dysfunction has also been reported to occur in the postoperative phase. Delayed paraplegia may be the result of reperfusion injury, although the exact mechanism of injury has not been proved.

e) Renal dysfunction
(1) The incidence of renal dysfunction after thoracoabdominal aortic resection is estimated to be between 30% and 50%; the possibility of permanent renal failure requiring hemodialysis is estimated to be between 2% and 12%.
(2) The cause of renal insufficiency is ischemia, which is related to aortic occlusion. Intraoperative hypotension has been identified as an independent predictor of postoperative renal dysfunction.
(3) Maintenance of intravascular volume and stable circulatory status appears to be the most reliable method of minimizing renal dysfunction.
(4) Preoperatively, volume status should be corrected with non–glucose-containing crystalloid solutions.
(5) Intraoperative volume replacement should be guided by invasive monitoring.
(6) Pharmacologic adjuncts to produce diuresis, such as mannitol and furosemide, should be administered approximately 20 to 30 minutes before clamp application.
(7) Low-dose dopamine is also advocated as a means of increasing renal perfusion but has not been shown to protect renal function.

3. Anesthetic technique

a) The principles of perioperative management of thoracic or thoracoabdominal aneurysms are similar to those previously discussed for abdominal aortic aneurysmectomies.

b) Anesthetic selection should be based on the presence of concomitant disease processes, with the objective of maintenance of cardiovascular stability and the minimization of morbidity and mortality.
c) Intraoperative monitoring should focus on detection of myocardial, neurologic, and renal ischemia. The hemodynamic consequences of aortic cross-clamping should be attenuated by the use of pharmacologic adjuncts.
d) Restoration of circulating blood volume, as guided by left-sided filling pressure, minimizes the hemodynamic alterations caused by the release of the aortic clamp.
e) Unique to thoracic aortic surgery is the use of one-lung ventilation. The highest degree of vigilance should be used to detect potential inadequacies in ventilation and oxygenation.
f) Extreme blood loss should be anticipated. Venous access and blood product availability should be confirmed during the preoperative phase. Methods of minimizing the use of homologous blood products, such as perioperative blood salvage, can be used.
g) Coagulopathy is a constant threat that results from the administration of blood products. The close monitoring of coagulation parameters and the administration of fresh-frozen plasma, platelets, or specific coagulation factors can minimize the incidence and severity of coagulopathies.

4. **Postoperative implications**
   a) After surgery is completed, if a double-lumen ETT was used, it should be replaced with a standard ETT to provide a secure airway because postoperative ventilatory assistance is usually required. Anatomic landmarks may have become edematous during surgery, causing difficulty with reintubation. Under these circumstances, the double-lumen ETT may be left in place. Replacement, guided by fiberoptic evaluation, can proceed in the postoperative period after the airway edema has dissipated.
   b) Close observation of circulatory and pulmonary status is warranted in the postoperative phase. Hemodynamic control is vital to maintain perfusion to vital organs without creating excessive demands on the heart or the aortic graft. Administration of dopamine may be continued during this time.
   c) Careful monitoring of respiratory status aided by arterial blood gas analysis is important. Epidural analgesia using local anesthetics, narcotics, or both can be administered for pain relief.

Complications

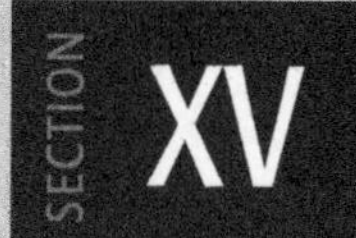

A. ADVERSE COGNITIVE IMPAIRMENT

1. Introduction

Impairments in cognitive functioning from disturbances in the brain's physiology can easily occur in the surgical patient. Neurologic impairment can be devastating in postanesthesia patients in terms of quality of life and activities of daily living. Cognitive functioning is a broad construct that includes a number of categories, including attention span, concentration, judgment, memory, orientation, perception, psychomotor ability, reaction time, and social adaptability. The prevalence of adverse neurologic impairment in surgical patients often results from organic brain disorders; the most common incidences are confusion, delirium, awareness, and (infrequently) coma.

2. Postoperative cognitive dysfunction

a) Postoperative cognitive dysfunction (POCD) is characterized by persistent and long-term deterioration of cognitive performance after anesthesia and surgery.

b) POCD is often associated with cardiac and orthopedic surgery, but it can also accompany other surgical procedures. Cognitive dysfunction in both cardiac and noncardiac surgery has largely focused on older adults, who might have a greater vulnerability to neurologic deterioration as a consequence of the aging process.

c) POCD is difficult to diagnose because it requires sophisticated neurophysiologic testing, including preoperative baseline tests.

d) Patient risk factors include age, lower levels of education, and history of stroke even without residual deficit.

e) Increased 1 year mortality is associated with patients who demonstrate cognitive decline at both hospital discharge and 3 months postop.

3. Confusion

a) The term *confusion* is used to describe the general affect and behaviors of patients; however, it is not specific and appears to have a great deal in common with delirium.

b) Confusion (a form of transient cognitive dysfunction) after anesthesia relates to disorders of orientation and is usually a relatively short-lived transient cognitive dysfunction.

c) Confusion after anesthesia is a normal occurrence, and it is suggested that patients refrain from engaging in activities requiring rapid responses for at least 48 hours postanesthesia.

4. Postoperative delirium

a) Delirium (or acute mental confusion) is transient, often abrupt and fluctuating, typically reversible, and related to increased risk of postoperative adverse reactions (i.e., pulmonary edema, myocardial infarction, respiratory failure, pneumonia, and death), increased length of hospital stay, increased health care cost, and poor functional and cognitive recovery. The onset occurs in hours to days after anesthesia and surgery.

b) Key symptoms include anxiety, incoherent or disorganized thinking and perceiving, reduced ability to sustain and shift attention to new external stimuli, and agitated behavior. There is sensory misperception; a disordered stream of thought; and difficulty in shifting, focusing, and sustaining attention to both external and internal stimuli. Irrelevant stimuli can easily distract the delirious individual.

c) The cause of postoperative delirium is multifactorial. Virtually any drug with central nervous system effects has been implicated, including narcotics (especially meperidine), benzodiazepines, and drugs that possess anticholinergic properties (except glycopyrrolate). Common are perceptual disturbances that result in misinterpretations, illusions, and hallucinations. Disturbances of sleep–wakefulness and psychomotor activity are present.

d) Precipitants are related to physical illness (e.g. cardiovascular disease), infection, hormone disorders, or nutritional deficiencies. Most frequent precipitants are metabolic disturbances; fluid and electrolyte imbalances; drug and alcohol toxicity; and unfamiliar and excessive sensory-environmental stimuli.

e) Delirium may be life threatening and is a medical emergency. Delirium occurs in about 20% of elderly surgical patients and is more common in patients undergoing orthopedic procedures (i.e., femoral fractures) with an incidence rate of 28% to 60% in this surgical population. Thirty-two percent of patients who had coronary artery bypass surgery reported postoperative delirium.

f) Early identification and prompt treatment of the causes of delirium prevent irreversible dementia and death, with interventions targeted at reversing physiologic disturbances and preventing sensory deprivation.

g) The choice of general anesthesia or regional anesthesia does not appear to be a factor, especially when sedation is used in conjunction with regional anesthesia (RA).

h) Management focuses on reversible risk factors such as current meds, pain management, and a better sleep environment. Haloperidol in doses no greater than 1.5 mg can be helpful, especially for agitated delirium. When administered prophylactically, it may reduce the severity of duration but not the incidence of delirium.

5. **Awareness**

a) Awareness, the unambiguous recall of events during general anesthesia, has an incidence of 0.18% in the United States. The term *recall,* the ensuing retention of an event after it occurs, is a better description of the phenomena; however, episodes of awareness are strong predictors of dissatisfaction with anesthesia care.

b) For every 1000 adult patients who receive a general anesthetic, as many as one or two will express the occurrence of awareness or recall; this figure is higher in children. Inadequate depths of anesthesia may lead to awareness and recall; accounts of awareness rely on patient recollection.

c) Although patient recollection of awareness or recall may be reported, most do not complain of recalling pain during the procedure. Instead, patients report "dreamlike" experiences and auditory remembrance during which they are not in distress.

d) Reports of intraoperative awareness should be addressed immediately and thoroughly evaluated to obtain information for quality assurance.

e) Management of awareness begins when patients are given an opportunity to discuss the causes of the event with the anesthesia provider to gain a clearer understanding of the circumstances surrounding the experience and follow-up consultation.

f) The awareness experience is certainly a distressing event and outside normal operative occurrences. These stressful events may lead to nightmares and sleep disturbances, intrusive memories and avoidance behavior, emotional numbing and forgetting, and other diagnostic criteria for posttraumatic stress disorder.

g) The causes of intraoperative awareness are diverse and are listed in the following box.

Situations Associated with Higher Incidences of Awareness Under Anesthesia

- Acute trauma with hypovolemia
- ASA Physical Status 3, 4, and 5
- Cardiac surgery, including off-pump
- Impaired cardiovascular status
- Cesarean section under general anesthesia
- Severe end-stage lung disease
- Bronchoscopy, laryngoscopy, or both
- History of awareness
- Expected intraoperative hypotension requiring treatment
- Chronic use of benzodiazepines or opioids requiring treatment, or both
- Anticipated difficult intubation
- Heavy alcohol intake
- Use of beta-blockers in conjunction with neuromuscular blockade

h) Awake paralysis, one of the most feared causes, is possibly the most preventable. Awake paralysis is related to lapses in practitioner vigilance and can lead to out-of-sequence neuromuscular blockade administration and medication error.

i) Prevention of awareness is the best treatment for awareness. The American Association of Nurse Anesthetists has an awareness policy that helps identify at-risk patients and measures to address and possibly avoid perioperative awareness. This anesthesia care plan to reduce the incidence and severity of awareness includes the fundamental practices listed in the box on pg. 600.

j) Although awareness and recall of some of the anesthesia experience are impossible to prevent in all patients, vigilance on the part of the anesthesia provider (i.e., close attention to monitoring modalities and to anesthetic levels) should decrease the incidence substantially.

Anesthesia Care Plan to Reduce the Incidence and Severity of Awareness

1. During preanesthesia evaluation, assess the risk of awareness. Incorporate the possibility of awareness as part of the informed consent for all high-risk scenarios.
2. Check all anesthesia equipment (anesthesia machine, vaporizer, infusion pumps) to ensure the ability to deliver adequate amounts of anesthetic agents.
3. Consider the use of brain function monitoring, particularly for high-risk scenarios, if available.
4. Consider premedication with amnestic agents.
5. Clearly label all drug syringes immediately when they are drawn up. Do not rely on recognition of syringe size to confirm its contents. Consider other methods of ensuring the correct drug given to avoid inadvertent paralysis of the awake patient.
6. Provide additional doses of hypnotic or initiate volatile agent administration for repeated intubation attempts.
7. Use an end-tidal agent monitor, with the low alarm set for a sufficient inhalation concentration to prevent awareness.
8. When using total intravenous anesthesia, ensure a patent intravenous line and periodically check the function of the syringe pump.
9. Avoid excessive muscle paralysis unless required for surgical indications. Routinely use a peripheral nerve stimulator to measure degree of paralysis.
10. Conduct postoperative assessment to determine if unintended awareness occurred. If appropriate, refer the patient to a healthcare professional for support and therapy.

Adapted from Ghoneim MM. Awareness during anesthesia. *Anesthesiology.* 2000; 92(2):597-602; Bergman, Kluger MT, Short TG, et al. Awareness during general anesthesia: a review of 81 cases from the Anaesthetic Incident Monitoring Study. *Anaesthesia.* 2002; 57(6):549-556.

B. EYE INJURY

1. **Corneal abrasion**
   a) Corneal injury is an infrequent occurrence during anesthesia. The cornea is a tough, transparent, dome-shaped surface covering the eyes that serves as a barrier to infection and trauma in this highly exposed organ.
   b) Corneal abrasions are superficial defects of the corneal epithelium. Application of a short-acting topical anesthetic before assessment facilitates an examination.
   c) Visual acuity is usually normal unless the abrasion includes the visual axis or if there is considerable edema. There may be miosis caused by ciliary spasm and blepharospasm (marked by an uncontrollable, forcible closure of the eyelids) of the affected eye as a result of photophobia.
   d) The cornea may also appear hazy if edema is present.
   e) A corneal abrasion, although infrequent, is the foremost injury after general anesthesia and may occur during other types of anesthesia (monitored anesthesia care and major conduction block) when something strikes the eye.
   f) Corneal abrasions cause tearing, sensations of a foreign body, photophobia, reduced visual acuity, and eye pain. Postoperative corneal injuries can lead to significant morbidity and lost productivity.

g) Drying of an exposed cornea or patient movement during ophthalmic surgery (e.g., coughing, turning) can lead to abrasion of the cornea with subsequent poor surgical outcomes.
h) Keratoconjunctivitis sicca, also called dry eye disease (DED) and dysfunctional tear syndrome, is a multifactorial disorder of the tear film and ocular surface involving multiple interacting mechanisms.
i) Pressure on the eye (e.g., prone position, leaning of the face) may result from occlusion of choroidal blood flow and reduction of blood flow to the cornea. Because the cornea contains no blood vessels, oxygen delivery is accomplished through diffusion.
j) As a result, reduced blood flow to the cornea leads to a reduction in oxygen availability with subsequent corneal edema. The avascular nature of the cornea, dry environment, pressure, and desquamation of the epithelium of the eye may lead to corneal abrasion.
k) The diagnosis of corneal abrasion is confirmed by green fluorescence in damaged areas of the cornea seen under Wood's lamp or cobalt blue light on slit lamp examination after the application of fluorescein.
l) The treatment of corneal abrasion varies; however, occlusion of the affected eye is often recommended. Occlusion of the affected eye is also frequently associated with topical application of antibiotic ointment of nonsteroidal medications.
m) Primary goals of therapy are pain control, prevention of infection, and rapid healing of the corneal epithelium. Most corneal abrasions heal within 1 to 3 days; however, defects involving greater than half of the corneal surface may require 4 to 5 days to fully heal.
n) Prevention of corneal abrasion is a primary focus during the course of anesthesia. Although no method is guaranteed to be 100% effective, care and vigilance are required to reduce the associated morbidity of this disturbing complication.
o) Methods to protect the eyes during general anesthesia are listed in the table on pg. 602.

2. **Blindness**
   a) Blindness as a complication of anesthesia during nonocular surgery is a rare but devastating surgical risk and a medicolegal concern for the surgical team (anesthesia provider, surgeon, and nursing staff).
   b) The incidence of perioperative blindness ranges from 0.002% of all surgeries to as high as 0.2% of cardiac and spine surgeries.
   c) Any portion of the visual pathways may be involved, but the most common site of permanent injury is the optic nerves. The most often presumed mechanism is ischemia. With more than 1.2 billion myelinated nerve fibers arising from the cell bodies of cells in the retina, ischemia can be an immense problem, resulting in axonal swelling of these fibers and blindness. Other potential causes of postoperative visual loss include: pressure on the eyes, anemia, prolonged hypotension and increased intraocular pressure.
   d) Treatment and prevention of perioperative blindness, especially as a complication of anesthesia, are difficult. Immediate consultation is imperative for patients with perioperative blindness. If an obvious ocular cause is not apparent, urgent neuroimaging should be obtained to rule out intracranial pathology.

Commonly Used Methods to Protect Eyes During General Anesthesia

Method	Strengths	Weaknesses
Manual closure	Prevents trauma to the globe and eyelids Prevents injury associated with the introduction of agents (ointments, tape) onto the eye	Inappropriate when surgery involves the head or neck Incompatible with the prone or lateral position; may cause greater harm to the eye
Taping the eyelids	Prevents exposure keratopathy and injury associated with the introduction of agents onto the eye	Incorrect placement leads to exposure keratopathy May cause corneal abrasion if tape is placed directly onto the cornea Inappropriate when surgery involves the head or neck Incompatible with the prone or lateral position; may cause greater harm to the eye May cause injury when removing tape at the end of the procedure
Ophthalmic ointments, methylcellulose, and hydrogels	Equally effective as taping to prevent corneal abrasion Prevent drying of the eyes for extended periods Permit continuous perioperative monitoring of the eyes during certain procedures	Postoperative sensation of foreign body in some patients Cause blurred vision and confusion in some patients May cause allergic reactions after the use of ointments containing methylparaben, chlorobutanol, and other preservatives May require reassessment during long procedures
Eye shields and pads	Reduce the risk of mechanical injury May be used in prone and lateral positions Equally effective as taping and ointments at preventing corneal abrasion	Must include taping eyelids or applying ointment

C. OPERATING ROOM FIRE

1. **Introduction**
   a) Fires in the operating room are a relatively rare event. The classic fire triangle requires the presence of three elements: fuel, an ignition source, and an oxidizing agent (gas that supports combustion).
   b) Of the approximately 100 surgical fires reported each year, approximately 20 cause major thermal injuries; however, one to two of these fires result in death.

c) The most common locations of these fires are in the airway (34%), about the head or face (28%), and several other areas of or in the patient's body (38%).
d) The most common ignition sources are electrosurgical equipment (68%) and lasers (13%). High-intensity light cords have also been reported to be a source of ignition.
e) Fuels commonly found in the operating room consist of alcohol, solvents, sheets and drapes (cloth and disposable paper), and plastic or rubber materials (including endotracheal tubes [ETTs]).
f) Oxygen is by far the most common oxidizing agent, although nitrous oxide can also support combustion. Materials that are only marginally combustible in air can produce a massive flame in the presence of high oxygen concentration.

2. **Fire precaution and prevention**
   a) The risk of ignition of combustible materials is progressively increased as oxidizing agents build in the operating room.
   b) Oxygen levels should be kept as low as can be safely done, and leaks to the ambient air should be kept to a minimum, with special attention to oxygen and nitrous oxide leaks from the anesthesia mask and nasal cannula.
   c) Providers should reduce the oxygen concentration when a heat-producing device, such as a cautery unit or fiberoptic light source, is used. Although fiberoptic light is often called "cool light," heat is generated.
   d) When an open oxygen source is used, excessive oxygen can accumulate under the patient drape or about the operative site creating an enriched oxygen environment. If a spark is created in these areas, a flash fire can rapidly spread out of control.
   e) Procedures near the head and neck are more likely to be associated with fires because of the frequent presence of enriched oxygen and nitrous oxide. The total oxygen liter per minute flow should be kept as low as possible and should be consistent with the patient's status and response as monitored by standard physiologic monitors, with special attention to SaO_2 values compared with the patient's baseline values.
   f) Avoid petroleum-based ointments in the vicinity of surgery. These include petroleum-based ophthalmic ointments when surgery is in the vicinity of the face.
   g) When electrocautery is used, cloth towels are wetted with sterile water to surround a surgical site that is above the xyphoid process when open oxygen is administered by nasal cannula or face mask. Wet surgical towels reduce the likelihood of a flash fire being precipitated by cautery.
   h) If possible, administer higher levels of inspired oxygen during the preparation and local anesthetic infiltration if needed and then reduce the inspired oxygen to the lowest possible level consistent with the patient's condition during the use of electrosurgery, electrocautery, or laser units (drills, defibrillators, static electricity).
   i) When surgical drapes are placed over the face (e.g., for eye surgery) during local or local and monitored anesthesia care (MAC) techniques, consider tenting the drapes to allow for O_2 escape and active evacuation of the ambient gases given off by nasal cannulas or face masks. This can be achieved by the placement of a funnel-like collection device that evacuates the gases by way of the hospital suction system.

j) Consider giving an oxygen-air blend with an Fio_2 of 0.3 or less. This can be done by administering nasal oxygen via oxygen tubing connected with an approximately 5-mm ETT connector placed at the Y-connection outlet from the circle system anesthesia circuit. In this manner, a mixture of oxygen and medical-grade air can be blended from the anesthesia machine flowmeters while using the oxygen analyzer to regulate the O_2 level of (ideally) 0.3 or less.
k) The use of an incise drape (clear vinyl drape that is placed over the proposed surgical site so that the incision is made through the clear drape) has been recommended by some sources to keep the oxygen concentrated below the incision. This should not be considered a totally effective method of keeping the oxygen concentration low in the surgical field.
l) Channeling of oxygen can occur through any small opening in the area between the incise drape and the skin.
m) The hot tip of an electrocautery unit laid on a drape can cause ignition of the drapes. The cautery hand unit should be placed in its holster when not in use. Activate heat sources only when the tip is in view and deactivate it before the tip leaves the surgical site.
n) When using an open O_2 source: If possible, stop oxygen administration for a minimum of 1 minute before the use of electrosurgical units (cautery) near the head, face, and neck.
o) Arrange drapes to allow ready access to the patient's face to facilitate observation and maximal exchange of ambient room air, increase communications with the patient, and have ready access for possible airway manipulations.
p) Oxygen and nitrous oxide are heavier than room air, so these gases gravitate down over the patient in a manner similar to that of water poured over a surface. Heavier-than-air gas tends to spread and become concentrated under the drapes. It also contributes to a phenomenon called surface fiber flame propagation (SFFP).
q) When oxygen coats the fine fibers of a surface (e.g., draping fabrics) or even fine facial hair (vellus) and other body hair surfaces, the flames can quickly spread when these fibers ignite rapidly in the presence of oxygen enrichment. Facial hair and any other hair should be coated with a water-soluble gel if it is in the area of surgery and cautery use is anticipated.

3. **Fire management**
   a) If a fire starts, immediately cut or tear off any burning drapes or other materials from the patient.
   b) Water should be readily available to extinguish fire, especially in the mouth or other open body cavities. Because many drapes (especially disposable ones) are liquid resistant, water will tend to bead up rather than soak the material to reduce flame propagation.
   c) If tearing the material away is difficult or ineffective, use a CO_2 fire extinguisher. Fire blankets should be available to smother flames if they occur. However, if there is a concern that the fire started under a surgical drape because of an oxygen-enriched environment, a fire blanket may not be able to smother the fire, and the fire could actually continue to thermally injure the patient.
   d) Sponges, gauze, pledgets, and strings should be wet and kept moistened when in use in the area of surgery to help prevent airway fires.

D. STROKE (BRAIN ATTACK)

1. **Introduction**
   a) Stroke has been defined as an acute neurologic deficit that persists for longer than 24 hours.
   b) The incidence of acute perioperative ischemic stroke is low and uncommon; however, the overall mortality rate is high, with roughly 80% occurring as a consequence of thromboembolic mechanisms.
   c) The major causes include combined cardiac procedures, vascular procedures, lacunar or cerebellar infarction, and hemorrhage. Risk factors include male gender, a history of transient ischemic attacks, and cigarette smoking.
   d) Perioperatively, the incidence depends mainly on the type and complexity of the surgical procedure. Slightly fewer than half of all perioperative strokes are recognized within the first day postsurgery, and the remaining cases occur after an uneventful postrecovery period, usually from the second postoperative day forward.
   e) The stress of surgery results in hypercoagulability and activation of the hemostatic system, which results in reduced fibrinolysis after surgery.
   f) Perioperative withholding of antiplatelet and anticoagulant agents can exacerbate surgery-induced hypercoagulability and add to the risk of perioperative stroke.
   g) The neurologic deficit may be mild and transient and may often go unnoticed, depending on the extent of the infarct.
   h) The American Heart Association guidelines suggest the use of systemic thrombolysis using alteplase (a recombinant tissue plasminogen activator) within 3 hours of the onset of stroke. Although the mortality rate is unchanged, the use of thrombolytic therapy has been shown to support carotid and vertebrobasilar recanalization in approximately 25% of cases when given within 3 hours of symptoms and to improve 3-month neurologic outcomes.
   i) Intraarterial thrombolysis has not been shown to be better than the intravenous (IV) route, and IV streptokinase is not indicated for acute ischemic stroke.
   j) Stroke in patients with sickle cell disease is often fatal, particularly in children between the ages of 4 and 15 years. There is a 300-fold increased risk of stroke in these patients, making it the most common cause of childhood stroke.
   k) The combination of surgery and anesthesia is an independent risk factor for the development of acute ischemic stroke perioperatively.
   l) Acute ischemic stroke has a high mortality rate, and in certain instances of intractable intracranial hypertension, hemicraniectomy or decompressive surgery of the posterior fossa could be lifesaving.
   m) Practitioner understanding of the pathologic mechanism of stroke after anesthesia and surgery is vital and requires additional investigation to prevent this overwhelming complication.

ACETAMINOPHEN (OFIRMEV)

Classification
Nonnarcotic analgesic; nonsteroidal anti-inflammatory drug

Indications
Mild to moderate analgesia for pain, antipyretic

Dose
The recommended dose of Ofirmev for patients 13 years old or older weighing 50 kg or more is 1000 mg every 6 hours or 650 mg every 4 hours intravenously; the maximum daily dose of acetaminophen by any route is 4000 mg. For patients older than 2 years old weighing less than 50 kg, the recommended dose is 15 mg/kg every 6 hours or 12.5 mg/kg every 4 hours intravenously.

Onset and Duration
Onset: 5 to 15 minutes. Duration: 4 to 6 hours

Ofirmev can be given directly from the 100-mL vial (10 mg/mL) without further dilution and should be infused over 15 minutes.

Adverse Effects
The antipyretic effect of acetaminophen may mask fever. In clinical trials of intravenous acetaminophen, adverse effects were minor and similar to those with placebo.

Precautions and Contraindications
Avoid use in patients with liver disease. Overdose can cause serious or fatal hepatic injury, particularly in patients who are fasting. Hepatic toxicity after acetaminophen overdose can be treated with *N*-acetylcysteine.

Anesthetic Considerations
Intravenous acetaminophen decreases pain and reduces fever in adults and children. It has an opioid-sparing effect. It is effective for mild to moderate pain.

ADENOSINE (ADENOCARD)

Classification
Antiarrhythmic

Indications
Supraventricular tachycardia

Dose
6-mg bolus administered over 1 to 2 seconds followed by normal saline line flush; may increase to 12-mg bolus if arrhythmia persists past 2 minutes. May repeat 12-mg bolus once.

Dosage forms: 3 mg/mL; 2- and 5-mL vials

Onset and Duration
Onset: 10 to 20 seconds; duration: 1 minute

Adverse Effects
Flushing, dyspnea, chest pain, headache, nausea, cough, malaise

Precautions and Contraindications
Adenosine should not be used in patients receiving methylxanthine therapy (i.e., aminophylline, theophylline). Dipyridamole (Persantine) inhibits cellular uptake of adenosine. Use it with caution in patients with asthma. It is contraindicated in patients with second- or third-degree heart block.

Anesthetic Considerations
This is an agent for use preoperatively and postoperatively. It is not used under anesthesia because it produces sinus arrest. It may be administered in lieu of or preceding administration of calcium channel blockers for long-term suppression.

ALBUTEROL SULFATE (PROVENTIL, VENTOLIN)

Classification
β_2-adrenergic agonist, sympathomimetic, bronchodilator

Indications
Treatment of asthma and other forms of bronchospasm

Dose
Inhaler (metered dose): two deep inhalations 1 to 5 minutes apart; may be repeated every 4 to 6 hours (daily dose should not exceed 16 to 20 inhalations; each metered aerosol actuation delivers approximately 90 mcg/puff). Oral: 2 to 4 mg three to four times daily (total dose not to exceed 16 mg). Syrup: 2 mg/5 mL is available.

Onset and Duration
Onset: inhalation: 5 to 15 minutes; oral: 15 to 30 minutes. Peak effect: inhalation: 0.5 to 2 hours; oral: 2 to 3 hours. Duration: inhalation: 3 to 6 hours; oral: 4 to 8 hours.

Adverse Effects
Tachycardia, arrhythmias, hypertension, tremors, anxiety, headache, nausea, vomiting, hypokalemia

Precautions and Contraindications
Safe use is not established during pregnancy. Use albuterol cautiously in patients with cardiovascular disease, hypertension, and hyperthyroidism. Monitor glucose and electrolyte levels.

Anesthetic Considerations
Tolerance or tachyphylaxis can develop with long-term use. It has additive effects with epinephrine and other sympathomimetics. It is antagonized by β-receptor antagonists.

ALFENTANIL HCL (ALFENTA)

Classification
Opioid agonist; produces analgesia and anesthesia

Indications
Perioperative analgesia

Dose
Induction: intravenous: 50 to 150 mcg/kg; infusion: 0.1 to 3 mcg/kg/min.

Onset and Duration
Onset: intravenous: 1 to 2 minutes; intramuscular: less than 5 minutes; epidural: 5 to 15 minutes. Duration: intravenous: 1 to 15 minutes; intramuscular: 10 to 60 minutes; epidural: 30 minutes.

Adverse Effects
Bradycardia, hypotension, arrhythmias, respiratory depression; euphoria, dysphoria, convulsions, nausea and vomiting, biliary tract spasm, delayed gastric emptying, muscle rigidity, pruritus

Precautions and Contraindications
Reduce the alfentanil dose in elderly, hypovolemic, or high-risk surgical patients and with the concomitant use of sedatives and other narcotics.

It crosses the placental barrier, and use in labor may produce respiratory depression in neonates. Resuscitation may be required; have naloxone available.

Anesthetic Considerations
Circulatory and ventilatory depressant effects are potentiated by narcotics, sedatives, volatile anesthetics, and nitrous oxide. Analgesia is enhanced by α_2-agonists. Muscle rigidity in the higher dose range can be sufficient to interfere with ventilation.

ALPROSTADIL, PGE_1 (PROSTIN VR)

Classification
Prostaglandin E

Indications
Neonates: to maintain temporary patency of the ductus arteriosus until corrective or palliative surgery can be performed

Dose
Children: continuous infusion into large vein: 0.05 to 0.1 mcg/kg/min initially; when a therapeutic response occurs, decrease to lowest possible dose to maintain response (maximum dose: 0.4 mcg/kg/min).

Dosage forms: 500 mcg/mL, 1-mL ampules (refrigerate at 2° to 8° C). Must be diluted in 5% dextrose in water (D_5W) or normal saline for continuous infusion to a final concentration of 5 to 20 mcg/mL.

Onset and Duration
Onset: 30 minutes; elimination half-life: 5 to 10 minutes; duration: 30 minutes to 2 hours

Adverse Effects
Apnea (10%-12%), fever (14%), flushing (10%), bradycardia and seizures (4%), thrombocytopenia (less than 1%), disseminated intravascular coagulation (1%), anemia, tachycardia, hypotension (4%), diarrhea (2%), gastric outlet obstruction secondary to antral hyperplasia (related to cumulative dose)

Precautions and Contraindications

Apnea is most frequent in infants weighing less than 2 kg within the first hour of alprostadil administration; ventilatory assistance may be required. It is contraindicated in neonates with respiratory distress syndrome. Use it with caution in patients with bleeding tendencies because of alprostadil's ability to inhibit platelet aggregation. In all neonates, monitor arterial pressure; if arterial pressure falls significantly, decrease the rate of infusion.

Anesthetic Considerations

Alprostadil is used to maintain a patent ductus arteriosus in newborns.

AMINOCAPROIC ACID (AMICAR)

Classification

Hemostatic agent; prevents the conversion of plasminogen to plasmin

Indications

Control of clinical bleeding in which hyperfibrinolysis is a contributing factor (hyperfibrinolysis should be confirmed by laboratory values such as prolonged thrombin time, prolonged prothrombin time, hypofibrinogenemia, or decreased plasminogen levels); also: open heart surgery; postoperative hematuria after transurethral prostatic resection, suprapubic prostatectomy, and nephrectomy; hematologic disorders such as aplastic anemia, abruptio placentae, cirrhosis, neoplastic diseases, and prophylaxis in patients with hemophilia before and after tooth extraction and other bleeding in the mouth and nasopharynx; reduction of blood loss in trauma and shock; possible prevention of ocular hemorrhaging and bleeding in subarachnoid hemorrhage

Dose

Acute bleeding: 5 g infused during the first hour followed by a continuous infusion of 1 g/hr for 8 hours or until bleeding is controlled

Chronic bleeding: 5 g preoperatively by intravenous piggyback over 1 hour; then 5 g by intravenous piggyback every 6 hours. Do not exceed 30 g in 24 hours. Decrease dose by 15% to 25% in patients with renal disease.

Children: 100 mg/kg intravenous piggyback over 1 hour; then 30 mg/kg/hr until bleeding is controlled (maximum dose: 18 g/m^2/day).

Dosage forms: 250 mg/mL, 20 mL parenteral vial (5 g)

Administration: Dilute each dose in a proper volume of D_5W normal saline or lactated Ringer's solution.

Onset and Duration

Onset: 1 to 72 hours; half-life 1 to 2 hours in patients with normal renal function. No single concentration fits all. It must be diluted. Consult the package insert, an intravenous reference, or the pharmacy. Duration: 8 to 12 hours.

Adverse Effects

Convulsions; myopathy; rarely muscle necrosis, nausea, vomiting; rapid infusion associated with hypotension, bradycardia, arrhythmias

Precautions and Contraindications

A definitive diagnosis of hyperfibrinolysis must be made before aminocaproic acid administration. Use caution in patients with cardiac, renal, or hepatic disease. Administration in the presence of renal or ureteral bleeding is not recommended because of ureteral clot formation and the possible risk of obstruction. Owing to the substantial risk of serious or fatal thrombus formation, aminocaproic acid is contraindicated in patients with disseminated intravascular coagulation unless heparin is administered concurrently.

Anesthetic Considerations

Do not administer without a definite diagnosis of laboratory findings indicative of hyperfibrinolysis.

AMINOPHYLLINE (THEODUR, OTHERS)

Classification

Bronchodilator

Indications

Long-term therapy for bronchial asthma; reversal of bronchospasm associated with chronic obstructive pulmonary disease

Dose

Loading dose: for patients not already receiving a theophylline preparation, intravenous: 5 to 6 mg/kg (administered over 20-30 minutes). Oral or rectal: 6 mg/kg. Maintenance: intravenous: 0.5 mg/kg/hr; oral: 2 to 4 mg/kg every 6 to 12 hours. Therapeutic range: 10 to 20 mcg/mL.

Dilution for infusion loading dose: dilute 500 mg in 500 mL D_5W or normal saline (1 mg/mL)

Children 9 to 16 years: 1 mg/kg/hr for 12 hours; then 0.8 mg/kg/hr; children 6 months to 9 years: 1.2 mg/kg/hr for 12 hours; then 1 mg/kg/hr

Dosage forms: injection: 25 mg/mL; tablets: 100, 200 mg; tablets (sustained release): 225 mg; oral solution: 105 mg/5 mL; rectal solution: 60 mg/mL (rectal solution not marketed in the United States); rectal suppositories: 250, 500 mg

Onset and Duration

Onset: intravenous: 2 to 5 minutes; oral: within 30 minutes. Duration: oral: 4 to 8 hours

Adverse Effects

Palpitations, sinus tachycardia, supraventricular and ventricular tachycardia, flushing, tachypnea, seizures, headache, irritability, nausea, vomiting, hyperglycemia

Elevated serum levels are noted in patients receiving cimetidine, quinolone antibiotics, and macrolide antibiotics and in patients with cardiac failure or liver insufficiency. Decreased serum levels are seen with phenobarbital, phenytoin, rifampin, and smokers. Toxicity occurs with plasma levels greater than 20 mcg/mL. Avoid rapid infusions, which may cause hypotension, arrhythmias, and possibly death.

Precautions and Considerations

Caution when used in patients with seizure disorders, hypertension, or ischemic heart disease.

Anesthetic Considerations

Aminophylline potentiates the pressor effects of sympathomimetics and may produce seizures, cardiac arrhythmias, cardiorespiratory arrest, and ventricular arrhythmias with excessive plasma levels or in patients receiving volatile anesthetics. Use isoflurane or sevoflurane in patients who must be administered aminophylline or other exogenous sympathomimetic drugs before or during surgery. Use of halothane may potentiate cardiac dysrhythmia.

AMIODARONE (CORDARONE)

Classification
Class III antiarrhythmic

Indications
Treatment of life-threatening ventricular arrhythmias that do not respond to other antiarrhythmics (i.e., recurrent ventricular fibrillation and hemodynamically unstable ventricular tachycardia); selective treatment of supraventricular arrhythmias

Dose
Loading: oral: 800 to 1600 mg/day for 1 to 3 weeks; maintenance: oral: 200 to 600 mg/day; therapeutic level: 1 to 2.5 mcg/mL

Dosage forms: tablets: 200 mg; intravenous: 100 to 300 mg

The recommended starting dose of intravenous amiodarone HCl is about 1000 mg over the first 24 hours of therapy delivered by the following infusion:

- Loading infusions: first rapid: 150 mg over the *first* 10 minutes (15 mg/min). Add 3 mL of amiodarone HCl intravenously (150 mg) to 100 mL D_5W (concentration = 1.5 mg/mL). Infuse 100 mL over 10 minutes.
- Followed by slow infusion: 360 mg over the next 6 hours (1 mg/min). Add 18 mL of amiodarone HCl intravenously (900 mg) to 500 mL D_5W (concentration = 1.8 mg/mL).
- Maintenance infusion: 540 mg over the remaining 18 hours (0.5 mg/min). Decrease the rate of the slow loading infusion to 0.5 mg/min.

Onset and Duration
Onset: 2 to 4 days. Half-life: between 2 weeks and 2 months (including active metabolites). Duration: 45 days

Adverse Effects
Arrhythmias, pulmonary fibrosis or inflammation, hepatitis or cirrhosis, corneal deposits, hyperthyroidism, hypothyroidism, peripheral neuropathy, cutaneous photosensitivity

Precautions and Contraindications
Amiodarone increases serum levels of digoxin, warfarin, quinidine, procainamide, phenytoin, and diltiazem. The likelihood of bradycardia, sinus arrest, and atrioventricular block increases with concurrent β-adrenergic antagonist and calcium channel blocker therapy.

Anesthetic Considerations
Antiadrenergic effects are enhanced in the presence of general anesthetics and manifest as sinus arrest, atrioventricular block, low cardiac output, or hypotension. Drugs that inhibit the automaticity of the sinus node such as halothane and lidocaine could accentuate the effects of amiodarone and increase the likelihood of sinus arrest. The potential need for a

temporary artificial cardiac (ventricular) pacemaker and administration of sympathomimetics such as isoproterenol should be considered in patients receiving this drug.

AMRINONE LACTATE (INOCOR)

Classification
Positive inotrope (phosphodiesterase inhibitor)

Indication
Short-term management of congestive heart failure

Dose
Loading dose: 0.75 mg/kg over 2 to 3 minutes. A second bolus may follow after 30 minutes. Maintenance is by continuous infusion of 5 to 10 mcg/kg/min (maximum dose: 10 mg/kg/day).

Dosage forms: injection: 5 mg/mL; dilution for infusion: 500 mg in 500 mL normal saline solution

Onset and Duration
Onset: within 5 minutes; duration: 30 minutes to 2 hours

Adverse Effects
Hypotension, arrhythmia, thrombocytopenia, abdominal pain, hepatic dysfunction

Precautions and Contraindications
Use amrinone with caution in hypotensive patients. Avoid exposure of the ampule to light. Do not mix in solutions containing dextrose or furosemide. Use it with caution in patients with allergies to bisulfites. Fluid balance, electrolyte concentrations, and renal function should be monitored carefully during treatment. Monitor platelet counts on a long-term basis. Amrinone contains sodium metabisulfite, a sulfite that may cause allergic-type reactions, including anaphylactic symptoms and life-threatening or less severe asthmatic episodes in susceptible patients. Sulfite sensitivity is seen more frequently in patients with asthma than in patients without asthma.

Anesthetic Considerations
This drug is an alternative to conventional inotropes. It is useful when both inotropic and vasodilating properties are desired or to lower pulmonary vascular resistance. Milrinone, another phosphodiesterase-3 inhibitor, is more commonly used.

APREPITANT (EMEND)

Classification
Antiemetic; neurokinin 1 (NK1) receptor antagonist

Indication
Postoperative nausea and vomiting

Dose
Oral 40-mg dose administered within 3 hours before the induction of anesthesia

Onset and Duration

Onset: 1 to 3 hours. Duration: up to 24 hours when used in multimodal therapy

Adverse Effects

The most frequent adverse events reported in clinical trials of aprepitant for postoperative nausea and vomiting were constipation, nausea, pruritus, pyrexia, hypotension, headache, and bradycardia.

Precautions and Contraindications

Aprepitant produces a dose-dependent inhibition of CYP3A4 and should be used with caution in patients receiving drugs that are primarily metabolized through CYP3A4. Weak inhibition of CYP3A4 by a single 40-mg dose is not expected to alter the plasma concentrations of these products to a clinically significant degree.

The efficacy of hormonal contraceptives may be reduced during coadministration with aprepitant for up to 28 days after the last dose.

Anesthetic Considerations

Aprepitant is most effective when used as a component of multimodal prophylaxis with a serotonin receptor blocker.

ATRACURIUM (TRACRIUM)

Classification

Nondepolarizing skeletal muscle relaxant

Indications

Relaxation of skeletal muscles during surgery; adjunct to general anesthesia or mechanical ventilation; facilitation of endotracheal intubation

Dose

Initially for paralyzing: intravenous: 0.3 to 0.5 mg/kg; maintenance: intravenous: 0.08 to 0.1 mg/kg

Dosage forms: injection: 10 mg/mL

Onset and Duration

Onset: less than 3 minutes. Duration: 30 to 45 minutes. Elimination: plasma (Hofmann elimination, ester hydrolysis). The primary metabolite is laudanosine (a cerebral stimulant) produced in low doses, excreted primarily in the urine.

Adverse Effects

Primarily resulting from histamine release: vasodilation, hypotension, sinus tachycardia, sinus bradycardia, hypoventilation, apnea, bronchospasm, laryngospasm, dyspnea, inadequate block, prolonged block, rash, and urticaria

Precautions and Contraindications

Use atracurium with caution in patients with conditions in which histamine release may prove hazardous, in patients with myasthenia gravis or other muscle disorders, and in patients with electrolyte disturbances.

Anesthetic Considerations

Monitor the patient's response with a peripheral nerve stimulator. Reverse the effects with anticholinesterase. Pretreatment doses may induce sufficient neuromuscular blockade to cause hypoventilation in some patients.

ATROPINE SULFATE

Classification

Competitive acetylcholine antagonist at muscarinic receptor

Indications

Symptomatic bradycardia, asystole, cardiopulmonary resuscitation (CPR); antisialagogue; for vagolytic effects to block bradycardia during surgery from stimulation of the carotid sinus, traction on abdominal viscera, or extraocular muscles; blockade of muscarinic effects of anticholinesterases; adjunctive therapy in the treatment of bronchospasm, peptic ulcer disease

Dose

Adults: sinus bradycardia. CPR: intravenous, intramuscular, subcutaneous, via endotracheal tube (diluted in 10 mL of sterile water or normal saline): 0.5 to 1 mg every 3 to 5 minutes as indicated (maximum dose: 40 mcg/kg/event). Preoperative: 0.4 mg intramuscular, subcutaneous, or oral: 30 to 60 minutes preinduction.

Blockade of muscarinic effects of anticholinesterases: 7 to 10 mcg/kg with edrophonium, 15 to 30 mcg/kg with neostigmine, 15 to 20 mcg/kg with pyridostigmine

Bronchodilation: inhalation: 0.025 mg/kg every 4 to 6 hours. Dilute to 2 to 3 mL in normal saline and deliver by compressed air nebulizer (maximum dose: 2.5 mg/dose). Pediatric bronchodilatory dose: 0.05 mg/kg diluted in normal saline three or four times daily.

Children: sinus bradycardia, CPR: intravenous, intramuscular, subcutaneous, or via endotracheal tube: 0.02 mg/kg every 5 minutes up to a maximum of 1 mg in children and 2 mg in adolescents (minimum dose, 0.1 mg). Preoperative: oral, intramuscular, subcutaneous: 0.02 mg/kg for neonates, 0.1 mg for children weighing 3 kg, 0.2 mg for those weighing 7 to 9 kg, and 0.3 mg for those weighing 12 to 16 kg.

Dosage forms: injection: 0.05, 0.1, 0.3, 0.4, 0.5, 0.8, and 1 mg/mL; inhalation solution: 0.2%, 0.5%; tablets: 0.4 mg, 0.6 mg

Onset and Duration

Inhibition of salivation occurs within 30 minutes to 1 hour and peaks in 1 to 2 hours after oral or intramuscular atropine administration. Increase in heart rate occurs within 3 to 10 minutes after intravenous or intramuscular administration. Duration: 15 to 45 minutes after intravenous administration and 2 to 4 hours after intramuscular administration.

Adverse Effects

Transient bradycardia resulting from a weak peripheral muscarinic cholinergic agonist effect in small doses (less than 0.5 mg in adults), tachycardia (high doses), urinary hesitancy, retention, mydriasis, blurred vision, increased intraocular pressure, decreased sweating, excitement, agitation, drowsiness, confusion, hallucinations, dry nose and mouth, allergic reactions, constipation.

Children and elderly patients are more susceptible to these adverse effects.

Precautions and Contraindications

Avoid atropine in situations in which tachycardia would be harmful (i.e., thyrotoxicosis, pheochromocytoma, coronary artery disease). Avoid in hyperpyrexial states because it inhibits sweating. It is contraindicated in acute-angle glaucoma, obstructive disease of the gastrointestinal tract, obstructive uropathy, paralytic ileus or intestinal atony, and acute hemorrhage in patients with unstable cardiovascular status. Use it with caution in patients with tachyarrhythmias, hepatic or renal disease, congestive heart failure, chronic pulmonary disease (because a reduction in bronchial secretions may lead to formation of bronchial plugs), autonomic neuropathy, hiatal hernia, gastroesophageal reflux, gastric ulcers, gastrointestinal infections, and ulcerative colitis.

Anesthetic Considerations

Additive anticholinergic effects may occur when atropine is administered concomitantly with meperidine, some antihistamines, phenothiazines, tricyclic antidepressants, and antiarrhythmic drugs that possess anticholinergic activity (e.g., quinidine, disopyramide, procainamide).

BUMETANIDE

Classification

Loop diuretic

Indications

Treatment of edema of cardiac, hepatic, or renal origin; hypertension, pulmonary edema; usually reserved for patients who do not respond to thiazide diuretics or in whom a rapid onset of diuresis is desired.

Dose

Initial dose: 0.5 to 1 mg intravenously over 1 to 2 minutes. If response is not adequate after the initial dose, a second or third dose may be administered at intervals of up to 2 to 3 hours, up to a maximum of 10 mg/day.

Children: intravenous, intramuscular, oral: 0.015 to 0.1 mg/kg. maximum, 2 mg/day

Onset and Duration

Onset: intravenous: few minutes. Peak effect: 15 to 30 minutes. Duration: 4 hours with normal doses of 1 to 2 mg and up to 6 hours with higher doses. Elimination half-life: 1 to 1.5 hours

Adverse Effects

Transient leukopenia, granulocytopenia, thrombocytopenia, hypotension, chest pain, dizziness; electrolyte abnormalities such as hyperuricemia, hypomagnesemia, hypokalemia, hypochloremia, azotemia, hyponatremia, or metabolic alkalosis; hyperglycemia; diarrhea; pancreatitis; nephrotoxicity; muscle cramps; arthritic pain; ototoxicity (less frequent than with furosemide)

Precautions and Contraindications

Patients may have anuria, hypersensitivity to bumetanide, severe fluid and electrolyte imbalances, and hepatic coma if an increase in blood urea nitrogen or creatinine occurs. Patients who are allergic to sulfonamides may have hypersensitivity to bumetanide.

Anesthetic Considerations

Loop diuretics may increase the neuromuscular blocking effect of nondepolarizing relaxants.

BUPIVACAINE HCL (MARCAINE, SENSORCAINE)

Classification

Amide-type local anesthetic

Indication

Regional anesthesia

Dose

Infiltration or peripheral nerve block: less than 150 mg (0.25%-0.5% solution). Epidural: 50 to 100 mg (0.25%-0.75% solution); children: 1.5 to 2.5 mg/kg (0.25%-0.5% solution). Caudal: 37.5 to 150 mg (15-30 mL of 0.25% or 0.5% solution); children: 0.4 to 0.7 mL/kg. Spinal bolus/infusion: 7 to 17 mg (0.75% solution); children: 0.5 mg/kg with minimum of 1 mg. Do not exceed 400 mg in 24 hours (maximum single dose, 175 mg).

Onset and Duration

Onset: infiltration: 2 to 10 minutes. Epidural: 4 to 7 minutes. Spinal: less than 1 minute. Peak effect: infiltration and epidural: 30 to 45 minutes. Spinal: 15 minutes. Duration: infiltration, spinal, epidural: 200 to 400 minutes (prolonged with epinephrine).

Adverse Effects

Hypotension, arrhythmias, cardiac arrest, respiratory impairment or arrest, seizures, tinnitus, blurred vision, urticaria, anaphylactoid symptoms; high spinal: urinary retention, lower extremity weakness and paralysis, loss of sphincter control, backache, palsies, slowing of labor

Precautions and Contraindications

Use bupivacaine with caution in patients with hypovolemia, severe congestive heart failure, shock, and all forms of heart block. It is not recommended for obstetric paracervical block or in concentrations higher than 0.5% because of the incidence of intractable cardiac arrest. It is contraindicated in patients with hypersensitivity to amide-type local anesthetics.

Anesthetic Considerations

Intravenous access is essential during major regional block. Toxic plasma levels of bupivacaine may cause cardiopulmonary collapse and seizures.

CHLOROPROCAINE HCL (NESACAINE)

Classification

Ester-type local anesthetic

Indications

Regional anesthesia; local anesthesia, including infiltration, epidural (including caudal), peripheral nerve block, sympathetic nerve block

Dose

Infiltration and peripheral nerve block: less than 40 mL (1%-2% solution). Epidural: bolus 10 to 25 mL (2%-3% solution), approximately 1.5 to 2 mL for each segment to be anesthetized. Repeat doses at 40- to 60-minute intervals. Infusion: 30 mL/hr (0.5% solution). Caudal: 10 to 25 mL (2%-3% solution); children: 0.4 to 0.7 mL/kg (L2-T10 level of anesthesia). Repeat doses at 40- to 60-minute intervals.

Onset and Duration

Rate of onset and potency of local anesthetic action may be enhanced by carbonation. Onset: infiltration or epidural: 6 to 12 minutes. Peak effect: infiltration or epidural: 10 to 20 minutes. Duration: infiltration or epidural: 30 to 60 minutes (prolonged with epinephrine).

Adverse Effects

Hypotension, arrhythmias, bradycardia, respiratory depression or arrest, seizures, tinnitus, tremors, urticaria, pruritus, angioneurotic edema; high spinal: backache; loss of perianal sensation and sexual function; permanent motor, sensory, autonomic (sphincter control) deficit in lower segments; slowing of labor

Precautions and Contraindications

Use with caution in patients with severe disturbances of cardiac rhythm, shock, heart block, or impaired hepatic function. Inflammation or infection may occur at the injection site. Elderly and pregnant patients are most at risk. It is contraindicated in patients with hypersensitivity to ester-type local anesthetics and to para-aminobenzoic acid or parabens. Do not use for spinal anesthesia.

Anesthetic Considerations

Reduce doses in obstetric, elderly, hypovolemic, and high-risk surgical patients and in those with increased intraabdominal pressure.

CIMETIDINE (TAGAMET)

Classification

Histamine (H_2) antagonist

Indications

Treatment of duodenal or gastric ulcers, gastroesophageal reflux disease; prophylaxis of aspiration pneumonitis in patients at high risk during surgery

Dose

Prophylaxis of aspiration pneumonitis: adults: 300 to 400 mg orally 1.5 to 2 hours before induction of anesthesia with or without a similar dose the preceding evening. When a more rapid onset of effect is needed, intravenous: dilute 300 to 400 mg in D_5W or normal saline to a volume of at least 20 mL and inject over a period not less than 5 minutes. A slower infusion, over 15 to 30 minutes, may be preferable owing to association of occasional severe bradycardia and hypotension with rapid infusion. Children younger than 12 years: use not indicated.

Dosage forms: tablets: 300, 400 mg; parenteral injection: 150 mg/mL

Onset and Duration

Onset: 15 to 45 minutes. Peak effect: 1 to 2 hours orally. Duration: 2 to 4 hours. Elimination half-life: 2 hours. Plasma cimetidine levels that suppress gastric acid secretion by 50% were maintained 4 to 5 hours after intravenous injection.

Adverse Effects

Mental status changes such as delirium, confusion, depression, primarily in elderly patients or those with hepatic or renal impairment; leukopenia, thrombocytopenia, and gynecomastia rarely (1%)

Hypotension and severe bradycardia are associated with rapid intravenous infusion. Serum creatinine and liver enzymes may rise during treatment, although hepatotoxicity and renal dysfunction are usually reversible.

Precautions and Contraindications

Caution is suggested in renal or hepatic insufficiency. Microsomal metabolism of many drugs may be inhibited. It is contraindicated in patients allergic to cimetidine or other H_2 antagonists.

Anesthetic Considerations

Cimetidine inhibits the hepatic mixed-function oxidase system; therefore, it may prolong the half-life of many drugs, including diazepam, midazolam, metoprolol, propranolol, theophylline, lidocaine, and other amide local anesthetics. Ranitidine may be the drug of choice in patients receiving lidocaine local or regional anesthesia.

CLEVIPREX (CLEVIDIPINE)

Classification

Intravenous calcium channel blocker; antihypertensive

Indication

Antihypertensive, when oral drugs are not feasible

Dose

Clevidipine is a milky white lipid emulsion. Titrate to achieve desired blood pressure reduction. Initial dose is 1 to 2 mg/hr. Double the dose every few minutes until blood pressure goals are met. Maintenance doses usually range from 4 to 6 mg/hr. Maximum doses are usually less than 16 mg/hr.

Onset and Duration

Onset: 2 to 4 minutes. Duration: 5 to 15 minutes after the infusion is stopped

Adverse Effects

Hypotension, tachycardia, negative inotropic effects in heart failure patients

Precautions and Contraindications

Contraindicated in patients with allergies to soybeans, soy products, eggs or egg products, defects in lipid metabolism such as pathologic hyperlipemia, lipoid nephrosis, or acute pancreatitis, and patients with severe aortic stenosis

Caution handling the lipid emulsion. Use aseptic technique and discard if not used in 12 hours. Caution in patients on beta-blocker therapy.

Anesthetic Considerations

Useful for titration to control blood pressure. Insertion of an arterial line advised to closely monitor pressures. Monitor for rebound hypertension for 8 hours after the infusion is discontinued.

CLONIDINE (CATAPRES, DIXARIT); EPIDURAL CLONIDINE (CATAPRES, DURACLON)

Classification

Central-acting α_2-adrenergic agonist; reduces sympathetic outflow by directly stimulating α_2-receptors in the medulla vasomotor center

Epidural action produces dose-dependent analgesia by preventing pain signal transmission at presynaptic and postjunctional α_2-adrenoreceptors in the spinal cord.

Indications

Hypertension; epidural and spinal anesthesia; symptomatic control of alcohol, opiate, nicotine, and benzodiazepine withdrawal; diagnosis of pheochromocytoma; growth hormone stimulation test; cancer-related pain; Tourette syndrome; attention deficit disorder; migraines.

The use of epidural clonidine in combination with epidural opiate agonists results in a decreased opiate requirement that treats neuropathic pain more effectively than visceral pain.

Dose

Maintenance: 0.2 to 0.6 mg/day orally in two divided doses. Hypertensive emergencies: 0.15 mg intravenously over 5 minutes. Transdermal patch: every 7 days (maximum dose: 0.6 mg/day). The same doses are used in renal impairment.

Epidural: must be preservative free. Postoperative pain: epidural clonidine combined with an opiate analgesic: 30 mcg/hr if added to fentanyl. Neuropathic pain: continuous epidural infusion combined with an opiate analgesic is 30 mcg/hr.

All dosages must be titrated to pain relief and the incidence of side effects.

The recommended starting dose of epidural clonidine HCl for continuous epidural infusion is 30 mcg/hr. Although dosage may be titrated up or down, depending on pain relief and occurrence of adverse events, experience with dosage rates above 40 mcg/hr is limited.

Familiarization with the continuous epidural infusion device is essential. Patients receiving epidural clonidine from a continuous infusion device should be closely monitored for the first few days to assess their response.

The 500 mcg/mL (0.5 mg/mL) strength product must be diluted before use in 0.9% sodium chloride for injection to a final concentration of 100 mcg/mL.

Onset and Duration

Onset: intravenous or oral: 30 to 60 minutes. Peak effect: 2 to 4 hours. May take too long for a true hypertensive crisis. Duration: antihypertensive: 6 to 10 hours, dose dependent.

Adverse Effects

Rebound hypertension, atrioventricular block, bradycardia, congestive heart failure, orthostatic hypotension, sedation, nightmares, constipation, dry mouth, pruritus, urinary retention, contact dermatitis

The most common noncardiovascular adverse reactions to epidural clonidine include anxiety, asthenia, chest pain, confusion, diaphoresis, dizziness, drowsiness, dyspnea, fever, nausea or vomiting, and xerostomia.

Precautions and Contraindications

- Avoid in conduction or sinoatrial disorders, hypersensitivity to clonidine, pregnancy, severe renal or hepatic disease. Concomitant administration of tricyclic antidepressants may increase the serum level.
- If the dose is held or when changing to transdermal application, watch for a rapid increase in blood pressure from unopposed α stimulation.
- It crosses the placenta easily and should be discontinued 8 to 12 hours before delivery.
- Epidural clonidine is not recommended for intrathecal administration or as an analgesic during labor and delivery or for postpartum or perioperative analgesia because of the risks of hemodynamic instability.

Anesthetic Considerations

- Severe rebound hypertension may result from abrupt withdrawal, with neurologic sequelae and myocardial infarction. Labetalol has been successfully used in treatment of hypertensive crisis. Continue on the day of surgery.
- Hepatic elimination is 50%.
- Clonidine reduces perioperative requirements of narcotics and volatile agents.
- Female patients and lower weight patients have an increased risk of the hypotensive effects of epidural clonidine (use cautiously in patients with severe cardiac disease or hemodynamic instability). More profound decreases in blood pressure may be seen if the drug is administered into the upper thoracic spinal segments.

COCAINE HCL (COCAINE)

Classification

Topical anesthetic and vasoconstrictor, ester-type local anesthetic

Indications

Topical anesthesia and vasoconstriction of mucous membranes (oral, laryngeal, and nasal)

Dose

Topical: 1.5 mg/kg (1%-4% solution). Nasal: 1 to 2 mL each nostril (1%-10% solution). Concentrations greater than 4% increase potential for systemic toxic reactions. Maximum dose: 1.5 mg/kg.

Onset and Duration

Onset: less than 1 minute. Peak effect: 2 to 5 minutes. Duration: 30 to 120 minutes. It is rapidly absorbed from all areas of application.

Adverse Effects

Seizures, sloughing of nasal mucosa, arrhythmias, tachycardia, hypertension

Precautions and Contraindications

Cocaine is for topical use only, not for intraocular or intravenous use. It potentiates other sympathomimetics; therefore, use reduced doses (if any at all) in patients receiving pressors or ketamine. Use it with caution in patients with nasal trauma.

Anesthetic Considerations

Hypertension, bradyarrhythmias, tachyarrhythmias, ventricular fibrillation, tachypnea, respiratory failure, euphoria, excitement, seizures, and sloughing of corneal epithelium may occur. Use it with caution in patients with a history of drug sensitivities or drug abuse (high addiction potential) and pregnancy. Prolonged use can cause ischemic damage to nasal mucosa. Cocaine is contraindicated for intraocular or intravenous use. It sensitizes the heart to catecholamines (epinephrine and monoamine oxidase inhibitors may increase cardiac arrhythmias, ventricular fibrillation, hypertensive episodes). It potentiates arrhythmogenic effects of sympathomimetics, and it has a high addiction potential.

CODEINE

Classification

Opioid agonist

Indications

Preoperative and postoperative analgesia

Dose

Oral: 15 to 60 mg every 4 hours; intramuscular or subcutaneous: 15 to 60 mg every 4 hours.

Onset and Duration

Onset: oral: 30 to 60 minutes; intramuscular or subcutaneous: 20 to 60 minutes. Duration: oral: 2 to 4 hours; intramuscular or subcutaneous: 2 to 3 hours.

Adverse Effects

Sedation, clouded sensorium, euphoria, dizziness, seizures with large doses, hypotension, bradycardia, nausea, vomiting, constipation, dry mouth, ileus, urinary retention, pruritus, flushing

Precautions and Contraindications

Use codeine with caution in patients with head injury, owing to respiratory depression and resulting increased intracranial pressure; in hepatic or renal disease; hypothyroidism; Addison disease; acute alcoholism; seizures; severe central nervous system depression; bronchial asthma; chronic obstructive pulmonary disease; respiratory depression; and shock. Use it with caution in patients with known hypersensitivity to the drug and in elderly patients. It may produce histamine release.

Anesthetic Considerations

General anesthetics, other narcotic analgesics, tranquilizers, sedatives, hypnotics, alcohol, tricyclic antidepressants, or monoamine oxidase inhibitors increase central nervous system depression.

CYCLOSPORINE (SANDIMMUNE, OTHERS)

Classification

Immunosuppressant

Indications

Prevention of rejection of organ or tissue (kidney, liver, heart) allograft in combination with steroid therapy

Dose

Initial: oral: 15 mg/kg as a single dose 4 to 24 hours before transplantation; continue for 1 to 2 weeks. Taper to maintenance dose: 5 to 10 mg/kg/day. Intravenous: 5 to 6 mg/kg/day as a single dose 4 to 12 hours before transplantation; continue until the patient is able to take oral medication.

Coadministration of a corticosteroid is recommended, as well as possibly azathioprine.

Onset and Duration

Onset: 1 to 6 hours (variable). Duration: 1 to 4 days. After oral administration, onset is variable. Elimination half-life: 10 to 27 hours.

Adverse Effects

Hypertension, hirsutism, tremor, acne, gum hyperplasia, headache, blurred vision, diarrhea, nausea, paresthesia, mild nephrotoxicity or hepatotoxicity

Precautions and Contraindications

History of hypersensitivity to cyclosporine or polyoxyethylated castor oil. Use it with caution in patients with impaired hepatic, renal, cardiac function, or malabsorption syndrome and in those who are pregnant.

Anesthetic Considerations

Altered laboratory values may occur. Cyclosporine may elevate blood urea nitrogen, serum creatinine, serum bilirubin, serum glutamic-oxaloacetic transaminase (aspartate aminotransferase), serum glutamic-pyruvic transaminase (alanine aminotransferase), and lactate dehydrogenase. It may prolong the duration of neuromuscular blockade by nondepolarizing muscle relaxants.

DANTROLENE SODIUM (DANTRIUM)

Classification

Skeletal muscle relaxant

Indications

Treatment of malignant hyperthermia (MHT); prophylaxis of MHT in patients with a family history; control of spasticity secondary to multiple sclerosis, spinal cord injury, cerebral palsy, or stroke

Dose

Adults: MHT: 1 mg/kg rapid intravenous bolus; repeat every 5 to 10 minutes until symptoms are controlled; the dose may be repeated to a cumulative dose of 10 mg/kg; oral doses of 4 to 8 mg/kg/day for 1 to 3 days may be administered in three or four divided doses to prevent recurrence of the manifestations. Prophylaxis of MHT: 2.5 mg/kg intravenous bolus 10 to 30 minutes preinduction; then 1.25 mg/kg intravenous bolus 6 hours later.

Dosage forms: capsules: 25, 50, 100 mg; parenteral injection: 20 mg. Administration: reconstitute by adding 60 mL of preservative-free sterile water for injection to each 20-mg vial and shake the vial until clear. Avoid diluent that contains a bacteriostatic agent. Protect from light and use within 6 hours. For direct intravenous injection. Avoid extravasation.

Onset and Duration

Effective blood concentrations: 100 to 600 ng/mL. Intravenous blood concentrations of the drug remain at approximately steady-state levels for 3 or more hours after infusion is completed. Mean half-life: 5 to 9 hours. Onset: oral: 1 to 2 hours; intravenous: less than 5 minutes. Duration: 8 to 12 hours.

Adverse Effects
Hepatotoxicity (hepatitis): 0.5%, with mortality reported as high as 10%; muscle weakness, tachycardia, erratic blood pressure, fatigue, central nervous system (CNS) depression, visual and auditory hallucinations, bowel obstruction, hematuria, crystalluria, urinary frequency, phlebitis, pericarditis, pleural effusion, postpartum uterine atony, myalgias

Precautions and Contraindications
Monitor liver function at the beginning of dantrolene therapy. Observe for hepatotoxicity, hepatitis. Owing to the increased risk of hepatotoxicity, use it with caution in patients with severely impaired cardiac or pulmonary function and in women or patients older than 35 years. It is contraindicated in active hepatic disease such as hepatitis or cirrhosis, when spasticity is used to maintain motor function, and in lactation.

Anesthetic Considerations
Enhanced CNS and respiratory depression occurs with other CNS depressants. Avoid the concomitant use of calcium channel blockers, which can precipitate hyperkalemia and cardiovascular collapse.

DESFLURANE (SUPRANE)

Classification
Inhalation anesthetic

Indication
General anesthesia

Dose
Titrate to effect for induction or maintenance of anesthesia. Minimum alveolar concentration: 6%.

Dosage forms: volatile liquid

Onset and Duration
Onset: loss of eyelid reflex: 1 to 2 minutes. Duration: emergence time: 8 to 9 minutes.

Adverse Effects
Hypotension, arrhythmia, respiratory depression, apnea, dizziness, euphoria, increased cerebral blood flow and intracranial pressure, nausea, vomiting, ileus, hepatic dysfunction, MHT

Precautions and Contraindications
Desflurane is contraindicated in patients with known or suspected genetic susceptibility to MHT. Changes in mental function may persist beyond the period of anesthetic administration and the immediate postoperative period.

Anesthetic Considerations
Abrupt onset of MHT may be triggered by desflurane; early signs include muscle rigidity, especially in the jaw muscles, and tachycardia and tachypnea unresponsive to increased depth of anesthesia. It crosses the placental barrier.

DESMOPRESSIN (DDAVP)

Classification
Synthetic vasopressin analog

Indications
Treatment of neurogenic diabetes insipidus; nocturnal enuresis; and, in hemophilia A or von Willebrand disease, to increase factor VIII activity; reduction of perioperative blood loss after cardiac surgery

Dose
Preoperative: 30 minutes before the procedure. Diabetes insipidus: 2 to 4 mcg intravenously or subcutaneously daily in two divided doses; intranasal: 10 to 40 mcg (0.1-0.4 mL) in one to three doses.

Pediatrics: 3 months to 12 years: hemophilia A or von Willebrand disease: 0.3 mcg/kg intravenously, diluted in saline and infused over 15 to 30 minutes. In children who weigh more than 10 kg, use 50 mL of diluent, and in children who weigh less than 10 kg, use 10 mL of diluent. Repeated doses in less than 48 hours may increase the possibility of tachyphylaxis.

Intranasal: 0.05 to 0.3 mL daily in single or divided doses. Doses should start at 0.05 mL or less and be individualized because an extreme decrease in plasma osmolarity in very young patients may produce convulsions.

Dosage forms: injection: 4 mcg/mL; desmopressin acetate for injection should be stored at 4° C; nasal: 10 to 40 mcg; may be divided into three doses; supplied as 10 mcg/0.1 mL or 100 mcg/mL

Onset and Duration
Onset: intranasal: 1 hour; intravenous: 30 minutes. Duration: 8 to 20 hours. Elimination half-life: 3.6 hours.

Adverse Effects
Hypotension, hypertension, transient headache (with higher doses), psychosis, seizures, water retention, hyponatremia, abdominal cramps, nasal congestion, rhinitis, facial flushing, hypersensitivity reactions

Precautions and Contraindications
This agent is contraindicated in hypersensitivity to desmopressin acetate and in children younger than 3 months. Patients with type IIB von Willebrand disease should not receive desmopressin because platelet aggregation may be reduced. Owing to an increased risk of thrombosis, use it with caution in patients with coronary artery disease. Fluid intake should be decreased in those who do not need the antidiuretic effects of desmopressin. Seizure activity may be related to rapid decreases in serum sodium concentrations secondary to desmopressin. Avoid overhydration; postoperative abdominal cramping may occur.

Anesthetic Considerations
None

DEXAMETHASONE (DECADRON)

Classification
Long-acting corticosteroid

Indications
Croup, septic shock, cerebral edema, respiratory distress syndrome including status asthmaticus, acute exacerbations of chronic allergic disorders, corticosteroid-responsive bronchospastic states, allergic or inflammatory nasal conditions, and nasal polyps

Dose
Initial: 0.5 to 9 mg, intramuscularly or intravenously daily, depending on the disease being treated. In less severe diseases, doses lower than 0.5 mg intramuscularly or intravenously may suffice, but in others, doses higher than 9 mg may be required.

Cerebral edema: 10 mg intravenously initially followed by 4 mg intramuscularly every 6 hours. Reduce dose after 2 to 4 days, then taper over 5 to 7 days.

Corticosteroid-responsive bronchospastic states: Respihaler: three inhalations three to four times daily (maximum dose: 12 inhalations/day).

Nasal conditions: Turbinaire: two sprays each nostril two to three times daily (maximum dose: 12 sprays/day)

Children: intramuscular or by intravenous push: 6 to 40 mcg/kg or 0.235 to 1.25 mg/m^2 administered one or two times daily. Must be administered slowly over 3 to 5 minutes by intravenous push.

Dosage forms: Respihaler inhalation: 0.1 mg/spray dexamethasone phosphate; Turbinaire intranasal: 0.1 mg/spray; solution for injection: 4, 10, 24 mg/mL; tablets: 0.25, 0.5, 0.75, 1, 1.5, 2, 4, 6 mg

Onset and Duration
Onset: intravenous or intramuscular: within 10 to 30 minutes; inhalation: within 20 minutes. Elimination half-life: 200 minutes; however, metabolic effects at the tissue level persist for up to 72 hours.

Adverse Effects
Cushing syndrome, adrenal suppression, hyperglycemia, hyperthyroidism, hypercalcemia, peptic ulcer, gastrointestinal hemorrhage, increased intraocular pressure, glaucoma, irritability, psychosis, osteoporosis

Precautions and Contraindications
Dexamethasone is contraindicated in patients with peptic ulcer, osteoporosis, psychosis or psychoneurosis, acute bacterial infections, herpes zoster, herpes simplex ulceration of the eye, and other viral infections. Use it with caution in patients with diabetes mellitus, chronic renal failure, or infectious disease and in elderly patients. Corticosteroids may increase the risk of developing tuberculosis in patients with a positive purified protein derivative test. They may increase the risk of development of serious or fatal infection in persons exposed to viral illnesses such as chickenpox.

Anesthetic Considerations
Short-term administration of intravenous or inhalation steroids may be helpful in shock and asthma. Dexamethasone may have some benefit in anaphylaxis. Toxicity after acute dosing is minimal.

DEXMEDETOMIDINE (PRECEDEX)

Classification
Adrenergic agonist; sedative hypnotic

Indications
A selective α_2-receptor agonist with sedative properties for short-term sedation in critical care settings. Patients are commonly intubated and mechanically ventilated. Administered by continuous infusion not exceeding 24 hours. Off-label use as an anesthesia adjunct.

Dose
Dexmedetomidine HCl should be administered using a controlled infusion device.

Dexmedetomidine HCl dosing should be individualized and titrated to the desired clinical effect. For adult patients, dexmedetomidine HCl is generally initiated with a loading infusion of 1 mcg/kg over 10 minutes followed by a maintenance infusion of 0.2 to 0.7 mcg/kg/hr. The rate of the maintenance infusion should be adjusted to achieve the desired level of sedation. Dexmedetomidine is not indicated for infusions lasting longer than 24 hours.

Dexmedetomidine HCl has been continuously infused in mechanically ventilated patients before extubation, during extubation, and after extubation. It is not necessary to discontinue dexmedetomidine HCl before extubation provided the infusion does not exceed 24 hours.

Onset and Duration
Onset: 10 to 30 minutes, depending on the dose. Duration: 15 minutes to 4 hours, depending on the dose and duration of infusion

Adverse Effects
Hypotension, bradycardia, hypertension, nausea, vomiting, and fever are most frequently reported.

Precautions and Contraindications
Because of the known pharmacologic effects of dexmedetomidine, patients should be continuously monitored while receiving dexmedetomidine. Clinically significant episodes of bradycardia and sinus arrest have been associated with dexmedetomidine administration in young, healthy volunteers with high vagal tone or with different routes of administration, including rapid intravenous or bolus administration.

Anesthetic Considerations
Adjunct to general and regional anesthesia, bridge to intensive care unit sedation and analgesia, supplement to regional block when avoiding respiratory depression is desirable, awake craniotomy

DIAZEPAM (VALIUM)

Classification
Central nervous system agent; benzodiazepine; anticonvulsant and anxiolytic

Indications
Anxiety, alcohol withdrawal, status epilepticus, preoperative sedation, sedation for cardioversion; used adjunctively for relief of skeletal muscle spasm associated with cerebral palsy, paraplegia, athetosis, stiff man syndrome, tetanus

Dose
Status epilepticus: adults: intramuscular or intravenous: 5 to 10 mg; repeat if needed at 10- to 15-minute intervals up to 30 mg; repeat if

needed in 2 to 4 hours. Children: intramuscular or intravenous: younger than 5 years: 0.2 to 0.5 mg slowly 2 to 5 minutes, up to 5 mg total dose. Children older than 5 years: 1 mg slowly 2 to 5 minutes up to 10 mg; repeat if needed in 2 to 4 hours.

Anxiety, muscle spasm, convulsions, alcohol withdrawal. Adults: oral: 2 to 10 mg two to four times daily; intramuscular or intravenous: 2 to 10 mg; repeat if needed in 3 to 4 hours. Children: oral: older than 6 months: 1 to 2.5 mg two to three times daily.

Dosage forms: tablets: 2, 5, 10 mg; capsules (sustained release): 15 mg; oral solution: 5 mg/5 mL and 5 mg/mL; injection: 5 mg/mL

Onset and Duration

Onset: oral: 30 to 60 minutes; intramuscular: 15 to 30 minutes; intravenous: 1 to 5 minutes. Peak effect: 1 to 2 hours orally. Duration: intravenous: 15 minutes to 1 hour; oral: up to 3 hours. Elimination half-life: 20 to 50 hours; excreted primarily in urine. It is metabolized in liver to active metabolites.

Adverse Effects

Drowsiness, fatigue, ataxia, confusion, paradoxical dizziness, vertigo, amnesia, vivid dreams, headache, slurred speech, tremor, muscle weakness, electroencephalogram changes, tardive dyskinesia, hypotension, tachycardia, edema, cardiovascular collapse, blurred vision, diplopia, nystagmus, xerostomia, nausea, constipation, incontinence, urinary retention, changes in libido

Precautions and Contraindications

Diazepam is contraindicated in acute narrow-angle glaucoma, untreated open-angle glaucoma, and during or within 14 days of monoamine oxidase inhibitor therapy. Safe use during pregnancy (category D) and lactation has not been established.

Anesthetic Considerations

Diazepam reduces requirements for volatile anesthetics. A potential for thrombophlebitis exists with intravenous administration. Elderly patients have decreased clearance and dosage requirements. Its effects are antagonized by flumazenil. It may cause neonatal hypothermia.

DIGOXIN (LANOXIN)

Classification

Inotropic agent

Indications

Treatment of supraventricular arrhythmias, heart failure, atrial fibrillation, flutter

Dose

Adults: loading: intravenous or oral: 0.5 to 1 mg in divided doses (administer 50% of loading dose as first dose; then 25% fractions at 4- to 8-hour intervals until adequate therapeutic response is noted, toxic effects occur, or the total digitalizing dose has been administered). Monitor clinical response before each additional dose. Maintenance: intravenous or oral: 0.0625 to 0.25 mg; dosages should be individualized. Elderly patients (older than

65 years): oral: 0.125 mg or less daily as maintenance dose. Small patients may require less.

Children older than 2 years: loading: oral: 0.02 to 0.06 mg/kg divided every 8 hours for 24 hours; intravenous: 0.015 to 0.035 mg/kg divided every 8 hours for 24 hours; maintenance: oral: 25% to 35% of digitalizing dose daily, divided into two doses

Children 1 month to 2 years: loading: oral: 0.035 to 0.060 mg/kg in three divided doses over 24 hours; intravenous: 0.02 to 0.05 mg/kg; maintenance: oral: 25% to 35% of digitalizing dose daily divided every 12 hours

Neonates younger than 1 month: loading: oral: 0.025 to 0.035 mg/kg divided every 8 hours over 24 hours; intravenous: 0.015 to 0.025 mg/kg; maintenance: oral: 25% to 35% of digitalizing dose daily divided every 12 hours

Premature infants: loading: intravenous: 0.015 to 0.025 mg/kg in three divided doses over 24 hours. Maintenance: intravenous: 0.01 mg/kg daily divided every 12 hours.

Dosage forms: tablets: 0.125, 0.25, 0.5 mg; capsules (Lanoxicaps): 0.05, 0.1, 0.2 mg; oral solution: 0.05 mg/mL; injection: 0.1 mg/mL, 1-mL ampule (100 mcg); 0.25 mg/mL, 2-mL ampule (500 mcg)

Onset and Duration

Onset: intravenous: 5 to 30 minutes; oral: 30 minutes to 2 hours. Duration: intravenous or oral: 3 to 4 days.

Adverse Effects

Enhanced toxicity in hypokalemia, hypomagnesemia, hypercalcemia; wide range of arrhythmias, atrioventricular block, headache, psychosis, confusion, nausea, vomiting, ocular changes, diarrhea, gynecomastia

Overdosage may cause complete heart block, atrioventricular dissociation, tachycardia, and fibrillation.

Precautions and Contraindications

Digoxin is contraindicated in ventricular fibrillation.

Anesthetic Considerations

Decrease the dosage in patients with impaired renal function and in elderly patients. Monitor serum potassium, calcium, and digoxin levels. The use of synchronized cardioversion in patients with digitalis toxicity should be avoided because it may initiate ventricular fibrillation.

Digoxin interacts with numerous drugs. Increased serum levels are seen with calcium channel blockers (e.g., verapamil, diltiazem, nifedipine), esmolol, flecainide, captopril, quinidine, amiodarone, benzodiazepines, anticholinergics, oral aminoglycosides, and erythromycin. Succinylcholine may cause arrhythmias in digitalized patients. Additive bradycardia may occur with cardiac depressant anesthetics.

DILTIAZEM (CARDIZEM)

Classification

Calcium channel blocker

Indications

Angina pectoris; supraventricular tachycardia

Dose

Bolus intravenous: 0.25 mg/kg over 2 minutes. If needed, follow after 15 minutes with 0.35 mg/kg over 2 minutes. Maintenance infusion: 5 to 15 mg/hr. Adults: oral: 30 mg three or four times daily before meals and at bedtime. Dosage may be gradually increased to a maximum of 360 mg/day in divided doses. Sustained-release capsules: 90 mg; oral: twice daily, titrate dosage to effect (maximum dose: 360 mg/day).

Dosage forms: oral: 30, 60, 90, 120 mg; sustained release: 60, 90, 120, 180, 240, 300 mg; intravenous: 5 mg/mL, 5- and 10-mL vials

Onset and Duration

Onset: oral: 30 minutes; intravenous: 1 to 3 minutes. Elimination half-life: 3 to 5 hours. Duration: 4 to 6 hours.

Adverse Effects

Hypotension, flushing, atrioventricular block, constipation, pruritus, bradycardia, edema, nausea, vomiting, diarrhea, depression, headache, fatigue, dizziness

Precautions and Contraindications

Hypotension occurs with coadministration with digoxin, β-blockers, and cimetidine. Diltiazem potentiates the cardiovascular depressant effects of volatile, injectable anesthetic agents.

Anesthetic Considerations

Intravenous infusions of diltiazem are useful for intraoperative treatment of atrial tachyarrhythmias.

DIPHENHYDRAMINE (BENADRYL)

Classification

Histamine (H_1) antagonist, ethanolamine class

Indications

Adjuvant with epinephrine in the treatment of anaphylactic shock and severe allergic reactions; treatment of drug-induced extrapyramidal effects, motion sickness; antiemetic

Dose

Antihistamine or antiemetic: 10 to 50 mg intramuscularly or intravenously every 2 to 3 hours (maximum dose: 400 mg/day).

Recommend increasing the dosing interval to every 6 to 12 hours in patients with moderate renal failure (glomerular filtration rate, 10-50 mL/min).

Children: 1 to 2 mg/kg up to 150 mg/m^2/day in up to four divided doses by slow intravenous push (3 to 5 minutes)

Dosage forms: injection: 10 mg/mL, 50 mg/1 mL Steri-dose syringe or ampule; capsules: 25, 50 mg; elixir and syrup: 12.5 mg/15 mL

Onset and Duration

Onset: oral: 1 hour. Duration: 4 to 6 hours. Elimination half-life: 4 to 8 hours

Adverse Effects

Sedation (most frequent); dizziness, tinnitus, tremors, euphoria, blurred vision, nervousness, palpitations, hypotension, psychotic reactions, hypersensitivity

Other side effects are probably related to the antimuscarinic actions of diphenhydramine and include dry mouth, cough, and urinary retention.

Precautions and Contraindications

Diphenhydramine is contraindicated in patients with a hypersensitivity to it and other antihistamines of a similar chemical structure. Antihistamines are contraindicated in patients taking monoamine oxidase inhibitor therapy. Avoid in patients with narrow-angle glaucoma.

Anesthetic Considerations

Concurrent central nervous system depressants may produce an additive effect with diphenhydramine.

DOBUTAMINE HCL (DOBUTREX)

Classification

β_1-Adrenergic agonist

Indications

Vasopressor; positive inotrope

Dose

Infusion: 0.5 to 30 mcg/kg/min. Note: Must be diluted, and an intravenous pump (syringe pump in pediatric patients) must be used.

Onset and Duration

Onset: 1 to 2 minutes. Duration: less than 10 minutes

Adverse Effects

Hypertension, tachycardia, arrhythmias, angina, shortness of breath, headache, phlebitis at injection site

Precautions and Contraindications

Arrhythmias and hypertension occur at high dobutamine doses. Use it with caution in patients with idiopathic hypertrophic subaortic stenosis. Do not mix dobutamine with sodium bicarbonate, furosemide, or other alkaline solutions; correct hypovolemia before or during treatment.

Anesthetic Considerations

Dobutamine is useful for short-term intraoperative therapy for shock and congestive heart failure. Arterial line monitoring is highly recommended.

DOLASETRON (ANZEMET)

Classification

Antiemetic; select serotonin antagonist

Indications

Postoperative nausea and vomiting

Dose

12.5 mg (intravenous) 15 minutes before the cessation of anesthesia or 100 mg (oral) within 2 hours before surgery

Onset and Duration
Onset: 20 to 60 minutes. Duration: 4 to 9 hours

Adverse Effects
Headache, asthenia, somnolence, diarrhea, and constipation

Dolasetron can cause ECT interval changes (PR, QTc, JT prolongation, and QRS widening). These changes are related in magnitude and frequency to blood levels of the active metabolite. These changes are self-limiting with declining blood levels. Some patients have interval prolongations for 24 hours or longer. Interval prolongation could lead to cardiovascular consequences, including heart block or cardiac arrhythmias.

Precautions and Contraindications
Caution when using in patients with ischemic heart disease or arrhythmias.

Anesthetic Considerations
Monitor cardiovascular status, especially in patients with a history of coronary artery disease.

DOPAMINE HCL (INTROPIN)

Classification
Naturally occurring catecholamine

Indications
Vasopressor; positive inotrope

Dose
Infusion: 1 to 5 mcg/kg low dose; pressor dose range: 5 to 20 mcg/kg, greater than 20 mcg/kg for extreme cases. Note: Must be diluted, and an intravenous pump must be used.

Onset and Duration
Onset: 2 to 4 minutes. Duration: less than 10 minutes after termination of infusion

Adverse Effects
Nausea, vomiting, tachycardia, angina, arrhythmias, dyspnea, headache, anxiety

Precautions and Contraindications
Caution administering through a peripheral line; may see excessive tachycardia at higher doses.

Anesthetic Considerations
Avoid dopamine or use it at greatly reduced dose if the patient has received a monamine oxidase inhibitor. Infuse it into a large vein; extravasation may cause sloughing. Treat extravasation by local infiltration of phentolamine (≈1 mg in 10 mL normal saline). Correct hypovolemia as quickly as possible before or during dopamine treatment.

EDROPHONIUM CHLORIDE (TENSILON)

Classification
Anticholinesterase agent

Indications

Reversal of neuromuscular blockade; diagnostic assessment of myasthenia gravis, and supraventricular tachycardia

Dose

Reversal: slow intravenous: 0.5 to 1 mg/kg (maximum dose: 40 mg), with atropine (0.007-0.015 mg/kg), administered before the edrophonium

Assessment of myasthenia or cholinergic crisis: slow intravenous: 1 mg every 1 to 2 minutes until change in symptoms (maximum dose: 10 mg); intramuscular: 10 mg.

Onset and Duration

Onset: intravenous: 30 to 60 seconds; intramuscular: 2 to 10 minutes. Duration: intravenous: 20 to 40 minutes; intramuscular: 20 to 60 minutes.

Adverse Effects

Bradycardia, tachycardia, atrioventricular block, nodal rhythm, hypotension; increased oral, pharyngeal, bronchial secretions; bronchospasm; respiratory depression; seizures; dysarthria; headaches; lacrimation; miosis; visual changes; nausea; emesis; flatulence; increased peristalsis; rash; urticaria; allergic reactions; anaphylaxis

Precautions and Contraindications

Use edrophonium with caution in patients with bradycardia, bronchial asthma, cardiac arrhythmias, peptic ulcer, peritonitis, or mechanical obstruction of the intestines or urinary tract.

Overdosage may induce a cholinergic crisis characterized by nausea, vomiting, bradycardia or tachycardia, excessive salivation and sweating, bronchospasm, weakness, and paralysis. Treatment involves discontinuation of edrophonium and administration of atropine, 10 mcg/kg intravenously every 10 minutes until muscarinic symptoms disappear.

Owing to the brief duration of action of edrophonium, neostigmine or pyridostigmine is generally preferred for reversal of the effects of nondepolarizing muscle relaxants.

Anesthetic Considerations

Administer with an anticholinergic to avoid cholinergic side effects (e.g., bronchoconstriction, bradycardia). Edrophonium is not recommended when deep block is present.

EMLA (MIXTURE OF LIDOCAINE AND PRILOCAINE)

Classification

Local anesthetic

Indication

Topical local anesthesia

Dose

Adults: A thick layer of lidocaine–prilocaine cream is applied to intact skin and covered with an occlusive dressing, or alternatively, a lidocaine–prilocaine anesthetic disc is applied to intact skin:

- Minor dermal procedures: For minor procedures such as intravenous cannulation and venipuncture, apply 2.5 g of lidocaine–prilocaine cream, half the 5-g tube) over 20 to 25 cm^2 of skin surface or 1 lidocaine–prilocaine anesthetic disc (1 g over 10 cm^2) for at least 1 hour. In controlled clinical trials using lidocaine–prilocaine cream, two sites were usually prepared in case there was a technical problem with cannulation or venipuncture at the first site.

- Major dermal procedures: For more painful dermatologic procedures involving a larger skin area, such as split-thickness skin graft harvesting, apply 2 g of lidocaine–prilocaine cream per 10 cm^2 of skin and allow it to remain in contact with the skin for at least 2 hours.

Pediatrics: age up to 3 months or weighing less than 5 kg: 1 g over 10 cm^2 of skin for up to 1 hour maximum; age 3 months up to 12 months and weighing more than 5 kg: 2 g over 20 cm^2 of skin for up to 4 hours maximum; age 1 to 6 years and weighing more than 10 kg: 10 g over 100 cm^2 of skin for up to 4 hours maximum; age 7 to 12 years and weighing more than 20 kg: 20 g over 200 cm^2 of skin for up to 4 hours maximum

Onset and Duration

The onset, depth, and duration of dermal analgesia on intact skin provided by EMLA depend primarily on the duration of application. To provide sufficient analgesia for clinical procedures such as venipuncture, EMLA should be applied under an occlusive dressing for at least 1 hour. To provide dermal analgesia for clinical procedures such as split-thickness skin graft harvesting, EMLA should be applied under occlusive dressing for at least 2 hours. Satisfactory dermal analgesia is achieved 1 hour after application, peaks at 2 to 3 hours, and persists for 1 to 2 hours after removal. Absorption from the genital mucosa is more rapid and onset time is shorter (5-10 minutes) than after application to intact skin. After a 5- to 10-minute application of EMLA to female genital mucosa, the average duration of effective analgesia to an argon laser stimulus (which produces a sharp, pricking pain) is 15 to 20 minutes (with individual variations in the range of 5-45 minutes).

Adverse Effects

During or immediately after treatment with lidocaine or prilocaine on intact skin, possible erythema, edema, or abnormal sensation of skin at treatment site

Systemic adverse reactions after appropriate use of EMLA are unlikely because of the small dose absorbed.

Precautions and Contraindications

Application of EMLA to larger areas or for longer times than those recommended could result in sufficient absorption of lidocaine and prilocaine to result in serious adverse effects. EMLA is contraindicated in patients who exhibit allergies to amide local anesthetics. EMLA should be used with care in patients with conditions or therapy associated with methemoglobinemia.

Anesthetic Considerations

EMLA is generally safe. When EMLA is used, the patient should be aware that the production of dermal analgesia may be accompanied by the block of all sensations in the treated skin. For this reason, the patient should avoid inadvertent trauma to the treated area caused by scratching, rubbing, or exposure to extreme hot or cold temperatures until complete sensation has returned.

ENALAPRILAT (VASOTEC IV)

Classification
Angiotensin-converting enzyme (ACE) inhibitor

Indication
Hypertension

Dose
Intravenous: 0.625 to 1.25 mg over 5 minutes every 6 hours.
Dosage forms: 1.25 mg/mL, 1- and 2-mL vials

Onset and Duration
Onset: 10 to 15 minutes. Duration: approximately 6 hours

Adverse Effects
Cough, hypotension, renal impairment, angioedema

Precautions and Contraindications
Patients taking diuretics may have to adjust the dose while they are receiving ACE inhibitors. Enalaprilat is contraindicated during pregnancy.

Anesthetic Considerations
This is a useful addition to antihypertensive drug choices for perioperative use.

ENOXAPARIN (LOVENOX, LOW-MOLECULAR-WEIGHT HEPARIN)

Classification
Anticoagulant (antithrombotic), inhibiting factors Xa and IIa and only slightly affecting clotting times

Indications
Prevention of postoperative pulmonary embolism (PE) or deep venous thrombosis (DVT); reduction of ischemic complications in patients with cardiovascular disease who have unstable angina and non–Q-wave myocardial infarctions

Dose
Immediately after surgery: 30 mg or 40 mg subcutaneously every 12 hours to prevent DVT or PE; 1 mg/kg subcutaneously every 12 hours with 100 to 325 mg oral aspirin daily to treat patients with unstable angina or non–Q-wave myocardial infarction.

Onset and Duration
Onset: subcutaneous: 20 to 60 minutes. Peak effect: 3 to 5 hours. Duration: 12 hours. Elimination half-life: 3 to 4.5 hours.

Adverse Effects
Hemorrhage; epidural or subarachnoid or injection site hematomas; thrombocytopenia; increased aspartate aminotransferase; alanine aminotransferase; liver enzymes; chills, fever, urticaria

Precautions and Contraindications
Avoid intramuscular injections of enoxaparin. Use it with caution in pregnant patients and those with a history of coagulopathies or gastrointestinal

bleeding. Enoxaparin is absolutely contraindicated in patients with active bleeding, thrombocytopenia, a history of heparin-induced thrombocytopenia, and pork or heparin sensitivities.

Anesthetic Considerations

Central axis blocks or removal of indwelling catheters should not occur at least 12 hours before or after the last administration of enoxaparin or, conservatively, not within the previous 24 hours. Coagulation tests do not need to be routinely ordered while the patient is taking enoxaparin. However, if coagulation test results are abnormal or bleeding occurs, anti–factor Xa is the most sensitive test to indicate therapeutic anticoagulation levels. Treat an overdose with protamine sulfate. Each milligram of protamine will neutralize 1 mg of enoxaparin.

EPHEDRINE SULFATE

Classification

Noncatecholamine sympathomimetic with mixed direct and indirect actions as well as central nervous system effects

Indications

Hypotension, bradycardia

Dose

Intravenous: 5 to 25 mg (or 100-300 mcg/kg); intramuscular: 25 to 50 mg; oral: 25 to 50 mg every 3 hours

Onset and Duration

Onset: intravenous: almost immediate; intramuscular: a few minutes. Duration: intravenous: 10 to 60 minutes.

Adverse Effects

Hypertension, tachycardia, arrhythmias, pulmonary edema, anxiety, tremors, hyperglycemia, transient hyperkalemia and then hypokalemia, necrosis at the site of injection, possible tolerance

Precautions and Contraindications

Use ephedrine cautiously in patients with hypertension and ischemic heart disease. It has an unpredictable effect in patients in whom endogenous catecholamines are depleted; it may produce central nervous system stimulation.

Anesthetic Considerations

Ephedrine is associated with an increased risk of arrhythmias. It is potentiated by tricyclic antidepressants and monoamine oxidase inhibitors.

EPINEPHRINE HCL (ADRENALINE CHLORIDE)

Classification

Endogenous catecholamine

Indications

Inotropic support; treatment of anaphylaxis; to increase duration of action of local anesthetic; hemostasis; cardiac arrest; bronchodilation

Dose

Cardiac arrest: 0.5 to 1 mg intravenous bolus every 5 minutes as necessary. Inotropic support: 2 to 20 mcg/min (0.1-1 mcg/kg/min). Anaphylaxis: 100 to 300 mcg intravenous push, depending on severity.

Onset and Duration

Onset: intravenous: immediate. Duration: intravenous: 5 to 10 minutes

Adverse Effects

Restlessness, fear, throbbing headache, tachycardia, tachydysrhythmias, premature ventricular contractions, ventricular tachycardia, ventricular fibrillation, severe hypertension, angina, extension of myocardial infarction, pulmonary edema

Precautions and Contraindications

Use epinephrine with caution in patients with coronary artery disease, hypertension, diabetes mellitus, or hyperthyroidism and in patients taking monoamine oxidase inhibitors.

Anesthetic Considerations

Epinephrine may be administered through the endotracheal tube.

ESMOLOL (BREVIBLOC)

Classification

Cardioselective β-blocker

Indications

Supraventricular tachycardia (SVT); perioperative hypertension

Dose

SVT: loading: 50 to 200 mcg/kg/min for 1 minute; follow by infusion of 50 mcg/kg/min for 4 minutes. If the desired effect is not achieved, repeat loading dose and increase infusion to 100 mcg/kg/min. May repeat the process up to a maximum of 300 mcg/kg/min.

Dosage forms: 10 mg/mL in 10-mL vial for direct intravenous injection; 250 mg/mL in 10-mL ampule for intravenous infusion

Onset and Duration

Onset: 1 to 2 minutes. Duration: 10 to 20 minutes. Peak effect: 5 to 6 minutes. Do not infuse for more than 48 hours.

Adverse Effects

Hypotension, bradycardia, congestive heart failure, bronchospasm, confusion, depression, urinary retention, nausea and vomiting, rash

Precautions and Contraindications

Use esmolol with caution in patients with asthma; chronic obstructive pulmonary disease; atrioventricular heart block, or cardiac failure not caused by tachycardia; and diabetes.

Anesthetic Considerations

Esmolol may have additive cardiovascular depressant effects when it is coupled with volatile or intravenous anesthetic agents. Use it with caution in bronchospastic patients, owing to minimal cardioselectivity.

ETHACRYNIC ACID (EDECRIN)

Classification

Loop diuretic

Indications

Edema of cardiac, hepatic, or renal origin; hypertension, pulmonary edema; usually reserved for patients who do not respond to thiazide diuretics or in whom a rapid onset of diuresis is desired

Dose

0.5 to 1 mg/kg slowly over several minutes up to a maximum of 100 mg in a single dose. The usual average dose is 50 mg. Children: 1 mg/kg over 20 to 30 minutes.

Dosage forms: 50-mg vial, powder for injection; reconstitute by adding 50 mL D_5W or normal saline; tablets: 25, 50 mg

Onset and Duration

Onset: intravenous: 5 to 15 minutes. Duration: intravenous: 2 hours but may last 6 to 7 hours. Elimination half-life: 1 to 4 hours.

Adverse Effects

Fluid and electrolyte imbalance, including hypomagnesemia, hypocalcemia, hypokalemia, hypochloremia, metabolic alkalosis, hyperuricemia; hypoglycemia and hyperglycemia; thrombocytopenia; agranulocytopenia; vertigo; ototoxicity (associated with rapid intravenous injection); pancreatitis; gastrointestinal hemorrhage; hepatotoxicity; hypotension; diarrhea

Precautions and Contraindications

Avoid rapid intravenous injection of ethacrynic acid. Use it with extreme caution in patients with impaired renal or hepatic function. It is contraindicated for use in patients after anuric renal failure is established, as well as in patients with hypotension; dehydration with low serum sodium or metabolic alkalosis with hypokalemia; nursing mothers; infants; and patients with severe watery diarrhea.

Anesthetic Considerations

Loop diuretics have been reported to increase the neuromuscular blocking effect of nondepolarizing relaxants, possibly because of their potassium-depleting effects.

ETOMIDATE (AMIDATE)

Classification

Central nervous system agent; nonbarbiturate hypnotic without analgesic activity

Indication

Induction of general anesthesia

Dose

Adult: intravenous: 0.2 to 0.3 mg/kg over 30 to 60 seconds.

Dosage forms: injection: 2 mg/mL, ampules and prefilled syringe.

Onset and Duration

Onset: 1 minute. Duration: 3 to 10 minutes. Metabolized in the liver. Half-life: 75 minutes; excreted primarily in the urine.

Adverse Effects
Myoclonus, tonic movements, eye movements, hypertension, hypotension, tachycardia, bradycardia, other arrhythmias, postoperative nausea and vomiting, hypoventilation, hyperventilation, transient apnea, laryngospasm, hiccups, snoring, adrenocortical suppression

Precautions and Contraindications
Use etomidate cautiously in immunosuppressed patients. Its safety during pregnancy, in nursing women, and in children younger than 4 years has not been established.

Anesthetic Considerations
Use etomidate with caution in patients with steroid deficiency. Use the large veins. Myoclonus is reduced by premedication with a benzodiazepine or an opioid.

FAMOTIDINE (PEPCID)

Classification
Histamine (H_2) antagonist

Indications
Treatment of duodenal or gastric ulcers and gastroesophageal reflux; prophylaxis of aspiration pneumonitis in patients at high risk during surgery

Dose
Prophylaxis of aspiration pneumonitis: adults: 20 to 40 mg orally the evening before surgery or the morning of surgery before induction of anesthesia (or both the evening before and the morning of surgery). If a more rapid onset is desired, 2 mL of intravenous famotidine (10 mg/mL) may be diluted to a concentration of 5 to 10 mL with D_5W, normal saline, or lactated Ringer's solution and administered over at least 2 minutes before induction.

Dosage forms: tablets: 20, 40 mg; parenteral injection: 10 mg/mL in 2- or 4-mL vials

Onset and Duration
Onset: 20 to 45 minutes. Peak effect: 1 to 3 hours orally. Duration: Plasma famotidine concentrations that suppress gastric acid secretion by 50% are maintained for 12 hours after an oral dose of 40 mg and 7 to 9 hours after a 20-mg dose.

Adverse Effects
Headache (2%-4.5%), constipation (1.4%), and drowsiness (most frequently reported); mental confusion in elderly patients (occasionally)

Potential bradydysrhythmias and hypotension may be associated with rapid infusion.

Precautions and Contraindications
Caution suggested in patients with hepatic or renal dysfunction (possible dose reductions required). This drug is contraindicated in patients with known hypersensitivity to famotidine or other H_2 antagonists.

Anesthetic Considerations

Famotidine is a safe alternative to gastric prophylaxis preoperatively.

FENOLDOPAM (CORLOPAM)

Classification

Antihypertensive (dopamine DA-1-receptor agonist)

Indications

A potent vasodilator that stimulates the postsynaptic dopamine DA receptors, thereby lowering blood pressure, peripheral vascular resistance, and renal vascular resistance and increasing cardiac hemodynamics; short-term use (up to 48 hours) for patients with severe hypertension or malignant hypertension

Dose

Administer fenoldopam as a continuous infusion; no loading dose is needed. The infusion range is 0.04 to 0.8 mcg/kg/min; titrate slowly for blood pressure reduction. Initial doses less than 0.1 mcg/kg/min are marginally antihypertensive but have less reflex tachycardia. Initial doses higher than 0.3 mcg/kg/min have been associated with reflex tachycardia.

Onset and Duration

Onset: 5 minutes. Peak effect: 15 minutes. Rapidly metabolized. Half-life: 5 minutes.

Adverse Effects

Reflex tachycardia with a higher initial dosing regimen possibly causing increased intraocular pressure, hypotension, hypokalemia (infusion time greater than 6 hours can cause potassium to fall to less than 3 mEq), headache, flushing, nausea

Precautions and Contraindications

Fenoldopam has no absolute contraindications. Use it with caution in patients with severe hepatic disease. It contains a metabisulfite compound, so do not use this drug in patients sensitive to sulfites (especially patients with asthma) because allergic reaction may result. The concomitant use of other antihypertensive agents (calcium channel blockers, nitrates, β_1-blockers, and α_2-blockers) may result in unexpected hypotension.

Anesthetic Considerations

Titrate the drug slowly to prevent reflex tachycardia. Check the patient's potassium level if titrating a long-term infusion (greater than 6 hours). Review for sulfite allergies, especially in patients with asthma. Use with caution in patients with open globe injuries or glaucoma because fenoldopam may increase intraocular pressure. It is generally used as an alternative to nitroprusside.

FENTANYL (SUBLIMAZE, DURAGESIC, ORALET)

Classification

Opioid agonist

Indications

Analgesia and anesthesia

Dose

Analgesia: intravenous: 1 to 2 mcg/kg

Induction: 30 mcg/kg; infusion: 0.2 mcg/kg/min. Epidural bolus: 1 to 2 mcg/kg; infusion: 2 to 60 mcg/hr. Spinal bolus: 0.1 to 0.4 mcg/kg. Dosage forms: injection: 0.05 mg/mL; transdermal patch: 100 mcg/hr. In conjunction with epidural administration: 1 to 2 mcg/kg. For infusion with epidural: 2 to 60 mcg/hr. In conjunction with spinal anesthesia: bolus dose of 0.1 to 0.4 mcg/kg.

Onset and Duration

Onset: intravenous: within 30 seconds; intramuscular: less than 8 minutes; epidural or spinal: 4 to 10 minutes. Duration: intravenous: 30 to 60 minutes; intramuscular: 1 to 2 hours; epidural or spinal; 4 to 8 hours.

Adverse Effects

Hypotension, bradycardia, respiratory depression, apnea, dizziness, blurred vision, seizures, nausea, emesis, delayed gastric emptying, biliary tract spasm, muscle rigidity

Precautions and Contraindications

Reduce fentanyl doses in elderly, hypovolemic, or high-risk surgical patients and with concomitant use of sedatives and other narcotics. It crosses the placental barrier and may produce depression of respiration in neonates. Prolonged depression may occur after cessation of transdermal patch use.

Anesthetic Considerations

Narcotic effects reversed by naloxone (0.2-0.4 mg intravenously). Circulatory and ventilatory depressant effects are potentiated by narcotics, sedatives, volatile anesthetics, nitrous oxide, and possibly monoamine oxidase inhibitors, phenothiazines, and tricyclic antidepressants; analgesia is enhanced by α_2-agonists. Muscle rigidity in higher dose range sufficient to interfere with ventilation.

FLUMAZENIL (ROMAZICON)

Classification

Benzodiazepine-receptor antagonist

Indication

Reversal of benzodiazepine-receptor agonist

Dose

Intravenous: 0.2 to 1 mg (4-20 mcg/kg); titrate to patient response; may repeat at 20-minute intervals (maximum single dose: 1 mg; maximum total dose: 3 mg in any 1 hour)

Dosage forms: injection: 0.1 mg/mL

Onset and Duration

Onset: 1 to 2 minutes. Duration: 30 to 90 minutes, depending on the dose of flumazenil and plasma concentration of benzodiazepine to be reversed.

Adverse Effects

Arrhythmia, tachycardia, bradycardia, hypertension, angina, flushing, reversal of sedation, seizures, agitation, emotional lability, nausea and vomiting, pain at injection site, thrombophlebitis

Precautions and Contraindications

Institute measures to secure airway, ventilation, and intravenous access before administering flumazenil. Resedation may occur and is more common with large doses of long-acting benzodiazepines.

Anesthetic Considerations

Do not use flumazenil until the effects of neuromuscular blockade have been fully reversed. Administer it in a large vein to minimize pain at the injection site. Monitor the patient for resedation.

FOSPROPOFOL (LUSEDRA)

Classification

Hypnotic sedative

Indications

Intravenous sedation

Dose

Loading dose: 6.5 mg/kg; initial dose not to exceed 16.5 mL
Maintenance dose: 1.6 mg/kg not to exceed 4 mL
Dosage forms: 35 mg/mL; 30 mL vial

Onset and Duration

Onset: 4 to 12 minutes. Duration: 21 to 45 minutes

Adverse Effects

Perineal paresthesias, pruritus, hypotension, apnea

Precautions and Contraindications

Dose should be reduced in patients older than 65 years of age and those with significant systemic disease. Continuous monitoring by qualified providers is mandatory.

Anesthetic Considerations

Fospropofol is a water-soluble prodrug of propofol. Upon administration, liver metabolism releases the active propofol. Proper airway equipment must be immediately available. Useful for sedation during nonoperating room procedures.

FUROSEMIDE (LASIX)

Classification

Loop diuretic

Indications

Edema of cardiac, hepatic, or renal origin; hypertension; pulmonary and cerebral edema; usually reserved for patients who do not respond to thiazide diuretics or in whom a rapid onset of diuresis is desired

Dose

Diuresis: adult: 20 to 40 mg intramuscularly or intravenously as a single dose. Intravenous doses should be injected slowly over 1 to 2 minutes. Additional doses of 20 mg greater than the previous dose may be administered every 2 hours until desired response is obtained. For intravenous bolus injections, do not exceed 1 g/day administered over 30 minutes. Acute pulmonary edema: 40 mg intravenously initially; may repeat in 1 hour with 80 mg if necessary. Children: intramuscular or intravenous: 1 mg/kg single dose initially, increasing by 1 mg/kg every 2 hours or more until desired response is obtained or to a maximum of 6 mg/kg/day.

Dosage forms: tablets: 20, 40, 80 mg; injection: 10 mg/mL; oral solutions: 10 mg/mL and 40 mg/5 mL.

Onset and Duration

Onset: intravenous: onset of diuresis usually occurs in 5 minutes. Duration: 2 hours. Elimination half-life: widely variable; normal is 0.5 to 1 hour, but a period of 11 to 20 hours has been reported in patients with hepatic or renal insufficiency.

Adverse Effects

Dehydration, hypotension, hypochloremic alkalosis, hypokalemia, hypomagnesemia, hyperglycemia, hyperuricemia

Ototoxicity has been reported with too rapid intravenous injection of large doses. Rarely reported are thrombocytopenia, neutropenia, jaundice, pancreatitis, and a variety of skin reactions.

Precautions and Contraindications

Furosemide is contraindicated in anuria (except for a single dose in acute anuria) and pregnancy. Use it with caution in patients with severe or progressive renal disease and hepatic disease. Discontinue it if renal function worsens. Use caution in patients who are allergic to sulfonamides and patients with severe electrolyte imbalance.

Anesthetic Considerations

Monitor electrolytes and fluid balance. Administer furosemide carefully in patients taking digitalis. It may be associated with enhancement of nondepolarizing neuromuscular blocking drugs.

GLUCAGON

Classification

Hormone; antidiabetic agent (antihypoglycemic); diagnostic agent

Indications

Treatment of hypoglycemia or β-blocker overdose; inotropic agent used to relax smooth muscle of gastrointestinal tract for radiologic studies; anaphylaxis resistant to epinephrine

Dose

Diagnostic aid for radiologic examination: intravenous or intramuscular: 0.25 to 2 mg before initiation of radiologic procedure. Hypoglycemia: intravenous, intramuscular, or subcutaneous: 0.5 to 1 mg.

Onset and Duration

Onset: less than 5 minutes. Peak effect: 5 to 20 minutes. Duration: 10 to 30 minutes

Adverse Effects

Hypertension, hypotension, respiratory distress, dizziness, lightheadedness, nausea and vomiting, urticaria, hypoglycemia, hyperglycemia

Precautions and Contraindications

Glucagon is contraindicated in patients with a hypersensitivity to the drug (owing to its protein nature). Use it cautiously in patients with history of insulinoma or pheochromocytoma. Safe use during pregnancy and in nursing women has not been established.

Anesthetic Considerations

Rapid intravenous administration may cause a decrease in blood pressure. It potentiates the hypoprothrombinemic effects of anticoagulants. Parenteral glucose must be administered because release of insulin may subsequently cause hypoglycemia.

GLYCOPYRROLATE (ROBINUL)

Classification

Competitive acetylcholine antagonist at muscarinic receptor

Indications

Vagolytic premedication to block bradycardia from stimulation of the carotid sinus or traction on abdominal viscera or extraocular muscles during surgery; blockade of muscarinic effects of anticholinesterases; adjunctive therapy in the treatment of bronchospasm and peptic ulcer disease

Compared with atropine, glycopyrrolate has twice the potent antisialagogue activity, less tachycardia, and no clinically significant increases in intraocular pressure at doses used preoperatively. It has no sedative effects.

Dose

Adults: Premedication or vagolysis: intravenous, intramuscular, subcutaneous: 0.1 to 2 mg (4-6 mcg/kg) administered 30 to 60 minutes preinduction; may repeat in 2- to 3-minute intervals for vagolysis up to 1 mg total. Blockade of muscarinic effects of anticholinesterase: 0.2 mg for each 1 mg of neostigmine or 5 mg of pyridostigmine. Bronchospasm: inhalation 0.4 to 0.8 mg every 8 hours; dilute injectate solution in 2 to 3 mL normal saline and deliver by compressed air nebulizer.

Children: preoperative 2 years or older: 4 mcg/kg. For oral administration, use injectable solution and dilute in 3 to 5 mL juice or carbonated cola beverage. Oral absorption is erratic. Intraoperative vagolysis: 0.01 mg/kg intravenously not to exceed 0.1 mg; may repeat in 2 to 3 minutes.

Dosage forms: injection: 0.2 mg/mL; tablets: 1, 2 mg

Onset and Duration

Onset: oral: 1 hour; intramuscular or subcutaneous: 15 to 30 minutes; inhalation: 3 to 5 minutes; intravenous administration: less than 1 minute. Duration: antisialagogue effect: 7 to 12 hours, depending on the route of administration and dose; vagal blockade: 2 to 3 hours intravenously, 8 to 12 hours orally.

Adverse Effects

Tachycardia (high doses), headache, urinary hesitancy, retention, decreased sweating, dry nose and mouth, constipation

Precautions and Contraindications

Avoid glycopyrrolate when tachycardia would be harmful (i.e., thyrotoxicosis, pheochromocytoma, coronary artery disease). Avoid it in hyperpyrexial states because it inhibits sweating. Use it with caution in patients with hepatic or renal disease, congestive heart failure, chronic pulmonary disease (because a reduction in bronchial secretions may lead to formation of bronchial plugs), hiatal hernia, gastroesophageal reflux, gastrointestinal infections, and ulcerative colitis. It is contraindicated in acute-angle glaucoma, obstructive disease of the gastrointestinal tract, obstructive uropathy, paralytic ileus, intestinal atony, and acute hemorrhage in patients whose cardiovascular status is unstable.

Anesthetic Considerations

Additive anticholinergic effects may occur with meperidine, some antihistamines, phenothiazines, tricyclic antidepressants, and antiarrhythmic drugs that possess anticholinergic activity (e.g., quinidine, disopyramide, procainamide). It is the preferred agent in pregnant patients over atropine and scopolamine because it does not cross the placental barrier.

GRANISETRON (KYTRIL)

Classification

Selective serotonin receptor antagonist

Indications

Effective single agent used to control nausea and vomiting induced by cisplatin and other cytotoxic agents and for postoperative nausea and vomiting

Dose

The recommended dosage for prevention of postoperative nausea and vomiting is 1 mg.

Onset and Duration

Onset: peak plasma concentrations demonstrate wide interindividual variation. After a 40-mcg/kg dose, nausea and vomiting subside within several minutes. Duration: serum levels decline to less than 10 ng/mL at 24 hours after a single 40-mcg/kg infusion. Antiemetic effects last up to 24 hours after intravenous infusion of 40 mcg/kg.

Adverse Effects

Headache and constipation (most common); also somnolence, dizziness, diarrhea, flushing, transient elevation of liver enzymes

Precautions and Contraindications

Previous hypersensitivity to granisetron or ondansetron, liver disease (owing to the noted elevation of liver enzymes after repeat administration of granisetron), pregnancy, and breastfeeding are contraindications.

Anesthetic Considerations

The injection should not be mixed in solution with other drugs. No specific antidote for overdose exists; give symptomatic treatment. Inducers or inhibitors of cytochrome P450 drug-metabolizing enzymes may change the clearance and duration of granisetron.

HEPARIN

Classification

Anticoagulant; accelerates the rate at which antithrombin III neutralizes thrombin and factors VII, IX, X, and XI

Indications

Prophylaxis and treatment of deep venous thrombosis (DVT) and pulmonary thromboembolism (PE); acute arterial occlusion, intracardiac mural thrombosis, after myocardial infarction after intravenous thrombolytic treatment, disseminated intravascular coagulation with gross thrombosis, anticoagulation during cardiopulmonary bypass (CPB), prophylaxis of thromboembolism in patients with mitral valve disease or atrial fibrillation; maintenance of patency of indwelling venipuncture devices (lock flush)

The value of this drug in transient ischemic attacks secondary to cerebral embolism has not been established.

Dose

Dosage is highly individualized and based on daily activated partial thromboplastin time (aPTT) compared with aPTT 6 hours after each dosage change. Obtain baseline aPTT and adjust the dose according to clinical state. For prophylaxis (i.e., hip surgery, atrial fibrillation, valve disease): the ratio of aPTT to baseline aPTT should be 1.2 to 1.5; for prosthetic heart valves, DVT, PE, recurrent embolism: 1.5 to 2. For CPB, monitor the activated clotting time (ACT) and maintain an ACT of 400 to 480 seconds. Baseline ACT values are 80 to 150 seconds. ACT should be determined 5 minutes after heparin administration. Adequate heparinization must be ensured before initiation of CPB.

CPB: before induction of anesthesia, 300 units/kg should be prepared in case emergency initiation of CPB is necessary. Intravenous bolus: 350 to 400 units/kg. Up to 500 units/kg may be required to maintain ACT greater than 400 seconds in heparin-resistant patients. Additional heparin is needed for prolonged CPB. A 100 unit/kg hourly reinforcement dose is administered starting 2 hours after the initial dose.

Prophylactic or low-dose subcutaneous therapy: 5000 units subcutaneously every 8 to 12 hours. Baseline aPTT is obtained because bleeding complications are occasionally discovered, but routine aPTT monitoring is not necessary. For surgical prophylaxis, ideally started 2 hours preoperatively.

Full-dose continuous intravenous infusion for treatment of DVT or PE is based on ideal body weight: intravenous bolus loading dose: 70 units/kg (3000-10,000 units); intravenous maintenance dose: continuous infusion 13 to 16 units/kg/hr (750-1300 units/hr). For continuous intravenous infusion, 25,000 units heparin may be mixed in 500 mL D_5W or normal saline. The resulting solution is 50 units/mL.

Dosage forms: injection: 1000, 2500, 5000, 7500, 10,000, 20,000, and 40,000 units/mL; lock flush solution: 10 units, 100 units/mL; premixed infusion in dextrose: 50 units/mL; premixed infusion in normal saline: 50 units, 100 units/mL

Onset and Duration

Onset: intravenous: immediate; subcutaneous: 20 to 30 minutes. Elimination half-life: 1 to 2 hours in healthy adults. Duration: half-life and duration increase with increasing doses; prolonged in liver and renal disease.

Adverse Effects

Hemorrhage, thrombocytopenia, white-clot syndrome (rare paradoxical thrombosis), necrotizing skin lesions, elevated liver enzymes, osteoporosis, priapism, hypersensitivity

Precautions and Contraindications

Avoid intramuscular injections of heparin. It is contraindicated in patients with hemophilia; thrombocytopenia; acute bleeding; peptic ulcer; esophagitis; diverticulitis; esophageal varices; arterial aneurysm; gastrointestinal or urinary tract malignancy; vascular retinopathy; recent liver or renal biopsy; acute pericarditis; threatened abortion; infective endocarditis; recent regional anesthesia; severe hypertension; recent cerebrovascular accident; recent surgery; or trauma to the brain, eye, or spinal cord.

Platelet counts, hematocrit, and occult blood in stool and urine should be monitored during the entire course of therapy. An increased risk of bleeding exists with the concomitant use of aspirin, nonsteroidal anti-inflammatory drugs, dipyridamole, thrombolytic agents, dextran, dihydroergotamine, and warfarin. Intravenous nitroglycerin may antagonize the effects of heparin and should be administered via a separate line if possible. Digoxin, nicotine, propranolol, antihistamines, and tetracycline may reduce heparin's effects.

Bleeding and heparin overdosage may be treated with protamine sulfate; 1 mg protamine neutralizes 100 units heparin.

Anesthetic Considerations

Regional anesthesia is contraindicated. A heparin continuous intravenous infusion should be discontinued 4 to 6 hours preoperatively, and the aPTT should be checked to ensure return to baseline.

HETASTARCH (HESPAN)

Classification

Plasma expander, anticoagulant

Indications

Adjunct for plasma volume expansion in shock resulting from hemorrhage, burns, sepsis, surgery, or other trauma; mild anticoagulant effects after vascular procedures

Dose

Plasma volume expansion from 500 to 1000 mL. Total dosage does not usually exceed 1500 mL/day (20 mL/kg/day). In acute hemorrhagic shock, rates approaching 20 mL/kg/hr have been used.

Dosage forms: 6% solution in 0.9% sodium chloride, 500-mL intravenous infusion bottle

Onset and Duration

Onset: 15 to 30 minutes. Duration: 24 to 48 hours. Average half-life: 17 days

Adverse Effects

Anaphylactic reactions (periorbital edema, urticaria, wheezing); peripheral edema of the lower extremities; chills; mild temperature elevation; muscle pain

Large volumes may alter coagulation times and may result in transient prolongation of prothrombin time, partial thromboplastin time, and bleeding; decreased hematocrit; and excessive dilution of plasma proteins.

Precautions and Contraindications
Hetastarch is contraindicated in patients with severe bleeding disorders, severe cardiac failure, and renal failure with oliguria or anuria. Hetastarch does not have oxygen-carrying capacity, nor does it contain plasma proteins such as coagulation factors. Therefore, it is not a substitute for blood or plasma.

Anesthetic Considerations
Infuse it slowly to avoid volume overload. Check the patient's coagulation profile.

HYALURONIDASE (VITRASE AND OTHERS)

Classification
Enzyme

Indications
Adjunct to increase absorption and dispersion of other injected drugs such as local anesthetics; hypodermoclysis; subcutaneous urography

Dose
Adjunct: 150 units to injection medium containing other medication. Hypodermoclysis (adults and children older than 3 years): 150 units injected subcutaneously before clysis or injected into clysis tubing near needle for each 1000-mL clysis solution. Subcutaneous urography (patient prone): 75 units subcutaneously over each scapula followed by injection of contrast medium at the same sites.

Onset and Duration
Onset: immediate. Duration: 30 to 60 minutes

Adverse Effects
Rash, urticaria, local irritation

Precautions and Contraindications
Use hyaluronidase with caution in patients with blood-clotting abnormalities or severe hepatic or renal disease. Avoid injecting it into diseased areas to prevent spread of infection.

Anesthetic Considerations
It is useful to prevent thrombus formation during vascular procedures as well as for volume expansion. It is also a useful addition for promoting the spread of local anesthetics.

HYDRALAZINE (APRESOLINE)

Classification
Direct-acting arterial vasodilator

Indications
Antihypertensive; vasodilator

Dose
Intravenous and intramuscular: 2.5 to 40 mg (0.1-0.2 mg/kg); oral: 10 to 100 mg four times daily

Dosage forms: injection: 20 mg/mL; tablets: 10, 25, 50, and 100 mg

Onset and Duration

Onset: intravenous: 5 to 20 minutes; intramuscular: 10 to 30 minutes; oral: 30 to 120 minutes. Duration: intravenous: 2 to 4 hours; intramuscular or oral: 2 to 8 hours.

Adverse Effects

Hypotension, paradoxical pressor response, tachycardia, palpitations, angina, dyspnea, nasal congestion, peripheral neuritis, depression, anxiety, headache, dizziness, nausea and vomiting, diarrhea, lupuslike syndrome, rash, urticaria, eosinophilia, hypersensitivity, leukopenia, splenomegaly, agranulocytosis

Precautions and Contraindications

Use hydralazine cautiously in patients with coronary artery disease and mitral valvular rheumatic heart disease, as well as in patients receiving monoamine oxidase inhibitors.

Anesthetic Considerations

One may see a reduced response to epinephrine. Enhanced hypotensive effects occur in patients receiving diuretics, monoamine oxidase inhibitors, diazoxide, and other antihypertensives. It primarily dilates the arterial vasculature.

HYDROCORTISONE SODIUM SUCCINATE (A-HYDROCORT, SOLU-CORTEF)

Classification

Corticosteroid (glucocorticoid and mineralocorticoid properties)

Indications

Treatment of choice for steroid-replacement therapy; also anti-inflammatory and immunosuppressive agent, although glucocorticoids (prednisone) are preferred for this use; adjunctive therapy in anaphylaxis to prevent prolonged antigen-antibody reactions; adjunctive treatment of ulcerative colitis (enema)

Dose

Adults: shock: 500 mg to 2 g (succinate) intravenously every 2 to 6 hours until the condition is stabilized. Not recommended beyond 48 to 72 hours. Adjunctive therapy in anaphylaxis: hydrocortisone phosphate or succinate intravenously 5 mg/kg initially; then 2.5 mg/kg every 6 hours. Adrenal insufficiency: acute, precipitated by trauma or surgical stress: If adrenocorticotropic hormone testing is not being performed, 200 to 300 mg intravenous hydrocortisone succinate over several minutes; then 100 mg intravenously every 6 hours for 24 hours. If the patient is stable, dosage tapering may begin on the second day. Consider steroid replacement in any patient who has received corticosteroid therapy for at least 1 month in the past 6 to 12 months, with 50 to 100 mg intravenously (succinate) before, during, and after surgery. For intraarticular, soft tissue, and intrasynovial injections, use acetate only (acetate is not for intravenous use): 10 to 50 mg combined with local anesthetic such as procaine. Injections may be repeated every 3 to 5 days (for bursae) to once every 1 to 4 weeks (for joints).

Children: 0.16 to 1 mg/kg or 6 to 30 mg/m^2 (phosphate or succinate) intramuscularly or intravenously one or two times daily. The dose depends on the disease being treated.

Onset and Duration

Onset: intravenous or intramuscular: 5 minutes. Duration: approximates the duration of hypothalamus-pituitary-adrenal axis suppression (i.e., 30-36 hours); after a single oral dose of hydrocortisone, this is 1.25 to 1.5 days.

Adverse Effects

Glaucoma and cataracts (long-term therapy); muscle weakness, sodium retention, edema, hypokalemic alkalosis, hyperglycemia, Cushing syndrome, peptic ulcer, increased appetite, delayed wound healing, psychotic behavior, congestive heart failure, hypertension, growth suppression, pancreatitis

Acute adrenal insufficiency may occur with abrupt withdrawal after long-term therapy. Withdrawal symptoms include rebound inflammation, fatigue, weakness, arthralgia, fever, dizziness, lethargy, depression, orthostatic hypotension, dyspnea, anorexia, and hypoglycemia.

Precautions and Contraindications

Hydrocortisone is contraindicated in patients with systemic fungal infections. It may mask or exacerbate infections. Use it with caution in patients with ocular herpes simplex or a history of peptic ulcer disease. In patients with myasthenia gravis, hydrocortisone interacts with anticholinesterase agents to produce severe weakness.

Anesthetic Considerations

Hypotension from the stress of anesthesia and surgery may occur if regular doses of steroids were taken within 2 months preceding surgery. Supplemental steroids are indicated commencing with preoperative dose and continuing for 3 days for major surgery, for 24 hours for minor surgery, and one dose for a very brief procedure and then tapered to normal therapy.

Because of adrenal suppression, etomidate should be avoided in patients with adrenal insufficiency.

IBUPROFEN (CALDOLOR)

Classification

Non-narcotic analgesic, antipyretic, nonsteroidal anti-inflammatory drug (NSAID)

Indications

Non-narcotic analgesic for treatment of mild to moderate pain

Dose

400 to 800 mg intravenous every 6 hours; 3200 mg maximum per day

Infuse over 30 minutes. Dilute the 400-mg vial in 100 mL; Dilute the 800-mg vial in 200 mL.

Onset and Duration

Onset: 5 to 15 minutes; duration 4 to 6 hours

Adverse Effects

Dizziness with higher doses. Ibuprofen inhibits platelet function and increases bleeding time, but no increase in bleeding was reported in clinical trials. NSAIDs are contraindicated in patients undergoing coronary artery bypass surgery. Extended use may produce gastrointestinal and renal toxicity. Some orthopedic surgeons have been reluctant to use ibuprofen postoperatively because of reports that it may interfere with bone healing.

Precautions and Contraindications

Contraindicated in aspirin-allergic patients with asthma

Anesthetic Considerations

Ibuprofen decreases pain and reduces fever in adults. It has an opioid-sparing effect. It is effective for mild to moderate pain.

IBUTILIDE FUMARATE (CORVERT)

Classification

Class III antiarrhythmic; cardiac action potential prolongation

Indications

Rapid conversion of atrial fibrillation or flutter of acute onset (less than 90 days) to sinus rhythm

Dose

Adults weighing more than 60 kg: 1 vial (1 mg) infused over 10 minutes (may be repeated once in 10 minutes after completion of first dose). Adults weighing less than 60 kg: 0.01 mL/kg infused over 10 minutes (may be repeated once in 10 minutes after completion of first dose). Not recommended for pediatric patients.

Onset and Duration

Onset: intravenous: immediate for antiarrhythmic properties. Peak effect: 10 minutes. Half-life: 6 hours. Atrial arrhythmias usually convert within 30 minutes after ibutilide therapy begins. Duration: 10 to 30 minutes.

Adverse Effects

Ventricular arrhythmias (often sustained torsades de pointes), heart block, congestive heart failure, bradycardia, tachycardia, hypotension, nausea, headache

Precautions and Contraindications

The drug is contraindicated in patients sensitive to ibutilide, those with second- or third-degree atrioventricular heart blocks or prolonged Q-T interval, and during pregnancy.

Anesthetic Considerations

The risk of proarrhythmias or polymorphic ventricular tachycardia is increased when ibutilide is used with other drugs that prolong the Q-T interval (phenothiazines, procainamide, quinidine, antihistamines). Electrocardiographic monitoring for 4 hours after drug therapy is mandatory because arrhythmias (premature ventricular contractions, ventricular tachycardia, tachycardia, bradycardia, varying degrees of heart blocks) can take place. Have emergency equipment available to perform overdrive pacing, defibrillate, or cardiovert the patient. Monitor serum potassium and magnesium because deficiencies in these electrolytes can precipitate polymorphic ventricular tachycardia.

INSULIN REGULAR (RAPID-ACTING) (HUMULIN R, NOVOLIN R, REGULAR ILETIN II)

Classification
Antidiabetic agent

Blood Glucose (mg/dL)	Insulin Regular
Less than	0 units
200-250	5 units subcut
250-300	10 units subcut
300-350	15 units subcut

Subcut, Subcutaneous.

Indications
Diabetic ketoacidosis, treatment of diabetes mellitus, hyperkalemia

Dose
Diabetes mellitus: in general, therapy is initiated with regular insulin, subcutaneously 5 to 10 units in adults and 2 to 4 units in children 15 to 30 minutes before meals and at bedtime. The dose and frequency are carefully individualized based on blood glucose monitoring every 4 to 6 hours. After satisfactory control is achieved, an intermediate form of insulin may be substituted; this is administered before breakfast in a dose approximately two-thirds to three-fourths that of the previous total daily dose established for regular insulin. Treatment plans are highly variable and patient dependent.

Perioperative management of patients with insulin-dependent diabetes: half the usual NPH-isophane insulin dose the morning of the day of surgery. It is critical for patients who are receiving nothing orally and receiving insulin also to receive an intravenous infusion of dextrose 5 to 10 g/hr (equal to 100-200 mL of a D_5W solution) to prevent hypoglycemia.

Postoperative: sliding scale every 4 to 6 hours. Individualize to the patient.

If blood glucose is greater than 350 mg/dL, administer insulin regular, 15 units subcutaneously plus intravenously 1 to 2 units/hr. Monitor blood glucose hourly. Correct electrolyte imbalances (hypokalemia, hypophosphatemia) and acidosis.

Diabetic ketoacidosis: requires insulin by continuous infusion; hourly blood glucose determination; and correction of acidosis, dehydration, and electrolyte imbalances. After renal function is established, potassium replacement therapy may be needed.

Dosage forms: injection: 100 units/mL. U500 Insulin (500 units/mL) is available but should be used only to fill implanted insulin pumps. It should never be stocked outside the pharmacy.

Onset and Duration

	Onset (hr)	Peak (hr)	Duration (hr)
Regular (rapid insulin)	0.5-1	1-5	5-8
Intermediate	1-4	4-12	18-24

Adverse Effects

Dose-related hypoglycemia; local allergic reactions, lipoatrophy, and resistance (overcome by switching to more highly purified sources); anaphylaxis

In general, human insulin is least antigenic, and pork is less antigenic than beef and pork or pure beef insulin.

Precautions and Contraindications

- Diabetic ketoacidosis is a life-threatening condition requiring prompt diagnosis and treatment.
- Changes in purity, strength, brand, type, or species source may result in the need for a change in insulin dosage.
- Treat hypoglycemia with 0.6 mL/kg 50% dextrose intravenously.
- Hypersensitivity may occur.
- Insulin requirements may increase dramatically with stress, sepsis, trauma, or pregnancy.
- Only regular insulins (clear insulins) may be administered intravenously. Intermediate insulins may only be administered subcutaneously.
- Hypoglycemic action is increased by the concomitant administration of alcohol, β-blockers, monoamine oxidase inhibitors, salicylates, and sulfonylureas.
- Hypoglycemic action is decreased by thyroid hormones, corticosteroids, dobutamine, epinephrine, furosemide, and phenytoin.

Anesthetic Considerations

Blood glucose levels of 120 to 180 mg/dL should be sought, and blood glucose should be monitored frequently intraoperatively. If it is necessary to administer insulin intraoperatively, continuous intravenous infusion may be the best method. If it is administered subcutaneously, variability of skin blood flow during anesthesia may cause unpredictable results.

Large intravenous boluses of insulin can put the patient at risk for dysrhythmias caused by intracellular shifts of potassium, phosphorus, and magnesium.

IPRATROPIUM BROMIDE (ATROVENT)

Classification

Anticholinergic, bronchodilator (parasympatholytic)

Indications

Treatment and prevention of bronchospasm resulting from chronic obstructive pulmonary disease (COPD), including emphysema and chronic bronchitis

Dose

Metered-dose inhaler in adults: two to four sprays (initially, 18 mcg/spray); then two sprays every 4 hours (maximum dose: 216 mcg or 12 sprays/day).

Oral nebulizer in adults: 500 mcg with 2.5 mL of normal saline mixed via oral nebulization every 6 to 8 hours; may mix with albuterol in nebulizer if used within 1 hour of mixing.

Onset and Duration

Onset: within 15 to 30 minutes. Peak effect: 1 to 2 hours. Duration: 4 to 5 hours

Adverse Effects
Local or systemic anticholinergic effects, angina, blurred vision, headache, dizziness

Precautions and Contraindications
Use ipratropium cautiously for patients with narrow-angle glaucoma, bladder obstruction, and benign prostatic hypertrophy. It is contraindicated in patients hypersensitive to soya lecithin or related food products such as soybean and peanut, as well as in patients hypersensitive to ipratropium bromide, atropine, and its derivatives.

Anesthetic Considerations
Do not use it for relief of bronchospasm in acute chronic obstructive pulmonary disease exacerbation as a first-line drug. Use drugs with a faster onset.

ISOFLURANE (FORANE)

Classification
Inhalation anesthetic

Indication
General anesthesia

Dose
Titrate to effect for induction or maintenance of anesthesia. Minimum alveolar concentration: 1.14%.

Dosage forms: volatile liquid: 100 mL

Onset and Duration
Onset: a few minutes, dose dependent. Duration: emergence time: 15 to 20 minutes.

Adverse Effects
Hypotension, tachycardia, arrhythmia, respiratory depression, respiratory irritation, apnea, dizziness, euphoria, increased cerebral blood flow and intracranial pressure, nausea and vomiting, malignant hyperthermia, glucose elevation

Precautions and Contraindications
Isoflurane is contraindicated in patients with known or suspected genetic susceptibility to malignant hyperthermia. Changes in mental function may persist beyond the period of anesthetic administration and the immediate postoperative period.

Anesthetic Considerations
Anesthetic requirements decrease with age. It crosses the placental barrier. Abrupt onset of malignant hyperthermia may be triggered by isoflurane; early signs include muscle rigidity, especially of the jaw muscles, tachycardia, and tachypnea unresponsive to increased depth of anesthesia.

ISOPROTERENOL HCL (ISUPREL)

Classification
Synthetic sympathomimetic, nonspecific β-agonist

Indications

- For mild or transient episodes of heart block that do not require electric shock or pacemaker therapy
- For serious episodes of heart block and Adams-Stokes attacks (except when caused by ventricular tachycardia or fibrillation)
- For use in cardiac arrest until electric shock or pacemaker therapy, the treatments of choice, is available
- For bronchospasm occurring during anesthesia
- As an adjunct to fluid and electrolyte replacement therapy and the use of other drugs and procedures in the treatment of hypovolemic and septic shock, low cardiac output (hypoperfusion) states, congestive heart failure, and cardiogenic shock

Dose

Intramuscular or subcutaneous: 0.2 mg; intravenous: 0.02 to 0.06 mg; infusion: 2 to 20 mcg/min.

Onset and Duration

Onset: intravenous: immediately. Duration: intravenous: 1 to 5 minutes.

Adverse Effects

Tachyarrhythmias, hypertension, angina, paradoxical precipitation of Adams-Stokes attacks, pulmonary edema, headache, dizziness, tremors, nausea and vomiting, anorexia; possible exacerbation of ischemia or hypertension (when used for chronotropic support)

Precautions and Contraindications

Isoproterenol is contraindicated in patients with tachyarrhythmias, tachycardia, or hypertension.

Anesthetic Considerations

It is useful as an intravenous infusion for the treatment of refractory bradycardic states. The bronchodilating effect is better achieved with more specific β_2-agonists.

KETAMINE HCL (KETALAR)

Classification

Intravenous general anesthetic

Indications

Sole anesthetic agent for diagnostic and surgical procedures of short duration; induction of anesthesia in critically ill patients; small doses for outpatient analgesia

Dose

Induction: adult: intravenous: 1 to 4.5 mg/kg slowly over 60 seconds; intramuscular: 4 to 6 mg/kg; oral: 6 to 8 mg/kg. Half of the initial dose may be repeated as needed.

Dosage forms: injection: 10, 50, 100 mg/mL

Onset and Duration

Onset: intravenous: 2 to 5 minutes; intramuscular: 3 to 8 minutes; oral: 15 to 20 minutes. Duration: intravenous: 5 to 10 minutes; intramuscular: 12 to 25 minutes; oral: 30 to 60 minutes.

Adverse Effects

Hypertension, tachycardia, arrhythmias, apnea with rapid administration, laryngospasm, tonic or clonic movements, emergence delirium, hypersalivation, nausea and vomiting, diplopia, nystagmus, slight elevation in intraocular tension, serious emergence reactions

Precautions and Contraindications

Ketamine is contraindicated in hypertension, coronary heart disease or increased intracranial pressure, history of cerebrovascular accident, increased intraocular pressure, and psychiatric disorders. It is contraindicated for surgery or diagnostic procedures of the pharynx, larynx, and bronchial tree. Use it cautiously in patients with convulsive disorders.

Anesthetic Considerations

Do not mix ketamine with barbiturates in the same syringe. Emergence reactions are common in adults with high doses and are reduced by medication with a benzodiazepine. Catecholamine-depleted patients may respond to ketamine with unexpected reductions in blood pressure and cardiac output.

KETOROLAC TROMETHAMINE (TORADOL)

Classification

Nonsteroidal anti-inflammatory agent

Indications

Short-term (less than 5 days) management of moderately severe, acute pain that requires analgesia; generally used in a postoperative setting

Patients should be switched to alternative analgesics as soon as possible. Ketorolac therapy is not to exceed 5 days because of the potential for increased frequency and severity of adverse reactions. The combined duration of use of ketorolac intravenously or intramuscularly and orally should not exceed 5 days. Oral ketorolac is indicated only for continuation therapy after intravenous or intramuscular ketorolac.

Dose

Intramuscular (administer slowly and deeply into the muscle): patients younger than 65 years: one dose of 60 mg; patients older than 65 years, renally impaired, or weighing less than 50 kg: one dose of 30 mg

Intravenous (intravenous bolus over no less than 15 seconds): patients younger than 65 years: one dose of 30 mg; patients older than 65 years, renally impaired, or weighing less than 50 kg: one dose of 15 mg

Multiple-dose treatment (intravenous or subcutaneous): patients younger than 65 years: 30 mg every 6 hours, not to exceed 120 mg/day

Patients older than 65 years, renally impaired, or weighing less than 50 kg: 15 mg every 6 hours, not to exceed 60 mg/day

Onset and Duration

Onset: intravenous or intramuscular: 15 to 30 minutes. Peak effect: 1 to 2 hours. Duration: 4 to 6 hours.

Adverse Effects

Gastrointestinal: peptic ulcers, gastrointestinal bleeding, or perforation; renal toxicity; risk of bleeding: inhibition of platelet function; hypersensitivity

Because ketorolac and its metabolites are eliminated primarily by the kidneys, clearance of the drug is diminished in patients with reduced creatinine clearance. Renal toxicity with ketorolac has been seen in patients with conditions leading to a reduction in blood volume or renal blood flow, in which renal prostaglandins have a supportive role in the maintenance of renal perfusion. In these patients, administration of ketorolac may cause a dose-dependent reduction in renal prostaglandin formation and may precipitate acute renal failure.

Hypersensitivity reactions ranging from bronchospasm to anaphylactic shock have occurred, and appropriate counteractive measures must be available when administering the first dose.

Precautions and Contraindications

Fluid retention, edema, retention of sodium, oliguria, and elevations of serum urea nitrogen and creatinine have been reported. Therefore, ketorolac should be used only with caution in patients with cardiac decompensation, hypertension, or similar conditions. Ketorolac is contraindicated in patients with active peptic ulcer disease or recent gastrointestinal bleeding or perforation and in patients with a history of peptic ulcer disease or gastrointestinal bleeding. Ketorolac is also contraindicated in patients with advanced renal impairment and in patients at risk for renal failure owing to volume depletion. It is contraindicated in patients with suspected or confirmed cerebrovascular bleeding, hemorrhagic diathesis, and incomplete hemostasis and those with a high risk of bleeding. It is contraindicated as a prophylactic analgesic before any major surgery and is contraindicated intraoperatively when hemostasis is critical. Ketorolac is also contraindicated in patients with previously demonstrated hypersensitivity to ketorolac tromethamine or allergic manifestations to aspirin (ASA) or other nonsteroidal anti-inflammatory drugs (NSAIDs). It is contraindicated for patients currently receiving ASA or NSAIDs because of the cumulative risk of inducing serious NSAID-related side effects. Ketorolac is contraindicated for intrathecal or epidural administration owing to its alcohol content. It is contraindicated in labor and delivery because it may adversely affect fetal circulation and inhibit uterine contractions. Because of the potential adverse effects of prostaglandin-inhibiting drugs on neonates, ketorolac is contraindicated in nursing mothers.

Anesthetic Considerations

Do not use ketorolac as prophylactic analgesia before any major surgery or intraoperatively when hemostasis is critical; in patients with suspected or confirmed cerebrovascular bleeding, hemorrhagic diathesis, incomplete hemostasis, and at high risk of bleeding; in patients currently receiving ASA or NSAIDs; for epidural or intrathecal administration; or concomitantly with probenecid.

The use of ketorolac is not recommended in children.

Ketorolac reduced the diuretic response to furosemide in normovolemic healthy subjects by approximately 20%. Hypovolemia should be corrected before treatment with ketorolac is initiated. Ketorolac possesses no sedative or anxiolytic properties. The concomitant use with opiate-agonist analgesics can result in reduced opiate analgesic requirements. Ketorolac is highly bound to human plasma protein (99.2%).

LABETALOL (NORMODYNE, TRANDATE)

Classification
β- and α-adrenergic antagonist

Indication
Hypertension

Dose
Intravenous bolus: 0.15 to 0.25 mg/kg administered over 2 minutes; may repeat every 5 minutes up to 300 mg. Continuous infusion: 2 mg/min; titrate to effect. Oral: 100 mg twice daily alone or with diuretic; may increase to 200 mg twice daily after 2 days; further dose increase may be made every 1 to 3 days to maximal response. Maintenance dose: 200 to 400 mg twice daily.

Onset and Duration
Onset: intravenous: 1 to 3 minutes; oral: 20 to 40 minutes. Duration: intravenous: 0.25 to 2 hours; oral: 4 to 12 hours.

Adverse Effects
Hypotension, bradycardia, ventricular arrhythmias, congestive heart failure, chest pain, bronchospasm, headache, diarrhea

Precautions and Contraindications
Use labetalol cautiously in patients with chronic bronchitis, emphysema, preexisting peripheral vascular disease, pheochromocytoma, and diabetes. It is contraindicated in bronchial asthma, overt heart failure, greater than first-degree heart block, and hepatic failure.

Anesthetic Considerations
Inhalation anesthetics may enhance the drug's hypotensive effects.

LANSOPRAZOLE (PREVACID)

Classification
Proton pump inhibitor

Indications
Ulcers and acid reflux

Dose
Oral: 15 to 60 mg daily before meals

Onset and Duration
Onset: within 1 hour; peak effect: 2 hours; duration: greater than 24 hours

Adverse Effects
Abdominal pain, nausea, diarrhea

Precautions and Contraindications
Lansoprazole slows the gastric emptying of solids. Reduce the dose in hepatic disease. It is contraindicated for patients hypersensitive to lansoprazole or similar proton pump inhibitors.

Anesthetic Considerations
It is highly protein bound and undergoes liver elimination.

LEVOBUPIVACAINE (CHIROCAINE)

Classification
Amide-type local anesthetic

Indication
Regional anesthesia

Dose
For infiltration or peripheral nerve block: 0.25%, 0.5%, 0.75%. Dosing similar to bupivacaine.

Onset and Duration
Onset: infiltration: 2 to 10 minutes; epidural: 4 to 7 minutes; spinal: less than 1 minute. Peak effect: infiltration and epidural: 30 to 45 minutes; spinal: 15 minutes. Duration: infiltration, spinal, or epidural: 200 to 400 minutes (prolonged with epinephrine).

Adverse Effects
Hypotension, arrhythmias, cardiac arrest, respiratory impairment or arrest, seizures, tinnitus, blurred vision, urticaria, anaphylactoid symptoms; high spinal, urinary retention, lower extremity weakness and paralysis, loss of sphincter control, backache, palsies, slowing of labor

Precautions and Contraindications
Use levobupivacaine with caution in patients with hypovolemia, severe congestive heart failure, shock, and all forms of heart block. It is contraindicated in patients with hypersensitivity to amide-type local anesthetics.

Anesthetic Considerations
Intravenous access is essential during major regional block. Toxic plasma levels of levobupivacaine may cause seizures and cardiopulmonary collapse.

LIDOCAINE HCL (XYLOCAINE, XYLOCAINE JELLY, XYLOCAINE VISCOUS ORAL SOLUTION)

Classification
Amide-type local anesthetic; topical anesthetic; antiarrhythmic agent

Indications
Regional anesthesia, topical anesthesia, treatment of ventricular arrhythmias, attenuation of sympathetic response to laryngoscopy or intubation

Dose
Caudal or epidural: 20 to 30 mL 1% solution (200-300 mg); may also use 1.5% and 2% solutions (maximum dose: 200-300 mg/hr [4.5 mg/kg]). With epinephrine for anesthesia other than spinal, maximum dose is 500 mg (7 mg/kg).

Antiarrhythmic: slow intravenous bolus: 1 mg/kg (1%-2% solution) followed by 0.5 mg/kg every 2 to 5 minutes (maximum dose: 3 mg/kg/hr);

infusion (0.1% solution): 1 to 4 mg/min (20-50 mcg/kg/min). Use only preservative-free forms for intravenous administration.

Local anesthesia: topical: 0.6 to 3 mg/kg (1%-4% solution); infiltration or peripheral nerve block: 0.5 to 5 mg/kg (0.5%-2% solution); transtracheal: 80 to 120 mg (2-3 mL of 4% solution); superior laryngeal nerve: 40 to 60 mg (2-3 mL of 2% solution on each side); stellate ganglion: 50 mg (5 mL of 1% solution); intravenous (regional): upper extremity: 200 to 250 mg (40-50 mL of 0.5% solution), lower extremity: 250 to 300 mg (100-120 mL of 0.25% solution)

Onset and Duration

Onset: intravenous (antiarrhythmic effects): 45 to 90 seconds; infiltration: 0.5 to 3 minutes; epidural: 5 to 25 minutes. Peak effect: intravenous (antiarrhythmic effects): 1 to 2 minutes; infiltration and epidural: less than 30 minutes. Duration: intravenous (antiarrhythmic effects): 10 to 30 minutes; infiltration: 0.5 to 1.5 hours, with epinephrine: 2 to 6 hours; epidural: 1 to 3 hours (prolonged with epinephrine).

Adverse Effects

Hypotension, bradycardia, arrhythmias, heart block, respiratory depression or arrest, anxiety, tinnitus, seizures, postspinal headache, palsies, urticaria, pruritus; high spinal, loss of bladder and bowel control.

Precautions and Contraindications

Use lidocaine with caution in patients with hypovolemia, severe congestive heart failure, shock, all forms of heart block, and pregnancy. It is contraindicated in patients with hypersensitivity to amide-type local anesthetics and those with supraventricular arrhythmias.

Anesthetic Considerations

The dosage should be reduced for elderly, debilitated, and acutely ill patients. Anesthetic solutions containing epinephrine should be used with caution in patients with peripheral or hypertensive vascular disease. Benzodiazepines increase the seizure threshold. Do not use preparations containing preservatives for spinal or epidural anesthesia or for intravenous administration. Do not inject solutions containing epinephrine intravenously. Transient neurologic symptoms have been reported after spinal use.

LORAZEPAM (ATIVAN)

Classification

Benzodiazepine, antianxiety agent, hypnotic, sedative

Indications

Premedication; amnesia; temporary relief of insomnia

Dose

Intravenous or deep intramuscular: 1 to 2 mg (0.05 mg/kg) (maximum dose: 4 mg), dilute with equal volume D_5W or normal saline solution; oral: 1 to 2 mg, two to three times daily. Preoperative medication: 0.05 mg/kg 2 hours before procedure (maximum dose: 4 mg).

Dosage forms: tablets: 0.5, 1, 2 mg; injection: 2 mg/mL, 4 mg/mL

Onset and Duration

Onset: intravenous: 1 to 5 minutes; intramuscular: 15 to 30 minutes; oral: 1 to 6 hours. Duration: 6 to 24 hours. Elimination half-life: 10 to 15 hours; metabolized to inactive compounds.

Adverse Effects

Hypotension, hypertension, bradycardia, tachycardia, respiratory depression, dizziness, weakness, depression, agitation, amnesia, hysteria, urticaria, visual disturbances, blurred vision, diplopia, nausea and vomiting, abdominal discomfort, anorexia

Precautions and Contraindications

Intraarterial lorazepam injection may cause arteriospasm; treat with local infiltration of phentolamine (5-20 mg in 10 mL of normal saline). Use it with caution in elderly and debilitated patients. It is contraindicated for patients with known hypersensitivity to benzodiazepines and narrow-angle glaucoma.

Anesthetic Considerations

Unexpected hypotension and respiratory depression may occur when lorazepam is combined with opioids. Use it with caution in elderly patients and in patients with limited pulmonary reserve. It is not for use in children younger than 12 years. Treat overdoses with flumazenil. Decreased requirements for volatile anesthetics are noted.

MAGNESIUM SULFATE

Classification

Replacement agent; anticonvulsant

Indications

Prevention and control of seizures in toxemia or eclampsia of pregnancy, epilepsy, nephritis, and hypomagnesemia; treatment of acute magnesium deficiency; tocolytic therapy; adjunctive therapy of acute myocardial infarction, torsades de pointes ventricular tachycardia, and hypokalemia-related arrhythmias; laxative

Dose

Preeclampsia or eclampsia: intravenous: 4 g in 250 mL D_5W or normal saline infused slowly followed by 2 to 3 g/hr by continuous infusion; blood level should not exceed 7 mEq/L. Hypomagnesemic seizures: mild: 1 g intravenously or intramuscularly every 6 hours for four doses. Total parenteral nutrition: intravenous: 8 to 24 mEq/day.

Onset and Duration

Onset: intravenous: immediate; intramuscular: less than 1 hour; oral: 1 to 2 hours. Peak effect: intravenous: few minutes; intramuscular: 1 to 3 hours. Duration: intravenous: 30 minutes; intramuscular: 3 to 4 hours.

Adverse Effects

Hypotension, circulatory collapse, heart block, respiratory paralysis, flaccid paralysis, depressed reflexes, hypocalcemia, flushing, sweating, hypothermia

Precautions and Contraindications

Magnesium sulfate is not for use in patients with heart block or extensive myocardial damage. Use it with caution in patients with impaired renal function, in digitalized patients, and with concomitant use of other central nervous system depressants or neuromuscular blocking agents. Intravenous administration is contraindicated during the 2 hours preceding delivery. Oral administration is contraindicated in patients with abdominal pain, nausea, vomiting, fecal impaction, or intestinal irritation, obstruction, or perforation.

Anesthetic Considerations

Magnesium sulfate potentiates both depolarizing and nondepolarizing muscle relaxants. Periodic monitoring of serum magnesium concentrations is essential during magnesium therapy. Maintain urine output at a minimum of 100 mL every 4 hours. Monitor deep tendon reflexes during magnesium therapy. Stop therapy as soon as the desired effect is reached. Monitor the patient's respiratory function.

MANNITOL (OSMITROL)

Classification

Osmotic diuretic

Indications

Reduction of intracranial pressure and intraocular pressure; protection of renal function during periods of hypoperfusion (shock, burn, open-heart surgery, kidney transplants, abdominal aortic aneurysm repair); transurethral prostate resection (TURP) irrigation (minimizes hemolytic effects of water and promotes rapid excretion of absorbed irrigants)

Dose

Adults: reduction of intracranial or intraocular pressure: 1.5 to 2 g/kg of 15% to 25% solution over 30 to 60 minutes. When used preoperatively, administer 1 to 1.5 hours preoperatively for maximum pressure reduction. Test dose: Marked oliguria or suspected inadequate renal function: 0.2 g/kg or 12.5 g over 3 to 5 minutes. If satisfactory response is not obtained, may repeat. If response is still not obtained, do not use mannitol. Prevention of oliguric renal failure: 50 to 100 g intravenously over 2 hours. TURP: 2.5% to 5% irrigation instilled into bladder.

Children: 2 g/kg or 60 g/m^2 as 15% to 20% solution over 2 to 6 hours to treat edema and ascites; over 30 to 60 minutes to treat cerebral or ocular edema

Dosage forms: parenteral injection: 5%, 10%, 15%, 20%, 25%; urogenital irrigation solution: 2.5% to 5%

Onset and Duration

Onset: diuresis in 30 minutes to 1 hour; reduction of intracranial and intraocular pressure in 15 to 30 minutes. Duration: 3 to 8 hours.

Adverse Effects

Most serious: fluid imbalance and electrolyte loss; less serious: pulmonary edema, hypertension, water intoxication, congestive heart failure, skin necrosis with extravasation

Precautions and Contraindications

Monitor serum osmolarity and electrolytes closely. Discontinue mannitol if there is low urine output. Mannitol may crystallize at low temperatures. Do not use a solution containing crystals; resolubilize in hot water with periodic shaking. The use of mannitol is contraindicated in patients with pulmonary edema, congestive heart failure, severe dehydration, impaired renal function not responsive to test dose, edema associated with capillary fragility, and acute intracranial bleeding (except during craniotomy).

Anesthetic Considerations

Mannitol disrupts the blood-brain barrier, enhancing penetration of other drugs into the central nervous system.

MEPERIDINE HCL (DEMEROL)

Classification

Synthetic opioid agonist

Indication

Analgesia

Dose

Intravenous or intramuscular: 25 to 100 mg; intravenous: infusion 1 to 20 mg/hr for short duration; then titrate to patient's need

Onset and Duration

Onset: oral or intramuscular: 20 to 45 minutes; intravenous: 1 to 5 minutes. Duration: oral, intravenous, or intramuscular: 2 to 4 hours

Adverse Effects

Hypotension, cardiac arrest, respiratory depression or arrest, laryngospasm, euphoria, dysphoria, sedation, seizures, dependence, constipation, biliary tract spasm, chest wall rigidity, urticaria, pruritus

Precautions and Contraindications

Reduce the meperidine dose in elderly, hypovolemic, or high-risk surgical patients and with the concomitant use of sedatives and other narcotics. Severe and occasionally fatal reactions can occur in patients who are receiving or have just received monoamine oxidase inhibitors; treat these patients with hydrocortisone. It is not for long-term use. The toxic metabolite of meperidine HCl (normeperidine) is hazardous, especially in elderly patients and those with renal compromise.

Use it with caution in elderly patients and in patients with asthma, chronic obstructive pulmonary disease, increased intracranial pressure, supraventricular tachycardia, or renal failure.

Meperidine crosses the placental barrier. Use during labor may produce respiratory depression in neonates. If it is used, resuscitation of the neonate may be required; therefore, have naloxone available.

Cerebral irritation and seizures can occur when meperidine is used in large doses. Meperidine potentiates the central nervous system and cardiovascular depression of narcotics, sedative-hypnotics, volatile anesthetics, and tricyclic antidepressants. There is a severe and sometimes fatal reaction with monoamine oxidase inhibitors. Analgesia is enhanced by α_2-agonists.

Meperidine aggravates adverse effects of isoniazid. It is chemically incompatible with barbiturates.

Anesthetic Considerations

Meperidine is used occasionally for preoperative or postoperative analgesia.

MEPIVACAINE HCL (CARBOCAINE, POLOCAINE)

Classification

Amide-type local anesthetic

Indications

Regional anesthesia: infiltration, brachial plexus block, epidural, caudal

Dose

Infiltration: 50 to 400 mg (0.5%-1.5% solution). Brachial plexus block: 300 to 400 mg (30-40 mL of 1% solution). Epidural: 150 to 400 mg (15-20 mL of 1% to 2% solution). Caudal: 150 to 400 mg (15-20 mL of 1% to 2% solution).

Children: 0.4 to 0.7 mL/kg (maximum dose: 7 mg/kg with epinephrine)

Onset and Duration

Onset: infiltration: 3 to 5 minutes; epidural: 5 to 15 minutes. Peak effect: infiltration or epidural: 15 to 45 minutes. Duration: infiltration: 0.75 to 1.5 hours, 2 to 6 hours with epinephrine; epidural: 3 to 5 hours (prolonged with epinephrine)

Adverse Effects

Myocardial depression, arrhythmias, cardiac arrest, respiratory depression or arrest, anxiety, apprehension, tinnitus, seizures, loss of hearing, urticaria, pruritus

Precautions and Contraindications

Use mepivacaine with caution in debilitated, elderly, or acutely ill patients, especially if there is severe disturbance in cardiac rhythm or heart block. Use it with caution in pregnant patients. It is contraindicated in patients with hypersensitivity to amide-type local anesthetics.

Anesthetic Considerations

Do not use solutions with preservatives for caudal or epidural block. Mepivacaine is not for use as spinal or obstetric anesthesia.

METHADONE HCL (DOLOPHINE HCL)

Classification

Synthetic narcotic

Indications

Analgesia; opiate recovery programs

Dose

Analgesia: subcutaneous, intramuscular, or oral: 2.5 to 10 mg (0.1 mg/kg) every 4 hours; epidural bolus: 1 to 5 mg. Narcotic abstinence syndrome: oral: 20 to 120 mg/day.

Onset and Duration

Onset: intravenous: 5 to 10 minutes; intramuscular: 20 to 60 minutes; oral: 30 to 60 minutes; epidural: 5 to 10 minutes. Duration: intravenous, intramuscular, or oral: about 6 hours; epidural: 6 to 10 hours.

Adverse Effects

Hypotension, circulatory depression, bradycardia, syncope, respiratory depression, euphoria, dysphoria, disorientation, urinary retention, biliary tract spasm, constipation, anorexia, rash, pruritus, urticarial

Precautions and Contraindications

Reduce the methadone dose in elderly, hypovolemic, or high-risk surgical patients or with use of narcotics and sedative-hypnotics.

Anesthetic Considerations

Do not administer pentazocine to heroin addicts receiving methadone. Methadone is ineffective for relief of general anxiety. Use it with caution in patients with asthma, chronic obstructive pulmonary disease, or increased intracranial pressure. Methadone can produce the drug effects of morphine solution.

METHYLENE BLUE (UROLENE BLUE)

Classification

Antidote; diagnostic agent

Indications

Treatment of idiopathic and drug-induced methemoglobinemia; dye effect for tissue staining; urinary antiseptic (oral route); antidote to cyanide poisoning

Dose

Intravenous: 1 to 2 mg/kg (inject over several minutes); oral: 65 to 130 mg three times daily with water

Onset and Duration

Onset: intravenous: almost immediate. Peak effect: intravenous: less than 1 hour. Duration: intravenous or oral: several hours

Adverse Effects

Tachycardia, hypertension, precordial pain, cyanosis, confusion, headache, nausea and vomiting, diarrhea, abdominal pain, bladder irritation, hemolytic anemia, methemoglobinemia, hyperbilirubinemia, blue staining of skin

Precautions and Contraindications

Safe use during pregnancy is not established. Methylene blue is contraindicated in patients with renal insufficiency, hypersensitivity to methylene blue, glucose-6-phosphate dehydrogenase deficiency (hemolysis), or for intraspinal injection.

Anesthetic Considerations

Methylene blue causes discoloration of urine and feces. It may cause artificial readings with pulse oximetry; inject it slowly to prevent a local high concentration from producing additional methemoglobinemia. Monitor intake, output, and hemoglobin.

METHYLERGONOVINE (METHERGINE)

Classification
Oxytocic (ergot alkaloid); adrenergic antagonist; sympatholytic

Indications
Prevention and treatment of postpartum hemorrhage caused by uterine atony or subinvolution

Dose
Intramuscular: 0.2 mg every 2 to 5 hours; intravenous: 0.2 mg/mL (over 1 minute while monitoring blood pressure and uterine contractions); oral: 0.2 to 0.4 mg every 6 to 12 hours for 2 to 7 days

Onset and Duration
Onset: intravenous: immediate; intramuscular: 2 to 5 minutes; oral: 5 to 15 minutes. Peak effect: 3 hours. Duration: intravenous: 45 minutes; intramuscular: 3 hours; oral: 3 or more hours.

Adverse Effects
Hypertension, chest pain, palpitations, dyspnea, headache, nausea, vomiting, tinnitus; high doses: possible signs of ergotism

Precautions and Contraindications
Use it with caution in patients with hypertension; sepsis; obliterative vascular disease; and hepatic, renal, or cardiac disease. Methylergonovine is contraindicated in patients with hypersensitivity to ergot preparations and in those with toxemia or untreated hypocalcemia.

Anesthetic Considerations
Monitor patients for hypertension or other adverse effects. Parenteral sympathomimetics or other ergot alkaloids add to pressor effect and may lead to hypertension. Intravenous administration is not routine because it can produce sudden hypertension and cerebrovascular accidents.

METOCLOPRAMIDE (REGLAN)

Classification
Dopamine-receptor antagonist; antiemetic; stimulant of upper gastrointestinal motility

Indications
Diabetic and postsurgical gastric stasis; prevention of chemotherapy-induced emesis; facilitation of small bowel intubation; treatment of gastroesophageal reflux; prevention of postoperative nausea and vomiting

Dose
Adults: 10 mg intravenously slowly over 1 to 2 minutes as a single dose; may repeat once. Children: 6 to 14 years: intravenous: 2.5 to 5 mg; children younger than 6 years: intravenous: 0.1 mg/kg.

Dosage forms: intravenous: 5 mg/mL in 2- and 10-mL vials; oral: tablets: 5 mg and 10 mg; syrup: 5 mg/5 mL

Onset and Duration

Onset: 1 to 3 minutes. Duration: 2 to 3 hours. Elimination half-life: 2.5 to 5 hours in patients with normal renal function.

Adverse Effects

Anxiety, restlessness, mental depression, gastrointestinal upset, urticaria, allergic reactions, diarrhea, frequent drowsiness

Extrapyramidal side effects such as opisthotonos, clonic convulsions, oculogyric crisis, facial grimacing, involuntary movement of limbs, and rarely stridor and dyspnea (possibly from laryngospasm) occur with a 0.2% or less frequency in the foregoing doses but are more common in children. Diphenhydramine may reverse the extrapyramidal effects. Butyrophenones and phenothiazines may potentiate the extrapyramidal side effects.

Precautions and Contraindications

Use it with caution in pregnant patients. Metoclopramide may exacerbate Parkinson's disease and hypertension and may increase pressure on suture lines following gut anastomosis or closure. Patients should be cautioned that metoclopramide may impair their ability to perform activities requiring mental alertness, including driving or operating machinery. Alcohol and other central nervous system depressants may enhance these effects.

Do not use metoclopramide with monoamine oxidase inhibitors, tricyclic antidepressants, or sympathomimetics. Metoclopramide should not be used in patients with pheochromocytoma; a history of seizure disorder; or gastrointestinal hemorrhage, obstruction, or perforation.

Anesthetic Considerations

Metoclopramide may increase the neuromuscular blocking effects of succinylcholine or mivacurium by inhibiting plasma cholinesterase.

MIDAZOLAM (VERSED)

Classification

Benzodiazepine; hypnotic; sedative

Indications

Preoperative sedation; induction of anesthesia; long-term sedation in intensive care unit; sedation before short diagnostic and endoscopic procedures

Dose

Should be individualized based on the patient's age, underlying pathologic features, and concurrent indications. Adolescents (younger than 12 years): intravenous: 0.5 mg; can be repeated every 5 minutes until desired effect is achieved. Adults: preoperative sedation: intramuscular: 0.07 to 0.08 mg/kg 30 to 60 minutes before surgery; usual dose: approximately 5 mg; intravenous: initial: 0.5 to 2 mg slowly over 2 minutes; usual total dose: 2 to 5 mg; decrease dose in elderly patients; reduce dose by 30% if other central nervous system depressants are administered concomitantly.

Dosage forms: injection: 1, 5 mg/mL

Onset and Duration
Onset: intravenous: 1 to 5 minutes; intramuscular: 15 minutes; oral or rectal: less than 10 minutes. Duration: 2 to 6 hours. Elimination half-life: 14 hours; excreted in urine.

Adverse Effects
Tachycardia, hypotension, bronchospasm, laryngospasm, apnea, hypoventilation, vasovagal episodes, euphoria, prolonged emergence, agitation, hyperactivity, pruritus, rash

Precautions and Contraindications
Midazolam is not for intraarterial injection. Its safe use in pregnancy, in labor and delivery, by nursing mothers, or by children is not established. Midazolam is contraindicated in patients with intolerance to benzodiazepines and in those with acute narrow-angle glaucoma, shock, coma, or acute alcohol intoxication.

Anesthetic Considerations
Use midazolam with caution in elderly patients and in patients with chronic obstructive pulmonary disease, chronic renal failure, or congestive heart failure. Reduce the doses in hypovolemia and with the concomitant use of other sedatives or narcotics. Hypotension and respiratory depression may occur when it is administered with opioids; consider smaller doses. Treat overdoses with flumazenil.

MILRINONE (PRIMACOR)

Classification
Inotropic agent; phosphodiesterase-3 inhibitor

Indications
Therapy for congestive heart failure; cardiac bypass procedures and heart transplants

Dose
Intravenous: loading dose: 50 mcg/kg over 10 minutes; maintenance dose: 0.375 mcg/kg/min, 0.5 mcg/kg/min, or 0.75 mcg/kg/min

Dosage forms: intravenous: 1 mg/mL

Onset and Duration
Onset: intravenous: 2 minutes; oral: 1 to 1.5 hours. Duration: 2 hours.

Adverse Effects
Thrombocytopenia, arrhythmia, angina, hypotension, headache, hyperthermia

Precautions and Contraindications
Use it with caution in patients with renal insufficiency and in those with aortic or pulmonic valvular disease. Milrinone is contraindicated in patients with hypersensitivity to milrinone or amrinone.

Anesthetic Considerations
Milrinone is an attractive alternative to conventional inotropics. It may be useful if both an inotropic effect and vasodilation are desirable.

MORPHINE SULFATE (ASTRAMORPH, DURAMORPH, MORPHINE, MS CONTIN)

Classification
Opioid agonist

Indications
Premedication; analgesia; anesthesia; treatment of pain associated with myocardial ischemia and dyspnea associated with left ventricular failure and pulmonary edema

Dose
Analgesia: intravenous: 2.5 to 15 mg; intramuscular or subcutaneous: 2.5 to 20 mg; oral: 15 to 30 mg every 4 hours as needed; oral extended release: 30 mg every 12 hours; rectal: 5 to 20 mg every 4 hours. Anesthesia induction: intravenous: 1 mg/kg; epidural bolus: 2 to 5 mg; epidural infusion: 0.1 to 1 mg/hr; spinal (preservative-free solution only): 0.2 to 1 mg.

Children: intravenous: 0.05 to 0.2 mg/kg; intramuscular or subcutaneous: 0.1 to 0.2 mg/kg.

Onset and Duration
Onset: intravenous: almost immediate; intramuscular: 1 to 5 minutes; oral: less than 60 minutes; epidural and spinal: 1 to 60 minutes. Duration: intravenous, intramuscular, or subcutaneous: 2 to 7 hours; epidural and spinal: 24 hours.

Adverse Effects
Hypotension, hypertension, bradycardia, arrhythmias, chest wall rigidity, bronchospasm, laryngospasm, blurred vision, syncope, euphoria, dysphoria, urinary retention, antidiuretic effect, ureteral spasm, biliary tract spasm, constipation, anorexia, nausea, vomiting, pruritus, urticarial

Precautions and Contraindications
Reduce the morphine dose in elderly, hypovolemic, or high-risk surgical patients and with the concomitant use of sedatives and other narcotics. Morphine sulfate crosses the placental barrier, so use in labor may produce depression of respiration in neonates. Resuscitation of the neonate may be required; therefore, have naloxone available.

Anesthetic Considerations
Central nervous system and cardiovascular depressant effects are potentiated by alcohol, sedatives, antihistamines, phenothiazines, butyrophenones, monoamine oxidase inhibitors, and tricyclic antidepressants. Morphine sulfate may decrease the effects of diuretics in patients with congestive heart failure. Analgesia is enhanced by α_2-agonists.

NALMEFENE HCL (REVEX)

Classification
Opiate antagonist

Indications
Complete or partial reversal of drug effects, respiratory depression, and overdose associated with natural or synthetic opioids

Dose

Reversal of opiate depression: titrate to the desired response at increments of 0.25 mcg/kg every 2 to 5 minutes; doses greater than 1 mg/kg give no additional therapeutic effects; titrate at a dose of 0.1 mcg/kg every 2 to 5 minutes in patients with increased cardiovascular risk.

Suspected opiate overdose: first dose 0.5 mg/70 kg; second dose 1 mg/70 kg if required 2 to 5 minutes later; doses greater than 1.5 mg/70 kg do not provide increased therapeutic effects.

Suspicion of opiate dependency: challenge dose of 0.1 mg/70 kg; if signs of withdrawal do not appear within 2 minutes, the recommended dosage guidelines should be followed.

Onset and Duration

Onset: intravenous: within 2 minutes; intramuscular or subcutaneous: 5 to 15 minutes; intravenous: administration of a 1-mg dose of nalmefene will block 80% of brain opiate receptors within 5 minutes. The duration of action and opiate receptor occupancy of nalmefene were shown to be significantly greater than those of naloxone, which has a half-life of 1.1 hour. Duration: equals that of most opioids. This provides the patient with added protection against possible renarcotization. Elimination half-life: 10.8 hours. It is metabolized in liver via glucuronide conjugation and excreted in the urine. Plasma clearance is reported to be 0.8 L/kg/hr.

Adverse Effects

Pulmonary edema, hypotension, hypertension, ventricular arrhythmias, bradycardia, dizziness, depression, agitation, nervousness, tremor, confusion, myoclonus, withdrawal syndrome, nausea and vomiting, diarrhea, dry mouth, headache, chills, pruritus, pharyngitis

A higher occurrence of adverse effects is reported with amounts exceeding recommended dosages.

Precautions and Contraindications

Nalmefene has decreased plasma clearance in patients with liver or renal disease. The dose of nalmefene should be delivered over 60 seconds in patients with renal failure to minimize associated hypertension and dizziness. Dosage need not be adjusted for one-time administration. Recurrence of respiratory depression is possible even after a positive response to initial administration. Use it with caution in patients at increased cardiovascular risk. Acute withdrawal symptoms are associated with administration to opiate-dependent patients. There is incomplete reversal of buprenorphine-induced depression. Animal studies have shown a potential for seizure induction. The potential risk of seizure increases with the coadministration of nalmefene and flumazenil. Nalmefene is contraindicated in persons who display an allergic response related to the drug's administration. Safety and effectiveness of nalmefene for neonates and children have not been established.

Anesthetic Considerations

No adverse reactions were noted in studies in which nalmefene was coadministered after benzodiazepines, volatile anesthetics, muscle relaxants, or muscle relaxant reversal agents.

NALOXONE HCL (NARCAN)

Classification
Opioid antagonist

Indication
Opiate reversal

Dose
Intravenous, intramuscular, or subcutaneous: 0.1 to 0.2 mg titrated to patient response; may repeat at 2- to 3-minute intervals; response should occur with a maximum dose of 1.0 mg. Children: 5 to 10 mcg/kg every 2 to 3 minutes as needed.

Onset and Duration
Onset: intravenous: 1 to 2 minutes; intramuscular or subcutaneous: 2 to 5 minutes. Duration: intravenous, intramuscular, or subcutaneous: 1 to 4 hours.

Adverse Effects
Tachycardia, hypertension, hypotension, arrhythmias, pulmonary edema, nausea and vomiting related to dose and speed of injection

Precautions and Contraindications
Use naloxone with caution in patients with preexisting cardiac disease.

Anesthetic Considerations
Titrate naloxone slowly to effect the desired results. Patients who have received naloxone should be carefully monitored because the duration of action of some opiates may exceed that of this drug.

NALTREXONE HCL (REVIA, TREXAN)

Classification
Opiate receptor antagonist

Indications
Reversal of toxic effects of opioid drugs; treatment of opiate and alcohol addiction, Tourette syndrome, tardive dyskinesia, Lesch-Nyhan disease, and dyskinesia associated with Huntington disease

Dose
Oral: 25 mg tablet followed by 25 mg in 1 hour if no signs of withdrawal present (withdrawal will begin 5 minutes after oral dose and may last up to 48 hours)

Dosage forms: tablet: 25, 50 mg

Onset and Duration
Onset: within 5 minutes. Peak effect: within 1 hour. Duration: 24 to 72 hours

Adverse Effects
Headache, nervousness, confusion, restlessness, hallucinations, paranoia, nightmares, nausea and vomiting, diarrhea, abdominal pain and cramping,

phlebitis, epistaxis, tachycardia, hypertension, edema, hepatotoxicity, joint or muscle pain, severe narcotic withdrawal

Precautions and Contraindications

Patients addicted to heroin or other opiates should be drug free for 10 days before initiation of naltrexone therapy to avoid precipitation of withdrawal syndrome. Naltrexone contraindication is absolute in patients dependent on narcotics, in patients in acute withdrawal, and in those with liver disease or acute hepatitis. Serious overdose may occur after attempts to overcome the blocking effects of naltrexone.

Anesthetic Considerations

Baseline liver function studies should be performed. The primary active metabolite is subject to glucuronide conjugation. Aspartate transaminase levels may be temporarily elevated after initiation of therapy. Patients taking naltrexone may not respond to opiates administered during anesthesia. Blockade of naltrexone may be overcome by large doses of opiates.

NEOSTIGMINE METHYLSULFATE (PROSTIGMIN)

Classification

Anticholinesterase agent

Indications

Reversal of nondepolarizing muscle relaxants; myasthenia gravis

Dose

Reversal: slow intravenous: 0.06 mg/kg (maximum dose: 6 mg), with atropine (0.015 mg/kg) or glycopyrrolate (0.01 mg/kg). Myasthenia gravis: oral: 15 to 375 mg daily (three divided doses); intramuscular or slow intravenous: 0.5 to 2 mg (dose must be individualized).

Onset and Duration

Onset: reversal: intravenous: 3 to 15 minutes. Myasthenia gravis: intramuscular: less than 20 minutes; oral: 45 to 75 minutes. Duration: 45 to 60 minutes.

Adverse Effects

Bradycardia, tachycardia, atrioventricular block, nodal rhythm, hypotension, bronchospasm; respiratory depression; seizures; dysarthria; headaches; nausea, emesis, flatulence, increased peristalsis; urinary frequency; rash, urticaria, allergic reactions, anaphylaxis; increased oral, pharyngeal, and bronchial secretions

Precautions and Contraindications

Use neostigmine with caution in patients with bradycardia, bronchial asthma, epilepsy, cardiac arrhythmias, peptic ulcer, peritonitis, or mechanical obstruction of the intestines or urinary tract. Overdosage may induce a cholinergic crisis characterized by nausea, vomiting, bradycardia or tachycardia, excessive salivation and sweating, bronchospasm, weakness, and paralysis; treatment includes discontinuation of neostigmine use and administration of atropine (10 mg/kg intravenously every 3 to 10 minutes until muscarinic symptoms disappear).

Anesthetic Considerations

Neostigmine may increase postoperative nausea and vomiting.

NESIRITIDE (NATRECOR)

Classification

Purified preparation of a new drug class, human B-type natriuretic peptide (hBNP), manufactured from *Escherichia coli* using recombinant DNA technology

Indications

Intravenous treatment of acutely decompensated congestive heart failure in patients who have dyspnea at rest or with minimal activity; reduction of pulmonary capillary wedge pressure; improvement of dyspnea

Dose

Intravenous: 2 mcg/kg bolus followed by a continuous infusion at a dose of 0.01 mcg/kg/min

Withdraw the bolus volume from the nesiritide infusion bag and administer it over approximately 60 seconds through an intravenous port in the tubing. Immediately after administration of the bolus, infuse nesiritide at a flow rate of 0.1 mL/kg/hr. This will deliver a nesiritide infusion dose of 0.01 mcg/kg/min.

To calculate the appropriate bolus volume and infusion flow rate to deliver a 0.01 mcg/kg/min dose, use the following formulas:

$$\text{Bolus volume (mL)}: 0.33 \times \text{Patient weight (kg)}$$

$$\text{Infusion flow rate (mL/hr)}: 0.1 \times \text{Patient weight (kg)}$$

Onset and Duration

Onset: 15 to 60 minutes. Duration: 1 to 2 hours after discontinuation of infusion

Adverse Effects

Hypotension. The rate of symptomatic hypotension may be increased in patients with a blood pressure lower than 100 mmHg at baseline, and nesiritide should be used cautiously in these patients. Combining nesiritide with other drugs that may cause hypotension such as nitroglycerin or an angiotensin-converting enzyme inhibitor may increase the potential for hypotension.

Precautions and Contraindications

Nesiritide should be administered only in settings where blood pressure can be monitored closely, and the dose of nesiritide should be reduced or the drug discontinued in patients who develop hypotension.

Anesthetic Considerations

Nesiritide is not recommended for patients for whom vasodilating agents are not appropriate (e.g., patients with significant valvular stenosis, restrictive or obstructive cardiomyopathy, constrictive pericarditis, pericardial tamponade, or other conditions in which cardiac output depends on venous return) or for patients suspected to have low cardiac filling pressures.

NICARDIPINE (CARDENE)

Classification
Calcium channel blocker

Indications
Hypertension; chronic stable angina; vasospastic angina

Dose
Angina: initially 20 mg orally three times daily; titrate dosage according to patient response; usual dosage 20 to 40 mg orally three times daily

Hypertension: initially 20 to 40 mg orally three times daily, increase dosage according to patient response; intravenous: 5 mg/hr, increased by 2.5 mg/hr increments every 15 minutes, up to 15 mg/hr

Onset and Duration
Onset: intravenous: 1 minute; oral: 30 minutes to 2 hours; sustained release: 1 to 4 hours. Duration: intravenous/oral: 3 hours.

Adverse Effects
Edema, dizziness, headache, flushing, hypotension

Precautions and Contraindications
Use it with caution in patients with hypersensitivity to nicardipine, other dihydropyridines, or other calcium channel antagonists and those with symptomatic hypotension or advanced aortic stenosis.

Anesthetic Considerations
Nicardipine is an intravenous calcium channel blocker. It may be useful in controlling perioperative hypertension.

NIFEDIPINE (ADALAT, PROCARDIA)

Classification
Calcium channel blocker

Indications
Hypertension; chronic stable angina; vasospastic angina

Dose
10 to 30 mg three times daily up to 90 mg/day

Onset and Duration
Onset: oral: 20 minutes; sublingual: 5 to 20 minutes. Duration: oral or sublingual: 12 hours.

Adverse Effects
Hypotension, palpitations, peripheral edema, bronchospasm, shortness of breath, nasal and chest congestion, headache, dizziness, nervousness, nausea, diarrhea, constipation, inflammation, joint stiffness, peripheral edema, pruritus, urticaria, fevers, chills, sweating

Precautions and Contraindications
Monitor patient's blood pressure carefully during initial administration and titration. Use nifedipine with caution in hypovolemic patients,

elderly patients, and those with acute myocardial infarction and unstable angina.

Anesthetic Considerations

Nifedipine potentiates the effects of depolarizing and nondepolarizing muscle relaxants and provides additive cardiovascular depressant effects with the use of volatile anesthetics or other antihypertensives. Nifedipine increases the toxicity of digoxin, carbamazepine, and oral hypoglycemics. It may bring about cardiac failure, atrioventricular conduction disturbances, and sinus bradycardia with concurrent use of β-blockers; severe hypotension and bradycardia may occur with bupivacaine. The concomitant use of intravenous verapamil and dantrolene may result in cardiovascular collapse.

NITROGLYCERIN (NITRO-BID, NITRO-DUR, NITROGARD, NITROSTAT, NITROL, TRIDIL, NITROCINE, TRANSDERM-NITRO, NITROGLYN, NITRODISC)

Classification

Peripheral vasodilator

Indications

Angina; controlled hypotension, treatment of pulmonary edema and congestive heart failure associated with acute myocardial infarction

Dose

Initially, titrate 5 to 20 mcg/min; thereafter, titrate by 10 mcg/min steps. Tablets: 0.15 to 0.6 mg every 5 minutes as needed to maximum of three doses in 15 minutes (sustained-release buccal, 1 to 2 mg every 3-5 hours); place tablet between the lip and gum above the incisors.

Dosage forms: injection: 0.5 and 5 mg/mL: tablets: sublingual: 0.15, 0.3, 0.4, 0.6 mg; sustained-release buccal: 1, 2, 3 mg; oral: 2.5, 6.5, 9 mg; capsules: 2.5, 6.5, 9 mg; aerosol translingual: 0.4 mg/metered dose; transdermal systems: 2.5, 5, 7.5, 10, 15 mg/24 hours; ointment: 2% (1 inch contains 15 mg nitroglycerin). Dilution for infusion: 8 mg diluted in 250 mL D_5W or normal saline (32 mcg/mL), 50 mg in 250 mL, 100 mg in 250 mL (400 mcg/mL).

Onset and Duration

Onset: intravenous: 1 to 2 minutes; sublingual: 1 to 3 minutes; oral sustained release: 20 to 45 minutes; transdermal: 40 to 60 minutes. Duration: 30 minutes to 2 hours, depending on route.

Adverse Effects

Orthostatic hypotension, tachycardia, flushing, palpitations, fainting, headache, dizziness, weakness, nausea and vomiting

Precautions and Contraindications

Use it with caution in patients with hypotension, uncorrected hypovolemia, inadequate cerebral circulation, increased intracranial pressure, head trauma, cerebral hemorrhage, or severe anemia. Nitroglycerin is contraindicated in patients with compensatory hypertension such as with arteriovenous shunts, coarctation of the aorta, and inadequate cerebral circulation.

Anesthetic Considerations

The hypotensive effects of nitroglycerin are potentiated by alcohol, phenothiazines, calcium channel blockers, β-blockers, other nitrates, and antihypertensives. Nitroglycerin may antagonize the anticoagulant effect of heparin. Methemoglobinemia may occur at high doses.

Attenuation of hypoxic pulmonary vasoconstriction may occur with nitroglycerin. Infusion rates of greater than 3 mcg/kg/min may result in decreased platelet aggregation. The hypotensive effects of nitroglycerin are potentiated by volatile anesthetics, ganglionic blocking agents, other antihypertensives, and circulatory depressants.

NITROPRUSSIDE SODIUM (NIPRIDE, NITROPRESS)

Classification

Peripheral vasodilator

Indications

Hypertension; controlled hypotension; treatment of cardiogenic pulmonary edema; treatment of cardiogenic shock

Dose

Infusion: 10 to 300 mcg/min (0.25-10 mcg/kg/min) (maximum dose: 10 mcg/kg/min for 10 minutes or long-term infusion of 0.5 mcg/kg/min). Because of light sensitivity, wrap the intravenous solution container in foil. Monitor plasma thiocyanate concentrations in patients receiving infusions for more than 48 hours.

Onset and Duration

Onset: 30 to 60 seconds. Duration: 1 to 10 minutes

Adverse Effects

Reflex tachycardia; cyanide toxicity possible even with low doses

Treatment of cyanide toxicity: immediately discontinue nitroprusside use, administer oxygen, treat acidosis with bicarbonate, and start sodium nitrate 3% solution 4 to 6 mg/kg over 3 minutes to produce 10% methemoglobin (which will reversibly bind free cyanide ion). Follow with an infusion of sodium thiosulfate (vitamin B_{12}), 150 to 200 mg/kg.

Precautions and Contraindications

Use nitroprusside with caution in patients with renal or hepatic failure, which may lead to increased risk of cyanide toxicity. There is a potential for fetal cyanide toxicity in pregnant patients.

Anesthetic Considerations

Titrate it carefully for short periods of deliberate hypotension. Monitor the patient for cyanide toxicity. Elevated mixed venous oxygen tension may also occur.

NITROUS OXIDE (N_2O)

Classification

Inhalation anesthetic

Indications

Component of balanced anesthesia or dental analgesia

Dose

Induction: 70% in an oxygen mixture. Maintenance: 50% to 70% in oxygen. Analgesia: 20% to 30%. Supplied in steel cylinders (blue) as a colorless liquid under pressure.

Onset and Duration

Onset: 1 to 5 minutes. Duration: 5 to 10 minutes after cessation of continuous inhalation

Adverse Effects

Primarily caused by lack of oxygen from improper administration technique: confusion, cyanosis, convulsions, possible bone marrow depression

Precautions and Contraindications

Caution the patient not to drive or operate other machinery until the effects of nitrous oxide have completely disappeared. Inform the patient that confusion, vivid dreams, dizziness, and hallucinations may occur on termination of the drug. Inspired oxygen concentrations of at least 30% should be administered.

Anesthetic Considerations

Nitrous oxide is nonflammable but will support combustion. There is a noticeable second-gas effect that initially hastens the uptake of other agents when high concentrations are used. Nitrous oxide diffuses into air-containing cavities 34 times faster than nitrogen can leave. This can cause a potentially dangerous pressure accumulation (i.e., middle ear perforation, bowel obstruction, pneumothorax, air embolism, endotracheal tube cuff).

NIZATIDINE (AXID)

Classification

Histamine (H_2)-receptor antagonist

Indications

Treatment of duodenal or gastric ulcers and gastroesophageal reflux disease; prophylaxis of aspiration pneumonitis in patients at high risk during surgery

Dose

For prophylaxis of aspiration pneumonitis in adults: 150 mg orally 2 hours before the induction of anesthesia; may be administered with or without a similar dose the preceding evening. For patients with impaired renal function as evidenced by serum creatinine level greater than 2.5 mg/dL, a single dose only is needed.

Dosage forms: 150-mg capsule.

Onset and Duration

Onset: 0.5 hour. Peak effect: 1 to 3 hours after oral administration and less than detectable limits in healthy patients 12 hours later. Elimination half-life: 1 to 2.8 hours.

Adverse Effects

Headache (most common), gastrointestinal effects and dizziness (4.5%); rarely, thrombocytopenia, leukopenia, anemia; somnolence (2%) and mental confusion possible in elderly patients

Precautions and Contraindications
Caution is suggested in patients with hepatic or renal dysfunction. Nizatidine is contraindicated in patients with known hypersensitivity to nizatidine or other H_2 antagonists.

Anesthetic Considerations
Nizatidine is safe for use during anesthesia.

NOREPINEPHRINE BITARTRATE (LEVOPHED)

Classification
Catecholamine

Indications
Vasoconstrictor; inotrope; potent peripheral vasoconstrictor of arterial and venous beds; potent inotropic stimulator of the heart (β_1-adrenergic action) but to a lesser degree than epinephrine or isoproterenol.

It does not stimulate β_2-adrenergic receptors of the bronchi or peripheral blood vessels except at high doses. It increases systolic and diastolic blood pressures and coronary artery blood flow. Cardiac output varies reflexly with systemic hypertension but is usually increased in hypotensive patients when blood pressure is raised to an optimal level. At low doses, increased baroreceptor activity reflexly decreases the heart rate. Norepinephrine reduces renal, hepatic, cerebral, and muscle blood flow.

Dose
Infusion: 8 to 12 mcg/min; use the lowest effective dose.

Onset and Duration
Onset: 1 minute. Duration: 2 to 10 minutes

Adverse Effects
Bradycardia, tachyarrhythmias, hypertension, decreased cardiac output, headache, plasma volume depletion

Administer into a large vein to minimize extravasation. Treat extravasation with local infiltration of phentolamine (10 mg in 10 mL of normal saline) or sympathetic block.

Precautions and Contraindications
Norepinephrine bitartrate is contraindicated in patients with mesenteric or peripheral vascular thrombosis.

Anesthetic Considerations
Norepinephrine causes an increased risk of arrhythmias with use of volatile anesthetics or bretylium or in patients with hypoxia or hypercarbia. The pressor effect is potentiated in patients receiving monoamine oxidase inhibitors, tricyclic antidepressants, guanethidine, or oxytocics. Norepinephrine may cause necrosis or gangrene with extravasation.

OMEPRAZOLE (PRILOSEC)

Classification
Proton pump inhibitor

Indication
Gastroesophageal reflux disease

Dose
Oral: 10 to 40 mg daily before meals

Onset and Duration
Onset: within 1 hour. Peak effect: 2 hours. Duration: up to 72 hours

Adverse Effects
Headache, diarrhea, abdominal pain, nausea and vomiting, rash, constipation, dizziness

Precautions and Contraindications
Omeprazole is contraindicated in patients with hypersensitivity to omeprazole or other similar proton pump inhibitors.

Anesthetic Considerations
Omeprazole is highly protein bound. It undergoes liver and renal elimination. Omeprazole may prolong the elimination of drugs metabolized by oxidation in the liver (i.e., diazepam, warfarin, phenytoin).

ONDANSETRON HCL (ZOFRAN)

Classification
Gastrointestinal agent; serotonin ($5HT_3$) receptor antagonist; antiemetic

Indications
Prevention of nausea and vomiting associated with cancer chemotherapy; postoperative nausea and vomiting

Dose
With chemotherapy: intravenous: three doses—0.15 mg/kg first dose 30 minutes before chemotherapy, then 4 to 8 hours after first dose (may administer as 8 mg bolus, then 1 mg/hr continuous infusion with maximum dose of 32 mg/day). Perioperative nausea and vomiting: 2 to 4 mg.

Onset and Duration
Onset: variable; most effective if therapy begins before emetogenic chemotherapy. Peak effect: 1 to 1.5 hours. Duration: 12 to 24 hours.

Adverse Effects
Tachycardia, angina, dizziness, lightheadedness, headache, sedation, diarrhea, constipation, dry mouth, rash, bronchospasm, hypersensitivity reactions

Precautions and Contraindications
Use ondansetron with caution in pregnant or nursing women and in children younger than 3 years. Ondansetron is contraindicated in patients with hypersensitivity to the drug.

Anesthetic Considerations
Monitor cardiovascular status, especially in patients with a history of coronary artery disease.

OXYTOCIN (PITOCIN)

Classification
Oxytocic; lactation stimulant

Indications
Initiation or improvement of uterine contraction at term or after dilation of cervix and delivery of fetus; stimulation of letdown reflex in nursing mothers to relieve pain from breast engorgement

Dose
Administration of oxytocin is always via continuous intravenous infusion. Augmentation of labor: 10 units (1 mL) diluted in 1000 mL of infusate; infusion rates vary from 1 to 10 milliunits/min.

Minimizing of postpartum bleeding: 20 to 100 milliunits/min; effects appear within 3 minutes, are maximal at about 20 minutes and disappear within 15 to 20 minutes after discontinuing the infusion. In practical terms, 20 to 40 units is usually added to 1000 mL of fluid and is administered to effect.

Promotion of milk ejection: nasal: 1 spray or drop in one or both nostrils 2 to 3 minutes before nursing or pumping the breasts

Onset and Duration
Onset: intravenous: immediate; nasal: a few minutes; intramuscular: 3 to 5 minutes. Peak effect: intravenous: less than 20 minutes; intramuscular: 40 minutes. Duration: intravenous: 20 minutes to 1 hour; nasal: 20 minutes; intramuscular: 2 to 3 hours.

Adverse Effects
Hypersensitivity leading to uterine hypertonicity, tetanic contractions, uterine rupture, cardiac arrhythmias, nausea and vomiting, hypertension, subarachnoid hemorrhage, seizures from water intoxication, hyponatremia

Precautions and Contraindications
Use it with caution with other vasoactive drugs. Oxytocin is contraindicated in patients with hypersensitivity to the drug. Oxytocin is also contraindicated in complications of pregnancy: significant cephalopelvic disproportion, fetal distress in which delivery is not imminent, prematurity, placenta previa, or past history of uterine sepsis or of traumatic delivery. The nasal preparation is contraindicated during pregnancy.

Anesthetic Considerations
Administration should follow delivery of the fetus. Oxytocin may increase the pressor effects of sympathomimetics. Prolonged intravenous infusion of oxytocin with excessive fluid volume may cause severe water intoxication with seizures, coma, and death. Infuse oxytocin intravenously only after dilution in large volume, preferably with an infusion pump.

PALONESETRON (ALOXI)

Classification
Antiemetic; serotonin receptor antagonist

Indication
Postoperative nausea and vomiting

Dose
The recommended dose of palonestron is 0.025 to 0.075 mg intravenously.

Onset and Duration
Onset: 5 to 15 minutes. Duration: 24 to 72 hours

Adverse Effects
Headache, constipation, diarrhea, or dizziness may occur. Cardiac effects are similar to placebo.

Precautions and Contraindications
Palonosetron is contraindicated in patients known to have hypersensitivity to the drug or any of its components.

Anesthetic Considerations
Palonosetron can be distinguished from older 5-HT_3 receptor antagonists (ondansetron, dolasetron, and granisetron) by its unique chemical structure and substantially longer half-life (≈40 hr) and duration. Useful for initial and delayed postoperative nausea past 24 hours.

PANCURONIUM (PAVULON)

Classification
Nondepolarizing skeletal muscle relaxant

Indications
Adjunct to general anesthesia; skeletal muscle relaxation during surgery

Dose
Intravenous paralyzing: 0.04 to 0.1 mg/kg; pretreatment or maintenance: 0.01 to 0.02 mg/kg.

Dosage forms: injection: 1 mg/mL in 10-mL vial; ampule: 2 mg/mL

Onset and Duration
Onset: 1 to 3 minutes. Duration: 40 to 65 minutes

Adverse Effects
Tachycardia, hypertension, hypoventilation, apnea, bronchospasm, salivation, flushing, anaphylactoid reactions, inadequate block, prolonged block

Precautions and Contraindications
Pancuronium is contraindicated in patients with myasthenia gravis, bromide hypersensitivity, and conditions in which tachycardia is undesirable.

Anesthetic Considerations
Pretreatment doses of pancuronium may cause hypoventilation in some patients. Monitor the patient's response with a peripheral nerve stimulator. Reverse the effects with anticholinesterase.

PHENTOLAMINE (REGITINE)

Classification
α-Adrenergic blocker

Indications

Controlled hypotension; treatment of perioperative hypertensive crisis that may accompany pheochromocytoma removal; prevention or treatment of dermal necrosis or sloughing after intravenous administration or extravasation of barbiturate or sympathomimetic

Dose

Antihypertensive: intravenous or intramuscular: 2.5 to 5 mg. Antisloughing infiltration: 5 to 10 mg (maximum dose: 10 mg); dilute in 10 mL normal saline.

Dosage forms: injection: 5 mg/mL; dilution for infusion 200 mg in 100 mL D_5W or normal saline

Onset and Duration

Onset: intravenous: 1 to 2 minutes; intramuscular: 5 to 20 minutes. Duration: intravenous: 10 to 15 minutes; intramuscular: 30 to 45 minutes.

Adverse Effects

Hypotension, tachycardia, arrhythmias, myocardial infarction, dizziness, cerebrovascular spasm and occlusion, flushing, diarrhea, nausea and vomiting

Precautions and Contraindications

Use it with caution in patients with ischemic heart disease. Phentolamine-induced α-receptor blockade will potentiate β_2-adrenergic vasodilation of epinephrine, ephedrine, dobutamine, or isoproterenol.

Anesthetic Considerations

Use it with epinephrine, ephedrine, dobutamine, or isoproterenol. Phentolamine may cause a fall in blood pressure.

PHENYLEPHRINE (NEO-SYNEPHRINE)

Classification

Synthetic noncatecholamine; α-adrenergic agonist

Indications

Vasoconstriction; treatment of hypotension, shock, supraventricular tachyarrhythmias; prolongation of duration of local anesthetics

Dose

Intravenous: 10 to 100 mcg; do not exceed 0.5 mg initial dose or repeat sooner than 15 minutes. Intravenous infusion: 20 to 50 mcg/min; titrate to effect.

Onset and Duration

Onset: immediate. Duration: 15 to 20 minutes

Adverse Effects

Reflex bradycardia, arrhythmias, hypertension, headache, restlessness, reflex vagal action

Precautions and Contraindications

Use phenylephrine with extreme caution in elderly patients and patients with hyperthyroidism, bradycardia, partial heart block, or severe arteriosclerosis.

Anesthetic Considerations

Infuse phenylephrine into a large vein; treat extravasation with phentolamine (5-10 mg in 10 mL of normal saline, or sympathetic block, or both).

PHENYTOIN (DILANTIN)

Classification

Anticonvulsant

Indications

Convulsions; treatment of cardiac arrhythmias from digitalis intoxication, ventricular tachycardia, and paroxysmal atrial tachycardia resistant to conventional methods; treatment of migraine or trigeminal neuralgia

Dose

- Anticonvulsant: intravenous: 10 to 15 mg/kg in 50 to 100 mL of normal saline at a rate not exceeding 50 mg/min or 1.5 g/24 hr. Maintenance: intravenous or oral: 100 mg every 6 to 8 hours or 300 to 400 mg once a day.
- Antiarrhythmic: intravenous: 1.5 mg/kg slow push every 5 minutes until arrhythmia is suppressed or undesirable effects appear (maximum dose: 10 to 15 mg/kg/day)
- Children: anticonvulsant: loading dose 10 to 15 mg/kg, 1 g intravenous piggyback in normal saline up to 20 mg/kg in 24 hours. Oral maintenance: 4 to 8 mg/kg daily in two to three equally divided doses.

Dosage forms: injection: 50 mg/mL; capsules and extended-release capsules: 30, 100 mg; chewable tablets: 50 mg; oral suspension: 30 mg/5 mL, 125 mg/5 mL

Onset and Duration

Onset: intravenous: 3 to 5 minutes. Therapeutic levels: 10 to 20 mcg/mL; can be attained in 1 to 2 hours after appropriate loading. Elimination half-life: highly variable; increases as plasma levels increase; ranges from 8 to 60 hours (average: 22 hours). Patients with liver disease may have highly variable clearance because of saturation kinetics. Duration: 8 to 24 hours, depending on dose.

Adverse Effects

Often dose related: nausea and vomiting, gum hyperplasia, megaloblastic anemia (from folate deficiency), osteomalacia (with long-term therapy), thrombocytopenia, granulocytopenia, toxic hepatitis; rarely, exfoliative dermatitis, Stevens-Johnson syndrome, systemic lupus erythematosus; nystagmus (blood level greater than 20 mcg/mL), ataxia (blood level greater than 30 mcg/mL), and somnolence (blood level greater than 40 mcg/mL)

At rates exceeding 50 mg/min, hypotension, cardiovascular collapse, and central nervous system depression may occur.

Precautions and Contraindications

- If a rash occurs during therapy, phenytoin should be discontinued; if the rash is exfoliative, purpuric, or bullous or if systemic lupus erythematosus or Stevens-Johnson syndrome is suspected, phenytoin should not be restarted.
- Phenytoin will precipitate in all solutions other than normal saline. Flush the line before and after administration. Do not mix phenytoin

with other drugs. Phenytoin must be administered within 1 hour of mixing owing to short stability.
- Plasma levels should be monitored during therapy after a steady state is achieved and whenever toxicity is suspected.
- Phenytoin should be administered intravenously only with extreme caution in patients with respiratory depression or myocardial depression. Intravenous use is contraindicated in patients with sinus bradycardia, sinoatrial block, second- or third-degree atrioventricular block, or Adams-Stokes syndrome. Phenytoin is not useful in infantile febrile seizures.
- Abrupt withdrawal in patients with epilepsy may precipitate status epilepticus.
- Phenytoin is highly protein bound and has multiple drug interactions. Serum levels may be increased by diazepam, theophylline, warfarin, cimetidine, acute alcohol intake, and halothane. Serum levels are decreased by chronic alcoholism.

Anesthetic Considerations

Phenytoin treatment may increase the dose requirements for all nondepolarizing muscle relaxants except atracurium. Dose-response curves are shifted to the right, and the duration is markedly reduced.

Phenytoin follows Michaelis-Menten kinetics. A small incremental dose can radically increase free drug levels at equilibrium.

PHYSOSTIGMINE SALICYLATE (ANTILIRIUM)

Classification

Anticholinesterase agent

Indications

Reversal of prolonged somnolence and anticholinergic poisoning

Dose

Intravenous or intramuscular: 0.5 to 2 mg (10-20 mcg/kg) at rate of 1 mg/min; repeat dosing at intervals of 10 to 30 minutes

Onset and Duration

Onset: intravenous or intramuscular: 3 to 8 minutes. Duration: intravenous or intramuscular: 30 minutes to 5 hours.

Adverse Effects

Bradycardia, bronchospasm, dyspnea, respiratory paralysis, seizures, salivation, nausea and vomiting, miosis

Precautions and Contraindications

High doses of physostigmine may cause tremors, ataxia, muscle fasciculations, and ultimately a depolarization block. Use it with caution in patients with epilepsy, parkinsonian syndrome, or bradycardia. Do not use it in the presence of asthma, diabetes, or mechanical obstruction of the intestine or urogenital tract or in patients receiving choline esters or depolarizing muscle relaxants.

Anesthetic Considerations

Rapid intravenous administration may cause bradycardia and hypersalivation, leading to respiratory problems or possibly seizures. Treatment of cholinergic crisis includes mechanical ventilation with repeated bronchial aspiration and intravenous administration of atropine, 2 to 4 mg every 3 to 10 minutes until muscarinic symptoms disappear or until signs of atropine overdose appear.

PRILOCAINE HCL (CITANEST)

Classification
Amide-type local anesthetic

Indications
Regional anesthesia: infiltration or peripheral nerve block, topical, epidural, intravenous regional

Dose
Infiltration or peripheral nerve block: 0.5 to 6 mg/kg (0.5%-2% solution); topical: 0.6 to 3 mg/kg (2%-4% solution); epidural: 200 to 300 mg (1%-2% solution); (maximum dose: 6 mg/kg without epinephrine; 9 mg/kg with epinephrine 1:200,000).

Onset and Duration
Onset: infiltration: 1 to 2 minutes; epidural: 5 to 15 minutes. Peak effect: infiltration or epidural: less than 30 minutes. Duration: infiltration: 0.5 to 1.5 hours without epinephrine, 2 to 6 hours with epinephrine; epidural: 1 to 3 hours (prolonged with epinephrine).

Adverse Effects
Hypotension, arrhythmia, collapse, respiratory depression, paralysis, seizures, tinnitus, blurred vision, urticaria, anaphylactoid reactions, methemoglobinemia; high spinal: urinary retention, lower extremity weakness and paralysis, loss of sphincter control, headache, backache, slowing of labor

Precautions and Contraindications
Use it with caution in patients with hypovolemia, severe congestive heart failure, shock, all forms of heart block, or pregnancy. Prilocaine is contraindicated in patients with hypersensitivity to amide-type local anesthetics and in infants younger than 6 months (low dose may cause methemoglobinemia).

Anesthetic Considerations
Treat methemoglobinemia with methylene blue (1-2 mg/kg injected over 5 minutes). In intravenous regional blocks, deflate the cuff after 40 minutes and not before 20 minutes.

PROCAINAMIDE (PROCAN SR, PRONESTYL)

Classification
Class Ia antiarrhythmic

Indications
Treatment of lidocaine-resistant ventricular arrhythmias; arrhythmia control in malignant hyperthermia; treatment of atrial fibrillation or paroxysmal atrial tachycardia

Dose
Loading: slow intravenous push: 100 mg every 5 minutes (maximum dose: 500 mg); do not exceed 50 mg/min; children: 3 to 6 mg/kg administered over

5 minutes. Dilute 1000 mg in 50 mL D_5W. Intramuscular: 100 to 500 mg in doses divided every 3 or 6 hours. Maintenance: infusion: 2 to 6 mg/min; children: 0.02 to 0.08 mg/kg/min. Therapeutic level: 3 to 10 mcg/mL.

Dosage forms: injection: 100 mg/mL, 500 mg/mL. Dilution for infusion: 2 g in 500 mL D_5W (4 mg/mL).

Onset and Duration

Onset: intravenous: immediate; intramuscular: 10 to 30 minutes. Duration: 2.5 to 5 hours.

Adverse Effects

Hypotension, heart block, arrhythmias, seizures, confusion, depression, psychosis, anorexia, nausea and vomiting, diarrhea, systemic lupus erythematosus, pruritus, fever, chills

Precautions and Contraindications

Use it with caution in patients with first-degree heart block or arrhythmias associated with digitalis toxicity. Reduce doses in patients with congestive heart failure or renal failure. Procainamide is contraindicated in patients with complete heart block, torsades de pointes, or systemic lupus erythematosus.

Anesthetic Considerations

Procainamide requires periodic monitoring of patient plasma levels, vital signs, and electrocardiogram (QRS widening greater than 25% may signify overdosage). Procainamide potentiates the effect of both nondepolarizing and depolarizing muscle relaxants.

PROCAINE HCL (NOVOCAIN)

Classification

Ester-type local anesthetic

Indications

Local anesthetic: infiltration, peripheral nerve block, sympathetic nerve block, regional anesthesia

Dose

Infiltration: less than 500 mg (0.5%-2% solution); epidural: less than 500 mg (1%-2% solution); spinal: 50 to 200 mg (10% solution with glucose 5%). Solutions with preservatives may not be used for epidural or spinal block.

Onset and Duration

Onset: infiltration or spinal: 2 to 5 minutes; epidural: 5 to 25 minutes. Peak effect: infiltration, epidural, or spinal: less than 30 minutes. Duration: infiltration: 0.25 to 0.5 hours (without epinephrine), 0.5 to 1.5 hours (with epinephrine); epidural or spinal: 0.5 to 1.5 hours (prolonged with epinephrine).

Adverse Effects

Hypotension, bradycardia, arrhythmias, heart block, respiratory depression or arrest, tinnitus, seizures, dizziness, restlessness, loss of hearing, euphoria, postspinal headache, palsies, urticaria, pruritus, angioneurotic edema; high spinal: loss of bladder and bowel control, and permanent motor, sensory, and autonomic (sphincter control) deficits of lower segments

Precautions and Contraindications

Use it with caution in patients with severe cardiac disturbances (heart block, arrhythmias) or inflammation or sepsis at the injection site. Procaine is contraindicated in patients with hypersensitivity to para-aminobenzoic acid or parabens or ester-type anesthetics.

Anesthetic Considerations

Central nervous system effects are generally dose dependent and of short duration. Vasopressors and oxytocics may cause hypertension. Preparations containing preservatives should not be used for epidural and spinal anesthesia.

PROCHLORPERAZINE MALEATE (COMPAZINE)

Classification

Antiemetic; psychotherapeutic; phenothiazine antipsychotic

Indications

Control of nausea and vomiting; management of manifestations of psychotic disorders of excessive anxiety, tension, and agitation

Dose

Antiemetic: oral: 5 to 10 mg three or four times daily; rectal: 25 mg twice daily; intravenous or intramuscular: 5 to 10 mg (5 mg/mL/min) (maximum dose: 40 mg/day). Do not administer subcutaneously because of local irritation.

Onset and Duration

Onset: intravenous: a few minutes; intramuscular: 10 to 20 minutes; oral: 30 to 40 minutes; rectal: 60 minutes. Peak effect: intravenous, intramuscular, or oral: 15 to 30 minutes. Duration: intravenous, intramuscular, oral, or rectal: 3 to 4 hours.

Adverse Effects

Extrapyramidal reactions, dystonia, central nervous system depression, hypotension

Precautions and Contraindications

Prochlorperazine maleate is contraindicated in pediatric patients and in patients with parkinsonian disease.

Anesthetic Considerations

Prochlorperazine maleate may produce an additive central nervous system depression when it is used with anesthetics. Avoid using prochlorperazine maleate with droperidol or metoclopramide because of extrapyramidal effects.

PROMETHAZINE HCL (PHENERGAN, PENTAZINE, PHENAZINE, PROTHAZINE)

Classification

Phenothiazine: antiemetic, antivertigo agent, antihistamine (H_1-receptor antagonist), sedative, or adjunct to analgesics

Indications

Motion sickness or nausea; rhinitis; allergy symptoms; sedation; routine preoperative or postoperative sedation; adjunct to analgesics

Dose

Intravenous: administer cautiously because of hazard of phlebitis, necrosis, and gangrene of extremities; must dilute with equal volume of compatible diluent and administer slowly. Children: administer no larger dose than 0.5 mg/kg; intramuscular, oral, rectal: 12.5 to 50 mg. Do not administer subcutaneously or intraarterially because of the risk of necrosis and gangrene of extremities.

Dosage forms: tablet: 12.5, 25, and 50 mg; syrup: 6.25 and 25 mg/5 mL; suppositories: 12.5, 25, and 50 mg; injection: 25 and 50 mg/mL

Onset and Duration

Onset: intravenous: 150 seconds; intramuscular, oral, rectal: 15 to 30 minutes. Duration: intravenous, intramuscular, oral, rectal: 2 to 5 hours.

Adverse Effects

Hypotension, bradycardia, bronchospasm, drowsiness, sedation, dizziness, confusion, extrapyramidal reactions, agranulocytosis, thrombocytopenia

Precautions and Contraindications

Use it with caution because the central nervous system and circulatory depressant actions of alcohol, sedative-hypnotics, and anesthetics are potentiated. Promethazine is contraindicated in patients with Parkinson's disease and in those receiving monoamine oxidase inhibitors.

Anesthetic Considerations

Anesthetic recovery may be prolonged. Do not use in children younger than 2 years.

PROPOFOL (DIPRIVAN; GENERIC FORMULATIONS ALSO AVAILABLE)

Classification

Anesthesia induction agent

Indications

Anesthesia induction and maintenance; intravenous sedation; prolonged sedation in critical care

Dose

Intravenous bolus: 1 to 2.5 mg/kg. Dilute in suitable intravenous fluid, preferably D_5W. Do not dilute the final solution to less than 2 mg/mL to protect the suspension. Do not use any filter with a pore size smaller than 5 mm. Infusion: 25 to 200 mcg/kg/min.

Dosage forms: 10 mg/mL in 20-mL ampules and 50- and 100-mL vials.

Onset and Duration

Onset: immediate; duration: 5 to 20 minutes, depending on dose

Adverse Effects

Hypotension, bradycardia, respiratory depression, prolonged somnolence, vivid dreams, burning on injection, hiccups, disinhibition, arrhythmias

Precautions and Contraindications

Reduce the propofol dose or avoid the drug in patients with cardiac compromise; in elderly patients; and in those with respiratory disease, hypotension, or increased intracranial pressure. Watch for respiratory and cardiac depression when coadministering other central nervous system or cardiac depressant drugs. Strict aseptic technique must be used when handling the drug to avoid bacterial growth in the emulsion vehicle. The generic formulation contains metabisulfate and should be avoided in patients sensitive to these compounds. Infusion of doses larger than 5 mg/kg/hr for longer than 48 hours may result in propofol emulsion syndrome.

Anesthetic Considerations

Minimize pain on injection by giving a small dose of plain lidocaine (1%) before propofol injection. Both convulsant and anticonvulsant effects have been reported, so do not use propofol in patients with a history of seizures. The antiemetic properties of propofol may be an advantage in patients at risk for postoperative nausea and vomiting.

PROPRANOLOL (INDERAL, OTHERS)

Classification

Nonselective β-adrenergic receptor antagonist

Indications

Hypertension; angina; ventricular and supraventricular arrhythmias; hyperthyroidism; migraines

Dose

Intravenous: 0.25-mg increments, up to 3 mg; oral: 10 to 80 mg every 6 to 8 hours or 80 to 240 mg/day sustained release

Dosage forms: injection: 1 mg/mL (1 mL); tablet: 10, 20, 40, 60, 80, 90 mg

Onset and Duration

Onset: intravenous: less than 2 minutes; oral: 30 to 60 minutes. Duration: intravenous: 1 to 4 hours; oral: up to 24 hours sustained release.

Adverse Effects

Bradycardia, hypotension, atrioventricular block, bronchospasm, hypoglycemia, claudication, diarrhea, nausea, vomiting, constipation, nightmares, mental depression, insomnia, increased plasma triglycerides and decreased high-density lipoproteins

Precautions and Contraindications

Propranolol is contraindicated in patients with asthma and in patients with reduced myocardial reserve, peripheral vascular disease, diabetes, congestive heart failure, or shock. If the drug is discontinued abruptly, withdrawal may be manifested as increased nervousness, increased heart rate, increased intensity of angina, or increased blood pressure (related to upregulation). The effects of propranolol may be potentiated by inhalational anesthetics and other cardiodepressant drugs.

Anesthetic Considerations

Esmolol is preferred over propranolol for intraoperative use because of its more controllable duration of action. Propranolol may be useful as an antiarrhythmic because of its membrane-stabilizing properties.

PROTAMINE SULFATE

Classification

Heparin antagonist

Indications

Treatment of heparin overdosage; heparin neutralization after extracorporeal circulation in arterial and cardiovascular surgery

Dose

Dosage is based on blood coagulation studies, usually 1 mg protamine for every 100 units of heparin remaining in the patient, administered slowly by intravenous over 10 minutes in doses not to exceed 50 mg.

Because heparin blood concentrations decrease rapidly, the required dose of protamine sulfate decreases based on the elapsed time. Half of the usual dose of protamine should be administered if 30 minutes have elapsed since heparin administration and one-fourth of the usual dose should be administered if 2 hours or more has elapsed.

Dosage forms: parenteral injection for intravenous use only: 10-mg/mL, 5-mL ampule or vial. Reconstitute a 50-mg vial by adding 5 mL of sterile water or bacteriostatic water containing 0.9% benzyl alcohol. The resultant solution contains 10 mg/mL. A protamine solution is intended for intravenous bolus use and not for further dilution. If further dilution is desired, however, 5% dextrose or 0.9% sodium chloride intravenous piggyback may be used and administered over 30 minutes.

Children: injections preserved with benzyl alcohol may cause toxicity in neonates.

Onset and Duration

Onset: neutralization of heparin occurs within 5 minutes. Duration: neutralization of heparin persists for approximately 2 hours.

Adverse Effects

Rapid intravenous injection: hypotension, bradycardia, flushing; other possible effects: hypersensitivity, anaphylaxis, dyspnea, noncardiac pulmonary edema, circulatory collapse, pulmonary hypertension, "heparin rebound" (in cardiopulmonary bypass).

A paradoxical anticoagulant effect may occur with total doses greater than 100 mg.

Precautions and Contraindications

Monitor the patient's activated partial thromboplastin time or the activated coagulation time at least 5 to 15 minutes after protamine administration to determine its effect. Have equipment readily available to treat shock. Patients with sensitivity to fish and patients who have previously received either protamine or insulins containing protamine are considered at higher risk for hypersensitivity. If protamine is used in these patients, pretreatment with a corticosteroid or antihistamine should be considered. Protamine is contraindicated in patients with a history of allergy to the drug.

Anesthetic Considerations

Rapid intravenous injection of protamine is associated with hypotension, bradycardia, and flushing.

PYRIDOSTIGMINE BROMIDE (MESTINON)

Classification

Anticholinesterase agent

Indication

Reversal of nondepolarizing muscle relaxants

Dose

Reversal: intravenous: 10 to 30 mg (0.1-0.25 mg/kg), preceded by atropine (0.015 mg/kg) or glycopyrrolate (0.01 mg/kg) intravenously. Myasthenia gravis: oral: 60 to 1500 mg/day; sustained release: 180 to 540 mg daily or twice daily. To supplement oral dosage preoperatively and postoperatively, during labor and postpartum, during myasthenic crisis, or when oral therapy is impractical: administer 1/30 the oral dose intramuscularly or very slowly intravenously.

Neonates of myasthenic mothers: 0.05 to 0.15 mg/kg intramuscularly. Differentiate between cholinergic and myasthenic crisis in neonates. Administration 1 hour before completion of the second stage of labor enables patients to have adequate strength during labor and provides protection to infants in the intermediate postnatal stage.

Onset and Duration

Onset: reversal: intravenous: 2 to 5 minutes; myasthenia: intramuscular: less than 15 minutes; oral: 20 to 30 minutes. Duration: reversal: intravenous: 90 minutes; myasthenia: oral: 3 to 6 hours; intramuscular: 2 to 4 hours.

Adverse Effects

Bradycardia, atrioventricular block, nodal rhythm, hypotension, increased bronchial secretions, bronchospasm, respiratory depression, nausea, vomiting, diarrhea, abdominal cramps, increased peristalsis, increased salivation, muscle cramps, fasciculations, weakness, miosis, diaphoresis

Precautions and Contraindications

Use pyridostigmine with caution in patients with bradycardia, bronchial asthma, cardiac arrhythmias, or peptic ulcer and in patients with peritonitis or mechanical obstruction of the intestines or urinary tract.

Anesthetic Considerations

Overdosage of pyridostigmine may induce a cholinergic crisis characterized by nausea, vomiting, bradycardia or tachycardia, excessive salivation and sweating, bronchospasm, weakness, and paralysis. Treatment of a cholinergic crisis includes discontinuation of pyridostigmine and administration of atropine (10 mg/kg intravenously every 3-10 minutes until muscarinic symptoms disappear).

RANITIDINE (ZANTAC)

Classification
Histamine (H_2)-receptor antagonist

Indications
Treatment of duodenal or gastric ulcers and gastroesophageal reflux; prophylaxis of aspiration pneumonitis in patients at high risk during surgery

Dose
For patients with normal renal function: 50 mg by intravenous piggyback diluted in at least 25 mL D_5W, normal saline, or suitable diluent, administered over 15 to 20 minutes at least 1 hour before induction of anesthesia. The drug may be administered with or without a similar dose the preceding evening. For patients with impaired renal function, as evidenced by creatinine clearance less than 50 mL/min: single dose only is needed 1 to 4 hours before induction of anesthesia.

Alternatively, 150 mg ranitidine orally may be substituted for 50 mg by intravenous piggyback. When administered orally, however, it is recommended to be administered 2 hours preinduction.

Children 2 to 18 years: 0.1 to 0.8 mg/kg/dose by intravenous piggyback at least 1 hour before induction infused over at least 5 minutes. Dilute to concentration of 0.5 to 2.5 mg/mL.

Dosage forms: 150-mg tablets; parenteral injection: 25 mg/mL in 2-mL or 10-mL multidose vials

Onset and Duration
Onset: mean gastric acid concentration significantly decreases 1 hour after intravenous infusion. Duration: gastric acid inhibitory effects persist 8 to 12 hours.

Adverse Effects
Most frequent: headache, fatigue, dizziness, mild gastrointestinal disturbances; infrequent: reversible hepatitis and potential hepatotoxicity; rarely: reversible leukopenia, thrombocytopenia, granulocytopenia, aplastic anemia

Bradydysrhythmias and hypotension may be associated with rapid intravenous infusion.

Precautions and Contraindications
Use ranitidine with caution in patients with hypersensitivity to ranitidine or other H_2-receptor antagonists. Caution is suggested in patients with hepatic insufficiency.

Anesthetic Considerations
Ranitidine is useful for gastric preparation in high-risk surgical patients prone to aspiration. Do not use in non–high-risk patients.

REMIFENTANIL (ULTIVA)

Classification
Opiate analgesic

Indication
Perioperative analgesia

Dose

Infusion only: induction: 0.5 to 1 mcg/kg/min; maintenance: 0.05 to 0.8 mcg/kg/min; postoperative pain in postanesthesia care unit: 0.025 to 0.2 mcg/kg/min

Supplemental bolus of 0.05 mcg/kg may be administered during induction and maintenance. Supplemental bolus is not recommended postoperatively because of the risk of apnea or significant respiratory depression. Changes in infusion rate take 2 to 5 minutes for clinical response to change.

Dosage forms: 1 mg powder in 3-mL vial; 2 mg powder in 5-mL vial; 5 mg powder in 10-mL vial

Onset and Duration

Onset: 1 to 5 minutes. Duration: continuous infusion effect ceases 5 to 15 minutes after infusion is stopped

Adverse Effects

Similar to those of other opiate agonists and include nausea and vomiting, hypotension, bradycardia, respiratory depression, apnea, muscle rigidity, pruritus

Precautions and Contraindications

Oxygen saturation should be continuously monitored throughout remifentanil administration. Resuscitative and airway management equipment must be immediately available. Remifentanil should not be mixed with lactated Ringer injection or lactated Ringer's/D_5W but can be coadministered with these solutions in a freely running intravenous line. Do not run remifentanil in the same line with blood because this drug is metabolized by esterase enzymes. The intravenous line should be cleared after discontinuation to prevent inadvertent administration. Remifentanil is contraindicated for epidural or intrathecal administration because of glycine in the vehicle formulation.

Anesthetic Considerations

The effects of remifentanil rapidly dissipate after discontinuation of the infusion, so preparation for postoperative care may include longer acting opiates or nonsteroidal anti-inflammatory agents. Because remifentanil is metabolized by nonspecific esterases, no change in kinetics has been noted in patients with cholinesterase deficiencies or renal or hepatic disease. Normal kinetics have been noted in pediatric, geriatric, and obese patients.

ROCURONIUM (ZEMURON)

Classification

Nondepolarizing neuromuscular blocking agent

Indications

Tracheal intubation and intraoperative skeletal muscle relaxation; in critical care, facilitation of mechanical ventilation

Dose

Adults and children: intubation: 0.6 to 1.0 mg/kg. Maintenance: adults: 0.1 to 0.2 mg/kg; children: 0.08 to 0.12 mg/kg intravenously.

Onset and Duration

Onset: 60 to 90 seconds with intubating doses of three to five times the 95% effective dose (0.9-1.5 mg/kg; 95% effective dose: 0.3 mg/kg). Duration: 30 to 120 minutes, depending on the dose.

Adverse Effects

Rare: prolonged effect in patients with hepatic disease

Precautions and Contraindications

Rocuronium is contraindicated in patients known to have hypersensitivity to the drug. Proper airway maintenance capabilities must be ensured before administration.

Anesthetic Considerations

Use of inhalation agents, antibiotics, and magnesium may prolong the duration of action of rocuronium. Many clinicians consider it the agent of choice for nondepolarizing rapid sequence induction when intubating doses are used. No significant cardiac or histamine-releasing effects occur with clinical doses of rocuronium.

ROPIVACAINE HCL (NAROPIN)

Classification

Amide-type local anesthetic

Indications

Regional anesthesia: epidural, peripheral nerve block; local infiltration

Dose

Epidural: 75 to 250 mg (0.2%-0.5% solution); obstetric: less than 150 mg (0.5% solution); infiltration: less than 200 mg (0.2%-0.5% solution); peripheral nerve block: less than 275 mg (0.5% solution). Spinal doses have not been established. Do not exceed 770 mg in 24 hours.

Onset and Duration

Onset: epidural: 5 to 13 minutes; obstetrics: 11 to 26 minutes; infiltration: 1 to 5 minutes; peripheral nerve block: 10 to 45 minutes. Duration: epidural: 3 to 5 hours; obstetrics: 1.7 to 3.2 hours; infiltration: 2 to 6 hours; peripheral nerve block: 3.7 to 8.7 hours.

Adverse Effects

Hypotension, nausea and vomiting, bradycardia, paresthesia, fetal bradycardia, back pain, chills, fever, headache, pain, dizziness, pruritus, urinary retention, arrhythmias, seizures

Precautions and Contraindications

Reduce ropivacaine doses in debilitated, elderly, or acutely ill patients and in children. Use it with caution in patients with hypotension, hypovolemia, or heart block. Ropivacaine is not for use in paracervical, retrobulbar, intravenous regional, or subarachnoid blocks. It is contraindicated in patients with hypersensitivity to amide-type local anesthetics.

Anesthetic Considerations

Considerations with ropivacaine are similar to those with bupivacaine but with less depth and duration of the motor blockade. Its use with epinephrine has only a minor effect on onset and duration.

SALMETEROL XINAFOATE (SEREVENT)

Classification

β_2-Adrenergic agonist, antiasthmatic, bronchodilator

Indications

Maintenance treatment of asthma and chronic obstructive pulmonary disease (COPD); prevention of bronchospasm

Dose

Powder: one inhalation (50 mcg) twice daily (morning and evening 12 hours apart); aerosol: two inhalations (42 mcg) twice daily (morning and evening 12 hours apart)

Onset and Duration

Asthma maintenance: onset to produce bronchodilation: 10 to 20 minutes. Duration: 12 hours. COPD: onset to bronchodilation: within 30 minutes. Duration: up to 12 hours.

Adverse Effects

Sympathomimetic cardiovascular effects, ventricular arrhythmias, electrocardiographic changes (flattening of the T wave, prolonged Q-T interval, ST-segment depression), laryngospasm, stridor, excitement, aggravation of diabetes mellitus and ketoacidosis

Precautions and Contraindications

Use it with caution in patients with hypersensitivity to salmeterol, acute deteriorating asthma, coronary insufficiency, arrhythmias, hypertension, convulsive disorders, or thyrotoxicosis. Safety of salmeterol during pregnancy and in children has not been established. Use it with extreme caution in patients taking monoamine oxidase inhibitors or tricyclic antidepressants—cardiovascular sympathomimetic effects may be potentiated under these circumstances.

Anesthetic Considerations

Use of β-antagonists may block the effects of salmeterol and may predispose patients to bronchospasm. Dosing intervals of less than 12 hours may induce bronchospasm.

SCOPOLAMINE (TRANSDERM SCŌP)

Classification

Competitive acetylcholine antagonist at muscarinic receptor, antiemetic

Indications

Prevention and treatment of nausea and vomiting induced by motion (motion sickness), premedication, amnesia, sedation, or vagolysis

It produces greater sedation and amnesia and has greater antisialagogue and ocular effects than does atropine with lesser effects on the heart, bronchial smooth muscle, and gastrointestinal tract.

Dose

For postoperative nausea and vomiting, apply one patch the evening before surgery or 1 hour before cesarean section. Keep in place for 24 hr. Apply patch to hairless area behind the ear. Do not cut patch in half.

Dosage forms: patch: 0.33 mg/24 hr

Onset and Duration

Transdermal systems are designed to provide an antiemetic effect within 4 hours of application with a duration of up to 72 hours.

Adverse Effects

Hallucinations, delirium coma in central anticholinergic syndrome (treatment: pyridostigmine, 15 to 60 mg/kg); other effects: paradoxical bradycardia in low doses, mydriasis, blurred vision, tachycardia, drowsiness, restlessness, confusion, anaphylaxis, dry nose and mouth, constipation, urinary hesitancy, retention, increased intraocular pressure, decreased sweating

Children and elderly patients are more susceptible to adverse effects.

Precautions and Contraindications

Use scopolamine with caution when tachycardia would be harmful (i.e., thyrotoxicosis, pheochromocytoma, coronary artery disease). Avoid using scopolamine in patients in hyperpyrexial states because it inhibits sweating. Use it with caution in patients with hepatic or renal disease, congestive heart failure, chronic pulmonary disease (because a reduction in bronchial secretions may lead to formation of bronchial plugs), hiatal hernia, gastroesophageal reflux, gastrointestinal infections, or ulcerative colitis. Scopolamine is contraindicated in patients with acute-angle glaucoma, obstructive disease of the gastrointestinal tract, obstructive uropathy, intestinal atony, or acute hemorrhage when cardiovascular status is unstable.

Anesthetic Considerations

Scopolamine potentiates the sedative effects of narcotics, benzodiazepines, anticholinergics, antihistamines, and volatile anesthetics.

SEVOFLURANE (ULTANE)

Classification

Inhalation anesthetic

Indication

General anesthesia

Dose

Titrate to effect for induction or maintenance of anesthesia. Minimum alveolar concentration: 2%.

Dosage forms: volatile liquid

Onset and Duration

Onset: loss of eyelid reflex: 1 to 2 minutes. Duration: emergence time: 8 to 9 minutes.

Adverse Effects

Hypotension; arrhythmia; respiratory depression; apnea; dizziness; euphoria; increased cerebral blood flow and intracranial pressure; nausea; vomiting; ileus; malignant hyperthermia

Precautions and Contraindications

Sevoflurane is contraindicated in patients with known or suspected genetic susceptibility to malignant hyperthermia. It causes significant increases in free fluoride ion. Some practitioners avoid it in patients with overt renal disease. Sevoflurane reacts with carbon dioxide granulates in the anesthesia machine to produce compound A. A rare fire hazard has been reported when using Sevoflurane under certain anesthesia machine conditions.

Anesthetic Considerations

Sevoflurane is the mostly commonly used inhalation anesthetic in pediatric patients. It is safe and effective for inhalation anesthetic induction. A short period of restlessness upon emergence may occur.

SODIUM CITRATE (BICITRA)

Classification

Nonparticulate neutralizing buffer

Indications

Prophylaxis of aspiration pneumonitis during anesthesia (metabolizes to sodium bicarbonate and thus acts as systemic alkalinizer)

When administered within 60 minutes of surgery, sodium citrate is effective in raising the gastric pH to more than 2.5 in most patients. Theoretically, this decreases the risk of pulmonary damage secondary to aspiration of gastric contents; however, this remains controversial.

Dose

Adults: 15 mL diluted in 15 mL water as a single dose; children: 5 to 15 mL diluted in 5 to 15 mL water as a single dose, or 1 mEq/kg as a single dose.

Dosage forms: sodium citrate dihydrate 500 mg (321.5 mg of citrate)/ 5 mL and citric acid monohydrate 334 mg/5 mL. Each 1 mL contains 1 mEq sodium and 1 mEq citrate.

Onset and Duration

Onset: 2 to 10 minutes. Duration: 60 to 90 minutes. Maximally effective when administered less than 60 minutes preoperatively.

Adverse Effects

Saline laxative effect (when sodium citrate is administered orally); metabolic alkalosis (in large doses in patients with renal dysfunction)

Precautions and Contraindications

Sodium citrate is contraindicated in patients with severe renal impairment with oliguria, azotemia, or anuria. It is also contraindicated in patients with

Addison disease, heat cramps, acute dehydration, adynamic episodica hereditaria, or severe myocardial disease.

Anesthetic Considerations

Sodium citrate is useful for patients at a high risk of aspiration.

SOMATOSTATIN (ZECNIL)

Classification

Synthetic somatostatin; growth hormone release–inhibiting factor; also inhibitor of glucagon, insulin, secretin, gastrin, and thyroid-stimulating hormone

Indications

Prophylaxis in preoperative management of patients with carcinoid syndrome and treatment of hypotensive episodes associated with surgical manipulation of carcinoid tumor, gastrointestinal bleeding, malignant diarrhea, enterocutaneous and pancreatic fistulas, and short bowel syndrome

Epidural somatostatin is effective in treating postoperative pain; intrathecal and intraventricular somatostatin were used for the pain of terminal cancer in limited studies.

Dose

Adults: continuous infusion required to sustain therapeutic effects; usual infusion rate: 250 mcg/hr with or without initial 250-mcg bolus. Dilute 3 mg somatostatin in 50 mL D_5W or normal saline and infuse continuously over 12 hours (250 mcg/hr) on a syringe pump. Octreotide (Sandostatin), a long-acting analog of somatostatin, may also be used; the initial dose is 50 mcg subcutaneously, but intravenous injection can be used during an emergency.

Dosage forms: somatostatin (Zecnil): 3-mg lyophilized ampules; octreotide (Sandostatin): 0.1, 0.05, 0.5 mg/mL injection

Somatostatin is currently designated as an "orphan drug" by the Food and Drug Administration.

Onset and Duration

Onset: 5 to 10 minutes after initiation of infusion. Duration: effects decrease rapidly after discontinuance of infusion to baseline in 1 hour; plasma half-life: 1 to 3 minutes. Half-life of octreotide: after intravenous: 45 minutes; after subcutaneous: 80 minutes.

Adverse Effects

Nausea, vomiting, diarrhea, and abdominal cramps during infusion; glucose intolerance in nondiabetic patients and reduced insulin requirements in insulin-dependent diabetic patients; less frequent: arrhythmias, hyponatremia

Precautions and Contraindications

Use somatostatin with caution in patients with diabetes. Rebound hypersecretion of growth hormone and other hormones usually occurs after infusion is discontinued. Monitor blood glucose levels during therapy. Rebound fistula output is also noted in patients with enterocutaneous fistulas. Somatostatin is contraindicated in patients with previous hypersensitivity to the drug or with octreotide.

Anesthetic Considerations

Sandostatin is indicated for the symptomatic treatment of patients with metastatic carcinoid tumors in which it suppresses or inhibits the severe diarrhea and flushing episodes associated with the disease.

SOTALOL HYDROCHLORIDE (BETAPACE, SOTAGARD)

Classification

Antiarrhythmic, nonselective β-adrenergic blocking agent

Indications

Life-threatening ventricular arrhythmias (i.e., sustained ventricular tachycardia); torsade de pointes or ventricular tachycardia or fibrillation from nonsupraventricular tachycardia or supraventricular tachycardia arrhythmias; atrial fibrillation

Dose

Treatment of sustained ventricular tachycardia: adults: initially, 80 mg orally twice daily (maximum dose: 320 mg/day, administered in two divided doses).

Conversion and maintenance of sinus rhythm in patients with atrial fibrillation: adults: 80 to 160 mg orally twice daily; children: safety and efficacy have not been established.

Onset and Duration

Onset of action after oral administration: approximately 1 hour. Peak effect: 2.5 to 4 hours. Low lipid solubility; does not cross the blood-brain barrier. Duration: 4 to 6 hours.

Adverse Effects

Fatigue, bradycardia, dyspnea, angina, palpitations, dizziness, nausea and vomiting, asthenia, lightheadedness, elevated liver function tests

Overdosage rarely results in death. Treat by hemodialysis because of low protein binding.

Precautions and Contraindications

Patients with impaired renal function require dosage reductions. Sotalol is contraindicated in patients with bronchial asthma, bronchitis, sinus bradycardia, second- and third-degree atrioventricular block (may use if patient has functioning pacemaker), uncontrolled congestive heart failure, or cardiogenic shock.

Safety and efficacy have not been established in children. Adequate evaluation for use during pregnancy has not been established.

Anesthetic Considerations

Use sotalol with caution when using lidocaine or calcium channel blockers because the additive electrophysiologic effect may cause a proarrhythmic event.

SUCCINYLCHOLINE (ANECTINE, QUELICIN, OTHERS)

Classification

Depolarizing skeletal muscle relaxant

Indications

Surgical muscle relaxation for short procedures; facilitation of endotracheal intubation

Dose

Adults: intravenous: 1 to 1.5 mg/kg. Children: intravenous: 1 to 2 mg/kg; intramuscular: 2 to 4 mg/kg. Pretreat with atropine because of the incidence of bradycardia.

Dosage forms: injection: 20 mg/mL; powder for infusion: 500 mg (mix in 500 mL for 1 mg/mL solution)

Onset and Duration

Onset: immediate. Duration: 5 to 10 minutes

Adverse Effects

Effects related to the skeletal muscle depolarizing action of the drug: hyperkalemia, postoperative muscle pain, increased gastric pressure, increased intraocular pressure; cardiac arrhythmias: sudden cardiac arrest and bradycardia with repeat dosing or with any dose in children.

Prolonged paralysis and inadequate recovery may occur with infusion doses. Masseter muscle spasm may be a premonitory sign of malignant hyperthermia along with sudden unexplained tachycardia or an abrupt increase in carbon dioxide elimination.

Precautions and Contraindications

Succinylcholine should not be used for routine intubation in children younger than 12 years because of reports of sudden cardiac arrest in children with undiagnosed Duchenne muscular dystrophy and with muscle disorders. Succinylcholine is contraindicated in patients with malignant hyperthermia, genetic variants of plasma cholinesterase or cholinesterase deficiencies, myopathies associated with elevated creatine phosphokinase values, muscle disorders or muscular dystrophies, acute narrow-angle glaucoma, severe muscle trauma or muscle wasting, neurologic injury (i.e., paraplegia, quadriplegia, spinal cord injury, or cerebrovascular accident), hyperkalemia, severe sepsis, electrolyte imbalances, or third-degree burns over more than 25% total body surface. Repeated doses at short intervals (less than 5 minutes) are associated with bradycardia.

Anesthetic Considerations

Side effects are usually short lived because of the short duration of action of the drug. More serious side effects are addressed symptomatically. Remains the drug of choice for rapid-sequence induction in patients without contraindications.

SUFENTANIL CITRATE (SUFENTA)

Classification

Opioid agonist; produces analgesia and anesthesia

Indication

Perioperative analgesia

Dose

Analgesia: intravenous or intramuscular: 0.2 to 0.6 mcg/kg. Induction: intravenous: 2 to 10 mcg/kg; infusion: 0.01 to 0.05 mcg/kg/min. Epidural: bolus: 0.2 to 0.6 mcg/kg; infusion: 5 to 30 mcg/hr (0.2-0.6 mcg/kg/hr). Spinal: 0.02 to 0.08 mcg/kg.

Onset and Duration

Onset: intravenous: immediate; epidural and spinal: 4 to 10 minutes. Duration: intravenous: 20 to 45 minutes; intramuscular: 2 to 4 hours; epidural and spinal: 4 to 8 hours.

Adverse Effects

Hypotension, bradycardia, respiratory depression, apnea, dizziness, sedation, euphoria, dysphoria, anxiety, nausea and vomiting, delayed gastric emptying, biliary tract spasm, muscle rigidity

Precautions and Contraindications

Reduce the sufentanil dose in elderly, hypovolemic, or high-risk surgical patients and in patients taking sedatives or other narcotics. Sufentanil crosses the placental barrier; if it is used during labor, respiratory depression may result in a neonate.

Anesthetic Considerations

The narcotic effect of sufentanil is reversed with naloxone (intravenously, 0.2-0.4 mg). The duration of reversal may be shorter than the duration of the narcotic effect. The circulatory and ventilatory depressant effects of sufentanil are potentiated by other narcotics, sedatives, nitrous oxide, and volatile anesthetics; its ventilatory depressant effects are potentiated by monoamine oxidase inhibitors, phenothiazines, and tricyclic antidepressants. Analgesia is enhanced by α_2-agonists. The skeletal muscle rigidity associated with higher doses of sufentanil is sufficient to interfere with ventilation. Increased incidences of bradycardia occur with the additional use of vecuronium.

TERBUTALINE SULFATE (BRETHINE, BRETHAIRE, BRICANYL)

Classification

β_2-Adrenergic agonist, bronchodilator

Indications

Bronchodilator for treatment of asthma; tocolytic agent

Dose

Bronchodilator: subcutaneous: 0.25 mg (may repeat in 15-30 minutes; maximum dose: 0.5 mg in 4-6 hours); inhalation: two breaths separated by 60 seconds every 4 to 6 hours; oral: 5 mg three times daily (2.5-5 mg every 6 hours; maximum dose: 15 mg/day).

Children younger than 12 years: oral: 0.05 mg/kg/dose three times daily (maximum dose: 0.15 mg/kg/dose or 5 mg/day); subcutaneous: 5 to 10 mcg/kg/dose every 20 minutes for three doses.

Dosage forms: injection: 1 mg/mL (1 mL); tablet: 2.5, 5 mg.

Onset and Duration

Onset: subcutaneous: 30 to 60 minutes; oral: 2 to 3 hours; inhalation: 1 to 2 hours. Duration: subcutaneous: 1 to 4 hours; oral: 4 to 8 hours; inhalation: 2 to 6 hours.

Adverse Effects

Similar to those of other β-agonists: hypertension, tachycardia, arrhythmias, tremors, dizziness, headache, nausea and vomiting, gastrointestinal upset, hypokalemia, hyperglycemia

Precautions and Contraindications

Use terbutaline with caution in patients with hypertension, ischemic heart disease, arrhythmias, congestive heart failure, diabetes mellitus, hyperthyroidism, or seizures. The action of terbutaline is antagonized by β-adrenergic blocking agents. Tolerance to terbutaline develops with repeated use.

Anesthetic Considerations

Patients may experience wide swings in vital signs secondary to β-receptor stimulation. Bradycardia and hypotension may occur after cessation of therapy. Glucose, insulin, and potassium levels are commonly altered during therapy and should be evaluated. Mild hypokalemia is usually not treated. Additive hypertension and tachycardia occur when terbutaline is administered with other sympathomimetics. The adverse effects of terbutaline may be antagonized by β-blocking agents.

TETRACAINE HCL (PONTOCAINE)

Classification

Ester-type local anesthetic

Indications

Local, spinal, and topical anesthesia

Dose

Spinal: 2 to 20 mg adjusted to height (rarely greater than 15 mg). Decrease usual dose in pregnant patients. Dilute with equal volume of sterile dextrose 10% (hyperbaric) to control height more easily. Apply topical spray 2% solution in short spurts of less than 2 seconds (maximum dose: 1.5 mg/kg). Inject slowly, not faster than 1 mL/5 seconds. Pediatric doses have not been established.

Dosage forms: injection: 1% (2 mL) for spinal anesthesia; ointment (ophthalmic): 0.5% (3.5 g); solution (ophthalmic): 0.5% (15 mL); topical: 2% (30 mL, 118 mL)

Onset and Duration

Onset: spinal: 5 to 10 minutes; fixing time: 20 to 30 minutes. Duration: 1 to 3 hours, possibly longer if epinephrine is added to spinal bolus.

Adverse Effects

Spinal use: hypotension, bradycardia, respiratory depression or apnea, high or total spinal with paralysis, headache

Precautions and Contraindications

Avoid the use of tetracaine in patients allergic to ester-type local anesthetics (i.e., procaine, chloroprocaine, and cocaine). Tetracaine contains para-aminobenzoic acid, so avoid its use in patients with an allergy to this sunscreen. Tetracaine is reserved for spinal or topical anesthesia only because other local anesthetic drugs are safer for injection or infiltration. Seizures may occur with toxic doses. Monitor vital signs carefully during the initial administration. Tetracaine is not for ocular use.

Anesthetic Considerations

Tetracaine is a long-standing agent for spinal anesthesia. Use amide local anesthetics such as lidocaine or bupivacaine if an allergy to tetracaine is suspected. Watch for a high spinal level in patients during use of this drug.

Tetracaine produces a stronger motor block and more relaxation than bupivacaine. Adequate hydration during use will minimize hypotension. Reduce the dose in morbidly obese, obstetric, or elderly patients, as well as in patients with increased abdominal pressure.

TORSEMIDE (DEMADEX)

Classification

Loop diuretic

Indications

Treatment of edema as a result of cardiac, hepatic, or renal dysfunction; hypertension

Dose

Congestive heart failure: 10 to 20 mg orally or intravenously once daily; may titrate to therapeutic effect. Safety has not been established for doses exceeding 200 mg/day.

Renal dysfunction: 20 mg orally or intravenously once daily; may titrate to effect. Safety has not been established in doses exceeding 200 mg/day.

Hypertension: 5 mg once daily; increase to 10 mg as needed; then add another antihypertensive medication if the desired effect has not been achieved.

Onset and Duration

Onset: intravenous: 10 minutes. Peak effect: within 1 to 2 hours. Duration: diuresis for all routes lasts 6 to 8 hours.

Adverse Effects

Dizziness, headache, nausea and vomiting, hyperglycemia, polyuria; additional effects: hyperuricemia, electrolyte or volume depletions, esophageal bleeding, salicylate toxicity, arrhythmias, dyspepsia

Precautions and Contraindications

Contraindicated in patients with hypersensitivity to this drug or sulfonylureas in patients with anuria. Use with caution in hepatic dysfunction. Torsemide can reduce lithium elimination. Safety is not established during pregnancy or in children.

Anesthetic Considerations

The patient's electrolyte and volume status should be monitored carefully during torsemide treatment. Electrolyte imbalances may predispose patients taking digitalis to toxicity.

TRIMETHAPHAN (ARFONAD)

Classification

Autonomic ganglion blocking agent; antihypertensive

Indications

Controlled hypotension during surgery; used during neurologic procedures and abdominal aneurysm repair

Dose

1% solution (500 mg in 500 mL); infuse 0.3 to 2 mg/min and adjust to effect.

Onset and Duration

Onset: immediate. Duration: 5 to 30 minutes, depending on the duration of the infusion

Adverse Effects

Hypotension, tachycardia, histamine release, mydriasis, urinary retention, dry mouth

Precautions and Contraindications

Avoid using trimethaphan in asthmatic patients because of frequent histamine release. Excessive hypotension and tachycardia may occur, especially in hypovolemic patients. Avoid using trimethaphan in patients with deficiencies of plasma cholinesterase.

Anesthetic Considerations

Trimethaphan should be used as a supplement for deliberate hypotensive techniques. Tachyphylaxis develops frequently and is minimized by infusing slowly for brief periods. Nitroprusside and nitroglycerin are more commonly used. Many believe it is the drug of choice for cocaine intoxication–induced hypertensive episodes.

VANCOMYCIN (VANCOCIN)

Classification

Antimicrobial agent

Indications

Treatment of documented or suspected methicillin-resistant *Staphylococcus aureus* or β-lactam–resistant coagulase-negative streptococcus; treatment of documented or suspected staphylococcal or streptococcal infections in penicillin- or cephalosporin-allergic patients; prophylaxis of bacterial endocarditis in high-risk surgical patients (rheumatic heart disease, mitral valve prolapse, valvular heart dysfunction, bioprosthetic and allograft valves) undergoing dental, oral, or upper respiratory procedures and who are penicillin or cephalosporin allergic; prophylaxis in penicillin-allergic patients undergoing gastrointestinal, biliary, or genitourinary tract surgery or instrumentation and who are at risk of developing enterococcal endocarditis; prophylactic therapy for potential infections related to ventricular-peritoneal shunt, vascular graft, or open-heart surgery in penicillin-allergic patients

Because vancomycin is not absorbed orally, the only indication for oral vancomycin is pseudomembranous colitis.

Dose

Initial intravenous dosage recommendation: adults: initial intravenous dose 15 mg/kg followed by 10 mg/kg every 12 hours in patients with normal renal function (maximum dose: 3 g/day). Patients with mild renal failure (creatinine clearance less than or equal to 50 mL/min) should receive vancomycin every 24 to 72 hours; patients with moderate renal failure (creatinine clearance of 10 to 50 mL/min) should receive vancomycin every 72 to 240 hours; patients with severe renal failure (creatinine clearance less than 10 mL/min) should receive vancomycin every 240 hours.

Children: children heavier than 5 kg and older than 7 days postnatal age and younger than 13 years: 10 mcg/kg every 6 hours. Children older than 13 years: dosed as adults.

Peak and trough serum levels should be monitored if therapy extends beyond 24 hours perioperative prophylaxis. Dosage and dosage interval should be adjusted to produce peak levels of 25 to 40 mcg/mL and trough levels of 5 to 10 mcg/mL.

Dosage forms: Parenteral injection for intravenous use: 500-mg or 1-g vials. Reconstitute sterile powder by adding 10 mL or 20 mL of sterile water to 500-mg or 1-g vials, respectively. Reconstituted solution containing 500 mg or 1 g must be further diluted with at least 100 mL or at least 250 mL D_5W or normal saline, respectively. Infuse through an intravenous piggyback over 1 to 1.5 hours.

Onset and Duration

Onset: 15 to 30 minutes. Duration: 8 to 12 hours. Half-life varies: 4 to 6 hours reported in patients with normal renal function. Usually administered 1 hour before procedure for prophylaxis of endocarditis. Some clinicians suggest that the dose be repeated 8 to 12 hours later in patients with normal renal function; however, the American Heart Association, American Academy of Pediatrics, and American Dental Association state that a second dose is unnecessary.

Adverse Effects

Rapid infusion: red-man syndrome (erythema, pruritus, and rash involving face, neck, upper trunk, and arms), hypertension, tachycardia; ototoxicity associated with prolonged serum concentrations greater than 40 mcg/mL; other effects: chills, fever, neutropenia, thrombocytopenia, agranulocytosis, phlebitis

Precautions and Contraindications

Monitor renal function tests frequently during vancomycin therapy. Use the drug with caution in patients with renal impairment or in patients receiving other nephrotoxic or ototoxic drugs. Vancomycin is contraindicated in patients with hypersensitivity to the drug. Avoid using vancomycin in patients with previous hearing loss.

Anesthetic Considerations

Vancomycin potentiation of succinylcholine-induced neuromuscular blockade has been reported. The drug may increase neuromuscular blockade by nondepolarizing muscle relaxants, whose dose should be titrated. Administer it slowly over a 30-minute period.

VASOPRESSIN (PITRESSIN)

Classification

Antidiuretic hormone

Indications

Treatment of diabetes insipidus; treatment of bleeding esophageal varices and other types of upper gastrointestinal bleeding; control of refractory operative bleeding in intrauterine procedures

Dose

- Diabetes insipidus or treatment of abdominal distention in postoperative patients: 5 to 10 units three to four times daily as needed
- Gastrointestinal hemorrhage: 0.2 to 1 unit/min infused intravenously. After 12 hours of hemorrhage control, decrease the dose by half and then stop within the next 12 to 24 hours. Intravenous nitroglycerin should be infused concomitantly to control side effects.

- Locally to operative site: 20 units in 30 mL normal saline as a gauze soak
- Children: for diabetes insipidus: intramuscular or subcutaneous: 2.5 to 5 units every 6 to 8 hours; titrate based on response
- Intravenous: infusion pump 0.01 to 0.04 unit/min, or 40 units once for resuscitation in septic shock or cardiac arrest
- Gastrointestinal bleeding: 0.01 unit/kg/min

Dosage forms: 20 pressor unit/mL aqueous injection; must be diluted for intravenous infusion in D_5W or normal saline to a concentration of 100 to 1000 units/L.

Onset and Duration
Onset: 15 to 30 minutes. Duration: antidiuretic action: intramuscular or subcutaneous: 2 to 8 hours after administration; the pressor effects last 30 to 60 minutes after intravenous injection. Elimination half-life: 10 to 35 minutes.

Adverse Effects
Tremor, sweating, vertigo, water intoxication, hyponatremia, metabolic acidosis, abdominal cramps, nausea and vomiting, urticaria, anaphylaxis, angina in patients with preexisting cardiovascular impairment

Precautions and Contraindications
Use vasopressin with extreme caution in patients who cannot tolerate rapid retention of extracellular water or who have coronary artery disease. For intravenous infusion, use a central vein, preferably, owing to the possibility of tissue necrosis with extravasation. Monitor patients with epilepsy, migraine, asthma, or heart failure closely. Use intravenous administration only for emergency treatment of gastrointestinal hemorrhage. Vasopressin is contraindicated in patients with anaphylaxis or hypersensitivity to the drug and in those with chronic nephritis with nitrogen retention until reasonable nitrogen blood levels are attained.

Anesthetic Considerations
Watch the patient carefully for abrupt cardiac changes after vasopressin injection. Urine monitoring is mandatory.

VECURONIUM (NORCURON)

Classification
Nondepolarizing muscle relaxant

Indications
Intraoperative muscle relaxation; endotracheal intubation; facilitation of mechanical ventilation in critical care

Dose
Intravenous: 0.05 to 0.2 mg/kg for paralysis

Dosage forms: powder for injection 10 mg (5, 10 mL)

Onset and Duration
Onset: 1 to 3 minutes; duration: 30 to 60 minutes

Adverse Effects
Prolonged paralysis in patients with hepatic disease; apnea immediately on administration (so appropriate airway management and resuscitative equipment must be immediately available); no significant cardiac effects

Precautions and Contraindications

Airway equipment must be on hand for intubation and controlled ventilation in conjunction with the use of vecuronium. The drug's duration of action may be prolonged in patients with liver disease.

Anesthetic Considerations

Monitor the patient's response with a nerve stimulator to avoid excessive dosing. Long-term vecuronium infusions in critical care may result in prolonged recovery and an inability to reverse the effects, owing to active metabolites. Corticosteroid therapy in patients with multiorgan failure may exacerbate this effect.

VERAPAMIL (ISOPTIN, CALAN, OTHERS)

Classification

Calcium channel blocker

Indications

Supraventricular arrhythmias; hypertension; angina

Dose

Intravenous: 2.5 to 10 mg slowly; may repeat in 30 to 60 minutes; oral: 120 to 480 mg/day in divided doses

Dosage forms: injection: 2.5 mg/mL (2 mL); tablet: 40, 80, 120 mg; sustained-release tablet: 120, 180, 240 mg

Onset and Duration

Onset: intravenous: 2 to 5 minutes; oral: 30 to 60 minutes. Duration: intravenous: 30 minutes to 2 hours; oral: 4 to 12 hours.

Adverse Effects

Hypotension, heart block, tachycardia, bradycardia; ankle edema and constipation with long-term oral use

Precautions and Contraindications

Significant hypotension may occur in patients with poor left ventricular function. Verapamil may exacerbate atrioventricular block or Wolff-Parkinson-White syndrome. Additive depression occurs with concomitant use of other cardiac depressants.

Anesthetic Considerations

Titrate verapamil slowly, owing to significant cardiac depressant effects, which are additive with anesthetics. Diltiazem infusion may be a better option for the treatment of intraoperative atrial arrhythmias. β-Blockers are superior for the treatment of sinus tachycardia.

VITAMIN K, PHYTONADIONE (AQUAMEPHYTON, MEPHYTON)

Classification

Water-soluble vitamin

Indications

Prevention and treatment of hypoprothrombinemia caused by drug- or anticoagulant-induced vitamin K deficiency or hemorrhagic diseases of the newborn

Dose

The intravenous route should be used for emergencies only. Inject slowly intravenously only, not faster than 1 mg/min.

Newborn hemorrhage: intramuscular, subcutaneous prophylaxis: 0.5 to 1 mg within 1 hour of birth. Treat with 1 to 2 mg/day.

Anticoagulant reversal: infants: 1 to 2 mg every 4 to 8 hours; adult: oral, intravenous, intramuscular, subcutaneous: 2.5 to 10 mg, may repeat intravenous, subcutaneous, intramuscular dose every 6 to 8 hours and oral dose in 12 to 48 hours.

Dosage forms: tablet: 5 mg; injection: 2 mg/mL in 0.5-mL ampule and 10 mg/mL in 1-mL ampule and 2.5- and 5-mL vials

Onset and Duration

Onset: intravenous, intramuscular, subcutaneous: 1 to 3 hours; oral: 4 to 12 hours. Duration: 6 to 48 hours, depending on the dose and route of administration.

Adverse Effects

Severe anaphylaxis possible with intravenous use; severe hemolytic anemia possible in neonates administered large doses (greater than 20 mg)

Precautions and Contraindications

Use the intravenous route in emergencies only owing to the possibility of severe anaphylaxis. Vitamin K is ineffective in hereditary hypoprothrombinemia or hypoprothrombinemia secondary to severe liver disease.

Anesthetic Considerations

Prothrombin time must be monitored. Transfusion of blood or fresh-frozen plasma may be necessary in severe hemorrhagic states.

WARFARIN (COUMADIN)

Classification

Anticoagulant; depresses formation of vitamin K–dependent clotting factors (II, VII, IX, X) in the liver

Indications

Treatment or prophylaxis of deep venous thrombosis or pulmonary thromboembolism; prophylaxis of thromboembolism in patients with atrial fibrillation who are undergoing cardioversion of atrial fibrillation, those who have prosthetic heart valves, after major surgery requiring prolonged immobilization (total knee or hip replacements), and after myocardial infarction in patients who are at high risk of embolism (those with congestive heart failure, atrial fibrillation, previous myocardial infarction, or history of thromboembolism)

Dose

Warfarin dosing is adjusted according to prothrombin time (PT). Standardization of PT results among laboratories is accomplished with the use of an international normalized ratio (INR) equation:

$$\text{INR} = (\text{PT patient}/\text{PT normal})^{\text{ISI}}$$

where ISI is the International Sensitivity Index

The typical goal INR is 2 to 3 except for patients with prosthetic valves, for whom 2.5 to 3.5 is the desired goal. Commonly, doses of 5 to 10 mg/day are tapered to 2 to 10 mg/day, as indicated by the PT. Consult the pharmacy for institutional guidelines. Multiple drug interactions may increase or decrease the response.

Dosage forms: 2-, 2.5-, 5-, 7.5-, 10-mg tablets; 50 mg for parenteral injection with 2-mL diluent

Onset and Duration

Onset: antithrombogenic effects may not occur for up to 5 to 7 days after initiation of therapy; many clinicians recommend that heparin be administered concurrently for 3 to 7 days until the desired PT is achieved. Duration: single oral dose: 2 to 5 days. Elimination half-life: 0.5 to 3 days.

Adverse Effects

Dose-dependent bleeding, ranging from minor local bleeding or ecchymosis (2%-10%) to major hemorrhagic complications occasionally resulting in death; major hemorrhage usually involving gastrointestinal or genitourinary tract but possibly involve hepatic, cerebral, or pericardial sites; additional effects: agranulocytosis, leukopenia, thrombocytopenia, necrosis of skin, purple-toe syndrome, neuropathy

Minor bleeding can be treated with vitamin K intramuscularly or intravenously 5 to 10 mg, up to 50 mg. Frank bleeding should be treated with administration of fresh whole blood or fresh-frozen plasma (15 mL/kg).

Precautions and Contraindications

Numerous drugs may affect patient response to warfarin, especially hepatic enzyme–inducing or –reducing drugs and highly protein-bound drugs; consultation with a pharmacist or physician regarding all drugs is recommended. Use warfarin with extreme caution in patients with protein C deficiency, congestive heart failure, carcinoma, liver disease, or poor nutritional state. Warfarin is contraindicated in bleeding patients or in patients with hemorrhagic blood dyscrasias, aneurysms, pericarditis or pericardial effusions, uncontrolled hypertension, recent or contemplated surgery of the eye, brain, or spinal cord (or any traumatic surgery resulting in large open surfaces), and in patients with recent cerebrovascular accident. Renal and hepatic function in these patients should be monitored periodically. PT should be monitored daily initially. After PT is stabilized, these patients should be monitored every 4 to 6 weeks. Warfarin is teratogenic and is contraindicated in pregnancy. Risks of hemorrhage may increase with concomitant use of aspirin, nonsteroidal antiinflammatory drugs, cimetidine, amiodarone, steroids, chloral hydrate, metronidazole, streptokinase, urokinase, antibiotics, and heparin. Discontinue warfarin promptly in patients with purple-toe syndrome or skin necrosis. Further use of warfarin is contraindicated in these patients.

Anesthetic Considerations

Regional anesthesia is contraindicated. If possible, barbiturates should be avoided because they may decrease warfarin's effect. When emergency surgery is necessary in patients receiving warfarin, fresh-frozen plasma (15 mL/kg) or whole blood can restore coagulation to normal.

Antibiotics

APPENDIX 1

TABLE 1 **Aminoglycoside Dosages**

Aminoglycoside	Usual Loading Doses	Expected Peak Serum Concentrations
Tobramycin	1-2 mg/kg	4-10 mcg/mL
Gentamicin	1-2 mg/kg	4-10 mcg/mL
Amikacin	5-7.5 mg/kg	15-30 mcg/mL
Kanamycin	5-7.5 mg/kg	15-30 mcg/mL

TABLE 2 **Macrolide Antibiotic Dosages**

Antibiotic	Doses
Erythromycin	250 mg q6h or 333 mg q8h PO
Erythromycin ethylsuccinate (EES)	400 mg q6h PO
Erythromycin gluceptate (Ilotycin)	15-20 mg/kg daily in divided doses q6h IV
Erythromycin lactobionate (Erythrocin)	15-20 mg/kg daily in divided doses q6h IV
Azithromycin (Zithromax)	500 mg single dose on first day followed by 250 mg/day IV or PO
Clarithromycin (Biaxin)	250-500 mg q12h PO
Dirithromycin (Dynabac)	500 mg/day PO
Troleandomycin (Tao)	250-500 mg q6h PO

IV, Intravenous; *PO,* oral.

TABLE 3 **Parenteral Cephalosporins**

Generic Name (Generation)	Usual Adult Dose	Adjust Dose for Renal Insufficiency	Comment
Cefazolin (1)	0.25-2 g q6-12h	Yes	Commonly used for surgical prophylaxis
Cefmetazole (2)	2 g q6-12h	Yes	Intraabdominal infections
Cefonicid (2)	0.5-2 g q24h	Yes	May be useful in outpatient therapy of endocarditis
Cefotetan (2)	1-2 g q12-24h	Yes	Covers GI anaerobes
Cefoxitin (2)	1-2 g q4-8h	Yes	Covers GI anaerobes
Cefuroxime (2)	0.75-1.5 g q8h	Yes	Crosses blood-brain barrier
Cefepime (3)	0.5-2 g q8-12h	Yes	

Continued

TABLE 3 Parenteral Cephalosporins—cont'd

Generic Name (Generation)	Usual Adult Dose	Adjust Dose for Renal Insufficiency	Comment
Cefoperazone (3)	1-2 g q8-12h	No	
Cefotaxime (3)	1-2 g q4-12h	Yes	Crosses blood-brain barrier
Ceftazidime (3)	0.5-2 g q8-12h	Yes	
Ceftizoxime (3)	1-2 g/day divided q4-8h	Yes	Crosses blood-brain barrier
Ceftriaxone (3)	1-2 g q12-24h	No	May be useful in outpatient therapy of endocarditis; single-dose (250 mg IM) therapy for gonococcal genital and pharyngeal infections; crosses blood-brain barrier

GI, Gastrointestinal; *IM,* intramuscular.

TABLE 4 Parenteral Penicillins

Generic Name	Brand Name	Usual IV Adult Dose	Available Dosage Forms	Comments
		Natural Penicillins		
Penicillin G benzathine	Bicillin L-A	Given IM and never IV; 1.2-2.4 million units as a single dose	300,000 units/mL	Provides low, long-lasting blood levels of penicillin G
Penicillin G benzathine and procaine combined	Bicillin C-R	Given IM and never IV; 2.4 million units as a single dose	300,00 units/mL (150,000 units each of penicillin G benzathine and penicillin G procaine)	Provides low, long-lasting blood levels of penicillin G
Penicillin G procaine	Wycillin	Given IM and never IV; 300,000-1,000,000 units/day as 1-2 doses/day	600,000 units/mL in 1, 2 mL syringes	Indicated for infections that respond to low, long-lasting penicillin G blood levels

TABLE 4 **Parenteral Penicillins—cont'd**

Generic Name	Brand Name	Usual IV Adult Dose	Available Dosage Forms	Comments
Penicillin G potassium	Pfizerpen	1-24 milliunits/day in divided doses q4h, depending on severity of infection and microbial sensitivity	Injection: 5 million units; frozen premixed bag: 1, 2, 3 million units: powder for injection, 1, 5, 10, 20 million units	Infuse over 1-2 h; Note: 250 mg = 400,000 units; sodium content of 1 million unit = 2 mEq; potassium content of 1 million unit = 1.7 mEq; often called "aqueous" penicillin
Broad-Spectrum Penicillins				
Ampicillin	Omnipen	1-12 g/day divided q4-6h	Powder for injection: 250, 500 mg, 1, 2, 10 g*	Infuse over at least 10-15 min
Ampicillin–sulbactam	Unasyn	1.5-3 g q6-8h (equivalent to 1-2 g of ampicillin)	Powder for injection: 1.5 g (ampicillin 1 g + sulbactam 0.5 g), 3 g (ampicillin 2 g + sulbactam 1 g); 10 g*	Infuse over 15-30 min
Ticarcillin	Ticar	4-24 g/day in divided doses q4-6h	Powder for injection: 1, 3, 5, 20, 30 g*	Infuse over at least 30 min; sodium content of 1 g = 5.2-6.5 mEq
Ticarcillin–clavulanate	Timentin	12-24 g/day in divided doses q4-6h	Powder for injection and frozen premixed bags; ticarcillin disodium 3 g + clavulanate potassium 0.1 g	Infuse over 30 min; sodium content of 1 g = 4.75 mEq; potassium content of 1 g = 0.15 mEq
Piperacillin	Pipracil	18-24 g/day divided q4-6h, depending on severity	Powder for injection: 2, 3, 4, 40 g*	Infuse over at least 20 min; sodium content = 1.85 mEq/g

Continued

TABLE 4 Parenteral Penicillins—cont'd

Generic Name	Brand Name	Usual IV Adult Dose	Available Dosage Forms	Comments
Piperacillin–tazobactam	Zosyn	3.375 g q6h or 4.5 g q8h	Powder for injection (piperacillin/tazobactam) 2 g/0.25 g, 3 g/0.375 g, 4 g/0.5 g, 36 g/4.5 g*	Infuse over 30 min
Penicillinase-Resistant Penicillins				
Nafcillin	Unipen	500 mg: 2 g q4-6h	Powder for injection: 500 mg, 1, 2, 4, 10 g*	Infuse over 30-60 min
Oxacillin	Bactocill, Prostaphlin	250 mg: 2 g q4-6h	Powder for injection: 250, 500 mg, 1, 2, 4, 10 g*	By direct IV injection over 10 min

*Bulk package intended for pharmacy use only.

IM, Intramuscular; *IV,* intravenous.

From *2007 Mosby's Drug Consult.* St. Louis: Mosby, 2007: IV-13.

TABLE 5 Parenteral Fluoroquinolones

Generic Name	Brand Name	Usual Intravenous Adult Dose	Available Dosage Forms	Comments
Ciprofloxacin	Cipro	200-400 mg q12h	Injection: 200, 400 mg, in glass vials and premixed bags	Infuse over 60 min
Gatifloxacin	Tequin	200-400 mg q24h	Injection: 200, 400 mg; premixed bags: 400 mg/250 mL	Infuse over 60 min
Levofloxacin	Levaquin	500 mg q24h (for urinary tract infection, 250 mg q24h)	Injection: (24 mg/mL) 500, 750 mg; premixed bags; (5 mg/mL) 250, 500, 750 mg	L-Isomer of the racemate ofloxacin (another commercially available fluoroquinolone antibiotic); infuse over 60 min

TABLE 5 **Parenteral Fluoroquinolones—cont'd**

Generic Name	Brand Name	Usual Intravenous Adult Dose	Available Dosage Forms	Comments
Moxifloxacin	Avelox IV	400 mg q24h	Premixed bags: 400 mg/250 mL	Infuse over 60 min
Ofloxacin	Floxin	200-400 mg q12h	Injection: 200, 400 mg	Not effective for syphilis; infuse over 60 min
Trovafloxacin	Trovan	200-300 mg/day	Injection (as alatrofloxacin mesylate): (5 mg/mL) 250, 300 mg	IV formulation contains alatrofloxacin, a trovafloxacin prodrug; infuse over 60 min; case reports of fatal hepatic reactions; use only in cases of life- or limb-threatening infections and begin therapy in inpatient setting

IV, Intravenous.

TABLE 6 **Parenteral Sulfonamides**

Generic Name	Brand Name	Usual Adult Dose	Available Dosage Forms	Comments
Sulfamethoxazole–trimethoprim (SMZ-TMP), co-trimoxazole	Bactrim IV; Septra IV	8-20 mg/kg/day of TMP in divided doses q6h, depending on type and severity of infection	Injection: 80 mg SMZ and 16 mg TMP per mL	Infuse over 60-90 min; first-line therapy for *Pneumocystis carinii* pneumonia; pay special attention to complaints of skin or mucosal rash, which could signify early Stevens-Johnson syndrome

IV, Intravenous.

APPENDIX

2 Antithrombotic Drugs

TABLE 1 Indication and Choice of Antithrombotic Drugs

Indication	Drugs
Primary prevention	
Risk factors	Aspirin
No risk factors	None*
Secondary prevention	
Recent MI	Aspirin†
Ischemic stroke	Aspirin ± dipyridamole; or clopidogrel
UA/NSTEMI	Aspirin ± Clopidogrel or prasugrel or ticagrelor ± UFH or LMWH or fondaparinux‡ ± GPIIb/IIIa inhibitor
Acute MI (STEMI)	Aspirin +clopidogrel or prasugrel or ticagrelor +UFH or LMWH or fondaparinux‡ + GPIIb/IIIa inhibitor
PCI	Aspirin + Clopidogrel or prasugrel or ticagrelor +UFH or LMWH or bivalirudin ± GPIIb/IIIa inhibitor
VTE treatment	LMWH or UFH or fondaparinux + warfarin
VTE prevention	
Hospitalized medical patients	Low-dose UFH, LMWH, or fondaparinux
General surgery	Low-dose UFH, LMWH, or fondaparinux
Orthopedic surgery	Fondaparinux, rivaroxaban, dabigatran,‡ LMWH, or warfarin
Atrial fibrillation	Aspirin,† § warfarin, dabigatran, rivaoxban,‡ or apixaban¶
Peripheral arterial disease	Aspirin

*Some clinicians offer aspirin to women older than 65 years old and men younger than 45 years old.
†Or if intolerant to aspirin, clopidogrel.
‡Not approved by the Food and Drug Administration for this indication.
§For patients at low risk.
¶Not yet available in the United States.
GP, Glycoprotein; *LMWH,* low-molecular-weight heparin; *MI,* myocardial infarction; *NSTEMI,* non–ST segment elevation myocardial infarction; *PCI,* percutaneous coronary intervention; *STEMI,* ST segment elevation myocardial infarction; *UA,* unstable angina; *UFH,* unfractionated heparin.
Adapted from Antithrombotic Drugs. In *Treatment Guidelines from the Medical Letter*. 2011: 9(110): 61-66.

TABLE 2 Pharmacological Properties of Common Antithrombotic Medications

Type	Name	Pharmacodynamics	Pharmacokinetic (Metabolism/ Plasma Half-life)	Clinical Indication(s)	Perioperative Management (Stop Before Procedure)	Reversal Methods
Antiplatelet	Aspirin	COX 1-2 inhibitor	Liver/20 minutes	Acute MI and stroke	7 days	None
	NSAIDS (e.g., Ketorolac and Ibuprofen)	COX 1-2 inhibitor	Liver/2-7 hr	Pain and inflammation	24-48 hr	None
	Rofecoxib	COX 1 inhibitor	Liver/10-17 hr	Pain and inflammation	None	None
	Celecoxib	COX 1 inhibitor	Liver/10-17 hr	Pain and inflammation	None	None
	Clopidogrel	ADP receptor antagonist (prodrug)	Liver/7 days	Coronary artery disease and peripheral vascular disease	7 days	None
	Ticlopidine	ADP receptor antagonist (prodrug)	Liver/4 days	Coronary artery disease and peripheral vascular disease	7 days	None
	Prasugrel	ADP receptor antagonist	Liver/5 days	ACS and PCI	2-3 days	None
	Ticagrelor	ADP receptor antagonist	Liver/2-3 days	ACS and PCI	24-48 hr	None
	Dipyridamole	Inhibition of platelet uptake of adenosine diphosphate (e.g., phosphodiesterase antagonist)	Liver/40 min	Peripheral vascular disease	24-48 hr	None

Continued

TABLE 2 Pharmacological Properties of Common Antithrombotic Medications—cont'd

Type	Name	Pharmacodynamics	Pharmacokinetic (Metabolism/ Plasma Half-life)	Clinical Indication(s)	Perioperative Management (Stop Before Procedure)	Reversal Methods
	Abciximab	GPIIb/IIIa receptor antagonist	Kidneys/3 min	ACS and PCI	72 hr	None
	Eptifibatide	GPIIb/IIIa receptor antagonist	Kidneys/2 hr	ACS and PCI	24 hr	None
	Tirofiban	GPIIb/IIIa receptor antagonist	Kidneys/2 hr	ACS	24 hr	Dialysis
Anticoagulant	Warfarin	Vitamin K antagonist	Liver/2-4 days	Thromboembolism and thromboprophylaxis	2-4 days	Vitamin K, recombinant factor VII, prothrombin complex concentrate, FFP
	Heparin	Antithrombin III catalyst (e.g., activated factor II, IX, X, XI, and XII antagonism)	Liver/1-2 hr	Thromboembolism and thromboprophylaxis	6 hr	Protamine
	LMWH (e.g., dalteparin, enoxaparin, and tinzaparin)	Antithrombin III catalyst (e.g., activated factor II and X antagonism)	Kidneys/4-5 hr	Thromboembolism and thromboprophylaxis	12-24 hr	Protamine (partial)
	Pentasaccharide (e.g., fondaparinux)	Antithrombin III catalyst (e.g., activated factor X antagonism)	Kidneys/14-17 hr	Thromboprophylaxis	4 days	None

	Rivaroxaban	Direct activated factor X antagonism	Kidneys/5-10 hr	Thromboembolism and thromboprophylaxis	24-48 hr	None
	Apixaban	Direct activated factor X antagonism	Kidneys/10-14 hr	Thromboembolism and thromboprophylaxis	24-48 hr	None
	Argatroban	Direct thrombin inhibitor	Liver/40-50 min	Type II HIT	4-6 hr	None
	Hirudin	Direct thrombin inhibitor	Kidneys/1-2 hr	Type II HIT	8 hr	Dialysis and polymethyl methacrylate
	Bivalrudin	Direct thrombin inhibitor	Kidneys/25 min	PCI in patients with history of HIT	2-3 hr	None
	Dabigatran	Direct thrombin inhibitor	Kidneys/14-17 hr	Stroke prevention in nonvalvular atrial fibrillation	1-4 days	None
	Drotrecogin alfa	Activated protein C	Liver/2 hr	Severe sepsis	12 hr	None
Fibrinolytic	t-PA	Plasminogen to plasmin conversion	Liver/1-5 minutes	Acute MI and pulmonary embolism	1 hr	Antifibrinolytics
	Streptokinase	Plasminogen to plasmin conversion	Liver/15-30 min	Acute MI and pulmonary embolism	3 hr	Antifibrinolytics

ACS, Acute coronary syndrome; *ADP,* adenosine diphosphate; *COX,* cyclooxygenase; *FFP,* fresh-frozen plasma; *GP,* glycoprotein; *HIT,* heparin-induced thrombocytopenia; *LMWH,* low-molecular weight heparin; *NSAID,* nonsteroidal anti-inflammatory drug; *MI,* myocardial infarction; *PCI,* percutaneous coronary intervention; *t-PA,* tissue plasminogen activator

TABLE 3 **Regional Anesthesia in the Patient Receiving Thromboprophylaxis**

Antiplatelet medications	No contraindication with aspirin or NSAIDs; discontinue ticlodipine (generic) 14 days, clopidogrel (Plavix) and prasugrel (Effient) 7 days before block; GPIIb/IIIa inhibitors tirofiban (Aggrastat) and eptifibatide (Integrilin) 8 hr; abciximab (ReoPro) 24-48 hr to allow return of normal platelet function
Unfractionated heparin	
Subcutaneous	No contraindication with twice-daily dosing of <10,000 units, consider delay until after block if technical difficulty anticipated; the safety of doses >10,000 units or more than twice daily dosing has not been established
Intravenous	Heparinize 1 hr after block; remove catheter 2-4 hr after last heparin dose; document normal aPTT; sustained heparinization with an indwelling catheter associated with an increased risk; monitor neurologic status aggressively
LMWH	Delay procedures at least 12-24 hr after last dose of LMWH; regardless of technique, remove all catheters 2 hr before first LMWH dose; no additional hemostasis-altering drugs
Warfarin	Normal INR before neuraxial technique (usually requires 4-5 days); remove catheter when INR ≤1.5
Thrombolytics	Absolute contraindication
Thrombin inhibitors	Bivalirudin (Angiomax); desirudin (Iprivask), avoid regional block, insufficient information
Fondaparinux (Arixtra)	Until additional clinical information is obtained, neuraxial techniques should only involve single needle pass, atraumatic needle placement, no indwelling catheters; if this is not feasible, an alternate method of prophylaxis should be used
Dabigatran (Pradaxa)	Discontinue 7 days before regional block; for shorter time periods, document normal TT or ECT; first postoperative dose 24 hr after needle placement and 6 hr after catheter removal, whichever is later
Herbal medicine	No evidence for discontinuation; be aware of potential drug interactions

aPTT, Activated partial thromboplastin time; *ECT,* Ecarin clotting time; *GP,* glycoprotein; *INR,* international normalized ratio; *LMWH,* low-molecular-weight heparin; *NSAID,* nonsteroidal anti-inflammatory drug; *TT,* thrombin time.

Adapted from Horlocker TT, Wedel DJ, Rowlingson JC, et al. Regional anesthesia in the patient receiving antithrombotic or thrombolytic therapy: American Society of Regional Anesthesia and Pain Medicine Evidence Based Guidelines. 3rd ed. *Reg Anesth Pain Med* 2010; 35(1):64-101; Horlocker TT. Regional anaesthesia in the patient receiving antithrombotic and antiplatelet therapy. *Br J Anaesth* 2011; 107(Suppl 1):i96-106; Chelly JE. Thromboprophylaxis and regional anesthesia in the ambulatory setting. *Int Anesthesiol Clin* 2011; 49(4):166-173.

Corticosteroid Replacement

APPENDIX 3

Guidelines for Perioperative Adrenal Supplementation Therapy

Type of Surgery	Hydrocortisone Dose
Superficial surgery	None
Dental	
Biopsies	
Minor surgery	25 mg IV
Inguinal hernia	
Colonoscopy	
Moderate surgery	50-75 mg IV; taper over 1 to 2 days
Nonlaparoscopic cholecystectomy	
Colon resection	
Total abdominal hysterectomy	
Total joint replacement	
Major surgery	100-150 mg IV; taper over 1 to 2 days
Cardiovascular	
Thoracic	
Liver	

IV, Intravenous.

APPENDIX 4

Diabetic Drugs

TABLE 1 Oral Drugs for Type 2 Diabetes

Drug	Usual Daily Dosage
DPP-4 Inhibitors	
Sitagliptin (Januvia)	100 mg once
Saxagliptin (Onglyza)	2.5-5 mg once
Linagliptin (Tiadjenta)	5 mg once
First-Generation Sulfonylureas	
Chlorpropamide (Diabinese)	250-375 mg once
Tolazamide (Tolinase)	250-500 mg once or divided
Tolbutamide	1000-2000 mg divided
Second-Generation Sulfonylureas	
Glimepiride (Amaryl)	1-4 mg once
Glipizide (Glucotrol)	10-20 mg once or divided
(Glucotrol XL sustained-release tab)	5-20 mg once
Glyburide (DiaBeta, Micronase)	5-20 mg once or divided
(Glynase micronized tab: Glynase Prestab)	1.5-12 mg once or divided
Alpha-Glucosidase Inhibitors	
Acarbose (Precose)	50-100 mg tid with meals
Miglitol (Glyset)	50-100 mg tid with meals
Thiazolidinediones	
Rosiglitazone (Avandia) (restricted availability after November 18, 2011)	4-8 mg once or divided
Pioglitazone (Actos)	15-45 mg once
Biguanides	
Metformin (Glucophage)	1500-2550 mg divided
(Glucophage XR)	1500-2000 mg once
Glumetza (SR)	500-2000 mg once
Fortamet (SR)	1500-2500 mg once
Riomet (liquid)	1500-2550 mg divided
Nonsulfonylurea Secretagogues	
Repaglinide (Prandin)	1-4 mg tid before meals
Nateglinide (Starlix)	60-120 mg tid before meals
GLP-1 Agonists	
Exenatide (Byetta)	5 or 10 mcg subcut bid before breakfast and dinner
Liraglutide (Victoza)	1.2 or 1.8 mg subcut once
Amylin Analogue	
Pramlintide (Symlin)	60-120 mcg subcut tid before main meals

TABLE 1 Oral Drugs for Type 2 Diabetes—cont'd

Drug	Usual Daily Dosage
Combination Drugs	
Metformin/glyburide (Glucovance)	500 mg/5 mg bid
Metformin/rosiglitazone (Avandamet)	500 mg/2 mg bid
Metformin/glipizide (Metaglip)	500 mg/2.5 mg bid
Metformin/pioglitazone (Actoplus Met)	500 mg/15 mg bid
(Actoplus Met XR SR)	1000 mg/15 mg once
Metformin/repaglinide (Prandimet)	500 mg/1-2 mg bid-tid
Metformin/sitagliptin (Janumet)	500 mg/50 mg bid
Metformin/saxagliptin (Kombiglyze XR)	1000-2000 mg/5 mg once
Glimepiride/rosiglitazone (Avandaryl)	4 mg/4 mg bid
Glimepiride/pioglitazone (Duetact)	4 mg/30 mg once

bid, Twice a day; *DPP-4 inhibitor*, dipeptidyl-peptidase-4 inhibitor; *GLP-1*, glucagon-like peptide; *tid,* three times a day; *SR,* sustained release; *subQ,* subcutaneous; *XR,* extended release.
Modified from Drugs for type 2 diabetes. *Treat Guidel Med Lett* 2011;9(108):47-54.

TABLE 2 Insulin Preparations: Pharmacokinetics of Insulin Preparations

Insulin Type	Onset	Peak	Duration	Route
Long Acting				
Insuling detemir—Levemir (Novo Nordisk)	1-4 hr	Relatively flat	12-20 hr	subcut
Insulin glargine—Lantus (Sanofiaventis)	1-4 hr	No peak	22-24 hr	subcut
Rapid Acting				
Insulin aspart—Novolog (Novo Nordisk)	10-30 min	30 min-3 hr	3-5 hr	subcut
Insulin lispro—Humalog (Lilly)	10-30 min	30 min-3 hr	3-5 hr	subcut
Insulin glulisine—Apidra (Sanofiaventis)	10-30 min	30 min-3 hr	3-5 hr	subcut
Short-Acting Regular Insulin				
Humulin R (Lilly)	30-60 min	2½-5 hr	4-12 hrs	IV, subcut, IM
Novolin R (Novo Nordisk)	30-60 min	2½-5 hr	4-12 hrs	IV, subcut, IM
Intermediate Acting				
NPH				
Humulin N	1-2 hr	4-8 hr	10-20 hr	subcut
Novolin N	1-2 hr	4-8 hr	10-20 hr	subcut
Premixed Analogues				
Novolin 70/30 (Novo, Nordisk) (70% NPH, human insulin isophane suspension and 30% regular human insulin)	30-60 min	2-12 hrs	18-24 hrs	subcut

Continued

TABLE 2 Insulin Preparations: Pharmacokinetics of Insulin Preparations—cont'd

Insulin Type	Onset	Peak	Duration	Route
Novolog 70/30 (Novo, Nordisk) (70% insulin aspart protamine suspension and 30% insulin aspart injection)	10-20 min	1-4 hrs	18-24 hrs	subcut
Humalog Mix 75/25 (Lilly) (75% insulin lispro protamine suspension and 25% insulin lispro)	10-30 min	1-6½ hrs	14-24 hrs	subcut

IM, Intramuscular; *IV*, intravenous; *NPH*, neutral protamine Hagedorn; *subcut*, subcutaneous. Time course is based on subcutaneous administration.
Adapted from Drugs for type 2 diabetes. *Treat Guidel Med Lett* 2011;9(108):47-54.

Hematology

APPENDIX 5

TABLE 1 **Blood Coagulation Factors**

Factor*	Synonym	Biologic Half-life (hr)	Blood Product Source
I	Fibrinogen	100-150	Cryoprecipitate (200-300 mg/bag)
II	Prothrombin	50-80	FFP, PCC
V	Proaccelerin	12-36	FFP
VII	Proconvertin	4-6	Recombinant VIIa, FFP, PCC
VIII	Antihemophilic factor	12-15	FFP, PCC, factor concentrates, cryoprecipitate
IX	Christmas factor	18-30	FFP, PCC, factor concentrates
X	Stuart-Prower factor	25-60	FFP, PCC
XI	Plasma thromboplastin antecedent	40-80	FFP
XII	Hageman factor	50-70	Not associated with bleeding diathesis
XIII	Fibrin-stabilizing factor	150	FFP, cryoprecipitate
VWF	Von Willebrand factor	8-12	FFP, cryoprecipitate, factor concentrate

*Coagulation factors are numbered with Roman numerals in order of their discovery. Factor III (tissue factor) and factor IV (calcium ions) have been omitted. There is no factor VI.

FFP, Fresh-frozen plasma; *PCC,* prothrombin-complex concentrate.

Modified from Bickert Poon B, Witmer C, Pruemer J. Coagulation disorders. In Dipiro JT, Talbert RL, Yee GC, et al, eds. *Pharmacotherapy: A pathophysiological approach.* 8th ed. New York: McGraw-Hill; 2011:1741.

TABLE 2 **Hematology Laboratory Procedures**

Procedure	Identifies	Causes of Prolonged Value	Clinical Manifestations
Bleeding time	Platelet number and function	Thrombocytopenia	Bleeding from the gums
		Acquired platelet disorders (uremia)	Easy bruising Bleeding after surgery or tooth extraction
		Vasculitis	Epistaxis
		Connective tissue disorder	Menorrhagia
		Thrombocytopenia	
		Inherited qualitative platelet defects	

Continued

TABLE 2 Hematology Laboratory Procedures—cont'd

Procedure	Identifies	Causes of Prolonged Value	Clinical Manifestations
		von Willebrand disease Antiplatelet drugs (e.g., aspirin) Factor V or XI deficiency Afibrinogenemia, dysfibrinogenemia	
Prothrombin time (PT)	Factors of common pathway: I, II, V, VII, X	Newborn Vitamin K deficiency	Bleeding after surgery, childbirth, trauma
	Factor of extrinsic pathway: VII	Inherited factor deficiencies Warfarin therapy Liver disease Lupus anticoagulant Afibrinogenemia	Easy bruising
Activated partial thromboplastin time (aPTT)	HMWK, prekallikrein	Inherited factor deficiencies	Increased incidence of thrombotic disease possible with factor XII deficiency
	Factors XI, XII	Lupus anticoagulant heparin therapy	Joint and muscle bleeding with factor deficiencies
	Factors I, II, V, VIII, IX, X	Liver disease Afibrinogenemia	Mucosal bleeding with von Willebrand disease
Thrombin time (TT)	Fibrinogen	Afibrinogenemia, dysfibrinogenemia	Lifelong hemorrhagic disease
	Inhibitors of fibrin aggregation	Heparin therapy	

HMWK, High-molecular-weight kininogen.

Modified from Bickert Poon B, Witmer C, Pruemer J. Coagulation disorders. In Dipiro JT, Talbert RL, Yee GC, et al, eds. *Pharmacotherapy: A pathophysiological approach.* 8th ed. New York: McGraw-Hill: 2011:1741.

Immunosuppressive Drugs

Drug	Description	Mechanism of Action	Nonimmune Toxicity and Comments
Prednisone	Corticosteroid	Binds nuclear receptor and enhances transcription of IκB, which inhibits NF-κB and T-cell activation	Diabetes, weight gain, psychological disturbances, osteoporosis, ulcers, wound healing, adrenal suppression
Cyclosporine	11-amino-acid cyclic peptide from *Tolypocladium inflaturn*	Binds to cyclophilin; complex inhibits calcineurin phosphatase and T-cell activation	Nephrotoxicity, hemolytic uremic syndrome, hypertension, neurotoxicity, gingival hyperplasia, skin changes, hirsutism, posttransplantation diabetes, hyperlipidemia
Tacrolimus (Prograf)	Macrolide antibiotic from *Streptomyces tsukubaensis*	Binds to FKBP12; complex inhibits calcineurin phosphatase and T-cell activation	Effects similar to cyclosporine but with lower incidences of hypertension, hyperlipidemia, skin changes, hirsutism, and gingival hyperplasia but higher incidences of posttransplantation diabetes and neurotoxicity
Sirolimus (rapamycin)	Triene macrolide antibiotic from *Streptomyces hygroscopicus* from Easter Island (Rapa Nui)	Binds to FKBP12; complex inhibits target of rapamycin and IL-2–dependent T-cell proliferation	Hyperlipidemia, increased toxicity of calcineurin inhibitors, thrombocytopenia, delayed wound healing, delayed graft function, mouth ulcers, pneumonitis, interstitial lung disease

Continued

Drug	Description	Mechanism of Action	Nonimmune Toxicity and Comments
Everolimus	Derivative of sirolimus; similar mechanism and toxicities		
Mycophenolate mofetil (Cellcept)	Mycophenolic acid from *Penicillium stoloniferum*	Inhibits synthesis of guanosine monophosphate nucleotides; blocks purine synthesis, preventing proliferation of T and B cells	GI symptoms (mainly diarrhea), neutropenia, mild anemia
Azathioprine (Imuran)	Prodrug that undergoes hepatic metabolism to form 6-mercaptopurine	Converts 6-mercaptopurine to 6-thioinosine-5'-monophosphate, which is converted to thioguanine nucleotides that interfere with DNA and purine synthesis	Leukopenia, bone marrow depression, liver toxicity (uncommon)
Antithymocyte globulin	Polyclonal IgG from rabbits or horses immunized with human thymocytes	Blocks T-cell membrane proteins (e.g., CD2, CD3, CD45), causing altered function, lysis, and prolonged T-cell depletion	Cytokine release syndrome, thrombocytopenia, leukopenia, serum sickness
Muromonab-CD3 (OKT3)	Anti-CD3 murine monoclonal antibody	Binds CD3 associated with the TCR, leading to initial activation and cytokine release, followed by blockade of function, lysis, T-cell depletion	Severe cytokine release syndrome, pulmonary edema, acute renal failure, CNS changes
Basiliximab	Anti-CD25 chimeric monoclonal antibody	Binds to high-affinity chain of IL-2R (CD25) on activated T cells, causing depletion and preventing IL-2–mediated activation	Hypersensitivity reaction, uncommon
Dacluzimab	Anti-CD25 humanized monoclonal antibody	Similar to that of basiliximab	Hypersensitivity reaction (uncommon)

Drug	Description	Mechanism of Action	Nonimmune Toxicity and Comments
Rituximab	Anti-CD20 chimeric monoclonal antibody	Binds to CD20 on B cells and causes depletion	Infusion or hypersensitivity reactions, uncommon
Alemtuzumab	Anti-CD52 humanized monoclonal antibody	Binds to CD52 expressed on most T and B cells, monocytes, macrophages, NK cells, causing lysis and prolonged depletion	Mild cytokine release syndrome, neutropenia, anemia, autoimmune thrombocytopenia, thyroid disease
FTY720	Sphingosine-like derivative of myriocin from the fungus *Isaria sinclairii*	Functions as antagonist for sphingosine-1-phosphate receptors on lymphocytes, enhancing homing to lymphoid tissues and preventing egress, causing lymphopenia	Reversible first-dose bradycardia, potentiated by general anesthetics and β-blockers, nausea, vomiting, diarrhea, increased liver enzyme levels
Belatacept (LEA29Y)	High-affinity homologue of CTLA-4 Ig	Binds to CD80-CD86 and prevents costimulation via CD28	Clinical trials—preliminary results suggest equal efficacy to CsA but improved GFR

CNS, central nervous system; *CsA,* cyclosprine; *GFR,* glomerular filtration rate; *GI,* gastrointestinal; *Ig,* immunoglobulin; *IL-2,* interleukin-2; *IκB,* inhibitor of kappa B protein; *N F-κB,* nuclear factor kappa-B; *NK,* natural killer; *TCR,* T-cell receptor.

Adapted from Abbas AK, Lichtman AH, Pillai S. *Cellular and molecular immunology.* 6th ed. Philadelphia: Saunders. 2010.

APPENDIX 7

Pediatric Considerations

TABLE 1 Pediatric Conversion Factors*

Age	Weight (kg) 50th Percentile	Respiratory Rate (breaths/min)	Heart Rate (beats/min)	Systolic Blood Pressure (mmHg)
Premature	<3	50-60	120-180	40-60
Newborn	3-4	35-40	100-180	50-70
1 mo	4	35-40	100-180	50-70
3 mo	5	24-30	100-180	60-110
6 mo	7	25-30	100-180	60-110
12 mo	10	20-25	90-150	65-115
2 yr	12	16-22	90-150	75-125
3 yr	15	16-22	90-150	75-125
5 yr	20	14-20	60-140	80-120
7 yr	30	14-20	60-140	90-120
10 yr	40	12-20	60-100	90-120
<1 yr: (age [mo]) × 0.5 + 3.5				
>1 yr: (age [yr]) × 2 + 1				

*Estimating weight in kilograms.

TABLE 2 Estimating Endotracheal Tube Size*

Age	ETT Size	Laryngoscope Blade	Distance (cm)
Premature	2.5	0 Miller	According to weight: 500 g at 6 cm 1000 g at 7 cm 2000 g at 8 cm 3000 g at 9 cm
Newborn	3-3.5	0 Miller	10
6 mo	3.5-4	1 Miller	10-11
1 yr	4	1 to 2 Miller/Mac	11
2 yr	4.5-5	1 or 2 Miller/Mac	12.5
>20 mo: 4 + age (yr) ÷ 4			
Length of insertion (>1 yr: 12 + age ÷ 2)			

*This is only a guide; prepare an ETT one size larger and one size smaller than the ETT size selected.
ETT, Endotracheal tube

TABLE 3 Estimated Blood Volume

Age	Volume (mL/kg)
Premature	90
Full-term	90
0-2 yr	80
2+ yr	70

TABLE 4 Maximum Allowable Blood Loss (MABL)*

Nothing by Mouth (NPO) Time		
Age (mo)	**Clear Liquids (hr)**	**Milk/Solids (hr)**
0-6	2	4
6-36	2-4	4-6
>36	2-4	6-8

$$^{*}(\text{MABL}) = \frac{\text{Estimated blood volume (EBV)} \times (\text{Initial hematocrit} - \text{Target hematocrit})}{\text{Initial hematocrit}}$$

TABLE 5 Calculation of Maintenance Fluid Requirements

Weight (kg)	Requirement
0-10	4 mL/kg/hr
10-20	40 mL + 2 mL/kg >10
>20	60 mL + 1 mL/kg >20

NPO deficit:

NPO hours × Maintenance: Replace 50% the first hour, 25% the second hour, and 25% the third hour.

TABLE 6 Pediatric Drug Doses

Drug	Route	Dose
	Emergency (Resuscitation) Drugs	
Atropine	IV	0.02 mg/kg/dose (minimum, 0.1 mg/dose; maximum, 1 mg)
Calcium chloride	IV	10-20 mg/kg
Calcium gluconate	IV	50-100 mg/kg
Epinephrine	IV	0.01 mg/kg (0.1 mg/kg via ETT)
Lidocaine	IV	1 mg/kg
Sodium bicarbonate	IV	1 mEq/kg/dose; 0.3/kg/base deficit

Continued

TABLE 6 Pediatric Drug Doses—cont'd

Drug	Route	Dose
		Opiates
Codeine	IM or PO	0.5-1 mg/kg
Meperidine	IV	0.2-1 mg/kg
	IM	1-2 mg/kg
Midazolam	IV	0.05-0.1 mg/kg
	IM	0.2-0.3 mg/kg
	PO	0.5-0.75 mg/kg
Morphine	IV	0.05-0.2 mg/kg
	IM/subcut	0.1-0.2 mg/kg
Remifentanil	Infusion	0.5-1 mcg/kg/min (induction) 0.05-0.08 mcg/kg/min (maintenance)
Sufentanil	IV	0.1-0.5 mcg/kg with nitrous oxide; 5-10 mcg/kg alone
Fentanyl	IV	1-5 mcg/kg
		Induction Agents
Propofol	IV	2-3 mg/kg
Ketamine	IV	1-2 mg/kg
	IM	5-10 mg/kg
Dexmedetomidine	IV	0.2-0.7 mcg/kg/hr
		Muscle Relaxants
Atracurium IV	IV	0.2-0.5 mg/kg
Cisatracurium	IV	0.1 mg/kg
Pancuronium	IV	0.04-0.15 mg/kg
Succinylcholine	IV	1-2 mg/kg
	IM	2.5-4 mg/kg
Rocuronium	IV	0.6-1 mg/kg (intubation); 0.08-0.12 mg/kg (maintenance)
Vecuronium	IV	0.04-0.2 mg/kg
		Reversal Agents
Edrophonium	IV	0.5-1 mg/kg
Neostigmine	IV	0.05-0.07 mg/kg
Naloxone	IV, IM, or subcut	5-10 mcg/kg
Nalmefene	IV	0.25 mcg/kg

ETT, Endotracheal tube *IM,* intramuscular; *IV,* intravenous; *PO,* oral; *subcut,* subcutaneous.

Preoperative Laboratory Tests

APPENDIX 8

Test	Normal Serum Values
Activated coagulation time	80-120 sec
Alanine aminotransferase, female	9-24 units/L
Male	10-32 units/L
Albumin, total	6.6-7.9 g/dL
Fractional	4.4-4.5 g/dL
Alkaline phosphatase	45-125 units/L
Ammonia	80-110 mcg/dL
Amylase	20-110 units/L
Anion gap	8-14 mEq/L
Arterial blood gases: pH	7.35-7.45
Carbon dioxide pressure	35-45 mmHg
Oxygen pressure	80-100 mmHg
Bicarbonate	22-26 mEq/L
Aspartate aminotransferase	8-20 units/L
Bilirubin, direct	0-0.4 mg/dL
Indirect	0.1-1.2 mg/dL
Blood urea nitrogen	8-20 mg/dL
Calcium	4.5-5.5 mEq/L
Chloride	100-108 mEq/L
Creatine kinase, total	
Female	15-57 units/L
Male	24-100 units/L
MB	0-7 units/L
MM	6-70 units/L
Creatinine	0.2-1.5 mg/dL
Fibrin split product/fibrin degradation product	<3 mcg/mL
Fibrinogen	195-365 mg/dL
Glucose, fasting	70-100 mg/dL
Hematocrit, female	37%-47%
Male	42%-52%
Hemoglobin, female	15-16 g/dL
Male	14-18 g/dL
Glycosylated	5.5%-9%
International Normalized Ratio	1
Lactate dehydrogenase (LDH), total	48-115 international units/L
LDH_1	17.5%-28.3% of total LDH
LDH_2	30.4%-36.4% of total LDH ($LDH_1 < LDH_2$)
Magnesium	1.5-2.5 mEq/L
Phosphorus	1.8-2.6 mEq/L
Platelets	130,000-370,000/mm^3
Potassium	3.8-5.5 mEq/L
Pseudocholinesterase	8-80 units/mL
Prothrombin time	11-13.2 sec
Partial thromboplastin time	22.5-32.2 sec
Red blood cell count, female	4.2-5.4 million/dL
Red blood cell count, male	4.7-6.2 million/dL
Sodium	134-145 mEq/L

Continued

Test	Normal Serum Values
Triiodothyronine	90-230 ng/dL
Thyroxine	5-13 mcg/dL
Thyroid-stimulating hormone	0.406 microunits/mL
White blood cell count	4100-10,900/μL
Therapeutic Drug Level	
Amitriptyline	160-240 ng/mL
Digoxin	0.8-2 ng/mL
Lidocaine	1-5 mcg/dL
Lithium	0.7-1.5 mEq/L
Phenobarbital	10-30 mcg/mL
Phenytoin	10-20 mcg/mL
Theophylline	5-20 mcg/mL

MB, muscle brain bands; *MM*, muscle muscle bands.

Pulmonary Function Test Values

APPENDIX 9

Test	Normal Values
Vital capacity (VC)	60-70 mL/kg
Tidal volume (VT) (spontaneous ventilation)	6-8 mL/kg
Minute ventilation (VE)	80 mL/kg
Functional residual capacity (FRC)	28-32 mL/kg
Forced expiratory volume in 1 second (FEV_1)	>75%
Forced vital capacity (FVC)	60-70 mL/kg
Volume of dead space (VDS)	2 mL/kg
VDS/VT	33%
FEV_1/FVC	>75%

Index

F

G

I

J

K

L

M

N

O

P

S

U

V

W

X

Z

Printed in the United States
By Bookmasters